T0234902

PROCESSED FOOD ADDICTION

FOUNDATIONS, ASSESSMENT, AND RECOVERY

PROCESSED FOOD ADDICTION

FOUNDATIONS, ASSESSMENT, AND RECOVERY

Edited by

Joan Ifland
Marianne T. Marcus
Harry G. Preuss

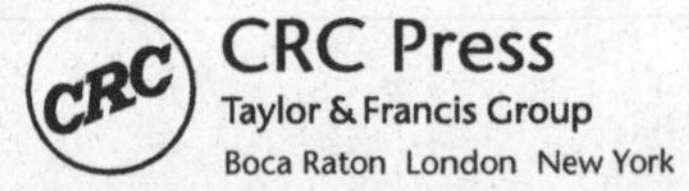

CRC Press is an imprint of the
Taylor & Francis Group, an **informa** business

CRC Press
Taylor & Francis Group
6000 Broken Sound Parkway NW, Suite 300
Boca Raton, FL 33487-2742

First issued in paperback 2020

ISBN-13: 978-1-4987-1996-4 (hbk)
ISBN-13: 978-0-367-50342-0 (pbk)

Library of Congress Cataloging-in-Publication Data

Names: Ifland, Joan, editor. | Marcus, Marianne T., editor. | Preuss, Harry G., editor.
Title: Processed food addiction : foundations, assessment, and recovery / edited by Joan Ifland, Marianne T. Marcus, Harry G. Preuss.
Description: Boca Raton, Florida : CRC Press, [2018] | Includes bibliographical references and index.
Identifiers: LCCN 2017031088 | ISBN 9781498719964 (hardback) | ISBN 9781315119922 (e-book) | ISBN 9781351646239 (e-book) | ISBN 9781498719971 (e-book) | ISBN 9781351636704 (e-book)
Subjects: LCSH: Compulsive eating--Treatment. | Food habits--Psychological aspects. | Processed foods--Psychological aspects. | Self-help techniques.
Classification: LCC RC552.C65.P76 2018 | DDC 616.85/26--dc23 LC record available at https://lccn.loc.gov/2017031088

Visit the Taylor & Francis Web site at
http://www.taylorandfrancis.com

and the CRC Press Web site at
http://www.crcpress.com

Contents

SECTION III Recovery from Processed Food Addiction

Editors

Joan Ifland is the chief executive officer of Food Addiction Training, LLC. She received her BA in economics and political science from Oberlin College, MBA from Stanford University, and PhD in interdisciplinary studies with a specialization in addictive nutrition from the Union Institute & University. She has innovated in the field of recovery from food addiction. She was the first chair of the Food Addiction Council for the American College of Nutrition. She is the author of the popular book *Sugars and Flours: How They Make Us Crazy, Sick, and Fat*. She founded Victory Meals in Houston, TX, which is the first prepared meal company to provide abstinent meals. She is currently developing online approaches to recovery at www.foodaddictionreset.com as well as the Facebook Group, Food Addiction Education. Her early career was spent at the Wisconsin State Legislature and the Continental Group, Stamford, CT.

Marianne T. Marcus is professor emerita at the University of Texas Health Science Center, School of Nursing, Houston, TX. She received her BSN from Columbia University, MA and MEd from Teachers College, Columbia University, and EdD from the University of Houston. Dr. Marcus served as chair of the Department of Nursing Systems, director of the Center for Substance Abuse Prevention, Education and Research, and was the John P. McGovern Distinguished Professor of Addiction Nursing. Her academic focus has been the education of interdisciplinary health professionals to deliver prevention, screening, and treatment services related to substance use disorders. She was the principal investigator for three successive faculty development grants funded by the Center for Substance Abuse Prevention (CSAP) and a federal grant to establish an Addictions Focus graduate subspecialty for nursing.

Dr. Marcus' research has focused on therapeutic community treatment for substance use disorders, including an NIH-funded behavioral therapies trial to determine the effect of mindfulness-based stress reduction on treatment in the therapeutic community setting. She has also conducted CSAP-funded community-based participatory research to test substance abuse prevention in vulnerable communities. Her professional honors include membership in the American Academy of Nursing, the University of Texas Academy of Health Science Education, and the Teachers College Nursing Education Alumni Association Hall of Fame.

Harry G. Preuss received his BA and MD from Cornell University, Ithaca, NY, and New York City; trained for three years in internal medicine at Vanderbilt University Medical Center; studied for two years as a fellow in renal physiology at Cornell University Medical; and spent two years in clinical and research training in nephrology at Georgetown University Medical Center. During his training years, he was a special research fellow of the National Institutes of Health (NIH). Following five years as an assistant and associate (tenured) professor of medicine at the University of Pittsburgh Medical Center where he became an established investigator of the American Heart Association, he returned to Georgetown Medical Center. He subsequently performed a six-month sabbatical in molecular biology at the NIH. Dr. Preuss is now a tenured professor in four departments at Georgetown University Medical Center—Biochemistry, Physiology, Medicine, and Pathology.

Contributors

Nicole M. Avena, PhD
Department of Neuroscience
Icahn School of Medicine at Mount Sinai
New York, NY

Kristen Criscitelli, MS, RD, CDN
Department of Pharmacological Sciences
Icahn School of Medicine at Mount Sinai
New York, NY

Jennifer M. Cross, MS, LPC, CHC
Authentic Living & Wellness - Life Coaching, Inc.,
Downers Grove, IL

Dennis M. Donovan, PhD
Psychiatry & Behavioral Sciences
University of Washington
Seattle, WA

Randall J. Ellis, BS
Biobehavioral Imaging and Molecular Neuropsychopharmacology Unit
National Institute on Drug Abuse Intramural Research Program
Baltimore, MD

Elaine Epstein, PsyD
Private Practice
Huntington Woods, MI

Rhona L. Epstein, PsyD
Private Practice
Philadelphia, PA

Natalie Gold, Hon BA Psych, RP
Ryerson University
Cert Gestalt Therapist
Gestalt Institute of Toronto
Toronto, ON, Canada

Joan Ifland, PhD, MBA
Food Addiction Training, LLC
Cincinnati, OH

Marianne T. Marcus, EdD, RN, FAAN
Department of Nursing Systems
University of Texas Health Science Center School of Nursing
Houston, TX

Adrian Meule, PhD
Department of Psychology
University of Salzburg
Salzburg, Austria

Michael Michaelides, PhD
Biobehavioral Imaging and Molecular Neuropsychopharmacology Unit
National Institute on Drug Abuse Intramural Research Program
and
Department of Psychiatry
Johns Hopkins Medicine
Baltimore, MD

Pamela M. Peeke, MD, MPH, FACP, FACSM
Department of Medicine
University of Maryland
Maryland, MD

Robin Piper, LMHC, MCAP, NCC, CCTP
Turning Point of Tampa
Tampa, FL

Harry G. Preuss MD, MACN, CNS
Department of Biochemistry
Georgetown University Medical Center
Washington, DC

Diane Rohrbach, NTP
Fare Nutrition
Seattle, WA

Kathleen M. Rourke, PhD, MSN, RD, RN
Department of Nursing
SUNY Polytechnic Institute
Utica, NY

Kathryn K. Sheppard, MA, LMHC
Private Practice
Palm Bay, FL

Eric Stice, PhD
Oregon Research Institute
Eugene, OR

Zack Stice
Oregon Research Institute
Eugene, OR

R. Sue Roselle, MS, CN, CNS
Roselle Center for Healing
Oakton, VA

Wendell C. Taylor, PhD, MPH
Department of Health Promotion and Behavioral Sciences
The University of Texas Health Science Center at Houston School of Public Health
Houston, TX

Gene-Jack Wang, MD
Laboratory of Neuroimaging
National Institute on Alcohol Abuse and Alcoholism
Bethesda, MD

Carrie L. Willey, PhD, LPC
Shades of Hope Treatment Center
Buffalo Gap, TX

H. Theresa Wright, MS, RD, LDN
Renaissance Nutrition
East Norriton, PA

Douglas M. Ziedonis, MD, MPH
University of California San Diego
UC San Diego Health System
San Diego, CA

Introduction: Learning about Processed Food Addiction

The epidemics of obesity and metabolic syndrome continue to spread globally even though 20 years have passed since the rate of obesity started to increase. In 2010, overweight and obesity were reported to cause 3.4 million deaths worldwide (Ng et al., 2014). Prevalence of the metabolic syndrome, a cluster of conditions that occurs together, increasing the risk of heart disease, stroke, and diabetes, has been estimated at between 20% and 30% (Grundy, 2008). The metabolic syndrome has grown to include central obesity, insulin resistance, dyslipidemia, hypertension, prothrombotic state, proinflammatory state, nonalcoholic fatty liver disease, reproductive disorders, cancer, and cognitive decline (Cornier et al., 2008; O'Neill & O'Driscoll, 2015; Panza et al., 2012). Traditional approaches to weight loss are now understood to be ineffective at curbing the epidemic (Turk et al., 2009). This textbook proposes that a new approach, of treating overeating as an addiction to processed foods, could provide an answer to the epidemic of obesity and the metabolic syndrome.

Recent research defines addiction in terms of compulsivity and impulsivity, i.e., loss of control. This quote from a recent review of addiction neurocircuitry describes the syndrome:

> A definition of *impulsivity* is "a predisposition toward rapid, unplanned reactions to internal and external stimuli without regard for the negative consequences of these reactions to themselves or others" (Moeller, Barratt, Dougherty, Schmitz, & Swann, 2001). A definition of *compulsivity* is the manifestation of "perseverative, repetitive actions that are excessive and inappropriate" (Berlin & Hollander, 2014). Impulsive behaviours are often accompanied by feelings of pleasure or gratification, but compulsions in disorders such as obsessive-compulsive disorder are often performed to reduce tension or anxiety from obsessive thoughts. In this context, individuals move from impulsivity to compulsivity, and the drive for drug-taking behaviour is paralleled by shifts from positive to negative reinforcement. However, impulsivity and compulsivity can coexist, and frequently do so in the different stages of the addiction cycle (Berlin & Hollander, 2014) in (Koob & Volkow, 2016).

As this textbook will describe, the compulsive use of processed foods conforms to these concepts. The loss of control for processed food addicts can be as profound and consuming as addiction to drugs and alcohol.

The processed food addiction (PFA) model is a fascinating, well-supported logical explanation for the obesity epidemic. Addictions in general are complex diseases with extensive consequences for the individual, people around the individual, and society as a whole. PFA is no exception. Attempts to classify chronic, compulsive abuse of processed foods as a weight-loss issue are now generally recognized as failures (Turk et al., 2009). PFA has a good chance of being an answer. A difficult, complicated answer, but an answer nonetheless.

It has taken the health community over 20 years to become experienced in the traditional answers for obesity, i.e., many variations of eat less, exercise more, as well as calories consumed versus calories expended. The research suggests that the field has come to the realization that these approaches are not working to achieve long-term weight normalization (Ochner, Barrios, Lee, & Pi-Sunyer, 2013). The pattern of failures points to the possibility of misdiagnosing and perhaps underestimating the problem on a widespread scale.

It is possible that the moment has arrived for the PFA model. Science has demonstrated similarities between chronic overeating and drug addiction to a point where the possibility of chronic overeating functioning as an addiction cannot be ignored (Schulte, Yokum, Potenza, & Gearhardt, 2016). There is good news in this development. Naming the correct diagnosis is certainly progress. However, the disheartening news is that addictions are stubborn relapsing conditions that are hard to treat.

Because of advances in the understanding of addictions, practitioners making the transition from the "calories in, calories out" model to the PFA model have a clearer path. Neurodysfunction dominates understanding of addiction as well as chronic overeating (Schulte et al., 2016). The anomalies can be seen to drive the manifestations of addiction that are found in the Diagnostic and Statistical Manual of Mental Disorders (DSM 5) Diagnostic Criteria for Substance-Related Addictive Disorders. And neurodysfunction informs core addiction recovery protocols of abstinence, cue avoidance, and cognitive restoration.

I.1 APPEAL OF THE MODEL

Why should a health practitioner pursue the PFA model? The reasons are compelling in the face of an epidemic of diet-related diseases now spreading around the globe (Ng et al., 2014). Although literally thousands of studies show the devastation of chronic overeating, a solution has not been found. The addiction model has gained recognition, but a means for implementing abstinence and cue-avoidance protocols has not been available. This textbook aims to fill that gap by methodically translating what is known about the addictive properties of chronic overeating into clinical practice.

Learning about PFA and techniques for helping clients to recover has appeal for a number of reasons. Westernized cultures are complex in terms of pressures to consume processed foods. Irrational food consumption as an addictive mechanism is a core premise of the PFA model. Learning how to defend against the pressure to overconsume processed foods derives from the model and includes abstinence from addictive foods as well as cue avoidance. The science is fascinating and the model is extensively supported by research. Practitioners have a responsibility to learn about such a well-supported approach. New approaches are urgently needed because traditional approaches have been shown to fail. The PFA approach can be adapted in different clinical settings. And learning about PFA helps practitioners to interpret the commercial and media environments that they live in and improve the quality of their clients' lives as well as their own. Learning about PFA is rewarding on many levels. It is a body of knowledge that can open practitioners' understanding of how to manage clients who suffer from chronic overeating. It gives practitioners a well-grounded basis from which to understand their clients' dysfunction and to guide them to a state of well-being.

I.2 PERSPECTIVES

For the reader, the textbook may present challenges of perspective. To fully grasp chronic overeating as an addiction to processed foods, assumptions about behavior, mental health, cultural norms, and business practices may benefit from reevaluation. Examples of shifts in perspective include:

- Clients are not weak-willed; rather they have a mental illness (VanderBroek-Stice, Stojek, Beach, vanDellen, & MacKillop, 2017).
- Biochemically, processed foods act more like recreational drugs than food (Chapter 6).
- Processing concentrates the natural opiates in plants into addictive substances (Chapter 6).
- Children can be addicted across a range of severity (Heerwagen, Miller, Barbour, & Friedman, 2010).
- Governments have abdicated their role in regulating processed foods (Amanzadeh, Sokal-Gutierrez, & Barker, 2015).
- There is substantial evidence supporting the concept of addiction to processed foods (VanderBroek-Stice et al., 2017).
- Media is not reporting on scientific advances in the field (Korownyk et al., 2014).
- PFA may be a more helpful diagnosis than eating disorder or obesity (Chapter 6).

- Symptoms of PFA such as the metabolic syndrome are not normal, although they are common (Olvera, Williamson, Fisher-Hoch, Vatcheva, & McCormick, 2015).
- Recovery from chronic overeating can be a long, slow process (Schulte et al., 2016).
- The etiology of chronic overeating is related more to environments than genetics (Watson, Wiers, Hommel, Ridderinkhof, & de Wit, 2016).
- PFA is a chronic relapsing condition similar to asthma or diabetes (Hsu et al., 2017).

All of these shifts in perception may take time, but they are worth pursuing. Compared to drug addiction, PFA may be harder to treat because of the young age of onset, the diversity of substances, the prevalence of cuing and availability, and deceptive media messages. Grounding in the appeal of the model, in spite of the challenges in perspective, is helpful.

I.3 ORGANIZATION OF THE TEXTBOOK

The textbook is organized into three parts: "Foundations," "Diagnosis and Assessment," and "Recovery from Processed Food Addiction." Section I, "Foundations," is designed to establish the scientific basis for the disease of PFA. The chapters are written by leading experts in research in chronic overeating and addiction. The chapters focus on the comparison of drug addiction to chronic overeating, neuroimaging work in the development of understanding of overeating, animal studies, food plans, and the biology of consequences. The goal of "Foundations" is to give practitioners confidence that the science supports the concept of PFA.

Section II, "Diagnosis and Assessment," is designed to enable the practitioner to identify PFA and severity in clients. The "Assessment" section can also serve to define the disease. As will be apparent, PFA is a disease that can extensively disrupt mental, emotional, behavioral, and physical well-being. The chapters describe overeating according to the 11 diagnostic criteria found in the DSM 5 for substance-related addiction disorders. These include unintended use, failure to cut back, time spent, cravings, failure to fulfill roles, interpersonal problems, activities given up, physically hazardous use, use in spite of consequences, tolerance, and withdrawal.

Each chapter gives information about the neurological dysfunction that underpins pathological behaviors. Further, food addicts may be misdiagnosed as presenting with obesity and a great deal of treatable neuropathology may be missed. The chapters are illustrated with examples of the dysfunction taken from the manuals of two 12-step fellowships, Food Addicts Anonymous, and Food Addicts in Recovery Anonymous. The "Assessment" section also includes a case study by Natalie Gold, a psychotherapist from Toronto, Canada.

Section III, "Recovery from Processed Food Addiction," is designed to give practitioners a step-by-step roadmap to recovery. It is based squarely on classic drug addiction recovery protocols. It covers avenues to success, the scientific premises of treatment, skill acquisition for adults, how to teach skills, and helping food-addicted children. "This section" emphasizes the need for patience, as food addiction is the only addiction that requires clients to learn a new way of preparing food as they wean themselves off of convenience foods. It is also the only recovery that requires the addict to be surrounded by relapse cues in the kitchen, grocery store, and possibly the workplace. Further, recovery can be complicated by the presence of addicted children in the household. Patience and pacing are offered as the keys to success in managing recovery from the severe mental illness that is food addiction.

I.4 WAYS TO USE THIS BOOK

This book is a first attempt to describe PFA scientifically and clinically. It combines science with what is known about clinical practice. Although PFA is a disease with extensive pathology, individual characteristics are readily understandable. Learning the pieces is a worthwhile but consuming endeavor. The book is meant to be accessible and adaptable by a range of health professionals, even possibly laypeople. The behaviors described in Section II, "Diagnosis and Assessment," are common behaviors. When assembled under the DSM 5 substance-related addiction diagnostic criteria, they reveal a complex picture, but the individual behaviors themselves are not difficult to recognize. The lessons in Section III, "Recovery from Processed Food Addiction," are also not difficult to understand. The material is readily accessible and readable. The challenge lies not in learning the materials. The challenge is to compassionately, consistently, and faithfully reinforce lessons with clients week after week, month after month, and year after year.

For counselors who have more time with each client, absorbing the three parts of the textbook to the point of being able to explain them to the client would be helpful. Taking the time to understand the manifestations of the disease in order to perform a comprehensive assessment would be valuable. The elements of the assessment support writing a comprehensive and accurate problem definition. The problem definition leads to motivating the client and identifying appropriate options for starting. For practitioners who intend to treat rather than refer, learning the characteristics of PFA in "Diagnosis and Assessment" and following the lessons laid out in "Approaches to Treatment" will allow the development of effective treatment of food addicts.

The textbook can be used on different levels to accommodate the nature of a health care practice. Given the depth of suffering experienced by food addicts and the apparent widespread nature of the disease, practitioners can justify taking the time to learn about PFA.

I.5 CONCLUSION

It is hoped that practitioners will be eager and excited to engage in a new disease description that is well-grounded in research and could provide an effective answer to the epidemic of chronic overeating.

Although evidence for PFA has been under development since the 1980s, this is the first time that the model has been academically translated into clinical practices. The PFA model is quite dynamic and it will undergo further development, refinement, and accessibility with experience and scientific findings.

The Introduction closes with this quote:

> If practitioners possess wide knowledge, both theoretical and practical, yet lack human qualities of compassion, caring, good faith, honesty, presence, realness, and sensitivity, they are more like technicians. I believe that those who function exclusively as technicians do not make a significant difference in the lives of their clients. It is essential that counselors explore their own values, attitudes, and beliefs in depth and work to increase their own awareness. (Cory, 2013, p. 4)

This textbook allows practitioners to explore their own relationship to the disease of PFA. The exploration opens the door to successfully treating food addicts with expertise and compassion.

Joan Ifland
Food Addiction Training, LLC
Cincinnati, OH

Marianne T. Marcus
The University of Texas Health Science Center at Houston
Houston, TX

Harry G. Preuss
Georgetown University Medical Center
Washington, DC

REFERENCES

Amanzadeh, B., Sokal-Gutierrez, K., & Barker, J. C. (2015). An interpretive study of food, snack and beverage advertisements in rural and urban El Salvador. *BMC Public Health, 15*, 521. doi:10.1186/s12889-015-1836-9.

Berlin, G. S., & Hollander, E. (2014). Compulsivity, impulsivity, and the DSM-5 process. *CNS Spectr, 19*(1), 62–68. doi:10.1017/S1092852913000722.

Cornier, M. A., Dabelea, D., Hernandez, T. L., Lindstrom, R. C., Steig, A. J., Stob, N. R., . . . Eckel, R. H. (2008). The metabolic syndrome. *Endocr Rev, 29*(7), 777–822. doi:10.1210/er.2008-0024.

Cory, G. (2013). *Theory and Practice of Counseling and Psychotherapy*. Boston, MA: Cengage.

Grundy, S. M. (2008). Metabolic syndrome pandemic. *Arterioscler Thromb Vasc Biol, 28*(4), 629–636. doi:10.1161/atvbaha.107.151092.

Heerwagen, M. J., Miller, M. R., Barbour, L. A., & Friedman, J. E. (2010). Maternal obesity and fetal metabolic programming: A fertile epigenetic soil. *Am J Physiol Regul Integr Comp Physiol, 299*(3), R711–R722. doi:10.1152/ajpregu.00310.2010.

Hsu, J. S., Wang, P. W., Ko, C. H., Hsieh, T. J., Chen, C. Y., & Yen, J. Y. (2017). Altered brain correlates of response inhibition and error processing in females with obesity and sweet food addiction: A functional magnetic imaging study. *Obes Res Clin Pract*. doi:10.1016/j.orcp.2017.04.011.

Koob, G. F., & Volkow, N. D. (2016). Neurobiology of addiction: A neurocircuitry analysis. *Lancet Psychiatry, 3*(8), 760–773. doi:10.1016/s2215-0366(16)00104-8.

Korownyk, C., Kolber, M. R., McCormack, J., Lam, V., Overbo, K., Cotton, C., . . . Allan, G. M. (2014). Televised medical talk shows-what they recommend and the evidence to support their recommendations: A prospective observational study. *BMJ, 349*, g7346. doi:10.1136/bmj.g7346.

Moeller, F. G., Barratt, E. S., Dougherty, D. M., Schmitz, J. M., & Swann, A. C. (2001). Psychiatric aspects of impulsivity. *Am J Psychiatry, 158*(11), 1783–1793. doi:10.1176/appi.ajp.158.11.1783.

Ng, M., Fleming, T., Robinson, M., Thomson, B., Graetz, N., Margono, C., . . . Gakidou, E. (2014). Global, regional, and national prevalence of overweight and obesity in children and adults during 1980–2013: A systematic analysis for the Global Burden of Disease Study 2013. *Lancet, 384*(9945), 766–781. doi:10.1016/s0140-6736(14)60460-8.

Ochner, C. N., Barrios, D. M., Lee, C. D., & Pi-Sunyer, F. X. (2013). Biological mechanisms that promote weight regain following weight loss in obese humans. *Physiol Behav, 120*, 106–113. doi:10.1016/j.physbeh.2013.07.009.

Olvera, R. L., Williamson, D. E., Fisher-Hoch, S. P., Vatcheva, K. P., & McCormick, J. B. (2015). Depression, obesity, and metabolic syndrome: Prevalence and risks of comorbidity in a population-based representative sample of Mexican Americans. *J Clin Psychiatry, 76*(10), e1300–e1305. doi:10.4088/JCP.14m09118.

O'Neill, S., & O'Driscoll, L. (2015). Metabolic syndrome: A closer look at the growing epidemic and its associated pathologies. *Obes Rev, 16*(1), 1–12. doi:10.1111/obr.12229.

Panza, F., Solfrizzi, V., Logroscino, G., Maggi, S., Santamato, A., Seripa, D., & Pilotto, A. (2012). Current epidemiological approaches to the metabolic-cognitive syndrome. *J Alzheimers Dis, 30*(2), S31–S75. doi:10.3233/jad-2012-111496.

Schulte, E. M., Yokum, S., Potenza, M. N., & Gearhardt, A. N. (2016). Neural systems implicated in obesity as an addictive disorder: From biological to behavioral mechanisms. *Prog Brain Res, 223*, 329–346. doi:10.1016/bs.pbr.2015.07.011.

Turk, M. W., Yang, K., Hravnak, M., Sereika, S. M., Ewing, L. J., & Burke, L. E. (2009). Randomized clinical trials of weight loss maintenance: A review. *J Cardiovasc Nurs, 24*(1), 58–80. doi:10.1097/01.jcn.0000317471.58048.32.

VanderBroek-Stice, L., Stojek, M. K., Beach, S. R., vanDellen, M. R., & MacKillop, J. (2017). Multidimensional assessment of impulsivity in relation to obesity and food addiction. *Appetite, 112*, 59–68. doi:10.1016/j.appet.2017.01.009.

Watson, P., Wiers, R. W., Hommel, B., Ridderinkhof, K. R., & de Wit, S. (2016). An associative account of how the obesogenic environment biases adolescents' food choices. *Appetite, 96*, 560–571. doi:10.1016/j.appet.2015.10.008.

Section I

Foundations

1 Overlap between Drug and Processed Food Addiction

Joan Ifland
Food Addiction Training, LLC
Cincinnati, OH

Pamela M. Peeke
University of Maryland
Maryland, MD

CONTENTS

1.1 INTRODUCTION

The processed food addiction (PFA) model is a relative newcomer to both the fields of eating disorders (ED) and substance use disorders (SUD). To ground the readers of this textbook in PFA, this chapter organizes the scientific evidence that demonstrates that the characteristics of overeating resemble those of drug addiction. With this evidence in mind, the reader may become more comfortable with the PFA concepts discussed in the textbook. A systematic review of the overlap between drug addiction and PFA helps develop the idea that commonly available processed food products could have addictive properties and be an agent in the loss of control over eating.

A number of review articles describe the evidence that overeating has acquired the drive of addiction in terms of motivation and incentive, craving, want, and liking (Volkow et al. 2008, 2012, 2013a, 2013b; Lutter and Nestler 2009; Liu et al. 2010; Morgan and Sizemore 2011; Marcus and Wildes 2014; Noori et al. 2016). Brain-imaging research consistently supports the core of evidence that overeating is a kind of addiction.

PFA is a debated concept in both the fields of ED and SUD. Subjects of debate include its role in the development of obesity (Chao et al. 2017; Davis 2017; Rogers 2017), its relationship with behavioral addiction (Frascella et al. 2010), its status as an eating disorder (Hebebrand et al. 2014; Goldschmidt 2017), and whether there is enough research to make conclusions (Ziauddeen et al. 2012; Hone-Blanchet and Fecteau 2014). Traditionally trained ED researchers may overlook it entirely (Heymsfield and Wadden 2017).

Reviewing the evidence for overeating as an addiction may help illuminate puzzling aspects of the obesity epidemic. The nature of addictive changes to the brain that are associated with both drug and processed food use may help clarify why overeaters cannot control their consumption of processed food products, just as drug addicts have lost control over drug use. Addictive neurological changes include downregulated reward pathways (Alsio et al. 2010; Karlsson et al. 2016), sensitized stress pathways (Cottone et al. 2009), and impaired cognitive functions. Learning about evidence for addictive properties for sugars, artificial sweeteners, gluten, flour, salt, caffeine, processed fats, and dairy products may help explain why overeaters lose control over these food products.

Further, the stubborn resistance of obesity to treatment may be better understood if addiction to processed food products is positioned as the core issue rather than excessive fat tissue. This could also be said for other consequences of chronic overeating such as diabetes, cardiovascular disease, hypertension, and dementia. Using PFA recovery approaches may lead to resolution of diet-related conditions.

Evaluating the evidence for PFA is important as an initial step in changing treatment of chronic overeating from a focus on eating behaviors to a focus on behaviors as they involve the consumption of addictive processed food products. For chronic overeaters, applying an addiction recovery approach could open the door to relief from cravings and loss of control. For example, a common denominator among addiction treatment programs is abstinence/reduced use of addictive substances. This includes abstinence from/reduced use of alcohol for the alcoholic, cocaine for the cocaine addict, tobacco for the smoker, and so forth. Even in the case of process addictions such as gambling, sex, shopping, and Internet addiction, recovery provides for refraining from or reducing the addictive behaviors as a tenet of the recovery process. In addition to the addictive substances or behaviors, the addict's exposure to cues (triggers) is limited. Cues have been shown to be instrumental in triggering cravings (Noori et al. 2016). If an addictive mechanism is at work in overeating, abstinence from addictive foods and associated cues could help reduce loss of control. The PFA model could be the basis for more effective treatment of chronic overeating and its consequences.

There are also parallels in industry practices between the global epidemic of tobacco addiction and the epidemic of overeating that may shed light on the complex factors perpetuating the obesity epidemic. These include marketing to children, cheap prices, easy availability, and intense advertising. Putting these at the center of public obesity policies can also help focus efforts to control the spread of obesity.

On the macro level, the PFA model could inform public education. Education about the addictive properties and consequences of processed food products could impact vast segments of obese cultures and encourage overeaters to change consumption patterns. Education about consequences was instrumental in curbing the use of tobacco. The effect of an educational effort about PFA could well impact the economic, social, and physical well-being of all segments of our society, obese and nonobese alike. Acceptance of the PFA model could also encourage adaptation of policies that are successful in curbing alcohol and tobacco use such as limits on advertising and availability as well as taxes (Nestle 2013).

Pathological overeating and chemical addictions are both physical and mental states with highly complex and extensive trait characteristics. Almost every aspect of the individual, family, and society at large is affected. As a result, the evidence for PFA can be approached from many angles. The literature for both addictions and obesity is extensive, which permits in-depth comparisons across a variety of dimensions. This chapter starts with similarities between overeaters and drug addicts, including neurofunctioning, cue reactivity, cognitive impairment, Pavlovian learning, genetics, conformance to DSM 5 SUD criteria, behavioral syndromes, muted sense of taste, and comorbidities. The "Family Systems" section covers family system patterns, child neglect and abuse, as well as fetal syndromes. The "Addictive Substances" section summarizes evidence for the psychoactive properties of processed foods, interchangeability of processed foods for drugs, polysubstance use, and abstinence in treatment. Finally, comparisons are made between macro factors found in both overeating and drug addiction, including epidemiological patterns, business practices, cost to society, and government subsidies.

Because the literature with respect to the topics of addiction and chronic overeating is vast, the evidence is summarized under each category. This is as opposed to a detailed discussion of each element, which would be beyond the scope of this chapter. The evidence presented is not intended to be exhaustive; rather it is representative of the kinds of research that demonstrate PFA.

Following the presentation of evidence, the "Discussion" section of this chapter reviews how the evidence can help the reader orient to the textbook. Although PFA is a highly complex and multifaceted disease, orienting to the evidence that processed foods have addictive properties could help readers absorb the information in the textbook more easily. Readers who are already oriented to general medicine, eating disorders, or substance use disorders can use their training as an underpinning to understand the textbook chapters.

Although the evidence is presented methodically, addiction syndromes in general, and especially PFA, are controversial. Because addicts can adjust their behavior when rewards are offered, even when addictive substances are available, some observers say loss of control does not exist (Peele 1992). There is also the concept that overeating occurs because of social and culture mores and not because of an addictive mechanism (Rogers and Smit 2000). Overeating has also been conceptualized as enhanced feeding instinct rather than a pathological syndrome (Ferrario 2017). Resolving this controversy is important because if overeating is found to emanate from addiction pathology, addiction treatment protocols and public policies could be adapted with much-needed improvements in outcomes.

1.2 METHODOLOGY

We searched PubMed; two handbooks of PFA, *Food Cravings and Addiction* (Hetherington 2001) and *Food and Addiction* (Brownell and Gold 2012); a book on the tobacco experience, *Cigarette Century* (Brandt 2007); a book on the politics of food, *Food Politics* (Nestle 1996, 2013); the 12-step literature; as well as popular books, *The Hunger Fix* (Peeke 2012), *The End of Overeating*

(Kessler 2009), and *Sugar, Fat, Salt* (Moss 2013), using the search terms *addiction, drug abuse, overeating, cueing, cravings, fast food,* and *obesity.*

1.3 RESULTS

A broad review of the addiction and overeating literature reveals that researchers have made similar findings in 20 types of research. The types of research are categorized into "Individuals," "Family Systems," "Psychoactive Properties," and "Macro Factors." Evidence discussed under the "Individuals" category includes neurofunctioning, cue reactivity, cognitive impairment, Pavlovian learning, genetics/epigenetics, conformance to DSM 5 SUD diagnostic criteria, behavioral syndromes, muted sense of taste, and comorbidities. The next category is "Family Systems" which includes inherited patterns of use, adverse childhood experiences, and a fetal syndrome. Similarities were also found in characteristics of substance use including psychoactive properties of processed foods, interchangeability of drugs and food, patterns of polysubstance use, and use of abstinence in treatment. Macro evidence was found in epidemiological patterns, business practices, cost to society, and government subsidies. These results are summarized as follows.

1.3.1 Individuals

1.3.1.1 Neurofunctioning

The neurological evidence for overeating as an addiction is extensive, as researchers were searching for ways to intervene in both addictions and overeating even before the advent of neuroimaging techniques in the late 1900s. In 2016 and 2017, several review articles described a model of addiction (Volkow et al. 2016a) and overeating (Stice and Yokum 2016; Moore et al. 2017) based largely on brain imaging research. The overlap between food and drug reactions in regions of brain activity has been described (Gearhardt et al. 2011; Kenny 2011; De Ridder et al. 2016) and has been shown to be more extensive in obesity than drug addiction (Tomasi and Volkow 2013). Similarities in attention bias have also been found (Field et al. 2016). Alterations in the morphology of dendrites have been found to follow binging in the prefrontal cortex for ethanol and nucleus accumbens for sucrose (Klenowski et al. 2016a, 2016b).

Key findings of the research are activation of the same reward/pleasure/addiction pathways for both addiction and overeating (Wang et al. 2011; Garcia-Garcia et al. 2014; Temple 2016). Downregulated pathways include dopamine (Blum et al. 2014; Wiss et al. 2016; Febo et al. 2017), opiate (Fields and Margolis 2015; Karlsson et al. 2015; Baldo 2016), serotonin (Fortuna 2012), and endocannabinoid (Watkins and Kim 2014; Volkow et al. 2017). In addition, reduced cognitive functioning has been found in both drug addicts and overeaters (Volkow and Wise 2005; Berthoud 2007; Morgenstern et al. 2013; Voon 2015). Specifically, impaired inhibition has been found for both alcohol in alcoholics and food in overeaters (Batterink et al. 2010; Filbey et al. 2012). Increased activation of stress pathways, particularly corticotropin releasing factor (CRF), has been found in drug addicts and in chronic consumption of high sugar/high fat foods (Cottone et al. 2009; Sinha and Jastreboff 2013; Zorrilla et al. 2014). Increased sensitization of reward pathways in response to food restriction is also found in both food and drug use (Carr 2016). This finding supports a role of increased stress in avoidance of withdrawal stress for both drug addiction and overeating.

The neurofunctioning literature is the strongest category of evidence that overeating can function as an addiction. The breadth and consistency of research supports the concept.

1.3.1.2 Cue Reactivity

A number of researchers have examined the brain's response to drug and food cues in laboratory animals as well as humans (Schroeder et al. 2001; Pelchat et al. 2004; Kelley et al. 2005; Cota et al. 2006; Cornier et al. 2007; Petrovich and Gallagher 2007; Petrovich et al. 2007; Anderson 2009; Claus et al. 2011; Stice et al. 2011; Tang et al. 2012; Jastreboff et al. 2013; Tomasi et al. 2015; Boswell and Kober 2016; Noori et al. 2016; Oginsky et al. 2016). The evidence shows that little exposure to either drug or processed food cues is required to stimulate a surge of neurotransmitter release in the reward pathways. It has been shown that mere thoughts of a food or drug can create an addictive response (Pelchat et al. 2004; Stice et al. 2008; Volkow et al. 2010).

Other characteristics of cueing that appear in both drug addiction and overeating include heightened response to compounded cues (Weiss 2005; Rolls and McCabe 2007), persistence of heightened reactivity after abstinence (Grimm et al. 2002, 2005), heightened reactivity in the early stages of abstinence (Lu et al. 2004; Grimm et al. 2005), heightened sensitivity in people with a history of misuse (Ranaldi et al. 2009), and place triggers (Schroeder et al. 2001; Hetherington 2007). Negative affect can also be a relapse cue (DiClemente and Delahanty 2016). Sensitivities to food cues but not drug cues are augmented by peripheral signaling in orexin, leptin, and insulin (Holland and Petrovich 2005; Blumenthal and Gold 2010). Leptin resistance is also a factor in uninhibited overeating in spite of satiety in response to cues (Berthoud 2007).

Like the neurofunctioning literature, the drug addiction and overeating cue-reactivity literature is broad and consistent. It functions to support cue avoidance in treatment, as well as public policy measures such as reduced advertising for processed food products. This would be especially applicable to advertising to children.

1.3.1.3 Cognitive Impairment

Chronic use of both addictive drugs and foods has been found to be associated with changes in cognitive function (Esch and Stefano 2004; Stefano et al. 2007). Volkow et al. found that neuropeptides may play a role in compromised cognitive functions (Volkow et al. 2011). Compromised thinking during cravings has also been observed (Kemps et al. 2008; Volkow et al. 2008). Noble et al. found that early life exposure to processed foods is associated with lifelong deficits in learning and memory (Noble and Kanoski 2016). Voon et al. found deficits in attention, memory, and inhibition in a population of binge eaters (Voon 2015). A number of studies have found that cognitive deficits associated with obesity in childhood and adolescence may persist into adulthood (Wang et al. 2014; Yau et al. 2014; Yesavage et al. 2014).

The body of evidence showing cognitive impairment in both habitual drug users and chronic overeaters has grown substantially in recent years. The evidence offers insight into why neither drug addicts nor overeaters make good decisions in drug- or food-cued environments. This is a useful body of evidence insofar as it helps guide treatment approaches. It suggests placing a greater emphasis on cue avoidance. It also supports focusing efforts on healing the frontal cortex. This is especially apparent in retraining decision-making and impulse-control functions.

Practitioners have justification for including greater guidance in their treatment blueprints for decision-making to avoid self-destructive choices. The evidence shows that the changes induced by drugs and processed foods extend well beyond reward pathway downregulation into frontal cortex metabolic impairment. The evidence is reflected in this textbook, which integrates restoration of cognitive pathways with desensitization of stress pathways and reductions in cue reactivity in a comprehensive approach.

1.3.1.4 Pavlovian Learning

There is evidence that repeated exposure to both drug and processed food use and cues leads to the development of both addiction and overeating (McAuliffe et al. 2006; Mahar and Duizer 2007; Corwin and Grigson 2009). This is thought to occur via the mechanism of Pavlovian conditioning of reward pathways to produce excessive neurotransmitters in response to cues and use (Petrovich and Gallagher 2007; Petrovich et al. 2007). Repeated cues and use heighten reward sensitivity and cravings in both addiction and overeating (Kelley et al. 2005). This body of literature contributes to the hypotheses that the etiology of the obesity epidemic is found in increased advertising and availability for obesogenic food as sources of repeat exposure to cues.

1.3.1.5 Genetics and Epigenetics

Researchers have found genetic anomalies in both drug addicts and overeaters at the TaqA1 allele (Noble et al. 1994; Blum et al. 1996; Stice and Dagher 2010). The TaqA1 allele has additionally been correlated with heightened reward sensitivity (Lee et al. 2007) and cravings (Yeh et al. 2016), as well as obesity and inflammation (Heber and Carpenter 2011). It also correlates with worse outcomes in weight-loss attempts (Benton and Young 2016). A study using the modified Yale Food Addiction Scale (YFAS) found genetic anomalies in regions of the genome that are not involved in eating (Cornelis et al. 2016). Polymorphisms found in leptin and opiomelanocortin genes may also play a role in both drug addiction and PFA (Heber and Carpenter 2011).

The overlap between drug and obesity genetic anomalies helps inform treatment as practitioners would know the genetic significance of a finding that an eating-disordered client had a history of drug or alcohol addiction. This would support a treatment recommendation that the overeating client with a history of drug abuse takes greater precautions against relapse.

This evidence for a genetic overlap between drug and PFA is strong, as the correlations are straightforward and repeated.

The field of epigenetics also contributes to evidence for an overlap between drug addiction and chronic overeating. By describing the role of environmental imprinting, epigenetics has provided evidence for similarities between for addictions (Blum et al. 2015) and obesity (Herrera et al. 2011). The evidence shows that although clients may have inherited addictive tendencies through their genetic profiles, such a vulnerability can be managed by controlling gene expressing through adjusting lifestyle, habits, and behavior as well as living environment. Therefore, DNA is not necessarily destiny. As is summarized in popular thinking, genetics may load the gun but lifestyle and environment pulls the trigger (Youngson and Morris 2013). This evidence gives practitioners the opportunity to educate processed food-addicted clients about the role of environment in curbing genetically drive behaviors. It can motivate clients to take action instead of succumbing to the idea that their fate is predetermined by their genetic makeup.

1.3.1.6 Conformance to DSM 5 SUD Criteria

Conformance with DSM 5 SUD diagnostic criteria is evidence that chronic overeaters are experiencing a range of dysfunctions that are similar to those found in drug addicts. These include unintended use, failed attempts to cut back, time spent, cravings, failure to fulfill roles, interpersonal problems, activities given up, physically hazardous use, use in spite of knowledge of consequences, progression, and withdrawal (Cassin and von Ranson 2007; Gearhardt and Corbin 2009; Ifland et al. 2009; Meule and Gearhardt 2014; Meule et al. 2016). The YFAS is derived from the DSM 5 SUD criteria. Part II of this textbook covers chronic overeating as it manifests according to the DSM 5 SUD diagnostic criteria. The similarities are quite extensive as control of eating gives way to cravings, and deterioration of employment, relationships, and activities progresses. The compulsivity and consequences distress drug and food addicts alike.

This category of evidence is consistent but not extensive. Nonetheless, it is an important body of evidence as the DSM 5 SUD criteria are the "gold standard" for diagnosing addictions.

1.3.1.7 Behavioral Syndromes

Both addicts and overeaters display a syndrome of behavior, including poor impulse control, numbing, blaming, shame, denial, minimizing, normalizing, and emotional avoidance (Barry et al. 2009; Mole et al. 2015; Volkow and Baler 2015; VanderBroek-Stice et al. 2017; Wang et al. 2017). Both addictions and overeating exhibit relapse and cravings (Rosenberg 2009; Krasnova et al. 2014; Joyner et al. 2015; Duarte et al. 2016). PFA, like drug addiction, is grounded in psychobiological pathology. The syndromes are not only psychological nor only biological. Both psychology and biology contribute to the pathology of self-destructive and inability to self-soothe. When taken with the neurofunction evidence, behavioral syndromes provide important corroborating evidence for the similarity between drug addiction and PFA.

1.3.1.8 Muted Sense of Taste

Both soft drink (Sartor et al. 2011) and tobacco use (Suliburska et al. 2004) result in a muted sense of taste. The muted sense of sweet taste could be a factor in recovery from PFA because vegetables have significantly lower levels of carbohydrate as compared to concentrated processed foods. The newly recovering food addict may not be able to taste the low level of carbohydrate and thus the vegetable may taste bitter. It will take some period of time for dopamine receptors to repair and support restoration of taste (Frank 2015). Clients may be more vulnerable to relapse during the process of restoration of dopamine functioning. For these reasons, it is beneficial to work to restore cognitive function and manage stress in early stage recovery.

1.3.1.9 Comorbidities

Both addictions and overeating are characterized by a range of dysfunctions as measured by the Addiction Severity Index (ASI) including a propensity for physical illnesses, mental illness, financial difficulties, relationship problems, social problems, and employment problems (McLellan et al. 1992, 2006; Ouyang et al. 2008; Lim et al. 2010; Lustig 2010; Nseir et al. 2010; Ifland et al. 2012). This research makes a case for the broad devastation of overeating and supports the idea that overeating is a kind of addiction. Chapter 22 of this textbook describes possible manifestations of PFA as organized by the ASI.

1.3.2 Family System Patterns

1.3.2.1 Inherited Patterns of Use

Researchers have shown that obesity and addictions both manifest in family systems. For example, children raised in alcoholic families are more likely to become alcoholics, children raised in families that abuse both drugs and alcohol are more likely to abuse both, and children raised by obese parents are more likely to become obese (Ellis et al. 1997; Raimo et al. 2000; Kampov-Polevoy et al. 2003; Krahnstoever Davison et al. 2005; Bayol et al. 2007; Seliske et al. 2009). Parents and children show similar PFA profiles (Merlo et al. 2009). Doba et al. found that a lack of social self-confidence was observed in patients with anorexia nervosa or with drug dependence disorder and their parents.

Families were characterized by disturbances, by low cohesion, and by emotional reliance on another person in both anorexia and drug addiction (Doba et al. 2014). Neurobiological markers found in adolescents and adults with a family history of alcoholism are similar to those found in the obese in terms of impaired impulse control, memory loss, and anomalies in reward and emotion processing (Cservenka 2016). The breastmilk of mothers consuming fructose has been found to have higher levels of fructose and to correlate with infant obesity (Goran et al. 2017).

Interestingly, women with a family history of alcoholism crave sugar more than women without this history (Pepino and Mennella 2007), and children of alcoholics crave sugar more than children of nonalcoholic parents (Mennella et al. 2010).

Family patterns constitute a body of ancillary evidence that processed foods can function similarly to addictive drugs, although processed food use may start at a younger age than drug use.

1.3.2.2 A Role for Adverse Childhood Experiences

Both drug addiction and PFA have been correlated with adverse childhood experiences (ACE). ACE include emotional, physical, and sexual abuse; a battered mother or witnessing violence; parental separation or divorce; and growing up with a substance-abusing, mentally ill, or incarcerated household member (Anda et al. 1999). ACE have been shown to correlate with adult smoking (Anda et al. 1999; Dong et al. 2005), alcoholism (Dube et al. 2001; Dong et al. 2005), and drug use (Dube et al. 2003). Similar results have been found for food addiction (Mason et al. 2013) and obesity (Felitti et al. 1998).

1.3.2.3 A Fetal Syndrome

Offspring of laboratory rats fed obesogenic foods develop the metabolic syndrome, including neuro-imprinting (Armitage et al. 2005) and fatty livers (Bayol et al. 2010). Babies of mothers who abuse alcohol and those who overeat to the point of obesity suffer from congenital defects (Stothard et al. 2009; Mattson et al. 2010; Riley et al. 2011) including fatty liver. The presence of a fetal syndrome supports the concept of chronic overeating as a kind of addiction.

1.3.3 Addictive Substances

1.3.3.1 Psychoactive Characteristics of Processed Foods

There is growing acceptance that foods high in sugar, fat, or salt are a factor in the obesity epidemic (Ifland et al. 2009; Harper and Mooney 2010; Berthoud 2012; Stice et al. 2013; Martinez Steele et al. 2016). Chapter 6 of this textbook covers the addictive properties of processed foods.

Recent research has shown neuroadaptations to high sugar/high fat foods in terms of downregulation of reward pathways, cognitive impairment, and sensitization of stress pathways (Moore et al. 2017). The evidence for sugar addiction has been demonstrated in rats, showing progressive use and a withdrawal syndrome (Avena et al. 2008). Sugar was also associated with opioid stimulation (Olszewski and Levine 2007) and numbs pain in children (Pepino and Mennella 2005). Higher-calorie soft drinks elicited a greater response in brain activity than lower-calories drinks in an adolescent population (Feldstein Ewing et al. 2016). However, addictive responses to sweetened condensed milk were extinguished more rapidly than similar responses to cocaine (Martin-Fardon et al. 2016).

Fat consumption in rats has been shown to be attenuated by pharmaceuticals used in drug treatment (Islam and Bodnar 1990; Rao et al. 2008). Fat cravings can be reduced by exercise (Beaulieu et al. 2017). A withdrawal syndrome for fat has been demonstrated (Sharma et al. 2013). Chocolate has been demonstrated to possess psychoactive elements, including methylxanthines, biogenic amines, and cannabinoid-like fatty acids (Bruinsma and Taren 1999). Similar findings have been made for caffeine (Hughes et al. 1992).

Moreover, the psychoactive element of theobromine in combination with caffeine has been shown to affect mood (Smit et al. 2004). Salt can be used addictively (Cocores and Gold 2009), and dairy products contain naturally occurring morphine (Meisel 1986; Teschemacher et al. 1997) that can produce a numbing effect in rats (Blass et al. 1989). The numbing reaction in rats is similar to wheat gluten, which contains an opioid peptide (Fanciulli et al. 2005). Food manufacturing processes are similar to drug and alcohol processing (Ifland et al. 2009) and include distillation, particle size reduction (powdering), extraction, concentration, and heating to high temperatures. Schulte et al. found that more highly processed foods are used more addictively (Schulte et al. 2015).

1.3.3.2 Interchangeability of Drugs and Food

In addiction recovery centers, clinicians have observed that when individuals withdraw from drugs abuse and alcohol, they substitute food (Hodgkins et al. 2004; Kleiner et al. 2004; Kendzor et al. 2008; Cocores and Gold 2009; Gearhardt and Corbin 2009). Smokers gain weight when they quit smoking (Epstein and Leddy 2006; Rupprecht et al. 2017). In an animal study, conditioned rats chose sugar over cocaine (Lenoir et al. 2007). Chocolate and nicotine are shown to activate similar prefrontal cortex and limbic regions (Schroeder et al. 2001). Research has shown the neurological basis for these clinical findings in overlapping brain circuits (Volkow et al. 2012).

Food restriction has been shown to increase the persistence of cocaine cravings in rats (Jung et al. 2016), while overfeeding of "junk food" sensitized obesity-susceptible rats to the locomotive effects of cocaine (Oginsky et al. 2016). Repeated exposure to heroin increases appetite for food rewards during extinction (Ranaldi et al. 2009). Bulimia nervosa has been shown to co-occur with drug misuse (Hadad and Knackstedt 2014). A rat study comparing Oreo and cocaine self-administration found shared vulnerability to acquiring behaviors motivated by incentives (Levy et al. 2013). This evidence for the interchangeability of drugs for processed foods is consistent as it is a widely observed clinical phenomenon.

1.3.3.3 Polysubstance Use Patterns

In both addiction and overeating, addictions are stronger when more than one substance is concurrently abused. Families that misuse both alcohol and drugs are more dysfunctional than families that are addicted to alcohol alone (Raimo et al. 2000). Polysubstance abusers have more substance problems than single-substance abusers (Schuckit et al. 2001). Polyaddictions are harder to treat than single-substance misuse (Connor et al. 2013, 2014).

Chocolate is thought to be addictive because of the presence of both sugar and fat (Bruinsma and Taren 1999), as it is known that combinations of sugar and fat activate endocannabinoid circuits (DiPatrizio and Simansky 2008) and encourage overeating in rats (Berner et al. 2008; Moore et al. 2017). Combinations of fat, sugar, salt, dairy, gluten, and caffeine are found in fast-food meals that have been implicated in the metabolic syndrome (De Vogli et al. 2014; Manzel et al. 2014; Rudelt et al. 2014). This category of evidence lacks research into the myriad of specific combinations of processed foods as they are offered commercially.

SUD are also found to correlate with process addictions. Cocaine and sex addiction are shown to co-occur. Risk of relapse from both food and smoking can be mitigated by exercise (Bernard et al. 2013). Overlapping neural substrates respond to drug, gambling, food, and sexual cues (Noori et al. 2016). Gamblers have been shown to use high sugar/high fat foods (Chamberlain et al. 2016). Food addicts may also be using cocaine and prescription drugs to control weight (Dennis and Pryor 2014).

1.3.3.4 Abstinence in Treatment

In both drug addiction and overeating, the same approaches to treatment are found. Both conditions respond to abstinence from the substances or foods associated with loss of control (Ries 2009; Food Addicts Anonymous 2010). While abused substances are fairly easy to identify in drug and alcohol treatment, in PFA the situation is more complex with a number of processed food products recommended for abstinence by food addiction professionals and 12-step recovery groups. These include sugar and all other sweeteners, flour, excessive salt, fatty foods, and caffeine. Treatment protocols for recovery from both addiction and overeating call for long-term support and avoidance of external triggers, such as people, places, and things (Ayyad and Andersen 2000; McNatt et al. 2007; Leombruni et al. 2009; McIver et al. 2009; Ries 2009; Food Addicts Anonymous 2010). Treatment of overeating through abstinence from particular processed foods has not been investigated. Evidence cited here is from self-endorsed food addiction recovery 12-step groups. This evidence needs further research.

The strength of the evidence in this category is uneven from substance to substance. It is perhaps strongest for sugar, fat, and caffeine; moderately strong for dairy and salt; and weakest for flour.

1.3.4 Macro Factors

1.3.4.1 Epidemiological Patterns

Similar to addictions, overeating and obesity are more likely to occur in undereducated, lower-income Hispanic and African-American populations, possibly through the mechanisms of stress (Olstad et al. 2016; Pateman et al. 2016) and advertising (Widome et al. 2013; Cassady et al. 2015). Analogous to tobacco use, obesity has reached about 2/3 of the population, but whereas 2/3 of smokers were men, obesity is fairly closely divided among men and women (Giovino et al. 1995; Ellis et al. 1997; Caetano and Clark 1998; Ogden et al. 2007; Ng et al. 2014). Most importantly, fast-food outlets are more highly clustered around low-income neighborhoods (Day and Pearce 2011), and the proximity of food outlets is more of a factor in obesity in low-income schools (Mellor et al. 2011). The epidemiological evidence shows parallels between overeating and drug addiction.

In both the tobacco and processed epidemics, children are affected. In the case of tobacco, the mechanism is secondhand smoke. In the case of pediatric PFA, children are target-marketed directly.

1.3.4.2 Business Practices

Processed food and tobacco corporations use deceptive advertising to impute social values and health to promote their products especially to younger audiences. Other processed food marketing practices include affordable pricing and availability through vending machines and numerous retail outlets (Nestle 1996; Lewin et al. 2006; Brandt 2007; Brownell and Warner 2009). Product formulation to increase addictive properties is also evident in both tobacco (Alpert et al. 2016) and processed foods (Moss 2013; Schulte et al. 2015). The evidence for these practices in the tobacco industry is strong (Brandt 2007; Glynn et al. 2010). Business practices of the food industry have been documented as well (Nestle 2013).

1.3.4.3 Cost to Society

Overeating, drug abuse, alcoholism, and tobacco create a significant cost to the societies in which these epidemics are present (Harwood et al. 1998; Wang et al. 2008). In 1998, obese patients cost 36% more to treat than lean patients in inpatient and outpatient spending and 77% more in medications. Smokers cost 21% more than nonsmokers in inpatient and outpatient spending and 28% more in medications (Sturm 2002). Research shows that diet-related diseases are the leading cause of increased health care spending in the United States, both because of the greater number of patients and the greater expense of treating diet-related disease (Thorpe 2013). In 2008, the cost of obesity in the United States was estimated to be $147 billion (Finkelstein et al. 2009). In 2015, the cost of tobacco was $295 billion, alcohol $224 billion, and illicit drugs $193 billion (National Institute of Drug Abuse 2015). This concept is well documented and provides peripheral evidence for overeating as an addiction.

1.3.4.4 Government Subsidies

Government subsidies were present in tobacco production and continue to be present in crops that support obesity, including wheat, corn, dairy products, and sugar (Tillotson 2004; Glynn et al. 2010). This evidence is straightforward and conclusive. It is somewhat central to the argument that overeating is an addiction because subsidies lower the price of processed foods. This makes processed food products easy to obtain and permits frequent use, which is tied to increased reward sensitivity and the development of loss of control (Petrovich 2013; Burger and Stice 2014).

1.3.5 Summary of Evidence

The results show consistent similarities between overeating and drug addiction in all features examined. There is a variety of evidence for the hypothesis that "overeating is like drug and alcohol addiction." There is evidence that individuals who habitually use drugs are functioning similarly to those who chronically overuse processed food in terms of neurofunctioning, including downregulated reward pathways and sensitized stress pathways. In both conditions, there is heightened cue reactivity as well as cognitive impairment in learning, decision-making memory, and impulse control. Evidence is also found for an overlap in Pavlovian learning of neurons and genetic/epigenetic anomalies. There is also similar conformance to the 11 DSM 5 SUD diagnostic criteria, behavioral syndromes, a muted sense of taste, and a constellation of comorbidities.

In addition, similarities arise in family systems in terms of inherited patterns of use, a role for adverse childhood experiences, and a fetal syndrome. Further, there is an overlap between psychoactive properties of processed foods, interchangeability of drugs for food and vice versa, patterns of polysubstance use in both drugs and processed foods, and use of abstinence in treatment for both drug addiction and PFA.

Macro factors are demonstrated in epidemiological patterns, business practices, cost to society, and government subsidies. Epidemiological studies found the same disadvantaged populations suffering disproportionately from both overeating and addictions. Worldwide, the same business practices for processed foods are present as for tobacco in terms of advertising, availability, and affordable pricing. We also found a great cost to society as well as government subsidies for both tobacco and the processed foods used in overeating.

Across a range of types of evidence, there is evidence that overeating manifests similarly to drug addiction.

1.4 DISCUSSION

The display of evidence showing the similarities between drug addiction and chronic overeating serves a number of purposes within the context of a growing pandemic of the metabolic syndrome.

1.4.1 Context

It is helpful to place the evidence in the context of the development of addiction disease concepts in the 1900s and the early 2000s. In that period of time, the perception of addiction has evolved from a moral failure or a vice (Vaillant 1995) to a dysfunctional adaptation of the brain to addictive substances (Volkow et al. 2016a). Neuroimaging has shown that receptors in the reward pathways are downregulated, while stress pathways are sensitized and cognitive functions are impaired. These neuroadaptations combine to perpetuate the addiction by creating the sensation of stress while minimizing compensating pleasure and increasing the distress of withdrawal. The research has prompted experts in the field to characterize addictions as lapsing diseases that are similar to other lapsing diseases such as asthma and diabetes (Volkow et al. 2016a). These findings of physical and functional changes in the brain help reduce the stigmatization of addicts and promote methods of recovery.

The research in drug addiction has comprehensively illuminated the nature of neuroadaptations to a variety of drugs including cocaine (Volkow et al. 2016b), heroin (Li et al. 2015), alcohol (Cservenka 2016), cannabis (Volkow et al. 2016b), and nicotine (Criscitelli and Avena 2016). Individual processed foods have not been researched as thoroughly and more evidence is based on animal than human studies. This is the case for sugar (Murray et al. 2015), fat (Tellez et al. 2013; Kuhn et al. 2014), and combinations of sugar and fat (Morgan and Sizemore 2011; Moore et al. 2017), while caffeine has been studied in humans (Juliano et al. 2014). Neuroadaptations for dairy and salt have not been established although evidence for dairy (Teschemacher et al. 1997) and salt (Cocores and Gold 2009) has been published.

The evolution of understanding of the neurodysfunctions associated with addictive drugs has been substantial in the years of brain-imaging research. The processes of neuroadaptations to a range of drugs have been established. This body of evidence is having an impact on treatment of addiction in terms of advances such as acceptance of lapsing as normal instead of as a failure (Volkow et al. 2016a), greater avoidance of cues (Michaelides et al. 2012), and greater emphasis on cognitive restoration (Rezapour et al. 2016).

Possibly because of these significant advances in understanding of neurodysfunction in drug addiction, food addiction research has grown out of that base. This is to say that there has not been a parallel, in-depth development of a body of research showing how processed food products derange brain function. In contrast, research has focused on obesity and a plethora of associated physical, mental, emotional, behavioral, family, and social correlates. Only sporadically and recently have researchers turned their attention to defining the progression of brain adaptations to specific processed foods. While drug addiction has been focused on the properties of specific drugs, PFA has only recently begun to illuminate the neuroimpact of specific processed food products.

The lack of food-specific research relative to drug-specific research could be the result of two distractions: (1) eating as the mode of absorption and (2) the consequence of excess fat tissue. It could be argued that these two distractions have delayed the focus on specific processed food products as productive objects of research in favor of research on eating behaviors and obesity.

As researchers turn their attention to delving into the properties of specific addictive foods, it can be expected that the field will generate findings that will help practitioners and food addicts abstain from or reduce use of these foods.

On the other hand, because of several decades of research into eating behaviors and the correlates of obesity, much has been shown about the behavior of food addicts as well as the consequences of chronic overuse of processed foods. It is this research that informs the DSM 5 SUD diagnostic criteria as applied to addictive eating. The wealth of findings means that practitioners can identify a range of behaviors related to overeating as meeting the criteria for addiction. Obesity and disordered eating research allows practitioners to categorize behaviors as loss of control including unintended use, failure to cut back, and time spent in the addiction. The behaviors also point to neurodysfunction in terms of progression, withdrawal, and use in spite of consequences. Without the extensive research into disordered eating and obesity, the picture of PFA would not be as robust and ready for application.

1.4.2 Application

The treatment of PFA has been undergoing a renaissance given the emerging science and medical research findings and discoveries within the neurological, biological, physiological, and psychological domains. The challenge has been, if there are similarities between substance addiction and addictive eating behavior, to determine whether the treatment modalities could be the same. The current evidence points to a variety of therapeutic options for chronic overeating and for drug addiction to include traditional 12-step fellowships, as well as the incorporation of exercise, meditation, mindfulness, lifestyle adaptations, ongoing lifestyle coaching, psychological counseling, pharmacotherapies, and bariatric surgery.

Drug and alcohol addiction professionals are finding that the traditional 28-day detox and rehab is woefully inadequate. This outdated treatment option has been replaced by a lifelong recovery-centric approach (Peeke 2016). Similarly, eating disorder professionals are finding that the short-term weight-loss approach also is woefully inadequate (Turk et al. 2009). The concept of a recovery-centric life for chronic overeaters is also applicable. The fields of both drug addiction and PFA are evolving in parallel in terms of understanding etiology, environmental influence, cuing, diagnosis, assessment, and treatment.

The translation of research into practice is the overall goal of this textbook. Because so much research has been accomplished in addictions, disordered eating, and obesity, this textbook emanates from a rich literature. It can be said that the textbook is organizing existing research through a new lens, i.e., that of chronic overeating as a substance use disorder.

The Table of Contents reflects the strength of the research. Findings in neuroscience form the bulk of the chapters in Part I, "Foundations." The neuroscience in both addictions and disordered eating is perhaps the strongest evidence for disordered eating as a kind of addiction. There are also chapters derived from the consequences and a chapter that organizes the evidence for the addictive properties of particular processed food products. The overlap of drug addiction and PFA forms the basis for Part I.

The overlap also forms the basis for the extensive discussion of addictive behaviors that occur in eating found in Part II, "Diagnosis and Assessment." For readers who are most comfortable with the DSM 5 SUD diagnostic criteria as the gold standard for measuring manifestations of addictions, the extensive diagnostic section of the textbook will be familiar and reassuring, perhaps even persuasive. This overlap between drug addiction and overeating will be familiar to followers of the YFAS, which is in part derived from the DSM 5 SUD diagnostic criteria. This section of the textbook is thoroughly embedded in research into eating behaviors as well as the consequences of obesity. In terms of behaviors and consequences, the DSM 5 SUD diagnostic criteria serve a function similar to that of the neuroscience. The similarities are so consistent that the evidence is hard to ignore. It is easiest to interpret the extensive conformance of eating to addiction diagnostic criteria as chronic overeating as a kind of addiction.

In Part III, "Approaches to Recovery," the overlap continues in terms of application of classic addiction treatment guidelines of abstinence or reduced harm in use, cue avoidance, cognitive restoration, and reclamation of relationships, career, education, etc. Again, the kinds of overlap described in the "Results" section of this chapter appear. Cue reactivity, cognitive impairment, and evidence for addictive neuroadaptations to processed food products drive PFA recovery guidelines.

The overlap of drug and chronic overeating/obesity is valuable to the field of PFA. The overlap makes possible the development of key concepts of diagnosis, assessment, and treatment. The overlap can give researchers and practitioners alike a roadmap to more effective knowledge and practice in the field of disordered eating.

1.5 LIMITATIONS

This chapter is about the evidence for PFA and is not a critical analysis of all of the literature. Thus, a limitation of this chapter is that it does not explore or attempt to explain the implications of the inconsistencies between drug addiction and overeating nor inconsistencies between the majority of research results and exceptions. Examples of the former include the role of peripheral signaling in response to food and food cues, which does not exist in drug signaling (Blumenthal and Gold 2010), and the finding of diminishing reward sensitivity in moderate and extreme obesity (Davis and Fox 2008). The latter includes a study that did not find a correlation between proximity of fast food and obesity in a high school (Crawford et al. 2008) and a study that found that dairy contributes to weight loss (Dougkas et al. 2011). Although an examination of these anomalies could well contribute to our understanding of PFA, they are beyond the scope of this chapter.

1.6 CONCLUSION

The evidence for overeating as an addiction is broad and consistently supportive of the concept. Similarities between overeating and drug abuse include neural anomalies in reward pathways, stress pathways, cue reactivity, and cognitive impairment through mechanisms of Pavlovian learning, genetics, and epigenetics. Overlaps are also found in behavior syndromes, conformance with addiction diagnostic criteria, a muted sense of taste, and extensive consequences. There are also findings for family patterns of use, the prevalence of adverse childhood experience in users, and a fetal syndrome in both chronic drug and processed food use. There is also the presence of addictive elements in processed foods, the interchangeability of food and drugs, a pattern of polysubstance use, and the use of abstinence in treatment.

Finally, there is evidence for the presence of similar macro forces such as epidemiological patterns of disproportionate use by disadvantaged populations, cost to society, corporate business practices, and crop subsidies for both processed foods and tobacco. This overlap between drug addiction and disordered eating forms the foundation for this textbook.

The overlap also gives practitioners a foundation for adopting treatment approaches based on concepts of classic drug addiction recovery. Given the severity of consequences of inadequate approaches, the numerous overlaps make it seem prudent to more aggressively protect vulnerable populations such as children, the elderly, the undereducated, the morbidly obese, and the mentally ill from processed food cueing, cheap prices, and easy availability. As the epidemic of obesity progresses, there are fewer plausible explanations for the lack of success in stemming the epidemic of chronic overeating (Lerma-Cabrera et al. 2016), which increasingly lends credence to the idea of PFA.

Public awareness of PFA may help promote a reduction of judgment of obese people (Lee et al. 2013) and support for public policies (Schulte et al. 2016). For the individual, the family, and society as a whole, policy approaches to protect the public from tobacco-style business practices related to processed food and processed food cueing would seem to be warranted (Gearhardt et al. 2012, 2013; Gearhardt and Brownell 2013), especially in lower- and middle-income countries (Lee and Gibbs 2013).

Further research will provide evidence to continue the debate. In the meantime, vigorous discussion and education are needed. Popular information channels, such as Internet educational sites and social media sites, as well as messages about the dangers of processed foods and techniques for achieving abstinence delivered by 12-step groups, may offer hope for educating people who suffer from overeating (Burrows et al. 2017).

REFERENCES

Alpert, H. R., I. T. Agaku and G. N. Connolly (2016) A study of pyrazines in cigarettes and how additives might be used to enhance tobacco addiction. *Tob Control* **25**: 4444–4450.

Alsio, J., P. K. Olszewski, A. H. Norback, Z. E. Gunnarsson, A. S. Levine, C. Pickering and H. B. Schioth (2010). Dopamine D1 receptor gene expression decreases in the nucleus accumbens upon long-term exposure to palatable food and differs depending on diet-induced obesity phenotype in rats. *Neuroscience* **171**(3): 779–787.

Anda, R. F., J. B. Croft, V. J. Felitti, D. Nordenberg, W. H. Giles, D. F. Williamson and G. A. Giovino (1999). Adverse childhood experiences and smoking during adolescence and adulthood. *JAMA* **282**(17): 1652–1658.

Anderson, P. (2009). Is it time to ban alcohol advertising? *Clin Med* **9**(2): 121–124.

Armitage, J. A., P. D. Taylor and L. Poston (2005). Experimental models of developmental programming: Consequences of exposure to an energy rich diet during development. *J Physiol* **565**(Pt 1): 3–8.

Avena, N. M., P. Rada and B. G. Hoebel (2008). Evidence for sugar addiction: Behavioral and neurochemical effects of intermittent, excessive sugar intake. *Neurosci Biobehav Rev* **32**(1): 20–39.

Ayyad, C. and T. Andersen (2000). Long-term efficacy of dietary treatment of obesity: A systematic review of studies published between 1931 and 1999. *Obes Rev* **1**(2): 113–119.

Baldo, B. A. (2016). Prefrontal cortical opioids and dysregulated motivation: A network hypothesis. *Trends Neurosci* **39**(6): 366–377.

Barry, D., M. Clarke and N. M. Petry (2009). Obesity and its relationship to addictions: Is overeating a form of addictive behavior? *Am J Addict* **18**(6): 439–451.

Batterink, L., S. Yokum and E. Stice (2010). Body mass correlates inversely with inhibitory control in response to food among adolescent girls: An fMRI study. *NeuroImage* **52**(4): 1696–1703.

Bayol, S. A., S. J. Farrington and N. C. Stickland (2007). A maternal "junk food" diet in pregnancy and lactation promotes an exacerbated taste for "junk food" and a greater propensity for obesity in rat offspring. *Br J Nutr* **98**(4): 843–851.

Bayol, S. A., B. H. Simbi, R. C. Fowkes and N. C. Stickland (2010). A maternal "junk food" diet in pregnancy and lactation promotes nonalcoholic fatty liver disease in rat offspring. *Endocrinology* **151**(4): 1451–1461.

Beaulieu, K., M. Hopkins, J. Blundell and G. Finlayson (2017). Impact of physical activity level and dietary fat content on passive overconsumption of energy in non-obese adults. *Int J Behav Nutr Phys Act* **14**(1): 14.

Benton, D. and H. A. Young (2016). A meta-analysis of the relationship between brain dopamine receptors and obesity: A matter of changes in behavior rather than food addiction? *Int J Obes (Lond)* **40**(Suppl 1): S12–21.

Bernard, P., G. Ninot, G. Moullec, S. Guillaume, P. Courtet and X. Quantin (2013). Smoking cessation, depression, and exercise: Empirical evidence, clinical needs, and mechanisms. *Nicotine Tob Res* **15**(10): 1635–1650.

Berner, L. A., N. M. Avena and B. G. Hoebel (2008). Bingeing, self-restriction, and increased body weight in rats with limited access to a sweet-fat diet. *Obesity (Silver Spring)* **16**(9): 1998–2002.

Berthoud, H. R. (2007). Interactions between the "cognitive" and "metabolic" brain in the control of food intake. *Physiol Behav* **91**(5): 486–498.

Berthoud, H. R. (2012). The neurobiology of food intake in an obesogenic environment. *Proc Nutr Soc* **71**(4): 478–487.

Blass, E. M., D. J. Shide and A. Weller (1989). Stress-reducing effects of ingesting milk, sugars, and fats. A developmental perspective. *Ann N Y Acad Sci* **575**: 292–305; discussion 305–296.

Blum, K., E. R. Braverman, R. C. Wood, J. Gill, C. Li, T. J. Chen, M. Taub, A. R. Montgomery, P. J. Sheridan and J. G. Cull (1996). Increased prevalence of the Taq I A1 allele of the dopamine receptor gene (DRD2) in obesity with comorbid substance use disorder: A preliminary report. *Pharmacogenetics* **6**(4): 297–305.

Blum, K., P. K. Thanos, R. D. Badgaiyan, M. Febo, M. Oscar-Berman, J. Fratantonio, Z. Demotrovics and M. S. Gold (2015). Neurogenetics and gene therapy for reward deficiency syndrome: Are we going to the promised land? *Expert Opin Biol Ther* **15**(7): 973–985.

Blum, K., P. K. Thanos and M. S. Gold (2014). Dopamine and glucose, obesity, and reward deficiency syndrome. *Front Psychol* **5**: 919.

Blumenthal, D. M. and M. S. Gold (2010). Neurobiology of food addiction. *Curr Opin Clin Nutr Metab Care* **13**(4): 359–365.

Boswell, R. G. and H. Kober (2016). Food cue reactivity and craving predict eating and weight gain: A meta-analytic review. *Obes Rev* **17**(2): 159–177.

Brandt, A. (2007). *The Cigarette Century: The Rise, Fall, and Deadly Persistence for the Product That Defined America.* New York: Basic Books.

Brownell, D. K. and M. S. Gold, Eds. (2012). *Food and Addiction: A Comprehensive Handbook.* Oxford: Oxford University Press.

Brownell, K. D. and K. E. Warner (2009). The perils of ignoring history: Big tobacco played dirty and millions died. How similar is big food? *Milbank Q* **87**(1): 259–294.

Bruinsma, K. and D. L. Taren (1999). Chocolate: Food or drug? *J Am Diet Assoc* **99**(10): 1249–1256.

Burger, K. S. and E. Stice (2014). Greater striatopallidal adaptive coding during cue-reward learning and food reward habituation predict future weight gain. *NeuroImage* **99**: 122–128.

Burrows, T., J. Skinner, M. A. Joyner, J. Palmieri, K. Vaughan and A. N. Gearhardt (2017). Food addiction in children: Associations with obesity, parental food addiction and feeding practices. *Eating Behaviors* **26**: 114–120.

Caetano, R. and C. L. Clark (1998). Trends in alcohol consumption patterns among whites, blacks and Hispanics: 1984 and 1995. *J Stud Alcohol* **59**(6): 659–668.

Carr, K. D. (2016). Nucleus Accumbens AMPA receptor trafficking upregulated by food restriction: An unintended target for drugs of abuse and forbidden foods. *Curr Opin Behav Sci* **9**: 32–39.

Cassady, D. L., K. Liaw and L. M. Miller (2015). Disparities in obesity-related outdoor advertising by neighborhood income and race. *J Urban Health* **92**(5): 835–842.

Cassin, S. E. and K. M. von Ranson (2007). Is binge eating experienced as an addiction? *Appetite* **49**(3): 687–690.

Chamberlain, S. R., S. A Redden and J. E. Grant (2016). Calorie intake and gambling: Is fat and sugar consumption "impulsive"? *J Gambl Stud*. Doi: 10.1007/s10899-016-9647-1.

Chao, A. M., J. A. Shaw, R. L. Pearl, N. Alamuddin, C. M. Hopkins, Z. M. Bakizada, R. I. Berkowitz and T. A. Wadden (2017). Prevalence and psychosocial correlates of food addiction in persons with obesity seeking weight reduction. *Compr Psychiatry* **73**: 97–104.

Claus, E. D., S. W. Ewing, F. M. Filbey, A. Sabbineni and K. E. Hutchison (2011). Identifying neurobiological phenotypes associated with alcohol use disorder severity. *Neuropsychopharmacology* **36**(10): 2086–2096.

Cocores, J. A. and M. S. Gold (2009). The salted food addiction hypothesis may explain overeating and the obesity epidemic. *Med Hypotheses* **73**(6): 892–899.

Connor, J. P., M. J. Gullo, G. Chan, R. M. Young, W. D. Hall and G. F. Feeney (2013). Polysubstance use in cannabis users referred for treatment: Drug use profiles, psychiatric comorbidity and cannabis-related beliefs. *Front Psychiatry* **4**: 79.

Connor, J. P., M. J. Gullo, A. White and A. B. Kelly (2014). Polysubstance use: Diagnostic challenges, patterns of use and health. *Curr Opin Psychiatry* **27**(4): 269–275.

Cornelis, M. C., A. Flint, A. E. Field, P. Kraft, J. Han, E. B. Rimm and R. M. van Dam (2016). A genome-wide investigation of food addiction. *Obesity (Silver Spring)* **24**(6): 1336–1341.

Cornier, M. A., S. S. Von Kaenel, D. H. Bessesen and J. R. Tregellas (2007). Effects of overfeeding on the neuronal response to visual food cues. *Am J Clin Nutr* **86**(4): 965–971.

Corwin, R. L. and P. S. Grigson (2009). Symposium overview—Food addiction: Fact or fiction? *J Nutr* **139**(3): 617–619.

Cota, D., M. H. Tschop, T. L. Horvath and A. S. Levine (2006). Cannabinoids, opioids and eating behavior: The molecular face of hedonism? *Brain Res Rev* **51**(1): 85–107.

Cottone, P., V. Sabino, M. Roberto, M. Bajo, L. Pockros, J. B. Frihauf, E. M. Fekete, L. Steardo, K. C. Rice, D. E. Grigoriadis, B. Conti, G. F. Koob and E. P. Zorrilla (2009). CRF system recruitment mediates dark side of compulsive eating. *Proc Natl Acad Sci U S A* **106**(47): 20016–20020.

Crawford, D. A., A. F. Timperio, J. A. Salmon, L. Baur, B. Giles-Corti, R. J. Roberts, M. L. Jackson, N. Andrianopoulos and K. Ball (2008). Neighbourhood fast food outlets and obesity in children and adults: The CLAN study. *Int J Pediatr Obes* **3**(4): 249–256.

Criscitelli, K. and N. M. Avena (2016). The neurobiological and behavioral overlaps of nicotine and food addiction. *Preventive Medicine* **92**: 82–89.

Cservenka, A. (2016). Neurobiological phenotypes associated with a family history of alcoholism. *Drug Alcohol Depend* **158**: 8–21.

Davis, C. (2017). A commentary on the associations among "food addiction," binge eating disorder, and obesity: Overlapping conditions with idiosyncratic clinical features. *Appetite* **115**: 3–8.

Davis, C. and J. Fox (2008). Sensitivity to reward and body mass index (BMI): Evidence for a non-linear relationship. *Appetite* **50**(1): 43–49.

Day, P. L. and J. Pearce (2011). Obesity-promoting food environments and the spatial clustering of food outlets around schools. *Am J Prev Med* **40**(2): 113–121.

De Ridder, D., P. Manning, S. L. Leong, S. Ross, W. Sutherland, C. Horwath and S. Vanneste (2016). The brain, obesity and addiction: An EEG Neuroimaging Study. *Sci Rep* **6**: 34122.

De Vogli, R., A. Kouvonen and D. Gimeno (2014). The influence of market deregulation on fast food consumption and body mass index: A cross-national time series analysis. *Bull World Health Organ* **92**(2): 99–107, 107A.

Dennis, A. B. and T. Pryor (2014). Introduction to substance use disorders for the eating disorder specialist. In: *Eating Disorders, Addictions, and Substance Use Disorders: Research, Clinical, and Treatment Perspectives.* T. D. Brewerton and A. B. Dennis, Eds., pp. 226–266. New York: Springer.

DiClemente, C. C. and J. Delahanty (2016). Homeostasis and change: A commentary on homeostatic theory of obesity by David Marks. *Health Psychol Open* **3**(1): 2055102916634366.

DiPatrizio, N. V. and K. J. Simansky (2008). Activating parabrachial cannabinoid CB1 receptors selectively stimulates feeding of palatable foods in rats. *J Neurosci* **28**(39): 9702–9709.

Doba, K., J. L. Nandrino, V. Dodin and P. Antoine (2014). Is there a family profile of addictive behaviors? Family functioning in anorexia nervosa and drug dependence disorder. *J Clin Psychol* **70**(1): 107–117.

Dong, M., R. F. Anda, V. J. Felitti, D. F. Williamson, S. R. Dube, D. W. Brown and W. H. Giles (2005). Childhood residential mobility and multiple health risks during adolescence and adulthood: The hidden role of adverse childhood experiences. *Arch Pediatr Adolesc Med* **159**(12): 1104–1110.

Dougkas, A., C. K. Reynolds, I. D. Givens, P. C. Elwood and A. M. Minihane (2011). Associations between dairy consumption and body weight: A review of the evidence and underlying mechanisms. *Nutr Res Rev* **24**(1): 72–95.

Duarte, C., J. Pinto-Gouveia, C. Ferreira and B. Silva (2016). Caught in the struggle with food craving: Development and validation of a new cognitive fusion measure. *Appetite* **101**: 146–155.

Dube, S. R., R. F. Anda, V. J. Felitti, J. B. Croft, V. J. Edwards and W. H. Giles (2001). Growing up with parental alcohol abuse: Exposure to childhood abuse, neglect, and household dysfunction. *Child Abuse Negl* **25**(12): 1627–1640.

Dube, S. R., V. J. Felitti, M. Dong, D. P. Chapman, W. H. Giles and R. F. Anda (2003). Childhood abuse, neglect, and household dysfunction and the risk of illicit drug use: The adverse childhood experiences study. *Pediatrics* **111**(3): 564–572.

Ellis, D. A., R. A. Zucker and H. E. Fitzgerald (1997). The role of family influences in development and risk. *Alcohol Health Res World* **21**(3): 218–226.

Epstein, L. H. and J. J. Leddy (2006). Food reinforcement. *Appetite* **46**(1): 22–25.

Esch, T. and G. B. Stefano (2004). The neurobiology of pleasure, reward processes, addiction and their health implications. *Neuro Endocrinol Lett* **25**(4): 235–251.

Fanciulli, G., A. Dettori, M. P. Demontis, P. A. Tomasi, V. Anania and G. Delitala (2005). Gluten exorphin B5 stimulates prolactin secretion through opioid receptors located outside the blood-brain barrier. *Life Sci* **76**(15): 1713–1719.

Febo, M., K. Blum, R. D. Badgaiyan, D. Baron, P. K. Thanos, L. M. Colon-Perez, Z. Demortrovics and M. S. Gold (2017). Dopamine homeostasis: Brain functional connectivity in reward deficiency syndrome. *Front Biosci (Landmark Ed)* **22**: 669–691.

Feldstein Ewing, S. W., E. D. Claus, K. A. Hudson, F. M. Filbey, E. Yakes Jimenez, K. M. Lisdahl and A. S. Kong (2016). Overweight adolescents' brain response to sweetened beverages mirrors addiction pathways. *Brain Imaging Behav.*

Felitti, V. J., R. F. Anda, D. Nordenberg, D. F. Williamson, A. M. Spitz, V. Edwards, M. P. Koss and J. S. Marks (1998). Relationship of childhood abuse and household dysfunction to many of the leading causes of death in adults. The Adverse Childhood Experiences (ACE) Study. *Am J Prev Med* **14**(4): 245–258.

Ferrario, C. R. (2017). Food addiction and obesity. *Neuropsychopharmacology* **42**(1): 361.

Field, M., J. Werthmann, I. Franken, W. Hofmann, L. Hogarth and A. Roefs (2016). The role of attentional bias in obesity and addiction. *Health Psychol* **35**(8): 767–780.

Fields, H. L. and E. B. Margolis (2015). Understanding opioid reward. *Trends Neurosci* **38**(4): 217–225.

Filbey, F. M., E. D. Claus, M. Morgan, G. R. Forester and K. Hutchison (2012). Dopaminergic genes modulate response inhibition in alcohol abusing adults. *Addict Biol* **17**(6): 1046–1056.

Finkelstein, E. A., J. G. Trogdon, J. W. Cohen and W. Dietz (2009). Annual medical spending attributable to obesity: Payer-and service-specific estimates. *Health Aff (Millwood)* **28**(5): w822–831.

Food Addicts Anonymous (2010). *Food Addicts Anonymous.* Port St. Lucie, FL: Food Addicts Anonymous, Inc.

Fortuna, J. L. (2012). The obesity epidemic and food addiction: Clinical similarities to drug dependence. *J Psychoactive Drugs* **44**(1): 56–63.

Frank, G. K. (2015). Advances from neuroimaging studies in eating disorders. *CNS Spectr* **20**(4): 391–400.

Frascella, J., M. N. Potenza, L. L. Brown and A. R. Childress (2010). Shared brain vulnerabilities open the way for nonsubstance addictions: Carving addiction at a new joint? *Ann N Y Acad Sci* **1187**: 294–315.

Garcia-Garcia, I., A. Horstmann, M. A. Jurado, M. Garolera, S. J. Chaudhry, D. S. Margulies, A. Villringer and J. Neumann (2014). Reward processing in obesity, substance addiction and non-substance addiction. *Obes Rev* **15**(11): 853–869.

Gearhardt, A., M. Roberts and M. Ashe (2013). If sugar is addictive...what does it mean for the law? *J Law Med Ethics* **41**(Suppl 1): 46–49.

Gearhardt, A. N., M. A. Bragg, R. L. Pearl, N. A. Schvey, C. A. Roberto and K. D. Brownell (2012). Obesity and public policy. *Annu Rev Clin Psychol* **8**: 405–430.

Gearhardt, A. N. and K. D. Brownell (2013). Can food and addiction change the game? *Biol Psychiatry* **73**(9): 802–803.

Gearhardt, A. N. and W. R. Corbin (2009). Body mass index and alcohol consumption: Family history of alcoholism as a moderator. *Psychol Addict Behav* **23**(2): 216–225.

Gearhardt, A. N., S. Yokum, P. T. Orr, E. Stice, W. R. Corbin and K. D. Brownell (2011). Neural correlates of food addiction. *Arch Gen Psychiatry* **68**(8): 808–816.

Giovino, G. A., J. E. Henningfield, S. L. Tomar, L. G. Escobedo and J. Slade (1995). Epidemiology of tobacco use and dependence. *Epidemiol Rev* **17**(1): 48–65.

Glynn, T., J. R. Seffrin, O. W. Brawley, N. Grey and H. Ross (2010). The globalization of tobacco use: 21 challenges for the 21st century. *CA Cancer J Clin* **60**(1): 50–61.

Goldschmidt, A. B. (2017). Are loss of control while eating and overeating valid constructs? A critical review of the literature. *Obes Rev* **18**(4): 412–449.

Goran, M. I., A. A. Martin, T. L. Alderete, H. Fujiwara and D. A. Fields (2017). Fructose in breast milk is positively associated with infant body composition at 6 months of age. *Nutrients* **9**(2): pii: E146.

Grimm, J. W., A. M. Fyall and D. P. Osincup (2005). Incubation of sucrose craving: Effects of reduced training and sucrose pre-loading. *Physiol Behav* **84**(1): 73–79.

Grimm, J. W., Y. Shaham and B. T. Hope (2002). Effect of cocaine and sucrose withdrawal period on extinction behavior, cue-induced reinstatement, and protein levels of the dopamine transporter and tyrosine hydroxylase in limbic and cortical areas in rats. *Behav Pharmacol* **13**(5–6): 379–388.

Hadad, N. A. and L. A. Knackstedt (2014). Addicted to palatable foods: Comparing the neurobiology of Bulimia Nervosa to that of drug addiction. *Psychopharmacology (Berl)* **231**(9): 1897–1912.

Harper, T. A. and G. Mooney (2010). Prevention before profits: A levy on food and alcohol advertising. *Med J Aust* **192**(7): 400–402.

Harwood, H. J., D. Fountain and G. Livermore (1998). Economic costs of alcohol abuse and alcoholism. *Recent Dev Alcohol* **14**: 307–330.

Hebebrand, J., O. Albayrak, R. Adan, J. Antel, C. Dieguez, J. de Jong, G. Leng, J. Menzies, J. G. Mercer, M. Murphy, G. van der Plasse and S. L. Dickson (2014). "Eating addiction," rather than "food addiction," better captures addictive-like eating behavior. *Neurosci Biobehav Rev* **47c**: 295–306.

Heber, D. and C. L. Carpenter (2011). Addictive genes and the relationship to obesity and inflammation. *Mol Neurobiol* **44**(2): 160–165.

Herrera, B. M., S. Keildson and C. M. Lindgren (2011). Genetics and epigenetics of obesity. *Maturitas* **69**(1): 41–49.

Hetherington, M., Ed. (2001). *Food Cravings and Addiction.* Leatherhead, Surrey, UK: Leatherhead Food Research Association.

Hetherington, M. M. (2007). Cues to overeat: Psychological factors influencing overconsumption. *Proc Nutr Soc* **66**(1): 113–123.

Heymsfield, S. B. and T. A. Wadden (2017). Mechanisms, pathophysiology, and management of obesity. *N Engl J Med* **376**(3): 254–266.

Hodgkins, C. C., K. S. Cahill, A. E. Seraphine, K. Frost-Pineda and M. S. Gold (2004). Adolescent drug addiction treatment and weight gain. *J Addict Dis* **23**(3): 55–65.

Holland, P. C. and G. D. Petrovich (2005). A neural systems analysis of the potentiation of feeding by conditioned stimuli. *Physiol Behav* **86**(5): 747–761.

Hone-Blanchet, A. and S. Fecteau (2014). Overlap of food addiction and substance use disorders definitions: Analysis of animal and human studies. *Neuropharmacology* **85**: 81–90.

Hughes, J. R., A. H. Oliveto, J. E. Helzer, S. T. Higgins and W. K. Bickel (1992). Should caffeine abuse, dependence, or withdrawal be added to DSM-IV and ICD-10? *Am J Psychiatry* **149**(1): 33–40.

Ifland, J., K. Sheppard and T. Wright (2012). From the front lines: The impact of refined food addiction on well-being. In *Handbook of Food And Addiction.* K. Brownell and M. Gold, Eds., pp. 348–353, Oxford University Press.

Ifland, J. R., H. G. Preuss, M. T. Marcus, K. M. Rourke, W. C. Taylor, K. Burau, W. S. Jacobs, W. Kadish and G. Manso (2009). Refined food addiction: A classic substance use disorder. *Med Hypotheses* **72**(5): 518–526.

Islam, A. K. and R. J. Bodnar (1990). Selective opioid receptor antagonist effects upon intake of a high-fat diet in rats. *Brain Res* **508**(2): 293–296.

Jastreboff, A. M., R. Sinha, C. Lacadie, D. M. Small, R. S. Sherwin and M. N. Potenza (2013). Neural correlates of stress- and food cue-induced food craving in obesity: Association with insulin levels. *Diabetes Care* **36**(2): 394–402.

Joyner, M. A., A. N. Gearhardt and M. A. White (2015). Food craving as a mediator between addictive-like eating and problematic eating outcomes. *Eat Behav* **19**: 98–101.

Juliano, L. M., S. Ferre and R. R. Griffiths (2014). The Pharmacology of Caffeine. *ASAM Principles of Addiction Medicine.* R. K. Ries, S. C. Miller, D. A. Fiellin and R. Saitz, Eds., pp. 182–198, Washington, DC: American Society of Addiction Medicine.

Jung, C., A. Rabinowitsch, W. T. Lee, D. Zheng, S. C. de Vaca and K. D. Carr (2016). Effects of food restriction on expression of place conditioning and biochemical correlates in rat nucleus accumbens. *Psychopharmacology (Berl)* **233**(17): 3161–3172.

Kampov-Polevoy, A. B., J. C. Garbutt and E. Khalitov (2003). Family history of alcoholism and response to sweets. *Alcohol Clin Exp Res* **27**(11): 1743–1749.

Karlsson, H. K., L. Tuominen, J. J. Tuulari, J. Hirvonen, R. Parkkola, S. Helin, P. Salminen, P. Nuutila and L. Nummenmaa (2015). Obesity is associated with decreased mu-opioid but unaltered dopamine D2 receptor availability in the brain. *J Neurosci* **35**(9): 3959–3965.

Karlsson, H. K., J. J. Tuulari, L. Tuominen, J. Hirvonen, H. Honka, R. Parkkola, S. Helin, P. Salminen, P. Nuutila and L. Nummenmaa (2016). Weight loss after bariatric surgery normalizes brain opioid receptors in morbid obesity. *Mol Psychiatry* **21**(8): 1057–1062.

Kelley, A. E., C. A. Schiltz and C. F. Landry (2005). Neural systems recruited by drug- and food-related cues: Studies of gene activation in corticolimbic regions. *Physiol Behav* **86**(1–2): 11–14.

Kemps, E., M. Tiggemann and M. Grigg (2008). Food cravings consume limited cognitive resources. *J Exp Psychol Appl* **14**(3): 247–254.

Kendzor, D. E., L. E. Baillie, C. E. Adams, D. W. Stewart and A. L. Copeland (2008). The effect of food deprivation on cigarette smoking in females. *Addict Behav* **33**(10): 1353–1359.

Kenny, P. J. (2011). Common cellular and molecular mechanisms in obesity and drug addiction. *Nat Rev Neurosci* **12**(11): 638–651.

Kessler, D. (2009). *The End of Overeating: Taking Control of the Insatiable American Appetite.* New York: Rodale.

Kleiner, K. D., M. S. Gold, K. Frost-Pineda, B. Lenz-Brunsman, M. G. Perri and W. S. Jacobs (2004). Body mass index and alcohol use. *J Addict Dis* **23**(3): 105–118.

Klenowski, P. M., M. J. Fogarty, M. Shariff, A. Belmer, M. C. Bellingham and S. E. Bartlett (2016a). Increased synaptic excitation and abnormal dendritic structure of prefrontal cortex layer V pyramidal neurons following prolonged binge-like consumption of ethanol. *eNeuro* **3**(6). Doi: 10.1523/ENEURO.0248-16.2016.

Klenowski, P. M., M. R. Shariff, A. Belmer, M. J. Fogarty, E. W. Mu, M. C. Bellingham and S. E. Bartlett (2016b). Prolonged consumption of sucrose in a binge-like manner, alters the morphology of medium spiny neurons in the nucleus accumbens shell. *Front Behav Neurosci* **10**: 54.

Krahnstoever Davison, K., L. A. Francis and L. L. Birch (2005). Reexamining obesigenic families: Parents' obesity-related behaviors predict girls' change in BMI. *Obes Res* **13**(11): 1980–1990.

Krasnova, I. N., N. J. Marchant, B. Ladenheim, M. T. McCoy, L. V. Panlilio, J. M. Bossert, Y. Shaham and J. L. Cadet (2014). Incubation of methamphetamine and palatable food craving after punishment-induced abstinence. *Neuropsychopharmacology* **39**(8): 2008–2016.

Kuhn, F. T., F. Trevizol, V. T. Dias, R. C. Barcelos, C. S. Pase, K. Roversi, C. T. Antoniazzi, K. Roversi, N. Boufleur, D. M. Benvegnu, T. Emanuelli and M. E. Burger (2014). Toxicological aspects of trans fat consumption over two sequential generations of rats: Oxidative damage and preference for amphetamine. *Toxicol Lett* **232**(1): 58–67.

Lee, A. and S. E. Gibbs (2013). Neurobiology of food addiction and adolescent obesity prevention in low- and middle-income countries. *J Adolesc Health* **52**(2 Suppl 2): S39–42.

Lee, N. M., J. Lucke, W. D. Hall, C. Meurk, F. M. Boyle and A. Carter (2013). Public views on food addiction and obesity: Implications for policy and treatment. *PLoS One* **8**(9): e74836.

Lee, S. H., B. J. Ham, Y. H. Cho, S. M. Lee and S. H. Shim (2007). Association study of dopamine receptor D2 TaqI A polymorphism and reward-related personality traits in healthy Korean young females. *Neuropsychobiology* **56**(2–3): 146–151.

Lenoir, M., F. Serre, L. Cantin and S. H. Ahmed (2007). Intense sweetness surpasses cocaine reward. *PLoS One* **2**(1): e698.

Leombruni, P., L. Lavagnino, F. Gastaldi, A. Vasile and S. Fassino (2009). Duloxetine in obese binge eater outpatients: Preliminary results from a 12-week open trial. *Hum Psychopharmacol* **24**(6): 483–488.

Lerma-Cabrera, J. M., F. Carvajal and P. Lopez-Legarrea (2016). Food addiction as a new piece of the obesity framework. *Nutr J* **15**: 5.

Levy, A., A. Salamon, M. Tucci, C. L. Limebeer, L. A. Parker and F. Leri (2013). Co-sensitivity to the incentive properties of palatable food and cocaine in rats; implications for co-morbid addictions. *Addict Biol* **18**(5): 763–773.

Lewin, A., L. Lindstrom and M. Nestle (2006). Food industry promises to address childhood obesity: Preliminary evaluation. *J Public Health Policy* **27**(4): 327–348.

Li, Q., W. Li, H. Wang, Y. Wang, Y. Zhang, J. Zhu, Y. Zheng, et al. (2015). Predicting subsequent relapse by drug-related cue-induced brain activation in heroin addiction: An event-related functional magnetic resonance imaging study. *Addict Biol* **20**(5): 968–978.

Lim, J. S., M. Mietus-Snyder, A. Valente, J. M. Schwarz and R. H. Lustig (2010). The role of fructose in the pathogenesis of NAFLD and the metabolic syndrome. *Nat Rev Gastroenterol Hepatol* **7**(5): 251–264.

Liu, Y., K. M. von Deneen, F. H. Kobeissy and M. S. Gold (2010). Food addiction and obesity: Evidence from bench to bedside. *J Psychoactive Drugs* **42**(2): 133–145.

Lu, L., J. W. Grimm, B. T. Hope and Y. Shaham (2004). Incubation of cocaine craving after withdrawal: A review of preclinical data. *Neuropharmacology* **47**(Suppl 1): 214–226.

Lustig, R. H. (2010). Fructose: Metabolic, hedonic, and societal parallels with ethanol. *J Am Diet Assoc* **110**(9): 1307–1321.

Lutter, M. and E. J. Nestler (2009). Homeostatic and hedonic signals interact in the regulation of food intake. *J Nutr* **139**(3): 629–632.

Mahar, A. and L. M. Duizer (2007). The effect of frequency of consumption of artificial sweeteners on sweetness liking by women. *J Food Sci* **72**(9): S714–718.

Manzel, A., D. N. Muller, D. A. Hafler, S. E. Erdman, R. A. Linker and M. Kleinewietfeld (2014). Role of "Western diet" in inflammatory autoimmune diseases. *Curr Allergy Asthma Rep* **14**(1): 404.

Marcus, M. D. and J. E. Wildes (2014). Disordered eating in obese individuals. *Curr Opin Psychiatry* **27**(6): 443–447.

Martin-Fardon, R., G. Cauvi, T. M. Kerr and F. Weiss (2016). Differential role of hypothalamic orexin/hypocretin neurons in reward seeking motivated by cocaine versus palatable food. *Addict Biol.* Doi: 10.1111/adb.12441. [Epub ahead of print].

Martinez Steele, E., L. G. Baraldi, M. L. Louzada, J. C. Moubarac, D. Mozaffarian and C. A. Monteiro (2016). Ultra-processed foods and added sugars in the US diet: Evidence from a nationally representative cross-sectional study. *BMJ Open* **6**(3): e009892.

Mason, S. M., A. J. Flint, A. E. Field, S. B. Austin and J. W. Rich-Edwards (2013). Abuse victimization in childhood or adolescence and risk of food addiction in adult women. *Obesity (Silver Spring)* **21**(12): E775–E781.

Mattson, S. N., S. C. Roesch, A. Fagerlund, I. Autti-Ramo, K. L. Jones, P. A. May, C. M. Adnams, V. Konovalova and E. P. Riley (2010). Toward a neurobehavioral profile of fetal alcohol spectrum disorders. *Alcohol Clin Exp Res* **34**(9): 1640–1650.

McAuliffe, P. F., M. S. Gold, L. Bajpai, M. L. Merves, K. Frost-Pineda, R. M. Pomm, B. A. Goldberger, R. J. Melker and J. C. Cendan (2006). Second-hand exposure to aerosolized intravenous anesthetics propofol and fentanyl may cause sensitization and subsequent opiate addiction among anesthesiologists and surgeons. *Med Hypotheses* **66**(5): 874–882.

McIver, S., P. O'Halloran and M. McGartland (2009). Yoga as a treatment for binge eating disorder: A preliminary study. *Complement Ther Med* **17**(4): 196–202.

McLellan, A. T., J. C. Cacciola, A. I. Alterman, S. H. Rikoon and D. Carise (2006). The addiction severity index at 25: Origins, contributions and transitions. *Am J Addict* **15**(2): 113–124.
McLellan, A. T., H. Kushner, D. Metzger, R. Peters, I. Smith, G. Grissom, H. Pettinati and M. Argeriou (1992). The fifth edition of the addiction severity index. *J Subst Abuse Treat* **9**(3): 199–213.
McNatt, S. S., J. J. Longhi, C. D. Goldman and D. W. McFadden (2007). Surgery for obesity: A review of the current state of the art and future directions. *J Gastrointest Surg* **11**(3): 377–397.
Meisel, H. (1986). Chemical characterization and opioid activity of an exorphin isolated from in vivo digests of casein. *FEBS Lett* **196**(2): 223–227.
Mellor, J. M., C. B. Dolan and R. B. Rapoport (2011). Child body mass index, obesity, and proximity to fast food restaurants. *Int J Pediatr Obes* **6**(1): 60–8.
Mennella, J. A., M. Y. Pepino, S. M. Lehmann-Castor and L. M. Yourshaw (2010). Sweet preferences and analgesia during childhood: Effects of family history of alcoholism and depression. *Addiction* **105**(4): 666–675.
Merlo, L. J., C. Klingman, T. H. Malasanos and J. H. Silverstein (2009). Exploration of food addiction in pediatric patients: A preliminary investigation. *J Addict Med* **3**(1): 26–32.
Meule, A. and A. N. Gearhardt (2014). Food addiction in the light of DSM-5. *Nutrients* **6**(9): 3653–3671.
Meule, A., A. Muller, A. N. Gearhardt and J. Blechert (2017). German version of the Yale Food Addiction Scale 2.0: Prevalence and correlates of "food addiction" in students and obese individuals. *Appetite* **115**: 54–61.
Michaelides, M., P. K. Thanos, N. D. Volkow and G. J. Wang (2012). Translational neuroimaging in drug addiction and obesity. *Ilar j* **53**(1): 59–68.
Mole, T. B., M. A. Irvine, Y. Worbe, P. Collins, S. P. Mitchell, S. Bolton, N. A. Harrison, T. W. Robbins and V. Voon (2015). Impulsivity in disorders of food and drug misuse. *Psychol Med* **45**(4): 771–782.
Moore, C. F., V. Sabino, G. F. Koob and P. Cottone (2017). Pathological overeating: Emerging evidence for a compulsivity construct. *Neuropsychopharmacology* **42**(7): 1375–1389.
Morgan, D. and G. M. Sizemore (2011). Animal models of addiction: Fat and sugar. *Curr Pharm Des* **17**(12): 1168–1172.
Morgenstern, J., N. H. Naqvi, R. Debellis and H. C. Breiter (2013). The contributions of cognitive neuroscience and neuroimaging to understanding mechanisms of behavior change in addiction. *Psychol Addict Behav* **27**(2): 336–350.
Moss, M. (2013). *Salt, Sugar, Fat: How the Food Giants Hooked Us.* Random House, New York.
Murray, S. M., A. J. Tulloch, E. Y. Chen and N. M. Avena (2015). Insights revealed by rodent models of sugar binge eating. *CNS Spectr* **20**(6): 530–536.
National Institute of Drug Abuse (2015). *Costs of Substance Abuse.* Retrieved March 10, 2017, from https://www.drugabuse.gov/related-topics/trends-statistics
Nestle, M. (1996). *Food Politics.* New York: Random House.
Nestle, M. (2013). *Food Politics.* Berkeley, CA: University of California Press.
Ng, M., T. Fleming, M. Robinson, B. Thomson, N. Graetz, C. Margono, E. C. Mullany, et al. (2014). Global, regional, and national prevalence of overweight and obesity in children and adults during 1980–2013: A systematic analysis for the Global Burden of Disease Study 2013. *Lancet* **384**(9945): 766–781.
Noble, E. E. and S. E. Kanoski (2016). Early life exposure to obesogenic diets and learning and memory dysfunction. *Curr Opin Behav Sci* **9**: 7–14.
Noble, E. P., R. E. Noble, T. Ritchie, K. Syndulko, M. C. Bohlman, L. A. Noble, Y. Zhang, R. S. Sparkes and D. K. Grandy (1994). D2 dopamine receptor gene and obesity. *Int J Eat Disord* **15**(3): 205–217.
Noori, H. R., A. Cosa Linan and R. Spanagel (2016). Largely overlapping neuronal substrates of reactivity to drug, gambling, food and sexual cues: A comprehensive meta-analysis. *Eur Neuropsychopharmacol* **26**(9): 1419–1430.
Nseir, W., F. Nassar and N. Assy (2010). Soft drinks consumption and nonalcoholic fatty liver disease. *World J Gastroenterol* **16**(21): 2579–2588.
Ogden, C. L., S. Z. Yanovski, M. D. Carroll and K. M. Flegal (2007). The epidemiology of obesity. *Gastroenterology* **132**(6): 2087–2102.
Oginsky, M. F., P. B. Goforth, C. W. Nobile, L. F. Lopez-Santiago and C. R. Ferrario (2016). Eating "junk-food" produces rapid and long-lasting increases in NAc CP-AMPA receptors: Implications for enhanced cue-induced motivation and food addiction. *Neuropsychopharmacology* **41**(13): 2977–2986.
Olstad, D. L., K. Ball, C. Wright, G. Abbott, E. Brown and A. I. Turner (2016). Hair cortisol levels, perceived stress and body mass index in women and children living in socioeconomically disadvantaged neighborhoods: The READI study. *Stress* **19**(2): 158–167.

Olszewski, P. K. and A. S. Levine (2007). Central opioids and consumption of sweet tastants: When reward outweighs homeostasis. *Physiol Behav* **91**(5): 506–512.

Ouyang, X., P. Cirillo, Y. Sautin, S. McCall, J. L. Bruchette, A. M. Diehl, R. J. Johnson and M. F. Abdelmalek (2008). Fructose consumption as a risk factor for non-alcoholic fatty liver disease. *J Hepatol* **48**(6): 993–999.

Pateman, K., P. Ford, L. Fizgerald, A. Mutch, K. Yuke, B. Bonevski and C. Gartner (2016). Stuck in the catch 22: Attitudes towards smoking cessation among populations vulnerable to social disadvantage. *Addiction* **111**(6): 1048–1056.

Peeke, P. (2012). *The Hunger Fix.* New York: Rodale.

Peeke, P. (2016). *How to Live a Recovery-Centric Life.* Retrieved March 3, 2017, from http://www.huffingtonpost.com/maria-rodale/how-to-live-a-recovery-ce_b_10940668.html

Peele, S. (1992). *The Truth about Addiction and Recovery.* New York: Fireside.

Pelchat, M. L., A. Johnson, R. Chan, J. Valdez and J. D. Ragland (2004). Images of desire: Food-craving activation during fMRI. *NeuroImage* **23**(4): 1486–1493.

Pepino, M. Y. and J. A. Mennella (2005). Sucrose-induced analgesia is related to sweet preferences in children but not adults. *Pain* **119**(1–3): 210–218.

Pepino, M. Y. and J. A. Mennella (2007). Effects of cigarette smoking and family history of alcoholism on sweet taste perception and food cravings in women. *Alcohol Clin Exp Res* **31**(11): 1891–1899.

Petrovich, G. D. (2013). Forebrain networks and the control of feeding by environmental learned cues. *Physiol Behav* **121**: 10–18.

Petrovich, G. D. and M. Gallagher (2007). Control of food consumption by learned cues: A forebrain-hypothalamic network. *Physiol Behav* **91**(4): 397–403.

Petrovich, G. D., C. A. Ross, M. Gallagher and P. C. Holland (2007a). Learned contextual cue potentiates eating in rats. *Physiol Behav* **90**(2–3): 362–367.

Petrovich, G. D., C. A. Ross, P. C. Holland and M. Gallagher (2007b). Medial prefrontal cortex is necessary for an appetitive contextual conditioned stimulus to promote eating in sated rats. *J Neurosci* **27**(24): 6436–6441.

Raimo, E. B., T. L. Smith, G. P. Danko, K. K. Bucholz and M. A. Schuckit (2000). Clinical characteristics and family histories of alcoholics with stimulant dependence. *J Stud Alcohol* **61**(5): 728–735.

Ranaldi, R., J. Egan, K. Kest, M. Fein and A. R. Delamater (2009). Repeated heroin in rats produces locomotor sensitization and enhances appetitive Pavlovian and instrumental learning involving food reward. *Pharmacol Biochem Behav* **91**(3): 351–357.

Rao, R. E., F. H. Wojnicki, J. Coupland, S. Ghosh and R. L. Corwin (2008). Baclofen, raclopride, and naltrexone differentially reduce solid fat emulsion intake under limited access conditions. *Pharmacol Biochem Behav* **89**(4): 581–590.

Rezapour, T., E. E. DeVito, M. Sofuoglu and H. Ekhtiari (2016). Perspectives on neurocognitive rehabilitation as an adjunct treatment for addictive disorders: From cognitive improvement to relapse prevention. *Prog Brain Res* **224**: 345–369.

Ries, R. K., S. C. Miller, D. A. Fiellin and R. Saitz, Eds. (2009). *Principles of Addiction Medicine.* Philadelphia, PA: Lippincott Williams & Wilkins.

Riley, E. P., M. A. Infante and K. R. Warren (2011). Fetal alcohol spectrum disorders: An overview. *Neuropsychol Rev* **21**(2): 73–80.

Rogers, P. J. (2017). Food and drug addictions: Similarities and differences. *Pharmacol Biochem Behav* **153**: 182–190.

Rogers, P. J. and H. J. Smit (2000). Food craving and food "addiction": A critical review of the evidence from a biopsychosocial perspective. *Pharmacol Biochem Behav* **66**(1): 3–14.

Rolls, E. T. and C. McCabe (2007). Enhanced affective brain representations of chocolate in cravers vs. non-cravers. *Eur J Neurosci* **26**(4): 1067–1076.

Rosenberg, H. (2009). Clinical and laboratory assessment of the subjective experience of drug craving. *Clin Psychol Rev* **29**(6): 519–534.

Rudelt, A., S. French and L. Harnack (2014). Fourteen-year trends in sodium content of menu offerings at eight leading fast-food restaurants in the USA. *Public Health Nutr* **17**(8): 1682–1688.

Rupprecht, L. E., T. T. Smith, E. C. Donny and A. F. Sved (2017). Self-administered nicotine differentially impacts body weight gain in obesity-prone and obesity-resistant rats. *Physiol Behav* **176**: 71–75.

Sartor, F., L. F. Donaldson, D. A. Markland, H. Loveday, M. J. Jackson and H. P. Kubis (2011). Taste perception and implicit attitude toward sweet related to body mass index and soft drink supplementation. *Appetite* **57**(1): 237–246.

Schroeder, B. E., J. M. Binzak and A. E. Kelley (2001). A common profile of prefrontal cortical activation following exposure to nicotine- or chocolate-associated contextual cues. *Neuroscience* **105**(3): 535–545.

Schuckit, M. A., G. P. Danko, E. B. Raimo, T. L. Smith, M. Y. Eng, K. K. Carpenter and V. M. Hesselbrock (2001). A preliminary evaluation of the potential usefulness of the diagnoses of polysubstance dependence. *J Stud Alcohol* **62**(1): 54–61.

Schulte, E. M., N. M. Avena and A. N. Gearhardt (2015). Which foods may be addictive? The roles of processing, fat content, and glycemic load. *PLoS One* **10**(2): e0117959.

Schulte, E. M., H. M. Tuttle and A. N. Gearhardt (2016). Belief in food addiction and obesity-related policy support. *PLoS One* **11**(1): e0147557.

Seliske, L. M., W. Pickett, W. F. Boyce and I. Janssen (2009). Density and type of food retailers surrounding Canadian schools: Variations across socioeconomic status. *Health Place* **15**(3): 903–907.

Sharma, S., M. F. Fernandes and S. Fulton (2013). Adaptations in brain reward circuitry underlie palatable food cravings and anxiety induced by high-fat diet withdrawal. *Int J Obes (Lond)* **37**(9): 1183–1191.

Sinha, R. and A. M. Jastreboff (2013). Stress as a common risk factor for obesity and addiction. *Biol Psychiatry* **73**(9): 827–835.

Smit, H. J., E. A. Gaffan and P. J. Rogers (2004). Methylxanthines are the psycho-pharmacologically active constituents of chocolate. *Psychopharmacology (Berl)* **176**(3–4): 412–419.

Stefano, G. B., E. Bianchi, M. Guarna, G. L. Fricchione, W. Zhu, P. Cadet, K. J. Mantione, F. M. Casares, R. M. Kream and T. Esch (2007). Nicotine, alcohol and cocaine coupling to reward processes via endogenous morphine signaling: The dopamine-morphine hypothesis. *Med Sci Monit* **13**(6): RA91–102.

Stice, E., K. S. Burger and S. Yokum (2013). Relative ability of fat and sugar tastes to activate reward, gustatory, and somatosensory regions. *Am J Clin Nutr* **98**(6): 1377–1384.

Stice, E. and A. Dagher (2010). Genetic variation in dopaminergic reward in humans. *Forum Nutr* **63**: 176–185.

Stice, E., S. Spoor, C. Bohon, M. G. Veldhuizen and D. M. Small (2008). Relation of reward from food intake and anticipated food intake to obesity: A functional magnetic resonance imaging study. *J Abnorm Psychol* **117**(4): 924–935.

Stice, E. and S. Yokum (2016). Neural vulnerability factors that increase risk for future weight gain. *Psychol Bull* **142**(5): 447–471.

Stice, E., S. Yokum, D. Zald and A. Dagher (2011). Dopamine-based reward circuitry responsivity, genetics, and overeating. *Curr Top Behav Neurosci* **6**: 81–93.

Stothard, K. J., P. W. Tennant, R. Bell and J. Rankin (2009). Maternal overweight and obesity and the risk of congenital anomalies: A systematic review and meta-analysis. *JAMA* **301**(6): 636–650.

Sturm, R. (2002). The effects of obesity, smoking, and drinking on medical problems and costs. *Health Aff (Millwood)* **21**(2): 245–253.

Suliburska, J., G. Duda and D. Pupek-Musialik (2004). Effect of tobacco smoking on taste sensitivity in adults. *Przegl Lek* **61**(10): 1174–1176.

Tang, D. W., L. K. Fellows, D. M. Small and A. Dagher (2012). Food and drug cues activate similar brain regions: A meta-analysis of functional MRI studies. *Physiol Behav* **106**(3): 317–324.

Tellez, L. A., J. G. Ferreira, S. Medina, B. B. Land, R. J. DiLeone and I. E. de Araujo (2013). Flavor-independent maintenance, extinction, and reinstatement of fat self-administration in mice. *Biol Psychiatry* **73**(9): 851–859.

Temple, J. L. (2016). Behavioral sensitization of the reinforcing value of food: What food and drugs have in common. *Prev Med* **92**: 90–99.

Teschemacher, H., G. Koch and V. Brantl (1997). Milk protein-derived opioid receptor ligands. *Biopolymers* **43**(2): 99–117.

Thorpe, K. E. (2013). Treated disease prevalence and spending per treated case drove most of the growth in health care spending in 1987–2009. *Health Aff (Millwood)* **32**(5): 851–858.

Tillotson, J. E. (2004). America's obesity: Conflicting public policies, industrial economic development, and unintended human consequences. *Annu Rev Nutr* **24**: 617–643.

Tomasi, D. and N. D. Volkow (2013). Striatocortical pathway dysfunction in addiction and obesity: Differences and similarities. *Crit Rev Biochem Mol Biol* **48**(1): 1–19.

Tomasi, D., G. J. Wang, R. Wang, E. C. Caparelli, J. Logan and N. D. Volkow (2015). Overlapping patterns of brain activation to food and cocaine cues in cocaine abusers: Association to striatal D2/D3 receptors. *Hum Brain Mapp* **36**(1): 120–136.

Turk, M. W., K. Yang, M. Hravnak, S. M. Sereika, L. J. Ewing and L. E. Burke (2009). Randomized clinical trials of weight loss maintenance: A review. *J Cardiovasc Nurs* **24**(1): 58–80.

Vaillant, G. E. (1995). *The Natural History of Alcoholism Revisited.* Cambridge MA: Harvard University Press.

VanderBroek-Stice, L., M. K. Stojek, S. R. Beach, M. R. vanDellen and J. MacKillop . (2017). Multidimensional assessment of impulsivity in relation to obesity and food addiction. *Appetite* **112**: 59–68.

Volkow, N. D. and R. D. Baler (2015). NOW vs LATER brain circuits: Implications for obesity and addiction. *Trends Neurosci* **38**(6): 345–352.

Volkow, N. D., A. J. Hampson and R. Baler (2017). Don't worry, be happy: Endocannabinoids and cannabis at the intersection of stress and reward. *Annu Rev Pharmacol Toxicol* **57**: 285–308.

Volkow, N. D., G. F. Koob and A. T. McLellan (2016a). Neurobiologic advances from the brain disease model of addiction. *N Engl J Med* **374**(4): 363–371.

Volkow, N. D., J. M. Swanson, A. E. Evins, L. E. DeLisi, M. H. Meier, R. Gonzalez, M. A. Bloomfield, H. V. Curran and R. Baler (2016b). Effects of cannabis use on human behavior, including cognition, motivation, and psychosis: A review. *JAMA Psychiatry* **73**(3): 292–297.

Volkow, N. D., G. J. Wang and R. D. Baler (2011). Reward, dopamine and the control of food intake: Implications for obesity. *Trends Cogn Sci* **15**(1): 37–46.

Volkow, N. D., G. J. Wang, J. S. Fowler and F. Telang (2008). Overlapping neuronal circuits in addiction and obesity: Evidence of systems pathology. *Philos Trans R Soc Lond B Biol Sci* **363**(1507): 3191–3200.

Volkow, N. D., G. J. Wang, J. S. Fowler, D. Tomasi and R. Baler (2012). Food and drug reward: Overlapping circuits in human obesity and addiction. *Curr Top Behav Neurosci* **11**: 1–24.

Volkow, N. D., G. J. Wang, J. S. Fowler, D. Tomasi, F. Telang and R. Baler (2010). Addiction: Decreased reward sensitivity and increased expectation sensitivity conspire to overwhelm the brain's control circuit. *Bioessays* **32**(9): 748–755.

Volkow, N. D., G. J. Wang, D. Tomasi and R. D. Baler (2013a). The addictive dimensionality of obesity. *Biol Psychiatry* **73**(9): 811–818.

Volkow, N. D., G. J. Wang, D. Tomasi and R. D. Baler (2013b). Obesity and addiction: Neurobiological overlaps. *Obes Rev* **14**(1): 2–18.

Volkow, N. D. and R. A. Wise (2005). How can drug addiction help us understand obesity? *Nat Neurosci* **8**(5): 555–560.

Voon, V. (2015). Cognitive biases in binge eating disorder: The hijacking of decision making. *CNS Spectr* **20**(6): 566–573.

Wang, G. J., A. Geliebter, N. D. Volkow, F. W. Telang, J. Logan, M. C. Jayne, K. Galanti, et al. (2011). Enhanced striatal dopamine release during food stimulation in binge eating disorder. *Obesity (Silver Spring)* **19**(8): 1601–1608.

Wang, H., B. Wen, J. Cheng and H. Li (2017). Brain structural differences between normal and obese adults and their links with lack of perseverance, negative urgency, and sensation seeking. *Sci Rep* **7**: 40595.

Wang, J., D. Freire, L. Knable, W. Zhao, B. Gong, P. Mazzola, L. Ho, S. Levine and G. M. Pasinetti (2014). Childhood/adolescent obesity and long term cognitive consequences during aging. *J Comp Neurol.* **523**(5): 757–768.

Wang, Y., M. A. Beydoun, L. Liang, B. Caballero and S. K. Kumanyika (2008). Will all Americans become overweight or obese? Estimating the progression and cost of the US obesity epidemic. *Obesity (Silver Spring)* **16**(10): 2323–2330.

Watkins, B. A. and J. Kim (2014). The endocannabinoid system: Directing eating behavior and macronutrient metabolism. *Front Psychol* **5**: 1506.

Weiss, F. (2005). Neurobiology of craving, conditioned reward and relapse. *Curr Opin Pharmacol* **5**(1): 9–19.

Widome, R., B. Brock, P. Noble and J. L. Forster (2013). The relationship of neighborhood demographic characteristics to point-of-sale tobacco advertising and marketing. *Ethn Health* **18**(2): 136–151.

Wiss, D. A., K. Criscitelli, M. Gold and N. Avena (2016). Preclinical evidence for the addiction potential of highly palatable foods: Current developments related to maternal influence. *Appetite* **115**: 19–27.

Yau, P. L., E. H. Kang, D. C. Javier and A. Convit (2014). Preliminary evidence of cognitive and brain abnormalities in uncomplicated adolescent obesity. *Obesity (Silver Spring)* **22**(8): 1865–1871.

Yeh, J., A. Trang, S. M. Henning, H. Wilhalme, C. Carpenter, D. Heber and Z. Li (2016). Food cravings, food addiction, and a dopamine-resistant (DRD2 A1) receptor polymorphism in Asian American college students. *Asia Pac J Clin Nutr* **25**(2): 424–429.

Yesavage, J. A., L. M. Kinoshita, A. Noda, L. C. Lazzeroni, J. K. Fairchild, J. Taylor, D. Kulick, et al. (2014). Effects of body mass index-related disorders on cognition: Preliminary results. *Diabetes Metab Syndr Obes* **7**: 145–151.

Youngson, N. A. and M. J. Morris (2013). What obesity research tells us about epigenetic mechanisms. *Philos Trans R Soc Lond B Biol Sci* **368**(1609): 20110337.

Ziauddeen, H., I. S. Farooqi and P. C. Fletcher (2012). Obesity and the brain: How convincing is the addiction model? *Nat Rev Neurosci* **13**(4): 279–286.

Zorrilla, E. P., M. L. Logrip and G. F. Koob (2014). Corticotropin releasing factor: A key role in the neurobiology of addiction. *Front Neuroendocrinol* **35**(2): 234–244.

2 Neurodysfunction in Addiction and Overeating as Assessed by Brain Imaging

Randall J. Ellis and Michael Michaelides
National Institute on Drug Abuse Intramural Research Program
Baltimore, MD

Gene-Jack Wang
National Institute on Alcohol Abuse and Alcoholism
Bethesda, MD

CONTENTS

2.1 INTRODUCTION

Food addiction is a growing global health concern implicated in the epidemic of obesity and overweight. The epidemic of obesity was declared by the World Health Organization and Centers for Disease Control and Prevention beginning in the late 1990s and early 2000s. Overweight people numbered over 1.9 billion in 2014, of which 39% were aged 18 and older. Overweight adults included 600 million obese or 13% of all adults (WHO 2015). In 2013, 42 million children under 5 years of age were overweight or obese, of which approximately 31 million resided in developing nations. Obesity more than doubled between 1980 and 2014. In the United States alone, the annual productive loss resulting from obesity absenteeism is between $3.38 billion and $6.38 billion (Trogdon et al., 2008).

Food addiction can be defined as the compulsive consumption of food despite a lack of hunger or a desire to stop eating (Meule and Gearhardt 2014). Excessive consumption of food can be defined as the consumption of calories beyond the body's requirement to function. The excess calories may be stored as fat, leading to weight gain and if uninterrupted, to overweight and obesity. Coinciding with public health and epidemiology research on the causes, effects, and strategies for dealing with the epidemic of obesity as well as the growing awareness of eating disorders, recent neuroimaging research is elucidating the neural mechanisms that underlie overeating and can help explain pathologies. Such work has demonstrated that the changes in brain mechanisms occurring in the context of overeating or obesity show significant similarities to the changes that occur in substance abuse and the development of addiction. In general, these studies have demonstrated that obesity/overeating and drug addiction show similar disruptions in the brain's reward systems.

2.2 SIMILARITIES BETWEEN OVEREATING AND ADDICTION

Conceptually, excess consumption of food and drugs can be thought of as the combination of three experiential components:

1. The first component is characterized by euphoria, reward, and pleasure, which reinforces consumption of food or drugs.
2. The second component is a strengthening of brain plasticity or sensitization regarding the incentive value of associated drug and food cues parallel to a weakening of inhibitory control mechanisms.
3. The third component pertains to negative affect and dysphoria, which occurs upon withdrawal from the food or drug, tolerance, and a stark craving and anticipation for the next instance when the food or drug will be consumed (Parylak, Koob, and Zorrilla 2011).

The positive and negative thought patterns and affect related to feeding rely on a complex network of neurotransmitters, hormones, neuropeptides, and other biological entities. Eating food, especially when hungry, is a normative, rewarding activity and rightfully so from an evolutionary standpoint. In primitive eras, where food availability was unpredictable, excess calories were rarely available. Hunter–gatherer societies had to expend significant energy to accumulate food. Calorie-dense food would be highly desirable because of the physically strenuous, and hence calorie-burning, nature of accumulating and maintaining food stores and other aspects of tribal life.

The scarcity of calorie-dense food in primitive eras is in stark contrast with modern conditions of industrialized living. Westernized cultures are marked by constant availability and low cost of high-calorie and hyperpalatable foods coupled with sedentary lifestyles. The drive to consume and accumulate calories and manage food uncertainty in the lives of primitive humans conflicts starkly with the proliferation of cheap processed foods that are available to consume very close to home.

Both high-calorie foods (e.g., refined sugars, processed fats, and their combinations) and addictive drugs (e.g., cocaine, heroin) can induce euphoria, reward sensitization, and withdrawal avoidance. An important difference is that drugs of abuse are not in any amount required for normative bodily functioning. By contrast, almost all animals require energy from exogenous food sources (e.g., protein, sugar, fat). Importantly, like the chronic use of drugs, chronic overconsumption of fat and sugar can alter the brain's natural reward systems (Volkow et al., 2013). As such, it is possible that repeated overconsumption of calorie-dense foods can lead to a state resembling that of addiction. Addiciton to food can cripple the health of the patient by hijacking healthy drives for food consumption. Neuroimaging modalities such as structural and functional magnetic resonance imaging (s/fMRI) and positron emission tomography (PET) have been used to demonstrate specific neurofunctional changes that are common to both drug abuse and overeating. Evidence from such studies is summarized in this chapter.

2.3 EVIDENCE FOR FOOD ADDICTION USING PET

2.3.1 Introduction

PET is a noninvasive imaging modality that requires the administration of radioactive substances or "tracers" (e.g., small molecules, peptides, antibodies, etc.) that emit positively charged particles (positrons) and whose distribution can be visualized inside the human brain (and other organs). Various PET radiotracers exist, but those that have been studied most extensively in the context of addiction and obesity are [^{18}F]fluorodeoxyglucose (FDG) and [^{11}C]raclopride, which respectively allow the measurement of brain glucose metabolism and dopamine D2 receptor binding and dopamine dynamics.

One major application of PET is the measurement of glucose metabolism in the brain using FDG. FDG is an analog of glucose, with a radioactive fluorine-18 atom substituting a hydroxyl group (-OH) in the 2' position of the glucose molecule. FDG is metabolized by the body similarly to glucose; however, the fluorine-18 atom emits positrons and this quality is exploited in the usage of PET to visualize glucose metabolism (Valls et al., 2016). The brain consumes approximately 20% of glucose-derived energy despite occupying only roughly 2% of the body's weight (Mergenthaler et al., 2013). Glucose is essential to neural physiology because it is required for producing adenine triphosphate (ATP). ATP is ubiquitous in myriad physiologicla processes because of its role in cellular metabolism. Additionally, glucose is imperative for the production of neurotransmitters, the maintenance of neuronal resting potentials, the regulation of cerebral blood flow, and apoptosis (cell death). Glucose uptake is therefore a crucial aspect of brain activity that indicates the distribution of limited energy resources in response to internal and external stimuli.

2.3.2 Glucose Anomalies in Drug and Food Abuse

When healthy subjects are presented with food (i.e., food stimulation), significant increases in glucose metabolism are observed in frontal cortical regions including the orbitofrontal cortex (OFC). These increases correlate with self-reported ratings of hunger and a desire to consume food (Wang et al., 2004). In addition, when fasted non-obese subjects were instructed to mentally regulate their craving responses to food cues, decreased glucose metabolism was seen in OFC as well as in other regions such as the hippocampus, amygdala, and striatum (Wang et al., 2009). The observation of an increase in OFC glucose metabolism when presented with food but decreased OFC metabolism during the control of food cravings is of particular relevance, as morbidly obese subjects have been shown to have lower baseline glucose metabolism in OFC and other prefrontal cortices (Volkow et al., 2008). It has been suggested that the overconsumption of food is a behavioral attempt to counterbalance this deficit in OFC glucose metabolism.

Similarly, in withdrawing cocaine abusers, OFC metabolism has been seen to increase during the first week of withdrawal, then steadily decline in the following weeks. OFC metabolism exhibits an inverse correlation to the number of days since the most recent cocaine consumption (Volkow et al., 1991). Additionally, OFC metabolic activity was increased in cocaine abusers in response to cocaine-related cues (Wang et al., 1999). Importantly, reduced baseline levels of OFC glucose metabolism have also been shown in methamphetamine abusers (Volkow et al., 2001). The research suggests similar patterns of OFC anomalies in food, cocaine, and methamphetamine abusers.

Another frontal cortical region affected in both food and drug addiction is the anterior cingulate cortex (ACC), known to play a significant role in cognitive control and decision-making (Shenhav, Botvinick, and Cohen 2013). Reductions of activity in the ACC have been shown to negatively correlate with errors in an auditory tone detection task in methamphetamine abusers (London et al., 2005). Coinciding with this, obese subjects have been shown to exhibit metabolic deficits in the ACC that correlate with receptor binding for the neurotransmitter dopamine, one of the most widely studied neurotransmitters in addiction research (Volkow et al., 2008).

2.3.3 Dopamine System Anomalies in Substance Abuse and Obesity

The cardinal neuromodulator associated with reward, motivation and heavily implicated in normal feeding, as well as in both drug addiction and obesity, is the catecholamine dopamine. There are three dopaminergic pathways relevant to addiction: the mesolimbic/mesoaccumbens, nigrostriatal, and mesocortical pathways (Kauer and Malenka 2007).

- The mesolimbic pathway is generally composed of neurons projecting from the ventral tegmental area (VTA) toward the nucleus accumbens (NAc) and other limbic structures. The mesolimbic pathway mediates reinforcement learning and reward.
- The nigrostriatal pathway, which plays an important role in motivation and habit formation, begins at the substantia nigra and projects to the dorsal striatum.
- The mesocortical pathway, mainly implicated in modulating decision-making and executive function, carries projections from the VTA to the frontal cortex. All drugs of abuse as well as food increase dopamine production in the NAc (Volkow et al., 2013). Mesolimbic pathway dopamine neurons become desensitized after the repeated administration of initially novel rewards, highlighting a mechanism for reward tolerance accompanied by self-administering larger amounts of the reward observed in both food and drug addiction (Volkow et al., 2013).

Rewards derived from both drugs and food are associated with the release of dopamine in these circuits. Reward has three crucial components: (1) the pleasurable or reinforcing effects of the reward, (2) the motivational drivers to subsequently pursue the reward, and (3) the external cues that become associated with the reward (Volkow et al., 2013). Mapping these three components of addiction onto neurochemical cascades and circuits in the brain demonstrates similar adaptations to both calorie-dense foods and drugs of abuse. The heterogeneity of disruptions of these systems can help explain the wide variety of manifestations of symptoms shared by both addiction and overeating.

In addition to changes in the reward system, deficits in the cognitive functions of addicts and overeaters, such as the degree to which someone can self-regulate craving, respond to stress, and make informed decisions, impact reward pathways (Volkow et al., 2010), along with the impulsive and habit-forming processes undergone in the development of addiction (Koob and Le Moal 1997). Importantly, disruptions in these systems have been associated with addictive symptoms and overeating in preclinical models as well as in humans.

2.3.4 Research Techniques

Dopamine release can be assessed in humans indirectly using [^{11}C]raclopride as a PET tracer. Volkow et al. were the first to show that methylphenidate and cocaine compete for the same dopamine binding sites (1995). Both cocaine and methylphenidate bind to and inhibit the dopamine transporter (DAT). DAT is the protein responsible for recycling dopamine from the synapse back into the cytosol of a presynaptic neuron, a process known as *reuptake* (Volkow et al., 2002). By inhibiting the action of DAT, synaptic dopamine is increased and this is thought to underlie in part the reinforcing and rewarding aspects of cocaine and other dopaminergic drugs. Dopamine displaces [^{11}C]raclopride at dopamine D2 receptors, and by assessing the binding of [^{11}C]raclopride to dopamine D2 receptors with PET before administering methylphenidate to these subjects, it can be deduced how much dopamine has been released. That is, if large quantities of dopamine are released in the brain, [^{11}C]raclopride will show low binding from being displaced at dopamine receptors. If dopamine levels decline, [^{11}C]raclopride will show high binding because of the greater availability of binding sites.

2.3.5 Dopamine Anomalies in Food and Drug Abuse

In studies utilizing [^{11}C]raclopride in PET, consumption of an artificial sweetener decreased dopamine release in ventral striatum in obese subjects, whereas it was increased in healthy controls (Wang et al., 2014). This demonstrates that these changes in dopamine release were inversely proportional to body mass index (BMI). That is, subjects with a higher BMI showed a decreased dopamine release in the ventral striatum, while subjects with a lower BMI showed increased dopamine release. This finding raises questions about the quality of reward experienced by the obese population and whether a reduced experience of reward preludes obesity or vice-versa.

Corroborating the association of dopamine release with the quality of a rewarding stimulus, healthy subjects show significantly increased dopamine release in the striatum subsequent to the consumption of a meal compared to a state of hunger (Small, Jones-Gotman, and Dagher 2003). These increases of dopamine release were correlated with verbally reported ratings of the pleasantness of the meal on a scale of 0–10. In healthy food-deprived subjects, presentation of food without consumption did not significantly increase dopamine release in dorsal striatum. However, an increase of striatal dopamine *was* observed after pretreatment with methylphenidate and this increase correlated with ratings of desire for food and hunger (Volkow et al., 2002). Overall, these findings may be indicative of a dysregulated or "blunted" reward response to caloric intake in obese study participants. The theory is that the experience of reward may require greater-than-normal food consumption in overweight and obese patients to achieve the same reward experienced by non-obese people.

Findings from amphetamine addiction research have shown similar anomalies in striatal dopamine dynamics. In a sample of healthy subjects, increased dopamine release following d-amphetamine administration was correlated with self-reported measures of "drug wanting" and "novelty-seeking exploratory excitability" after administration (Leyton, 2002). This study highlights the association of dopamine release not only with the rewarding effects of drugs, but also the exploration of novel stimuli, which may serve as an endophenotype for the impulsive, risky behaviors often seen in drug addiction (Ersche et al., 2010). In another study of healthy subjects, increased dopamine release resulting from amphetamine administration correlated with ratings of euphoria (Drevets et al., 2001).

Tetrahydrocannabinol, the psychoactive constituent of cannabis, also increases limbic striatal dopamine release in healthy subjects (Bossong et al., 2015). Marijuana abusers do not exhibit lower baseline dopamine receptor binding; however, their response to methylphenidate is significantly reduced relative to controls and this reduction correlates with negative emotionality (Volkow et al., 2014).

In a pilot study, smokers showed a significant increase in striatal dopamine binding after nicotine administration compared to placebo, but nonsmokers did not (Takahashi et al., 2008). In this study, both smokers and nonsmokers showed similar levels of dopamine binding after nicotine administration. Smokers showed an increase in striatal dopamine binding between the placebo and nicotine conditions while the nonsmokers did not. This finding shows that smokers, before being administered nicotine, show a lower baseline level of dopamine activity in the striatum compared to nonsmokers.

Heroin-addicted subjects show significantly less dopamine release and receptor binding in the striatum in comparison to healthy control subjects both before and after administration of methylphenidate (Martinez et al., 2012).

In addition to reward dysfunction, cognitive impairment is also found in both drug addicts and obese patients. Research on the neural correlates of self-control show the prime importance of the mesocortical pathway and dopamine D2 receptor functioning in its constituent brain regions, primarily the OFC and other frontal cortices, for both food and drug addiction (Nader et al., 2006; Volkow et al., 2008; de Weijer et al., 2011). D2 receptor deficits are accompanied by hypometabolism (lower glucose metabolism) in frontal cortical regions and correlate with disruptions of cognitive faculties in abusers of methamphetamine (Volkow et al., 2001), cocaine (Volkow et al., 1993), and alcohol (Volkow et al., 2007). Similar striatal deficits of D2 receptors and prefrontal hypometabolism are seen in obese subjects (Volkow et al., 2007). Cognitive impairment is found is both drug and food abusers.

It is not known whether the development of an addiction to food or drugs causes this reduction in D2 receptors in the midbrain and frontal lobes or if a preexisting deficit of D2 receptors in these regions potentiates a susceptibility to become addicted to food or drugs. There is some evidence for the latter explanation—patients with a family history of alcoholism who were not compulsive drinkers themselves were shown to have significantly higher D2 receptor binding in the striatum and normal glucose metabolic function in the prefrontal cortex (PFC) (Volkow et al., 2006). Furthermore, animal studies highlight that D2 receptor binding can predict both future body weight and sensitivity to cocaine reward (Michaelides et al., 2012).

2.4 EVIDENCE FOR FOOD ADDICTION USING MAGNETIC RESONANCE IMAGING TECHNIQUES

2.4.1 Introduction

Magnetic resonance imaging (MRI) is a noninvasive imaging modality based on the principles of nuclear magnetic resonance discovered by Bloch and Purcell in the 1940s (Grover et al., 2015). All atomic nuclei have a magnetic orientation known as a *spin*, based on the number of positively charged protons in the atom. In an MRI scanner, an external magnetic field is applied and the atoms in the brain (or another organ) assume an orientation either parallel (low-energy) or perpendicular (high-energy) to the applied magnetic field based on how much energy is absorbed. Beyond a threshold of absorbed energy, atoms change from a high-energy state to a low-energy state. This absorbed magnetic energy produces an electrical voltage in the nuclei of interest, and this signal can be read, manipulated, and visualized to produce structural information about the region of interest.

MRI can be used to examine brain regional volumetric changes in drug and food abusers. Obese subjects show reduced gray matter volume in the PFC (Mathar et al., 2016) and this is also seen in subjects suffering from alcoholism (Asensio et al., 2015). Asensio et al. showed that prefrontal gray matter volume was inversely correlated with impulsivity, which is thought to underlie certain aspects of drug abuse vulnerability. Cortical thinning in frontal nuclei has been shown in obese subjects (Marques-Iturria et al., 2013), as well as young adult smokers (Li et al., 2015) and amphetamine and ecstasy users (Koester et al., 2012).

In older females (age 52–92), higher BMI was associated with lower grey matter volume in left OFC, right inferior frontal, right precentral, and other brain regions (Walther et al., 2010). Similarly, in cocaine addicts, lower grey matter volume in the ACC and insular cortices, along with the inferior frontal gyrus, was associated with years of abuse (Connolly et al., 2013). In obese women given an executive function task, lower activation of inferior frontal gyrus, middle frontal gyrus, and other areas predicted future weight gain in the subsequent 1.3–2.9 years (Kishinevsky et al., 2012).

2.4.2 fMRI in Drug vs. Food Abuse

fMRI is derived from traditional MRI technology to detect magnetic changes in blood oxygen metabolism as a physiological measure of neural activity. The underlying principle is that changes to blood oxygenation correlate with activity in neuronal structures. The hemodynamic response across milli- or micrometer-sized voxels is measured as a magnetic contrast and has been termed the *blood-oxygen-level dependent contrast*, or BOLD contrast.

Stoeckel et al. discovered that, after being shown images of high-calorie foods, obese women exhibit significantly greater neural activation than controls in various brain regions including the ventral striatum or NAc, amygdala, OFC, medial PFC (mPFC), ACC, hippocampus, and others (2008). Additionally, the activation difference after being shown images of high-calorie foods vs. low-calorie foods was greater in obese subjects than controls for all of these and other areas but not the putamen. Rothemund et al. showed that higher BMI predicted higher levels of neural activation in the dorsal striatum, anterior insula, posterior cingulate, postcentral and lateral OFC, and other areas subsequent to viewing images of high-calorie foods (2007). Of particular interest are the associations of BMI with neural activation of the anterior insula and lateral OFC, as these two areas have previously been shown to be involved in gustatory processing (Rolls, 1990, 2015). These findings demonstrate the dysregulation of reward responses to food cues in the food-addicted brain and the correlation of this dysregulation with BMI.

These same activation differences have been shown in studies where subjects consumed food as opposed to being shown food cues (Dimitropoulos et al., 2012). In this study, obese and healthy normal subjects were scanned and presented visual cues for either high-calorie food, low-calorie food, or neutral objects before and after a meal. Results are presented as interactions between weight, group, and cue. Before consuming a meal, obese subjects as compared to controls showed greater differential activation in multiple prefrontal regions after being presented cues for high-calorie food vs. neutral cues, and low-calorie food vs. neutral cues. This is fairly intuitive, as food addicts tend to have heightened reward responses to high-calorie food and food cues as described above. Curiously, however, the control group showed greater differential activation in the postcentral gyrus, insula, and cerebellum after presentation of high-calorie vs. low-calorie food cues. Important to note, subjective ratings of hunger before the meal did not differ between groups. Perhaps the larger difference in activation between high-calorie and low-calorie food cues in the control group signifies greater salience of the presentation of a high-calorie food over a low-calorie food than the obese group, which exhibited relatively similar levels of activation in the insula between high and low-calorie food cues.

After consuming the meal, the obese group continued to show increased activation in ACC, OFC, and caudate after presentation of high-calorie food cues. By contrast, the healthy controls showed *decreased* activation in these areas after presentation of high-calorie food cues. Importantly, postmeal ratings of hunger did not differ between groups, eliminating the possibility that the obese subjects were simply still hungry after the meal. These differing activation profiles demonstrate dysfunctional reward anticipation mechanisms present in obese people even after consuming a meal and not feeling hungry.

Drug addiction fMRI studies have shown similar activation profiles in response to substances of abuse. Cocaine administration increases activation in NAc, caudate, insula, lateral prefrontal areas, and the cingulate in heavy cocaine abusers (Breiter et al., 1997). Additionally, abstinent cocaine users (1.9–574.2 weeks; mean = 44.9) exhibited right ventral striatal activity that correlated with self-reported compulsivity scores after presentation of cocaine cues (Bell et al., 2014). Cocaine also increases activation in prefrontal cortical areas, not limited to the OFC (Kufahl et al., 2005, 2008).

Heroin users show increased activation in areas previously implicated in food addiction that correlate with multiple verbal self-reports after presentation of drug-related cues. "Verbal self-reports of craving" correlate with activation of the bilateral ACC. Drug use imagination correlates with activation of the bilateral cerebellum. "Negative affect" correlates with activation of the right putamen (Hassani-Abharian et al., 2015). Self-reports of craving have also been shown to correlate with bilateral NAc and cerebellar activity after the presentation of heroin cues in heroin users who had used in the prior year but were maintaining abstinence with methadone (Li et al., 2015). Upon 1–3 month follow-up, those patients who relapsed showed greater accumbal and cerebellar responses to heroin-related cues than the nonrelapsing patients. There were no enhanced activations seen in the nonrelapsed groups relative to the relapsed group. In a study where heroin-related cues were presented before or after heroin administration, OFC responses to cues were blunted in the post-dose condition compared to the pre-dose condition (Langleben et al., 2008).

In non-treatment-seeking smokers who were abstinent overnight, smoking-related cues increased activity in the bilateral ventral striatum and left amygdala (Xu et al., 2014), and it has been shown that nicotine administration increases activation in the NAc, the cingulate, amygdala, and frontal cortices in current smokers (Stein et al., 1998).

MRI research has illuminated a range of similarities between drug and food abusers in terms of neurodysfunction. This is important support for the model of chronic overeating as a kind of addiction. Where PET can illuminate the effects of food, drugs, and their respective cues on brain metabolism and receptor binding, structural and functional MRI can elucidate the changes in structure and oxygenation resulting from these manipulations. Similar findings in drug and food addicts are made all the more robust and clinically tractable when verified using two distinct neuroimaging modalities.

2.5 CONCLUSION

This chapter provides a brief survey of the research methods and findings relevant to neurodysfunction in overeating, obesity, substance abuse, and drug addiction. These findings highlight overlapping functional and neurobiological circuits between drug addicts and the obese as evidenced via PET and MRI studies. The complementary findings suggest promising future therapies for each condition.

As substantial portions of the population are exhibiting higher rates of excessive food consumption, obesity, and other food-related disorders, so the need grows for clinical action informed by salient biological, psychological, and societal research. In terms of biology, recent technological advances in neuromodulation may hold promise for alleviating some of the symptoms associated with overeating and drug abuse. Neurostimulation and neuromodulation modalities are novel in this respect. Noninvasive techniques such as transcranial magnetic stimulation (TMS) and transcranial direct-current stimulation (tDCS) have been tested in subjects with eating disorders, with real-time fMRI neurofeedback showing potential value as well (Val-Laillet et al., 2015). TMS involves the application of magnetic fields to specific brain regions according to various parameters (e.g., depth, focality, intensity), and tDCS refers to the application of electrical currents to targeted regions along similar parameters (e.g., voltage). TMS of the motor cortex has been shown to induce striatal dopamine release in the striatum (Strafella et al., 2003), and the same lab previously showed that stimulation of PFC induces dopamine release in the caudate nucleus (Strafella et al., 2001).

The remote induction of dopamine release may serve as a potential therapeutic intervention for some of the neurofunctional deficits observed in obese and food and drug addiction populations. Den Eynde et al. were able to significantly reduce craving and bingeing behaviors in subjects with "bulimic-type eating disorders" after repeated TMS (rTMS) of the dorsolateral prefrontal cortex (DLPFC) (2013). De Ridder et al. also reduced alcohol craving with rTMS of the ACC (2013). tDCS of the DLPFC has been shown to decrease caloric intake in subjects with recurrent food cravings (three or more per day) (Lapenta et al., 2014).

In a study of healthy subjects, decreased cravings came from less carbohydrate consumption and were accompanied by a general decrease in appetite (Jauch-Chara et al., 2014). This is consistent with classic addiction treatment protocols of abstinence.

The next generation of addiction treatment specialists have the advantage of utilizing a growing body of research elucidating the neurobiological mechanisms underlying different addictions, from food to drugs, sex to gambling. While it has been estimated that it takes 17 years before 30% of scientific advances reach the clinic (Peterson 2005), it is these advances and support for them that may quell the exorbitant costs of addiction, in all of its forms, on society.

This chapter provides an integrative, coherent foundation for the biological understanding of PET and MRI modalities for assessing neurobiological correlates of obesity, overeating and drug addiction as it has been studied in humans. While the study of food addiction extends backward about 60 years (Randolph 1956), there is a tremendous amount of work ahead for researchers and clinicians alike to understand the interrelated biological, psychological, and social nuances of the addictive process. The addicted human brain is a highly complex organ, but with brain-imaging technology it seems to be within the grasp of science to understand it. And further, health professionals could use this understanding to heal and prevent ailments of neurological and psychiatric dysfunction as well as fuel the incremental creation of a healthier and more capable human condition.

ACKNOWLEDGMENTS

This work was supported by National Institutes of Health/National Institute on Alcohol Abuse and Alcoholism intramural grant Y1AA-3009 to GJW and NIH/National Institute on Drug Abuse.

REFERENCES

Asensio, S., Morales, J. L., Senabre, I., Romero, M. J., Beltran, M. A., Flores-Bellver, M., Romero, F. J. (2015). Magnetic resonance imaging structural alterations in brain of alcohol abusers and its association with impulsivity. *Addiction Biology*, *21*(4), 962–971. doi:10.1111/adb.12257.

Bell, R. P., Garavan, H., & Foxe, J. J. (2014). Neural correlates of craving and impulsivity in abstinent former cocaine users: Towards biomarkers of relapse risk. *Neuropharmacology*, *85*, 461–470. doi:10.1016/j.neuropharm.2014.05.011.

Bossong, M. G., Mehta, M. A., van Berckel, B. N., Howes, O. D., Kahn, R. S., & Stokes, P. R. (2015). Further human evidence for striatal dopamine release induced by administration of Δ 9-tetrahydrocannabinol (THC): Selectivity to limbic striatum. *Psychopharmacology*, *232*(15), 2723–2729.

Breiter, H. C., Gollub, R. L., Weisskoff, R. M., Kennedy, D. N., Makris, N., Berke, J. D., ... Hyman, S. E. (1997). Acute effects of cocaine on human brain activity and emotion. *Neuron*, *19*(3), 591–611.

Connolly, C. G., Bell, R. P., Foxe, J. J., & Garavan, H. (2013). Dissociated grey matter changes with prolonged addiction and extended abstinence in cocaine users. *PLoS One*, *8*(3). doi:10.1371/journal.pone.0059645.

De Ridder, D., Vanneste, S., Kovacs, S., Sunaert, S., & Dom, G. (2011). Transient alcohol craving suppression by rTMS of dorsal anterior cingulate: An fMRI and LORETA EEG study. *Neuroscience Letters*, *496*(1), 5–10.

De Weijer, B. A., van de Giessen, E., van Amelsvoort, T. A. A., Boot, E., Braak, B., Janssen, I. M., ... Booij, J. (2011). Lower striatal dopamine D2/3 receptor availability in obese compared with non-obese subjects. *EJNMMI Research*, *1*(1), 37. doi:10.1186/2191-219X-1-37.

Dimitropoulos, A., Tkach, J., Ho, A., & Kennedy, J. (2012). Greater corticolimbic activation to high-calorie food cues after eating in obese vs. normal-weight adults. *Appetite*, *58*(1), 303–312. doi:10.1016/j.appet.2011.10.014.

Drevets, W. C., Gautier, C., Price, J. C., Kupfer, D. J., Kinahan, P. E., Grace, A. A., ... & Mathis, C. A. (2001). Amphetamine-induced dopamine release in human ventral striatum correlates with euphoria. *Biological Psychiatry*, *49*(2), 81–96.

Ersche, K. D., Turton, A. J., Pradhan, S., Bullmore, E. T., & Robbins, T. W. (2010). Drug addiction endophenotypes: Impulsive versus sensation-seeking personality traits. *Biological Psychiatry*, *68*(8), 770–773. doi:10.1016/j.biopsych.2010.06.015.

Grover, V. P., Tognarelli, J. M., Crossey, M. M., Cox, I. J., Taylor-Robinson, S. D., & Mcphail, M. J. (2015). Magnetic resonance imaging: Principles and techniques: Lessons for clinicians. *Journal of Clinical and Experimental Hepatology*, *5*(3), 246–255. doi:10.1016/j.jceh.2015.08.001.

Hassani-Abharian, P., Ganjgahi, H., Tabatabaei-Jafari, H., Oghabian, M. A., Mokri, A., & Ekhtiari, H. (2015). Exploring neural correlates of different dimensions in drug craving self-reports among heroin dependents. *Basic and Clinical Neuroscience*, *6*(4), 271.

Jauch-Chara, K., Kistenmacher, A., Herzog, N., Schwarz, M., Schweiger, U., & Oltmanns, K. M. (2014). Repetitive electric brain stimulation reduces food intake in humans. *The American Journal of Clinical Nutrition*, *100*(4), 1003–1009.

Kauer, J. A., & Malenka, R. C. (2007). Synaptic plasticity and addiction. *Nature Reviews Neuroscience*, *8*(11), 844–858.

Kishinevsky, F. I., Cox, J. E., Murdaugh, D. L., Stoeckel, L. E., Cook, E. W., & Weller, R. E. (2012). fMRI reactivity on a delay discounting task predicts weight gain in obese women. *Appetite*, *58*(2), 582–592. doi:10.1016/j.appet.2011.11.029.

Koester, P., Tittgemeyer, M., Wagner, D., Becker, B., Gouzoulis-Mayfrank, E., & Daumann, J. (2012). Cortical thinning in amphetamine-type stimulant users. *Neuroscience*, *221*, 182–192. doi:10.1016/j.neuroscience.2012.06.049.

Koob, G., & Moal, M. (1997). Drug abuse: Hedonic homeostatic dysregulation. *Science*, *278*(5335), 52–58. doi:10.1126/science.278.5335.52.

Kufahl, P. R., Li, Z., Risinger, R. C., Rainey, C. J., Piacentine, L., Wu, G., ... & Li, S. J. (2008). Expectation modulates human brain responses to acute cocaine: A functional magnetic resonance imaging study. *Biological Psychiatry*, *63*(2), 222–230.

Kufahl, P. R., Li, Z., Risinger, R. C., Rainey, C. J., Wu, G., Bloom, A. S., & Li, S. J. (2005). Neural responses to acute cocaine administration in the human brain detected by fMRI. *NeuroImage*, *28*(4), 904–914.

Langleben, D. D., Kosha Ruparel, M. S. E., Elman, I., Samantha Busch-Winokur, B. A., Ramapriyan Pratiwadi, B. S. E., Loughead, J., ... & Childress, A. R. (2008). Acute effect of methadone maintenance dose on brain fMRI response to heroin-related cues. *American Journal of Psychiatry*, *165*(3), 390–394.

Lapenta, O. M., Di Sierve, K., de Macedo, E. C., Fregni, F., & Boggio, P. S. (2014). Transcranial direct current stimulation modulates ERP-indexed inhibitory control and reduces food consumption. *Appetite*, *83*, 42–48.

Leyton, M. (2002). Amphetamine-induced increases in extracellular dopamine, drug wanting, and novelty seeking a PET/[11C]Raclopride study in healthy men. *Neuropsychopharmacology*, *27*(6), 1027–1035. doi:10.1016/s0893-133x(02)00366-4.

Li, Q., Li, W., Wang, H., Wang, Y., Zhang, Y., Zhu, J., ... & Yan, X. (2015). Predicting subsequent relapse by drug-related cue-induced brain activation in heroin addiction: An event-related functional magnetic resonance imaging study. *Addiction Biology*, *20*(5), 968–978.

Li, Y., Yuan, K., Cai, C., Feng, D., Yin, J., Bi, Y., ... Tian, J. (2015). Reduced frontal cortical thickness and increased caudate volume within fronto-striatal circuits in young adult smokers. *Drug and Alcohol Dependence*, *151*, 211–219. doi:10.1016/j.drugalcdep.2015.03.023.

London, E. D., Berman, S. M., Voytek, B., Simon, S. L., Mandelkern, M. A., Monterosso, J., ... & Hayashi, K. M. (2005). Cerebral metabolic dysfunction and impaired vigilance in recently abstinent methamphetamine abusers. *Biological Psychiatry*, *58*(10), 770–778.

Marqués-Iturria, I., Pueyo, R., Garolera, M., Segura, B., Junqué, C., García-García, I., ... Jurado, M. Á. (2013). Frontal cortical thinning and subcortical volume reductions in early adulthood obesity. *Psychiatry Research: Neuroimaging*, *214*(2), 109–115. doi:10.1016/j.pscychresns.2013.06.004.

Martinez, D., Saccone, P. A., Liu, F., Slifstein, M., Orlowska, D., Grassetti, A., ... Comer, S. D. (2012). Deficits in dopamine D2 receptors and presynaptic dopamine in heroin dependence: Commonalities and differences with other types of addiction. *Biological Psychiatry*, *71*(3), 192–198. doi:10.1016/j.biopsych.2011.08.024.

Mathar, D., Horstmann, A., Pleger, B., Villringer, A., & Neumann, J. (2016). Is it worth the effort? Novel insights into obesity-associated alterations in cost-benefit decision-making. *Frontiers in Behavioral Neuroscience*, *9*, 360. doi:10.3389/fnbeh.2015.00360.

Mergenthaler, P., Lindauer, U., Dienel, G. A., & Meisel, A. (2013). Sugar for the brain: the role of glucose in physiological and pathological brain function. *Trends in neurosciences*, *36*(10), 587–597.

Meule, A., & Gearhardt, A. N. (2014). Food addiction in the light of DSM-5. *Nutrients*, *6*(9), 3653–3671.

Michaelides, M., Thanos, P. K., Kim, R., Cho, J., Ananth, M., Wang, G. J., & Volkow, N. D. (2012). PET imaging predicts future body weight and cocaine preference. *NeuroImage*, *59*(2), 1508–1513.

Nader, M. A., Morgan, D., Gage, H. D., Nader, S. H., Calhoun, T. L., Buchheimer, N., ... Mach, R. H. (2006). PET imaging of dopamine D2 receptors during chronic cocaine self-administration in monkeys. *Nature Neuroscience*, *9*(8), 1050–1056. doi:10.1038/nn1737.

Parylak, S., Koob, G., & Zorrilla, E. (2011). The dark side of food addiction. *Physiology & Behavior*, *104*(1), 149–156. doi:10.1016/j.physbeh.2011.04.063.

Peterson, K. (2005). Practice-based primary care research–translating research into practice through advanced technology. *Family Practice*, *23*(2), 149–150. doi:10.1093/fampra/cmi126.

Randolph, T. G. (1956). The descriptive features of food addiction; Addictive eating and drinking. *Quarterly Journal of Studies on Alcohol*, *17*, 198–224.

Rolls, E. T. (1990). A theory of emotion, and its application to understanding the neural basis of emotion. *Cognition & Emotion*, *4*(3), 161–190. doi:10.1080/02699939008410795.

Rolls, E. T. (2015). Functions of the anterior insula in taste, autonomic, and related functions. *Brain and Cognition*, *110*, 4–19. doi:10.1016/j.bandc.2015.07.002.

Rothemund, Y., Preuschhof, C., Bohner, G., Bauknecht, H., Klingebiel, R., Flor, H., & Klapp, B. F. (2007). Differential activation of the dorsal striatum by high-calorie visual food stimuli in obese individuals. *NeuroImage*, *37*(2), 410–421. doi:10.1016/j.neuroimage.2007.05.008.

Shenhav, A., Botvinick, M. M., & Cohen, J. D. (2013). The expected value of control: An integrative theory of anterior cingulate cortex function. *Neuron*, *79*(2), 217–240.

Small, D. M., Jones-Gotman, M., & Dagher, A. (2003). Feeding-induced dopamine release in dorsal striatum correlates with meal pleasantness ratings in healthy human volunteers. *NeuroImage*, *19*(4), 1709–1715. doi:10.1016/s1053-8119(03)00253-2.

Stein, E. A., Pankiewicz, J., Harsch, H. H., Cho, J. K., Fuller, S. A., Hoffmann, R. G., ... Bloom, A. S. (1998). Nicotine-induced limbic cortical activation in the human brain: A functional MRI study. *The American Journal of Psychiatry*, *155*(8), 1009–1115. doi:10.1176/ajp.155.8.1009.

Stoeckel, L. E., Weller, R. E., Cook, E. W., Twieg, D. B., Knowlton, R. C., & Cox, J. E. (2008). Widespread reward-system activation in obese women in response to pictures of high-calorie foods. *NeuroImage*, *41*(2), 636–647. doi:10.1016/j.neuroimage.2008.02.031.

Strafella, A. P., Paus, T., Barrett, J., & Dagher, A. (2001). Repetitive transcranial magnetic stimulation of the human prefrontal cortex induces dopamine release in the caudate nucleus. *Journal of Neuroscience*, *21*(15), 1–4.

Strafella, A. P., Paus, T., Fraraccio, M., & Dagher, A. (2003). Striatal dopamine release induced by repetitive transcranial magnetic stimulation of the human motor cortex. *Brain*, *126*(12), 2609–2615.

Takahashi, H., Fujimura, Y., Hayashi, M., Takano, H., Kato, M., Okubo, Y., ... & Suhara, T. (2008). Enhanced dopamine release by nicotine in cigarette smokers: A double-blind, randomized, placebo-controlled pilot study. *International Journal of Neuropsychopharmacology*, *11*(3), 413–417.

Trogdon, J. G., Finkelstein, E. A., Hylands, T., Dellea, P. S., Kamal-Bahl, S. J. (2008). Indirect costs of obesity: A review of the current literature. *Obesity Reviews*, *9*(5), 489–500. doi:10.1111/j.1467-789x.2008.00472.x.

Val-Laillet, D., Aarts, E., Weber, B., Ferrari, M., Quaresima, V., Stoeckel, L. E., ... & Stice, E. (2015). Neuroimaging and neuromodulation approaches to study eating behavior and prevent and treat eating disorders and obesity. *NeuroImage: Clinical*, *8*, 1–31.

Valls, L., Badve, C., Avril, S., Herrmann, K., Faulhaber, P., O'Donnell, J., & Avril, N. (2016). FDG-PET imaging in hematological malignancies. *Blood reviews*, *30*(4), 317–331.

Van den Eynde, F., Guillaume, S., Broadbent, H., Campbell, I. C., & Schmidt, U. (2013). Repetitive transcranial magnetic stimulation in anorexia nervosa: A pilot study. *European Psychiatry*, *28*(2), 98–101.

Volkow, N. D., Chang, L., Wang, G. J., Fowler, J. S., Ding, Y. S., Sedler, M., ... & Gifford, A. (2001). Low level of brain dopamine D2 receptors in methamphetamine abusers: Association with metabolism in the orbitofrontal cortex. *American Journal of Psychiatry*, *158*(12), 2015–2021.

Volkow, N. D., Ding, Y. S., Fowler, J. S., Wang, G. J., Logan, J., Gatley, J. S., ... & Wolf, A. P. (1995). Is methylphenidate like cocaine? Studies on their pharmacokinetics and distribution in the human brain. *Archives of General Psychiatry*, *52*(6), 456–463.

Volkow, N. D., Fowler, J. S., Wang, G. J., Hitzemann, R., Logan, J., Schlyer, D. J., ... & Wolf, A. P. (1993). Decreased dopamine D2 receptor availability is associated with reduced frontal metabolism in cocaine abusers. *Synapse*, *14*(2), 169–177.

Volkow, N. D., Fowler, J. S., Wolf, A. P., Hitzemann, R., Dewey, S., Bendriem, B., ... & Hoff, A. (1991). Changes in brain glucose metabolism in cocaine dependence and withdrawal. *The American Journal of Psychiatry*, *148*(5), 621–626.

Volkow, N. D., Wang, G. J., Begleiter, H., Porjesz, B., Fowler, J. S., Telang, F., ... & Alexoff, D. (2006). High levels of dopamine D2 receptors in unaffected members of alcoholic families: Possible protective factors. *Archives of General Psychiatry*, *63*(9), 999–1008.

Volkow, N. D., Wang, G. J., Fowler, J. S., Logan, J., Franceschi, D., Maynard, L., ... & Swanson, J. M. (2002). Relationship between blockade of dopamine transporters by oral methylphenidate and the increases in extracellular dopamine: Therapeutic implications. *Synapse*, *43*(3), 181–187.

Volkow, N. D., Wang, G. J., Fowler, J. S., Logan, J., Jayne, M., Franceschi, D., ... & Pappas, N. (2002). "Nonhedonic" food motivation in humans involves dopamine in the dorsal striatum and methylphenidate amplifies this effect. *Synapse*, *44*(3), 175–180.

Volkow, N. D., Wang, G. J., Telang, F., Fowler, J. S., Alexoff, D., Logan, J., ... & Tomasi, D. (2014). Decreased dopamine brain reactivity in marijuana abusers is associated with negative emotionality and addiction severity. *Proceedings of the National Academy of Sciences*, *111*(30), E3149–E3156.

Volkow, N. D., Wang, G. J., Telang, F., Fowler, J. S., Logan, J., Jayne, M., ... & Wong, C. (2007). Profound decreases in dopamine release in striatum in detoxified alcoholics: Possible orbitofrontal involvement. *The Journal of Neuroscience*, *27*(46), 12700–12706.

Volkow, N. D., Wang, G. J., Telang, F., Fowler, J. S., Thanos, P. K., Logan, J., ... Pradhan, K. (2008). Low dopamine striatal D2 receptors are associated with prefrontal metabolism in obese subjects: Possible contributing factors. *NeuroImage*, *42*(4), 1537–1543. doi:10.1016/j.neuroimage.2008.06.002.

Volkow, N. D., Wang, G. J., Tomasi, D., & Baler, R. D. (2013). Obesity and addiction: Neurobiological overlaps. *Obesity Reviews*, *14*(1), 2–18. doi:10.1111/j.1467-789X.2012.01031.x.

Walther, K., Birdsill, A. C., Glisky, E. L., & Ryan, L. (2010). Structural brain differences and cognitive functioning related to body mass index in older females. *Human Brain Mapping*, *31*(7), 1052–1064. doi:10.1002/hbm.20916.

Wang, G. J., Tomasi, D., Convit, A., Logan, J., Wong, C. T., Shumay, E., ... & Volkow, N. D. (2014). BMI modulates calorie-dependent dopamine changes in accumbens from glucose intake. *PloS One*, *9*(7), e101585.

Wang, G. J., Volkow, N. D., Fowler, J. S., Cervany, P., Hitzemann, R. J., Pappas, N. R., ... Felder, C. (1999). Regional brain metabolic activation during craving elicited by recall of previous drug experiences. *Life Sciences*, *64*(9), 775–784.

Wang, G. J., Volkow, N. D., Telang, F., Jayne, M., Ma, J., Rao, M., ... Fowler, J. S. (2004). Exposure to appetitive food stimuli markedly activates the human brain. *NeuroImage*, *21*(4), 1790–1797. doi:10.1016/j.neuroimage.2003.11.026.

Wang, G. J., Volkow, N. D., Telang, F., Jayne, M., Ma, Y., Pradhan, K., ... Fowler, J. S. (2009). Evidence of gender differences in the ability to inhibit brain activation elicited by food stimulation. *Proceedings of the National Academy of Sciences of the United States of America*, *106*(4), 1249–1254. doi:10.1073/pnas.0807423106.

World Health Organization. (2015). Obesity and overweight. Fact sheet No 311. 2015. Ref Type: Online Source.

Xu, X., Clark, U. S., David, S. P., Mulligan, R. C., Knopik, V. S., McGeary, J., ... & Sweet, L. H. (2014). The effects of nicotine deprivation and replacement on BOLD-fMRI response to smoking cues as a function of DRD4 VNTR genotype. *Nicotine & Tobacco Research*, *16*(7), 939–947, ntu010.

3 Neural Vulnerability Factors for Overeating

Treatment Implications

Eric Stice and Zack Stice
Oregon Research Institute
Eugene, OR

CONTENTS

3.1 OVERVIEW OF THE CHAPTER

Nearly 70% of US adults are overweight or obese, causing 300,000 deaths and $150 billion in health-related expenses in the United States yearly (Flegal et al., 2012). Yet, extant treatments almost never result in lasting weight loss (Turk et al., 2009). An improved understanding of neural vulnerability factors that predict overeating and subsequent weight gain has the potential to improve treatment.

Scholars have proposed several neural vulnerability factors that may increase risk for overeating. Because eating high-fat/high-sugar food increases activation in regions implicated in reward processing, including the striatum, midbrain, amygdala, and orbitofrontal cortex (OFC; Kringelbach et al., 2003; Small et al., 2001; Stice, Burger, & Yokum, 2013), and causes dopamine release in the dorsal striatum, with the amount released correlating with meal pleasantness ratings (Small et al., 2003) and caloric density of the food (Ferreira et al., 2012), etiologic theories have focused on reward regions. In contrast, anticipated palatable food intake (O'Doherty, Deichman, Critchley, & Dolan, 2002; Small, Veldhuizen, Felsted, Mak, & McGlone, 2008; Stice, Yokum, Burger, Epstein, & Smolen, 2012) and exposure to food images and cues (Frank et al., 2010; Van Meer, van der Laan, Adan, Viergever, & Smeets, 2015) activates regions implicated in incentive valuation, such as the OFC and amygdala. These findings have prompted a focus on incentive valuation regions in etiologic theories for obesity. It is important to note that palatable food intake, anticipated intake, and food cues also activate regions implicated in visual processing/attention (inferior parietal lobe, posterior cingulate cortex), gustatory processing (insula and overlying operculum), motor response (precentral gyrus, cerebellum), somatosensory processing (postcentral gyrus), and inhibitory behavior (inferior frontal gyrus, ventrolateral prefrontal cortex) (Huerta, Sarkar, Duong, Laird, & Fox, 2014; Stice et al., 2012; Tang et al., 2012; Van Meer et al., 2015).

This chapter reviews the primary theories relating aberrations in responsivity of brain reward and incentive valuation regions, as well as regions that affect activation in these regions (e.g., inhibitory regions), to overeating, as well as evidence that is consistent or inconsistent with these theories, focusing primarily on prospective and experimental data. It concludes by translating these findings into implications for the more effective management of overeating.

3.2 REWARD SURFEIT THEORY OF OBESITY

Individuals who show greater reward region responsivity to food intake, which is presumably an inborn characteristic, are theoretically at elevated risk for overeating and consequent weight gain (Davis, Strachan, & Berkson, 2004; Stice et al., 2008b). Apparently consistent with this reward surfeit theory, healthy weight adolescents at high versus low risk for future weight gain based on parental obesity status showed greater activation of regions implicated in reward (caudate, putamen, OFC) in response to receipt of high-calorie food and monetary reward (Stice, Yokum, Burger, Epstein, & Small, 2011). Elevated midbrain and medial OFC response to high-calorie food receipt also predicted higher subsequent *ad lib* milkshake consumption (Nolan-Poupart, et al., 2013). These results converge with evidence that individuals who rate high-calorie foods as high versus low in pleasantness show elevated future weight gain (e.g., Salbe et al., 2004). Critically, elevated response to high-calorie milkshake tastes in the midbrain, thalamus, hypothalamus, ventral pallidum, and nucleus accumbens predicted future weight gain at 1-year follow-up (Geha et al., 2013), though other studies did not find a main effect between reward region response to high-calorie food receipt and future weight gain (Stice, Spoor, Bohon, & Small, 2008a; Stice, Burger, & Yokum, 2015; Sun et al., 2015).

Non–substance-using adolescents at high versus low risk for future substance use disorders, based on parental substance use disorder, showed greater activation of a key reward region (midbrain) in response to high-calorie food taste (Stice & Yokum, 2014), and elevated reward region responsivity (caudate, putamen) in response to monetary reward predicted future substance use onset (Stice, Yokum, & Burger, 2013). Results suggest that reward region hyperresponsivity increases risk for a range of appetitive problems and that there may be parallels in neural vulnerability factors that increase risk for obesity and substance use.

Two studies found significant interactions wherein elevated caudate response to milkshake receipt predicted future weight gain for adolescents with a genetic propensity for greater dopamine signaling by virtue of possessing the *TaqIA* A2/A2 allele, but lower caudate response predicted weight gain for adolescents with a genetic propensity for lower dopamine signaling by virtue of possessing one or more *TaqIA* A1 alleles (Stice et al., 2008a; Stice et al., 2015). A third found a significant interaction wherein elevated amygdala response to milkshake receipt predicted future weight gain for adults with a genetic propensity for greater dopamine signaling by virtue of possessing the *TaqIA* A2/A2 allele, but lower amygdala response predicted weight gain for adults with a genetic propensity for lower dopamine signaling by virtue of possessing one or more *TaqIA* A1 alleles (Sun et al., 2015). The evidence that elevated reward region response to high-calorie food receipt predicted future weight gain for individuals with a genetic propensity for greater dopamine signaling appears consistent with the reward surfeit theory.

Additional genetic findings appear consistent with the reward surfeit theory. Specifically, individuals with a genetic propensity for elevated dopamine signaling in reward circuitry showed elevated future weight gain in three samples, as well as less weight loss in response to obesity treatment (Yokum, Marti, Smolen, & Stice, 2015). That study examined a multilocus score because it relates more strongly to reward region responsivity than the individual alleles used to calculate the composite genetic risk score (Nikolova, Ferrel, Manuck, & Hariri, 2011; Stice et al., 2012). Theoretically, this is because the greater the number of these genotypes, regardless of the particular combination, the greater the dopamine signaling. The multilocus composite was scored as follows: *TaqIA* A1/A1, *DRD2*-141C Ins/Ins, *DRD4*-L, *DAT1* 10R/10R, and *COMT* Met/Met genotypes were scored 0 (low); *TaqIA* A2/A2, *DRD2*-141C Ins/Del and Del/Del, *DRD4*-S, *DAT1* 9R, and *COMT* Val/Val genotypes were scored 1 (high), and *TaqIA* A1/A2 and *COMT* Met/Val genotypes were scored 0.5 (scores were summed to create the composite). Humans with the A2/A2 allele versus an A1 allele of the *Taq1A* polymorphism and the Del allele versus Ins/Ins genotype of the *DRD2*-141C Ins/Del polymorphism show more D2 receptors (Jönsson et al., 1999). Humans with the shorter than 7 allele (*DRD4*-S) versus 7-repeat or longer allele (*DRD4*-L) of the *DRD4* genotype show greater *in vitro* dopamine functioning and stronger response to dopamine agonists (Asghari et al., 1995; Seeger et al., 2001). Humans with the 9-repeat allele (*DAT1-S*) versus homozygous for the 10-repeat allele (*DAT1*-L) of the *DAT1* show lower *DAT1* expression (Heinz et al., 2000), theoretically increasing synaptic dopamine clearance, producing lower basal dopamine levels, and increasing phasic dopamine release (van Dyck et al., 2005). Val homozygotes versus Met homozygotes of the *Catechol-O-methyltransferase* (*COMT* val^{158}met) gene putatively have lower basal striatal dopamine levels and greater phasic dopamine release (Lachman et al., 1996).

In sum, healthy weight adolescents at high-risk for future weight gain by virtue of parental obesity showed greater reward region responsivity to palatable food receipt; individuals who evidenced elevated reward region responsivity to palatable food receipt showed greater future weight gain, though this finding did not replicate; and youth with a genetic propensity for greater dopamine signaling showed greater future weight gain. Further, the evidence that individuals who showed greater reward region response to palatable food receipt and who have a genetic propensity for elevated dopamine signaling showed greater future weight gain is also apparently consistent with the reward surfeit theory. Thus, results provide moderate support for this etiologic theory.

3.3 INCENTIVE SENSITIZATION THEORY OF OBESITY

The incentive sensitization model posits that repeated intake of high-calorie palatable foods results in an elevated responsivity of regions involved in incentive valuation to cues that are associated with palatable food intake via conditioning, which prompts craving and overeating when these cues are encountered (Berridge et al., 2010). Animal experiments indicate that firing of striatal and ventral pallidum dopamine neurons initially occurs in response to receipt of a novel palatable food but that, after repeated pairings of palatable food intake and cues that signal impending receipt of that food, dopamine neurons begin to fire in response to food-predictive cues and no longer fire in response to food receipt (Schultz et al., 1997; Tobler et al., 2005). This theory implies that a period of overeating palatable foods contributes to the conditioning process that results in hyperresponsivity of reward regions to food cues.

Obese versus lean humans show greater responsivity of brain regions associated with reward and motivation (striatum, amygdala, OFC) to pictures of high-calorie foods versus low-calorie foods and control images (e.g., Frankort et al., 2011; Stice, Yokum, Bohon, Marti, & Smolen, 2010b; Stoeckel et al., 2008). Similarly, humans with versus without a range of various substance use disorders show greater activation of regions implicated in reward and motivation in response to substance use images (e.g., Due, Huettel, Hall, & Rubin, 2002; Myrick et al., 2004; Tapert et al., 2003). Elevated responsivity in the ventral striatum (Lawrence, Hinton, Parkinson, & Lawrence, 2012) and amygdala (Mehta et al., 2012) during exposure to food images also predicted greater subsequent *ad lib* high-calorie food intake. Healthy weight adolescents who were eating beyond objectively measured basal metabolic needs showed greater response during cues predicting impending palatable food receipt in regions that encode visual processing and attention (visual and anterior cingulate cortices), salience (precuneus), and reward and motivation (striatum), as well as a region in the primary gustatory cortex (frontal operculum; Burger & Stice, 2013). These findings suggest that overeating, even if it has not yet resulted in excess body fat, is accompanied by elevated responsivity of reward, attentional, and gustatory regions to food cues, which may drive future overeating.

Obese versus lean individuals also show greater recruitment of motor response regions when exposed to high-calorie food images (Brooks et al., 2013; Jastreboff et al., 2013), suggesting an elevated motor approach tendency. Obese versus lean individuals likewise show attentional bias for high-calorie food images (Braet & Crombez, 2003; Castellanos et al., 2009; Graham et al., 2011; Nijs et al., 2010a).

Critically, prospective functional MRI studies have found that elevated nucleus accumbens response to high-calorie palatable food images, elevated OFC response to cues that signal impending presentation of palatable food images, elevated striatal response to commercials for high-calorie foods, and elevated OFC response to cues signaling impending milkshake receipt predicted future weight gain (Demos et al., 2012; Stice et al., 2015; Yokum, Gearhardt, Harris, Brownell, & Stice, 2014; Yokum et al., 2011). Obese individuals who evidenced greater versus weaker reward and attention region response to high-calorie food images showed poorer response to behavioral weight loss treatment (Murdaugh et al., 2012). These results converge with evidence that individuals who work longer to earn high-fat/high-sugar snack foods, which presumably reflects greater anticipatory food reward, also show elevated future weight gain (Epstein, Yokum, Feda, & Stice, 2014). One study found an increase in striatal response to palatable food cues for originally healthy weight adolescents who gained weight relative to those who showed weight stability (Stice & Yokum, 2016a), providing evidence of the emergence of elevated incentive sensitization that occurs as a result of overeating.

There is also evidence that attentional bias for high-calorie food predicts greater *ad lib* food intake (Nijs, Muris, Euser, & Franken, 2010b; Werthmann, Field, Roefs, Nederkoorn, & Jansen, 2014) and future weight gain (Calitri, Pothos, Tapper, Brunstrom, & Rogers, 2010).

The evidence that elevated reward and attention region responsivity predicts future weight gain dovetails with evidence from controlled trials that weight loss reduces reward region (e.g., parahippocampal gyrus, parietal cortices, putamen, insula, visual cortex) responsivity to high-calorie food images (Cornier, Melanson, Salzberg, Bechtell, & Tregellas, 2012; Deckersbach et al., 2014; Rosenbaum, Pavlovich, Leibel, & Hirsch, 2008). Weight loss has also been associated with concurrent reductions in food preference ratings for high-calorie foods relative to weight stable controls (Deckersbach et al., 2014).

Echoing evidence that elevated dopamine signaling capacity amplified the predictive relation between elevated reward region response to palatable food receipt and future weight gain, the relation of reward region response to food images and future weight gain was moderated by a genetic propensity for greater dopamine signaling capacity in reward regions. Adolescents who showed elevated striatal and OFC response to palatable food images and who had a genetic propensity for greater dopamine signaling due to possessing an A2/A2 *TaqIA* allele showed elevated future weight gain (Stice et al., 2010b).

Experiments have also generated findings that appear consistent with the incentive sensitization theory. Young adults randomly assigned to consume high-calorie foods daily over 2–3 week periods showed an increased willingness to work for their assigned food relative to controls (Clark et al., 2010; Temple et al., 2009), echoing findings with rodents (Teegarden et al., 2009), as well as increased *ad lib* consumption of the snack foods after consuming the snack food on a daily basis (Tey et al., 2012).

The above findings imply that some individuals may show an elevated propensity to associate reward from palatable food intake with cues repeatedly paired with such food rewards, which drives elevated responsivity of reward regions to food cues. Using functional MRI, Burger and Stice (2014) documented an increase in caudate response to cues predicting impending milkshake receipt over repeated pairings of the predictive cues and milkshake receipt, demonstrating a direct measure of *in vivo* cue–reward learning in humans. Further, that study found a simultaneous decrease in putamen and ventral pallidum response during milkshake receipt that occurred over repeated pairings of the cue and milkshake receipt, mirroring the reduction in dopamine release in response to food reward after it is repeatedly paired with a cue that signals impending food receipt (Zellner & Ranaldi, 2010). The reduction in putamen and ventral pallidum signal may reflect reinforcer satiation. Critically, participants who exhibited the greatest escalation in ventral pallidum responsivity to cues and those individuals that showed the greatest decrease in caudate response to milkshake receipt showed larger increases in BMI at 2-year follow-up ($r = 0.39$ and –0.69, respectively). These data suggest that there are individual differences in food cue–reward learning and food reinforcer satiation that may give rise to elevated reward region responsivity that underlies incentive sensitization. These individual difference factors may explain why certain people have shown obesity onset in response to the obesogenic environment in Western cultures, whereas others have not.

In sum, heightened reward region responsivity to food cues or anticipated receipt predicted future weight gain and poorer response to a weight loss intervention. Studies found that weight loss was associated with a reduction in reward region responsivity to high-calorie food images. In addition, one study found that the predictive effects between reward region response to food images and future weight gain are stronger for individuals with a genetic propensity for elevated dopamine signaling. Experiments indicated that habitual intake of high-calorie snack foods resulted in greater subsequent intake of the snack food and a greater willingness to work for the snack foods. Further, individuals who showed the most potent reward–cue learning and food reinforcer satiation showed elevated future weight gain. These findings provide strong support for the incentive sensitization theory of obesity.

3.4 REWARD DEFICIT THEORY OF OBESITY

The reward deficit model of obesity posits that individuals with lower sensitivity of dopamine-based reward regions overeat to compensate for this reward deficiency (Wang et al., 2002). This theory was largely based on evidence that drugs that block dopamine D2 receptors increase appetite and result in weight gain, whereas drugs that increase brain dopamine concentrations reduce appetite and produce weight loss (Wang et al., 2001). Yet there are questionable aspects of this logic. First, all drugs that produce euphoria, including stimulants, barbiturates, benzodiazepines, opioids, and marijuana, increase dopamine signaling in reward circuitry (Wise & Rompre, 1989), but only stimulants produce weight loss. Second, "dopaminergic" drugs, such as amphetamine, increase neurotransmission of dopamine, serotonin, norepinephrine, epinephrine, histamine, acetylcholine, opioids, and glutamate (Loseth, Ellingsen, & Leknes, 2014; Miller, 2011), making it difficult to conclude that it is the increase in dopaminergic signaling that causes weight loss. Third, "antidopaminergic" drugs (aka, antipsychotics) affect neurotransmission of dopamine and serotonin and also show affinity for adrenergic, opioidergic, and glutamate receptors (Meltzer, 2002; Miller, 2009), making it difficult to conclude that it is the decrease in dopamine signaling that cause weight gain. Indeed, a randomized trial that directly compared the effects of haloperidol, an antipsychotic with very high affinity for dopamine D2 receptors, to clozapine and olanzapine, atypical antipsychotic medications with lower affinity for dopamine D2 receptors, found that only the atypical antipsychotics produced weight gain (Krakowski, Czobor, & Citrome, 2009).

Obese versus lean humans showed lower striatal dopamine D2 receptor availability (de Weijer et al., 2011; Haltia et al., 2007; Kessler et al., 2014; Volkow et al., 2008), though this finding was not replicated in other studies (Eisenstein et al., 2013; Haltia et al., 2008; Karlsson et al., 2015; Steele et al., 2010). Obese versus lean humans also had lower μ-opioid receptor availability in the ventral striatum, dorsal caudate, orbitofrontal cortex, anterior cingulate cortex, insula, and thalamus (Karlsson et al., 2015), as well as lower capacity of nigrostriatal neurons to synthesize dopamine (Wilcox et al., 2010). Obese versus lean humans showed less striatal responsivity to tastes of high-calorie beverages (Babbs et al., 2013; Frank et al., 2012; Green et al., 2011; Stice et al., 2008a, b). One study found a positive correlation between BMI and dopamine release in the dorsal striatum and substantia nigra in response to amphetamine (Kessler et al., 2014), suggesting that D2 receptor availability may not be closely coupled with phasic dopamine response from rewarding experiences. Obese versus lean individuals also showed greater tyrosine and phenylalanine availability, amino acid precursors used in the production of dopamine (Frank et al., 2015), which likewise implies that obese individuals may have greater endogenous dopamine availability.

However, prospective and experimental findings indicate that overeating contributes to reward region hyporesponsivity. Young women who gained weight over a 6-month period showed a reduction in striatal responsivity to palatable food receipt relative to women who remained weight stable (Stice, Yokum, Blum, & Bohon, 2010a). This finding converges with overfeeding experiments with animals; rats randomized to overeating conditions that resulted in weight gain versus control conditions showed downregulation of postsynaptic D2 receptors and reduced D2 sensitivity, extracellular dopamine levels in the nucleus accumbens and dopamine turnover, and lower sensitivity of dopamine reward circuitry to food intake, electrical stimulation, and amphetamine and potassium administration (Bello et al., 2002; Davis et al., 2008; Geiger et al., 2009; Johnson & Kenny et al., 2010; Kelley et al., 2003; Thanos et al., 2008). In one experiment, rats were randomized to a 40-day period of unlimited access to a high-fat/high-sugar diet, to limited access to a high-fat/high-sugar diet, or unlimited access to rat chow; rats in each of these conditions were subsequently randomized to exposure to a light cue that was associated with a foot shock or the light cue only (Johnson & Kenny, 2010). This study found that on a subsequent test day, exposure to the light cue that had been paired with the shock reduced caloric intake in rates that had experienced limited access to the high-fat/high-sugar diet or unlimited access to the chow diet but not in those that had previously had unlimited access to the high-fat/high-sugar diet, suggesting that habitual intake of energy dense diets induces a compulsive style of eating. The reduced dopamine signaling capacity appears to occur because habitual intake of high-fat diets decreases synthesis of oleoylethanolamine, a gastrointestinal lipid messenger (Tellez et al., 2013). People who report elevated intake of particular foods show reduced striatal response during intake of that food, independent of BMI (Burger & Stice, 2012; Green & Murphy, 2012; Rudenga & Small, 2012). Converging with these results, young adults randomly assigned to consume high-calorie foods daily over 2–12 week periods reported reduced "liking" of the foods relative to baseline and control high-calorie foods not consumed daily (Clark et al., 2010; Hetherington et al., 2000; 2002; Temple et al., 2009; Tey et al., 2012).

The finding that weight gain is associated with downregulation of dopamine-based reward circuitry dovetails with evidence that weight loss increases D2 receptor availability in humans (Steele et al., 2010) and rats (Thanos et al., 2008) and responsivity of reward circuitry to food cues (Cornier et al., 2012; Deckersbach et al., 2014; Rosenbaum et al., 2008). This literature seems consistent with the thesis that habitual overeating results in downregulation of reward circuitry and that reducing overeating can reverse this process.

Interestingly, an experiment found that intake of high-fat/high-sugar food resulted in downregulation of striatal D1 and D2 receptors in rats relative to isocaloric intake of low-fat/low-sugar rat chow (Aliso et al., 2010), implying that it is intake of energy-dense foods versus a positive energy balance *per se* that causes plasticity of reward circuitry. Mice that received chronic intragastric infusion of fat showed reduced striatal dopamine signaling from food intake relative to chow fed weight-matched control mice (Tellez et al., 2013), providing further evidence that habitual consumption of fat can reduce dopamine response to food intake, independent of weight gain. These results prompted a test of whether habitual ice cream intake was associated with reduced reward region responsivity to ice cream–based milkshake (Burger & Stice, 2012). Ice cream intake was inversely related to activation in the striatum (bilateral putamen: right $r = -0.31$; left $r = -0.30$; caudate: $r = -0.28$) and insula ($r = -0.35$) in response to milkshake receipt. Yet total kcal intake over the previous 2 weeks did not correlate with striatal or insula response to milkshake receipt, providing additional evidence that it may be intake of energy-dense food, rather than overall caloric intake, that reduces responsivity of reward circuitry.

The evidence that overeating results in downregulation of dopamine-based reward circuitry converges with data suggesting that habitual substance use, which also causes acute increases in dopamine signaling, likewise leads to downregulated reward circuitry. For instance, lower dopamine release in the nucleus accumbens in response to methylphenidate has been observed in cocaine-dependent and alcohol-dependent individuals relative to healthy controls (Volkow et al., 1997, 2007). Indeed, even adolescents with a short history of substance use showed less caudate response to monetary reward relative to adolescents who had not initiated substance use (Stice et al., 2013).

Geiger et al. (2009) speculated that rats that have experienced diet-induced downregulation of dopamine circuitry may similarly overeat to increase dopamine signaling. However, a study found that mice in which reduced striatal dopamine signaling from food intake was experimentally induced through chronic intragastric infusion of fat worked *less* for acute intragastric infusion of fat and consumed *less* rat chow *ad lib* than control mice (Tellez et al., 2013). These results converge with evidence that experimentally induced dopamine depletion resulted in decreased hunger ratings and less *ad lib* caloric intake relative to the control condition (Hardman, Herbert, Brunstrom, Munafo, & Rogers, 2014). Further, genetically engineered dopamine-deficient mice are unable to sustain appropriate levels of feeding, and dysregulation of dopamine signaling in the dorsal striatum in particular is sufficient to induce hypophagia (Sotak et al., 2005; Zhou & Palmiter, 1995). These results converge with the finding that experimental administration of 6-hydroxydopamine, a neurotoxin that selectively destroys dopaminergic and noradrenergic neurons, at several points along the nigrostriatal dopamine pathway between the substantia nigra and caudate–putamen results in severe aphasia (Robbins & Everitt, 1999). These results seem incompatible with the notion that an induced downregulation of dopamine reward circuitry leads to compensatory overeating.

Further, none of the prospective studies that examined the relation of the blood oxygen level dependent (BOLD) response to high-calorie palatable food images/cues, anticipated palatable food receipt, and palatable food receipt to future weight gain reviewed above found a main effect between reduced reward region responsivity to these food stimuli and greater future weight gain (Demos et al., 2012; Geha et al., 2013; Stice et al., 2008a, 2010b, 2015; Sun et al., 2015; Yokum et al., 2011, 2014). Likewise, lean youth at risk for future obesity by virtue of parental obesity showed hyper-responsivity of reward regions to palatable food receipt and monetary reward and no evidence of hyporesponsivity or reward regions (Stice et al., 2011).

However, a weaker striatal response to receipt of high-calorie chocolate milkshake predicted future weight gain for participants with a genetic propensity for lower dopamine signaling in reward circuitry, by virtue of possessing the *TaqIA* A1 allele (Stice et al., 2008a, 2015). Likewise, a weaker amygdala response to milkshake receipt predicted future weight gain for adults with a genetic propensity for lower dopamine signaling capacity by virtue of possessing a *TaqIA* A1 allele (Sun et al., 2015). Further, weaker putamen and OFC response to palatable food images predicted future weight gain for adolescents at genetic risk for lower dopamine signaling by virtue of possessing the *TaqIA* A1 allele (Stice et al., 2010b). The interactive effects suggest the possibility of qualitatively distinct reward surfeit and reward deficit pathways to obesity. It appears that the reward surfeit model may apply to individuals with a genetic propensity for greater dopamine signaling capacity and that the reward deficit model may apply to those with a genetic propensity for weaker dopamine signaling. Findings may imply that too much or too little dopamine signaling capacity and reward region responsivity may both increase risk for overeating, potentially because each perturbs homeostatic processes that maintain a balance between caloric intake and caloric expenditure. There are other examples of inverted U-shaped relations between neurotransmitters and neural function, such as the evidence that too little or too much epinephrine and norepinephrine impair memory formation (Eichenbaum et al., 1999). Future studies should test whether genotypes that affect dopamine signaling moderate the relations between reward region responsivity and future weight gain.

In sum, research has provided little prospective or experimental support for the thesis that individuals who show low responsivity of reward circuitry to food stimuli overeat to compensate for this deficit. Adolescents at high versus low risk for future weight gain showed elevated reward region responsivity to food and no evidence of blunted reward region response, and none of the prospective studies found a main effect wherein low reward region response to food stimuli predicted future weight gain. Indeed, most of these prospective studies found that *elevated* responsivity of reward circuitry to food images/cues, anticipated palatable food receipt, and palatable food receipt predicted future weight gain. Moreover, experimentally induced downregulation of dopamine response to fat intake in mice reduced caloric intake and the motivational value of high-calorie food compared to control mice, experimentally induced dopamine depletion was associated with less *ad lib* food intake in humans, and dopamine-deficient mice were unable to sustain adequate caloric intake. Yet interactions suggest that the reward surfeit model might operate for individuals with a genetic propensity for greater dopamine signaling capacity and the reward deficit model might operate for individuals with a genetic propensity for lower dopamine signaling capacity. Thus, although most findings from the prospective and experimental studies provided results that do not support the reward deficit theory, select results can be interpreted as providing support for this theory. This pattern of findings suggest that it would be useful if additional independent labs tested whether the *TaqIA* polymorphism moderates the relation between reward region response and future weight gain before the reward deficit theory is set aside.

3.5 INHIBITORY CONTROL DEFICIT THEORY OF OVEREATING

It has been proposed that individuals with inhibitory control deficits, and by extension lower responsivity of brain regions implicated in inhibitory control, are more sensitive to food cues and more vulnerable to the pervasive temptation of appetizing foods in our environment, which increases overeating (Diergaarde et al., 2009; Nederkoorn et al., 2006a).

Consistent with the inhibitory control deficit theory, obese versus lean individuals showed response inhibition deficits on go/no-go and stop-signal tasks (Nederkoorn, Jansen, Mulkens, & Jansen, 2006b; Nederkoorn et al., 2006a). Response inhibition deficits on a stop-signal task also correlated positively with *ad lib* caloric intake (Guerrieri et al., 2007). Rats that showed behavioral disinhibition in response to food reward on a serial reaction time task exhibited greater future sucrose-seeking behavior and enhanced sensitivity to sucrose-associated stimuli after extinction, relative to rats that exhibited behavioral inhibition (Diergaarde et al., 2009). Obese versus lean individuals showed a preference for immediate food and monetary reward versus larger delayed rewards (e.g., Epstein, Dearing, Temple, & Cavanaugh, 2008; Jasinska et al., 2012; Weller, Cook, Avsar, & Cox, 2008).

Critically, inhibitory control deficits in response to high-calorie foods in delay discounting tasks, which reflects an immediate reward bias, has reliably predicted future weight gain (e.g., Evans, Fuller-Rowell, & Doan, 2012; Francis & Susman, 2009; Schlam, Wilson Shoda, Mischel, & Ayduk, 2013). Low reported inhibitory control likewise predicts future weight gain (Anzman & Birch, 2009; Duckworth, Tsukayama, & Geier, 2010; Sutin, Ferrucci, Zonderman, & Terracciano, 2011). Further, individuals with inhibitory control deficits show poorer response to weight loss treatment (Nederkoorn et al., 2007; Weygandt et al., 2013).

In terms of neuroimaging findings, obese versus lean teens showed less activation of prefrontal regions (dorsolateral prefrontal cortex [dlPFC], ventral lateral prefrontal cortex) when trying to inhibit responses to high-calorie food images and behavioral evidence of reduced inhibitory control (Batterink et al., 2010), though low recruitment of inhibitory regions did not predict future weight gain. Low recruitment of inhibitory control regions (inferior, middle, and superior frontal gyri) during difficult versus easy choices on a delay-discounting task predicted future weight gain in another study ($r = 0.71$; Kishinevsky et al., 2012). Further, low recruitment of inhibitory control regions (dlPFC) during a delay discounting task predicted less weight loss in response to weight loss treatment (Weygandt et al., 2013). These results converge with evidence that obese versus lean adults showed less grey matter volume in the prefrontal cortex (Pannacciulli et al., 2006), a region that modulates inhibitory control, and with a marginal trend for reduced grey matter volume in the prefrontal cortex to predict future weight gain (Yokum, Ng, & Stice, 2012). Adolescents who showed less prefrontal inhibitory region recruitment during a go/no-go task were more likely to show onset of heavy alcohol use (Norman et al., 2011). Interestingly, obese versus lean humans also showed less recruitment of inhibitory regions (ventral medial prefrontal cortex) in response to high-calorie food images (Silvers et al., 2014) and high-calorie food TV commercials (Gearhardt et al., 2014). Further, lower dlPFC response to high-calorie food images predicted greater *ad lib* food intake over the next 3 days (Cornier et al., 2010), and individuals reporting chronic stress showed less recruitment of frontal regions in response to images of high-calories foods and showed greater *ad lib* caloric intake (Tryon, Carter, DeCant, & Laugero, 2013). The findings from the latter four studies are of note because they emerged in paradigms lacking a behavioral response component. These findings may be explained by the fact that the primary motor area receives a dense innervation from dopamine-containing fibers originating in the midbrain (Berger, Gaspar, & Verney, 1991). Indeed, participants have shown activation of motor regions, as assessed via electromyography, in response to palatable food images (Gupta & Aron, 2011).

In sum, individuals with a preference for immediate food reward, as assessed by behavioral paradigms, showed elevated weight gain, with similar results emerging from studies that used self-report measures of inhibitory control. Individuals with inhibitory control deficits also showed a poorer response to weight loss treatment and poorer maintenance of weight loss after treatment. Individuals who show less recruitment of inhibitory control regions in tasks that require inhibition showed elevated future weight gain, but this effect did not replicate in a second study that used a different inhibitory control paradigm. Individuals that showed less recruitment of inhibitory control regions during a delay discounting task showed less weight loss in response to a short-term diet and less weight loss maintenance over longer-term follow-up. Collectively, these results provide prospective support for the inhibitory control deficit theory of obesity, though many of the predictive effects were small and the findings were somewhat mixed. Interestingly, there is emerging evidence that obese individuals show less recruitment of inhibitory control regions in response to food stimuli. However, only two prospective brain imaging studies examined the relation of reduced responsivity of inhibitory control regions to future weight gain, making it difficult to draw firm inferences regarding the relation of inhibitory control deficits to future weight gain.

3.6 DYNAMIC VULNERABILITY MODEL OF OBESITY

According to the revised dynamic vulnerability model (Stice & Yokum, 2016b; Figure 3.1), which attempts to synthesize the above theories into a unifying etiologic model regarding neural vulnerability factors that increase risk for overeating and changes in neural responsivity that result from overeating that may contribute to future escalations in caloric intake, individuals who show elevated reward region responsivity to palatable food receipt are more likely to overeat and show consequent weight gain, based on the finding from Geha et al. (2013). We hypothesize that the relation of reward region responsivity to future weight gain is moderated by genotypes that impact dopamine signaling, wherein individuals who show stronger reward region responsivity to food intake will exhibit greater weight gain if they have a genetic propensity for elevated dopamine signaling, but individuals who show a weaker reward region responsivity to food intake will exhibit greater weight gain if they have

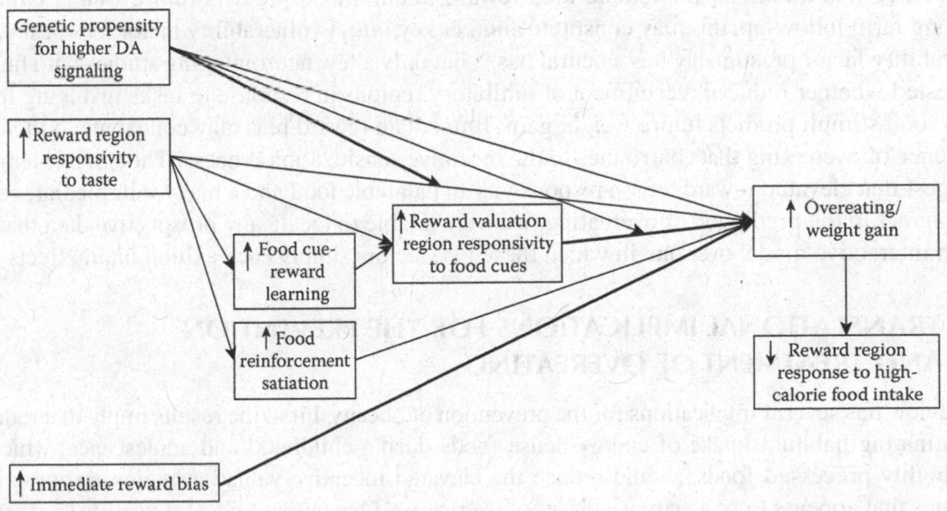

FIGURE 3.1 The refined version of the dynamic vulnerability model of obesity. The thick black arrows represent well-established relations and the thinner black arrows represent relations with a more provisional degree of empirical support.

a genetic propensity for weaker dopamine signaling. This prediction is based on interactions observed in three studies (Stice et al., 2008a; Stice et al., 2015; Sun et al., 2015) that imply that there may be two qualitatively distinct pathways to obesity that conform to the reward surfeit and reward deficit models. Data imply that having too little or too much DA signaling and reward region responsivity may both increase risk for overeating, suggesting that homeostatic mechanisms that regulate feeding may operate optimally when there is moderate dopamine signaling and reward region responsivity.

Elevated reward region responsivity to palatable food receipt is also hypothesized to contribute to more potent food cue–reward learning, based on findings from Burger and Stice (2014). And more potent food cue reward learning is thought to increase risk for future weight gain, also based on the findings from Burger and Stice (2014). Theoretically, greater food cue–reward learning results in elevated incentive valuation region responsivity to food cues, which drives overeating when the ubiquitous food cues are encountered in the environment, consistent with the incentive sensitization model. This hyperresponsivity of reward valuation regions to food cues appears to be a more potent driver of overeating than the initial hyperresponsivity of reward regions to palatable food intake, based on results from the prospective studies reviewed previously (Demos et al., 2012; Geha et al., 2013; Stice et al., 2015; Yokum et al., 2011; Yokum et al., 2014), implying that obesity can be conceptualized as resulting from aberrant learning.

In addition, data suggest that elevated reward region responsivity appears to contribute to greater food reinforcer satiation, which predicts future weight gain (Burger & Stice, 2014). Yet the mechanism by which greater food reinforcement satiation drives overeating is unclear, and it may be an artifact of an initial elevated reward region response to palatable food intake.

Overeating is hypothesized to result in a reduction in reward region responsivity to palatable food, based primarily on results from overfeeding experiments with animals (Bello et al., 2002; Davis et al., 2008; Geiger et al., 2009; Johnson & Kenny et al., 2010; Kelley et al., 2003; Thanos et al., 2008) but also on evidence that overeating seems to reduce reward region response to palatable food receipt (Stice et al., 2010a). Yet reduced reward region response to palatable food appears to decrease overeating on an acute basis, rather than increasing overeating. There is also evidence that genotypes that impact dopamine signaling moderate the relation of reward region responsivity to food cues and future weight gain (Stice et al., 2010b).

Further, data suggest that a bias for immediate reward also constitutes a risk factor for overeating and subsequent weight gain (Evans et al., 2012; Francis & Susman, 2009; Schlam et al., 2013). Given the evidence that a bias for immediate food reward in childhood predicts future weight gain over very long-term follow-up, this may constitute another key initial vulnerability factor for obesity. This vulnerability factor presumably has a neural basis, but only a few neuroimaging studies with humans have tested whether reduced recruitment of inhibitory regions in response to tasks involving inhibition to food stimuli predicts future weight gain. Immediate reward bias may contribute to the initial emergence of overeating that contributes to the incentive sensitization process. Though it is tempting to suggest that elevated reward region responsivity to palatable food and a bias for immediate reward may interact in the prediction of overeating, we were unable to locate any prospective data that support an interactive model over one in which these two factors simply each exhibit main effects.

3.7 TRANSLATIONAL IMPLICATIONS FOR THE PREVENTION AND TREATMENT OF OVEREATING

This review has several implications for the prevention of obesity. First, the results imply that reducing or eliminating habitual intake of energy-dense foods during childhood and adolescence, which are often highly processed foods, should reduce the elevated incentive valuation region responsivity to food cues that appears to be a primary driver of overeating. One obvious way for parents to effect this change is to avoid keeping high-calorie, processed foods in the home, instead purchasing high-fiber foods such as whole grain products, fruits, and vegetables. Second, prevention programs that promote the development of stronger executive function and inhibitory control, which includes resisting temptation (e.g., Diamond, Barnett, Thomas, & Munro, 2007), may reduce the immediate reward bias that increases risk for the emergence of overeating. More broadly, given the numerous changes that occur in response to overeating that maintain overeating, including increased sensitivity of reward and attention circuitry to food cues and damage to circuitry that governs homeostatic feeding, it would appear that preventing overeating might be more effective than treating it once it is established.

This review also has several implications for the treatment of overeating. First, given the evidence that habitual consumption of high-calorie foods promotes and maintains hyperresponsivity of reward and attention regions to cues for those unhealthy foods, a primary treatment goal should be to reduce or eliminate intake of high-calorie processed foods and instead promote intake of the whole foods noted above. Consumption of lower-calorie nonprocessed foods should result in extinction that reduces elevated reward and attention region responsivity to unhealthy food cues that maintains overeating. Results from this review suggest that intake of high-calorie foods, rather than caloric intake *per se*, plays a critical role in neural plasticity that maintains overeating. Second, acute dietary restriction, which also increases the reward value of food, particularly high-calorie foods (Leidy et al., 2011; Stice et al., 2013), should be avoided. Instead, obese individuals should consume three healthy meals daily and avoid periods of caloric restriction. Third, findings also suggest that reducing stress, which increases the reward value of food and decreases inhibitory control (Tryon et al., 2013), should also reduce hyperreward region responsivity to food cues. Fourth, reducing the presence of cues for high-calorie processed foods (cue avoidance), such pictures of and advertisements for such foods, should also reduce overeating (e.g., reducing exposure to unhealthy food commercials for youth). By extension, not having high-calorie processed foods in the home is another obvious way to reduce exposure to food cues. Fifth, it may be possible to capitalize on the fact that motor circuitry has direct inputs into reward valuation regions. Emerging evidence suggests that completing computer-based tasks in which participants are repeatedly cued to inhibit a motor response when high-calorie foods are presented and make motor responses to other stimuli (e.g., low-calorie foods) reduces valuation of such foods (Lawrence et al., 2014; Veling, Koningsbruggen, Aarts, & Stroebe, 2014), reward region responsivity to such foods (Stice, Lawrence, Kemps, & Veling, 2016), and produces weight loss.

Although these translational implications for the prevention and treatment of obesity are speculative and only a few have been investigated in randomized trials, continued research into neural vulnerability factors that predict future overeating and weight gain and subsequent randomized trials should lead to important breakthroughs in the prevention and treatment of overeating, reducing the elevated morbidity and mortality associated with obesity.

REFERENCES

Alsio, J., Olszewski, P., Norback, A., Gunnarsson, Z., Levine, A., Pickerings, C., & Schioth, H. (2010). Dopamine D1 receptor gene expression decreases in the nucleus accumbens upon long-term exposure to palatable food and differs depending on diet-induced obesity phenotype in rats. *Neuroscience, 171,* 779–787.

Anzman, S., & Birch, L. (2009). Low inhibitory control and restrictive feeding practices predict weight outcomes. *Journal of Pediatrics, 155,* 651–656.

Asghari, V., Sanyal, S., Buchwaldt, S., Paterson, A., Jovanovic, V., & Van Tol, H. (1995). Modulation of intracellular cyclic AMP levels by different human dopamine D4 receptor variants. *Journal of Neurochemistry, 65,* 1157–1165.

Babbs, R., Sun, X., Felsted, J., Chouinard-Decorte, F., Veldhuizen, M., & Small, D. (2013). Decreased caudate response to milkshake is associated with higher body mass index and greater impulsivity. *Physiology & Behavior, 121,* 103–111.

Batterink, L., Yokum, S., & Stice, E. (2010). Body mass correlates inversely with inhibitory control in response to food among adolescent girls: An fMRI study. *NeuroImage, 52,* 1696–1703.

Bello, N., Lucas, L., & Hajnal, A. (2002). Repeated sucrose access influences dopamine D2 receptor density in the striatum. *Neuroreport, 13,* 1575–1578.

Berger, B., Gaspar, P., & Verney, C. (1991). Dopaminergic innervation of the cerebral cortex: Unexpected differences between rodent and primate. *Trends in Neuroscience, 14,* 21–27.

Berridge, K., Ho, C., Richard, J., & DiFeliceantonio, A. (2010). The tempted brain eats: Pleasure and desire circuits in obesity and eating disorders. *Brain Research, 1350,* 43–64.

Braet, C., & Crombez, G. (2003). Cognitive interference due to food cues in childhood obesity. *Journal of Clinical Child and Adolescent Psychology, 32,* 32–39.

Brooks, S., Cedernaes, J., & Schiöth, H. (2013). Increased prefrontal and parahippocampal activation with reduced dorsolateral prefrontal and insular cortex activation to food images in obesity: A meta-analysis of fMRI studies. *PLoS One, 8,* e60393.

Burger, K., & Stice, E. (2012). Frequent ice cream consumption is associated with reduced striatal response to receipt of an ice cream-based milkshake. *American Journal Clinical Nutrition, 95,* 810–817.

Burger, K., & Stice, E. (2013). Elevated energy intake is correlated with hyperresponsivity in attentional, gustatory, and reward brain regions while anticipating palatable food receipt. *American Journal of Clinical Nutrition, 97,* 1188–1194.

Burger, K., & Stice, E. (2014). Greater striatopallidal adaptive coding during cue-reward learning and food reward habituation predict future weight gain. *NeuroImage, 99,* 122–128.

Calitri, R., Pothos, E., Tapper, K. Brunstrom, J., Rogers, P. (2010). Cognitive biases to healthy and unhealthy food words predict change in BMI. *Obesity, 18,* 2282–2287.

Castellanos, E., Charboneau, E., Dietrich, M., Park, S., Bradley, B., Mogg, K., et al., (2009). Obese adults have visual attention bias for food cue images: Evidence for altered reward system function. *International Journal of Obesity, 33,* 1063–1073.

Clark, E., Dewey, A., Temple, J. (2010). Effects of daily snack food intake on food reinforcement depend on body mass index and energy density. *American Journal of Clinical Nutrition, 91,* 300–308.

Cornier, M., Melanson, E., Salzberg, A., Bechtell, J., & Tregellas, J. (2012). The effects of exercise on the neuronal response to food cues. *Physiology & Behavior, 105,* 1028–1034.

Cornier, M., Salzberg, A., Endly, D., Bessesen, D., & Tregellas, J. (2010). Sex-based differences in the behavioral and neuronal responses to food. *Physiology & Behavior, 99,* 5538–5543.

Davis, C., Strachan, S., & Berkson, M. (2004). Sensitivity to reward: Implications for overeating and overweight. *Appetite, 42,* 131–138.

Davis, J., Tracy, A., Schurdak, J., Tschop, M., Lipton, J., Clegg, D., et al., (2008). Exposure to elevated levels of dietary fat attenuates psychostimulant reward and mesolimbic dopamine turnover in the rat. *Behavioral Neuroscience, 122,* 1257–1263.

Deckersbach, T., Das, S.K., Urban, L.E., Salinardi, T., Batra, P., Rodman, A. M. et al. (2014). Pilot randomized trial demonstrating reversal of obesity-related abnormalities in reward system responsivity to food cues with a behavioral intervention. *Nutrition and Diabetes, 4,* e129.

Demos, K., Heatherton, T., & Kelley, W. (2012). Individual differences in nucleus accumbens activity to food and sexual images predict weight gain and sexual behavior. *Journal of Neuroscience, 32,* 5549–5552.

de Weijer, B., van de Giessen, E., van Amelsvoort, T., Boot, E., Braak, B., Janssen, I., et al., (2011). Lower striatal dopamine D2/3 receptor availability in obese compared with non-obese subjects. *EJNMMI Research, 1,* 37.

Diamond, A., Barnett, W., Thomas, J., & Munro, S. (2007). Preschool program improves cognitive control. *Science, 318,* 1387–1388.

Diergaarde, L., Pattij, T., Nawijn, L., Schoffelmeer, A.N., & Vries, T.J. (2009). Trait impulsivity predicts escalation of sucrose seeking and hypersensitivity to sucrose-associated stimuli. *Behavioral Neuroscience, 123,* 794–803.

Duckworth, A., Tsukayama, E., & Geier, A. (2010). Self-controlled children stay leaner in the transition to adolescence. *Appetite, 54,* 304–308.

Due, D., Huettel, S., Hall, W., & Rubin, D. (2002). Activation in mesolimbic and visuospatial neural circuits elicited by smoking cues: Evidence from functional magnetic resonance imaging. *American Journal of Psychiatry, 159,* 954–960.

Eichenbaum, H., Cahill, L., Gluck, M., Hasselmo, M., Keil, F., Martin, A., et al., (1999). Learning and memory: Systems analysis. In M. Zigmond, F. Bloom, S. Landis, J. Roberts, & L. Squire (eds). *Fundamental Neuroscience* (pp. 1455–1486). Academic Press: San Diego, CA.

Eisenstein, S., Antenor-Dorsey, J., Gredysa, D., Koller, J., Bihum, E., Ranck, S., et al., (2013). A comparison of D2 receptor specific binding in obese and normal-weight individuals using PET with (N-[^{11}C]methyl) benperidol. *Synapse, 67,* 748–756.

Epstein, L., Dearing, K., Temple, J., & Cavanaugh, M. (2008). Food reinforcement and impulsivity in overweight children and their parents. *Eating Behaviors, 9,* 319–327.

Epstein, L., Yokum, S., Feda, D., & Stice, E. (2014). Parental obesity and food reinforcement predict future weight gain in non-obese adolescents. *Appetite, 82,* 138–142.

Evans, G., Ruller-Rowell, R., & Doan, S. (2012). Childhood cumulative risk and obesity: The mediating role of self-regulatory ability. *Pediatrics, 129,* e68.

Ferreira, J., Tellez, L., Ren, X., Yeckel, C., & da Araujo, I. (2012). Regulation of fat intake in the absence of flavour signaling. *Journal of Physiology, 590,* 953–972.

Flegal, K., Carroll, M., Kit, B., & Ogden, C. (2012). Prevalence of obesity and trends in the distribution of body mass index among US adults, 1999–2010. *JAMA, 307,* 491–497.

Francis, L., & Susman, E. (2009). Self-regulation failure and rapid weight gain in children from age 3 to 12 years. *Archives of Disease in Children and Adolescents, 163,* 297–302.

Frank, S., Laharnar, N., Kullmann, S., Veit, R., Canova, C., Hegner, Y., et al., (2010). Processing of food pictures: Influence of hunger, gender, and calorie content. *Brain Research, 1350,* 159–166.

Frank, G., Reynolds, J., Shott, M., Jappe, L., Yang, T., Tregellas, J., & O'Reilly, R. (2012). Anorexia nervosa and obesity are associated with opposite brain reward response. *Neuropsychopharmacology, 307,* 2031–2046.

Frank, S., Veit, R., Sauer, H., Enck, P., Friederich, H., Unholzer, T., et al., (2015). *Dopamine depletion reduced food-related reward activity independent of BMI.* Under review.

Frankort, A., Roefs, A., Siep, N., Roebroeck, A., Havermans, R., & Jansen, A. (2011). Reward activity in satiated overweight women is decreased during unbiased viewing but increased when imaging taste: An event-related fMRI study. *International Journal of Obesity, 36,* 1–11.

Gearhardt, A., Yokum, S., Stice, E., Harris, J., & Brownell, K. (2014). Relation of obesity to neural activation in response to food commercials. *Social Cognitive and Affective Neuroscience, 9,* 932–938.

Geha, P., Aschenbrenner, K., Felsted, J., O'Malley, S., & Small, D. (2013). Altered hypothalamic response to food in smokers. *American Journal of Clinical Nutrition, 97,* 15–22.

Geiger, B., Haburcak, M., Avena, N., Moyer, M., Hoebel, B., & Pothos, E. (2009). Deficits of mesolimbic dopamine neurotransmission in rat dietary obesity. *Neuroscience, 159,* 1193–1199.

Graham, R., Hoover, A., Ceballos, N., & Komogortsev, O. (2011). Body mass index moderates gaze orienting biases and pupil diameter to high and low calorie food images. *Appetite, 56,* 577–586.

Green, E., Jacobson, A., Haase, L., & Murphy, C. (2011). Reduced nucleus accumbens and caudate nucleus activation to a pleasant taste is associated with obesity in older adults. *Brain Research, 1386,* 109–117.

Green, E., & Murphy, C. (2012). Altered processing of sweet taste in the brain of diet soda drinkers. *Physiology Behavior, 107,* 560–567.

Guerrieri, R., Nederkoorn, C., Stankiewicz, K., Alberts, H., Geschwind, N., Martijn, C., et al., (2007). The influence of trait and induced state impulsivity on food intake in normal-weight healthy women. *Appetite, 49,* 66–73.

Gupta, N., & Aron, A. (2011). Urges for food and money spill over into motor system excitability before action is taken. *European Journal of Neuroscience, 33,* 183–188.

Haltia, L., Rinne, J., Helin, S., Parkkola, R., Nagren, K., & Kaasine, V. (2008). Effects of intravenous placebo with glucose expectation on human basal ganglia dopaminergic function. *Synapse, 62,* 682–688.

Haltia, L., Rinne, J., Merisaari, H., Maguire, R., Savontaus, E., Helin, S., et al., (2007). Effects of intravenous glucose on dopaminergic function in the human brain in vivo. *Synapse, 61,* 748–756.

Hardman, C., Herbert, V., Brunstrom, J., Munafo, M., & Rogers, P. (2014). Dopamine and food reward: Effects of acute tyrosine/phenylalanine depletion on appetite. *Physiology and Behavior, 105,* 1202–1207.

Heinz, A., Goldman, D., Jones, D. W., Palmour, R., Hommer, D., Gorey, J. G., et al., (2000). Genotype influences in vivo dopamine transporter availability in human striatum. *Neuropsychopharmacology, 22,* 133–139.

Hetherington, M., Bell, A., & Rolls, B. (2000). Effects of repeat consumption on pleasantness, preference, and intake. *British Food Journal, 102,* 507–521.

Hetherington, M., Pirie, L., & Nabb, S. (2002). Stimulus satiation: Effects of repeated exposure to foods on pleasantness and intake. *Appetite, 38,* 19–28.

Huerta, C., Sarkar, P., Duong, T., Laird, A., & Fox, P. (2014). Neural bases of food perception: Coordinate-based meta-analyses of neuroimaging studies in multiple modalities. *Obesity (Silver Spring), 22,* 1439–1446.

Jasinska, A., Yasuda, M., Burant, C., Gregor, N., Khatri, S., Sweet, M. et al., (2012). Impulsivity and inhibitory control deficits are associated with unhealthy eating in young adults. *Appetite, 59,* 738–747.

Jastreboff, A., Sinha, R., Lacadie, C., Small, D., Sherwin, R., & Potenza, M. (2013). Neural correlates of stress- and food cue-induced food craving in obesity: Association with insulin levels. *Diabetes Care, 36,* 394–402.

Johnson, P., & Kenny, P. (2010). Dopamine D2 receptors in addiction-like reward dysfunction and compulsive eating in obese rats. *Nature Neuroscience, 13,* 635–641.

Jönsson, E., Nöthen, M., Grünhage, F., Farde, L., Nakashima, Y., Propping, P., et al., (1999). Polymorphisms in the dopamine D2 receptor gene and their relationships to striatal dopamine receptor density of healthy volunteers. *Molecular Psychiatry, 4,* 290–296.

Karlsson, H., Tuominen, L., Tuulari, J., Hirvonen, J., Parkkola, R., Helin, S., et al., (2015). Obesity is associated with decreased μ-opioid but unaltered dopamine D_2 receptor availability in the brain. *Journal of Neuroscience, 35,* 3959–3965.

Kelley, A., Will, M., Steininger, T., Zhang, M., & Haber, S. (2003). Restricted daily consumption of a highly palatable food (chocolate Ensure(R)) alters striatal enkephalin gene expression. *European Journal of Neuroscience, 18,* 2592–2598.

Kessler, R., Zald, D., Ansari, M., Li, R., & Cowan, R. (2014). Changes in dopamine release and dopamine D2/3 receptor levels with the development of mild obesity. *Synapse, 68,* 317–320.

Kishinevsky, F., Cox, J., Murdaugh, D., Stoeckel, L., Cook, E., & Weller, R. (2012). fMRI reactivity on a delay discounting task predicts weight gain in obese women. *Appetite, 58,* 582–592.

Krakowski, M., Czobor, P., & Citrome, L. (2009). Weight gain, metabolic parameters, and the impact of race in aggressive inpatients randomized to double-blind clozapine, olanzapine or haloperidol. *Schizophrenia Research, 110,* 95–102.

Kringelbach, M., O'Doherty, J., Rolls, E., & Andrews, C. (2003). Activation of the human orbitofrontal cortex to a liquid food stimulus is correlated with its subjective pleasantness. *Cerebral Cortex, 13,* 1064–1071.

Lachman, H., Papolos, D., Saito, T., Yu, Y., Szumlanski, C., & Weinshilboum, R. (1996). Human catechol-O-methyltransferase pharmacogenetics: Description of a functional polymorphism and its potential application to neuropsychiatric disorders. *Pharmacogenetics, 6,* 243–250.

Lawrence, N., Hinton, E., Parkinson, J., & Lawrence, A. (2012). Nucleus accumbens response to food cues predicts subsequent snack consumption in women and increased body mass index in those with reduced self-control. *NeuroImage, 63,* 415–422.

Lawrence, N., Verbruggen, F., Morrison, S., Parslow, D., O'Sullivan, J., Javaid, M., et al., (2014) Training response inhibition to food to reduce overeating. *Journal of Psychopharmacology, 28,* A130.

Leidy, H., Lepping, R., Savage, C., & Harris, C. (2011). Neural responses to visual food stimuli after a normal vs. higher protein breakfast in breakfast-skipping teens: A pilot fMRI study. *Obesity, 19,* 2019–2025.

Loseth, G., Ellingsen, D., & Leknes, S. (2014). State-dependent μ-opioid modulation of social motivation. *Frontiers in Behavioral Neuroscience, 8,* 1–15.

Mehta, S., Melhorn, S., Smeraglio, A., Tyagi, V., Grabowski, T., Schwartz, M. et al., (2012). Regional brain response to visual food cues is a marker of satiety that predicts food choice. *American Journal of Clinical Nutrition, 96,* 989–999.

Meltzer, H. (2002). Mechanism of action of atypical antipsychotic drugs (pp. 819–831). In K. Davis, J. Coyle, & C. Nemeroff (eds.). *Neuropsychopharmacology: The Fifth Generation of Progress.* American College of Neuropscyhopharmacology, Lippincott, Williams, & Wilkins, Philadelphia, Pennsylvania.

Miller, G. (2011). The emerging role of trace amine-associated receptor 1 in the functional regulation of monoamine transporters and dopaminergic activity. *Journal of Neurochemistry, 116,* 164–176.

Miller, R. (2009). Mechanisms of action of antipsychotic drugs of different classes, refractoriness to therapeutic effects of classical neuroleptics, and individual variation in sensitivity to their actions. *Current Neuropharmacology, 7,* 302–314.

Murdaugh, D., Cox, J., Cook, E., & Weller, R. (2012). fMRI reactivity to high-calorie food pictures predicts short- and long-term outcome in a weight-loss program. *NeuroImage, 59,* 2709–2721.

Myrick, H., Anton, R., Li, X., Henderson, S., Drobes, D., Voronin, K., et al., (2004). Differential brain activity in alcoholics and social drinkers to alcohol cues: Relationship to craving. *Neuropsychopharmacology, 29,* 393–402.

Nederkoorn, C., Braet, C., Van Eijs, Y., Tanghe, A., & Jansen, A. (2006a). Why obese children cannot resist food: The role of impulsivity. *Eating Behaviors, 7,* 315–322.

Nederkoorn, C., Smulders, F., Havermans, R., Roefs, A., & Jansen, A. (2006b). Impulsivity in obese women, *Appetite, 47,* 253–256.

Nederkoorn, C., Jansen, E., Mulkens, S., & Jansen, A. (2007). Impulsivity predicts treatment outcome in obese children. *Behaviour Research and Therapy, 45,* 1071–1075.

Nijs, I., Franken, I., & Muris, P. (2010a). Food-related stroop interference in obese and normal-weight individuals: Behavioral and electrophysiological indices. *Eating Behaviors, 11,* 258–265.

Nijs, I., Muris, P., Euser, A., & Franken, I. (2010b). Differences in attention to food and food intake between overweight/obese and normal-weight females under conditions of hunger and satiety. *Appetite, 54,* 243–254.

Nikolova, Y., Ferrell, R., Manuck, S., & Hariri, A. (2011). Multilocus genetic profile for dopamine signaling predicts ventral striatum reactivity. *Neuropsychopharmacology, 36,* 1940–1947.

Nolan-Poupart, S., Veldhuizen, M. G., Geha, P., & Small, D. (2013). Midbrain response to milkshake correlates with ad libitum milkshake intake in the absence of hunger. *Appetite, 60,* 168–174.

Norman, A., Pulido, C., Squeglia, L., Spadoni, A., & Paulus, M. (2011). Neural activation during inhibition predicts initiation of substance use in adolescence. *Drug Alcohol Depend, 119,* 216–223.

O'Doherty, J., Deichmann, R., Critchley, H., & Dolan, R. (2002). Neural responses during anticipation of a primary taste reward. *Neuron, 33,* 815–826.

Pannacciulli, N., Del Parigi, A., Chen, K., Le, D., Reiman, E., & Tataranni, P. (2006). Brain abnormalities in human obesity: A voxel-based morphometric study. *NeuroImage, 31,* 1419–25.

Robbins, T., & Everitt, B. (1999). Motivation and reward (pp. 1245–1260). In M. Zigmond, F. Bloom, S. Landis, J. Roberts, & L. Squire (eds). *Fundamental Neuroscience.* San Diego, CA, Academic Press.

Rosenbaum, M., Sy, M., Pavlovich, K., Leibel, R. L., & Hirsch, J. (2008). Leptin reverses weight loss-induced changes in regional neural activity responses to visual food stimuli. *Journal of Clinical Investigation, 118,* 2583–2591.

Rudenga, K., & Small, D. (2012). Amygdala response to sucrose consumption is inversely related to artificial sweetener use. *Appetite, 58,* 504–507.

Salbe, A., DelParigi, A., Pratley, R., Drewnowski, A., & Tataranni, P. (2004). Taste preferences and body weight changes in an obesity-prone population. *American Journal of Clinical Nutrition, 79,* 372–378.

Schlam, T., Wilson, N., Shoda, Y., Mischel, W., & Ayduk, O. (2013). Preschoolers' delay of gratification predicts their body mass 30 years later. *Journal of Pediatrics, 162,* 90–93.

Schultz, W., Dayan, P., & Montague, P. R. (1997). A neural substrate of prediction and reward. *Science, 275,* 1593–1599.

Seeger, G., Schloss, P., & Schmidt, M. H. (2001). Marker gene polymorphisms in hyperkinetic disorder-predictors of clinical response to treatment with methylphenidate? *Neuroscience Letters, 313,* 45–48.

Silvers, J., Insel, C., Powers, A., Franz, P., Weber, J., Mischel, W., Casey, B.J., & Ochsner, K. (2014). Curbing craving: Behavioral and brain evidence that children regulate craving when instructed to do so but have higher baseline craving than adults. *Psychological Science, 10,* 1932–1942.

Small, D., Jones-Gotman, M., & Dagher, A. (2003). Feeding-induced dopamine release in dorsal striatum correlates with meal pleasantness ratings in healthy human volunteers. *NeuroImage, 19,* 1709–1715.

Small, D., Veldhuizen, M., Felsted, J., Mak, Y., &, McGlone, F. (2008). Separable substrates for anticipatory and consummatory food chemosensation. *Neuron, 57,* 786–797.

Small, D., Zatorre, R., Dagher, A., Evans, A., & Jones-Gotman, M. (2001). Changes in brain activity related to eating chocolate: From pleasure to aversion. *Brain, 124,* 1720–1733.

Sotak, B., Hnasko, T., Robinson, S., Kremer, E., & Palmiter, R. (2005). Dysregulation of dopamine signaling in the dorsal striatum inhibits feeding. *Brain Research, 1061,* 88–96.

Steele, K., Prokopowicz, G., Schweitzer, M., Magunsuon, T., Lidor, A., Kuwabawa, H., et al., (2010). Alterations of central dopamine receptors before and after gastric bypass surgery. *Obesity Surgery, 20,* 369–374.

Stice, E., & Yokum, S. (2014). Brain reward region responsivity of adolescents with and without parental substance use disorder. *Psychology of Addictive Behaviors, 28,* 805–815.

Stice, E., & Yokum, S. (2016a). Gain in body fat associated with increased striatal response to palatable food cue whereas body fat stability is associated with decreased striatal response. *Journal of Neuroscience, 36,* 6949–6956.

Stice, E., Yokum, S., & Burger, K. (2013). Elevated reward region responsivity predicts future substance use onset but not overweight/obesity onset. *Biological Psychiatry, 73,* 869–876.

Stice, E., Burger, K. S., & Yokum, S. (2013). Relative ability of fat and sugar tastes to activate reward, gustatory, and somatosensory regions. *American Journal of Clinical Nutrition, 98,* 1377–1384.

Stice, E., Burger, K. S., & Yokum, S. (2015). Reward region responsivity predicts future weight gain and moderating effects of the *TaqIA* allele. *Journal of Neuroscience, 35,* 10316–10324.

Stice, E., Burger, K., & Yokum, S. (2013). Caloric deprivation increases responsivity of attention and reward regions to intake, anticipated intake, and images of palatable foods. *NeuroImage, 67,* 322–330.

Stice, E., Lawrence, N., Kemps, E., & Veling, H. (2016). Training motor responses to food: A novel treatment for obesity targeting implicit processes. *Clinical Psychology Review, 49,* 16–27.

Stice, E., Spoor, S., Bohon, C., & Small, D. (2008a). Relation between obesity and blunted striatal response to food is moderated by TaqIA A1 allele. *Science, 322,* 449–452.

Stice, E., & Yokum, S. (2016b). Neural vulnerability factors that increase risk for future weight gain. *Psychological Bulletin, 142,* 447–471.

Stice, E., Spoor, S., Bohon, C., Veldhuizen, M., & Small, D. (2008b). Relation of reward from food intake and anticipated food intake to obesity: A functional magnetic resonance imaging study. *Journal of Abnormal Psychology, 117,* 924–935.

Stice, E., Yokum, S., Blum, K., & Bohon, C. (2010a). Weight gain is associated with reduced striatal response to palatable food. *Journal of Neuroscience, 30,* 13105–13109.

Stice, E., Yokum, S., Bohon, C., Marti, N., & Smolen, A. (2010b). Reward circuitry responsivity to food predicts future increases in body mass: Moderating effects of DRD2 and DRD4. *NeuroImage, 50,* 1618–1625.

Stice, E., Yokum, S., Burger, K. S., Epstein, L., & Smolen, A. (2012). Multilocus genetic composite reflecting dopamine signaling capacity predicts reward circuitry responsivity. *Journal of Neuroscience, 32,* 10093–10100.

Stice, E., Yokum, S., Burger, K., Epstein, L., & Small, D. (2011). Youth at risk for obesity show greater activation of striatal and somatosensory regions to food. *Journal of Neuroscience, 31,* 4360–4366.

Stoeckel, L., Weller, R., Cook, E., Twieg, D., Knowlton, R., & Cox, J. (2008). Widespread reward-system activation in obese women in response to pictures of high-calorie foods. *NeuroImage, 41,* 636–647.

Sun, X., Kroemer, N., Veldhuizen, M., Babbs, A., de Araujo, I., Gitelman, D. et al., (2015). Basolateral amygdala response to food cues in the absence of hunger is associated with weight gain susceptibility. *Journal of Neuroscience, 35,* 7964–7976.

Sutin, A., Ferrucci, L., Zonderman, A., & Terracciano, A. (2011). Personality and obesity across the adult life span. *Journal of Personality and Social Psychology, 101,* 579–592.

Tang, D., Fellows, L., Small, D., & Dagher, A. (2012). Food and drug cues activate similar brain regions: A meta-analysis of functional MRI studies. *Physiology & Behavior, 106,* 317–324.

Tapert, S., Cheung, E., Brown, G., Frank, L., Paulus, M., Schweinsburg, A., Meloy, M., & Brown, S. (2003). Neural response to alcohol stimuli in adolescents with alcohol use disorder. *Archives of General Psychiatry, 60,* 727–735.

Teegarden, S., Scott, A., & Bale, T. (2009). Early life exposure to a high fat diet promotes long-term changes in dietary preferences and central reward signaling. *Neuroscience, 162,* 924–932.

Tellez, L., Medina, S., Han, W., Ferreira, J., Licona-Limon, P., Ren, X., et al., (2013). A gut lipid messenger links excess dietary fat to dopamine deficiency. *Science, 341,* 800–802.

Temple, J., Bulkley, A., Badawy, R., Krause, N., McCann, S., & Epstein, L. (2009). Differential effects of daily snack food intake on the reinforcing value of food in obese and nonobese women. *American Journal of Clinical Nutrition, 90,* 304–313.

Tey, S., Brown, R., Gray, A., Chisholm, A., & Delahunty, C. (2012). Long-term consumption of high energy-dense snack foods on sensory-specific satiety and intake. *American Journal of Clinical Nutrition, 95,* 1038–1047.

Thanos, P., Michaelides, M., Piyis, Y., Wang, G., & Volkow, N. (2008). Food restriction markedly increases dopamine D2 receptor (D2R) in a rat model of obesity as assessed with in-vivo muPET imaging ([11C] raclopride) and in-vitro ([3H] spiperone) autoradiography. *Synapse, 62,* 50–61.

Tobler, P., Fiorillo, C., & Schultz, W. (2005). Adaptive coding of reward value by dopamine neurons. *Science, 307,* 1642–1645.

Tryon, M. S., Carter, C. S., DeCant, R., & Laugero, K. D. (2013). Chronic stress exposure may affect the brain's response to high calorie food cues and predispose to obesogenic eating habits. *Physiology & Behavior, 120,* 233–242.

Turk, M., Yang, K., Hravnak, M., Sereika, S., Ewing, L., & Burke, L. (2009). Randomized clinical trials of weight loss maintenance: A review. *Journal of Cardiovascular Nursing, 24*(1), 58–80.

van Dyck, C. H., Malison, R. T., Jacobsen, L. K., Seibyl, J. P., Staley, J. K., Laruelle, M., ... Gelernter, J. (2005). Increased dopamine transporter availability associated with the 9-repeat allele of the SLC6A3 gene. *Journal of Nuclear Medicine, 46,* 745–751.

Van Meer, F., van der Laan, L. N., Adan, R. A. H., Viergever, M. A., & Smeets, P. A. M. (2015). What you see is what you eat: An ALE meta-analysis of the neural correlates of food viewing in children and adolescents. *NeuroImage, 104,* 35–43.

Veling, H., Koningsbruggen, G., Aarts, H., & Stroebe, W. (2014). Targeting impulsive processes of eating behavior via the Internet. Effects on body weight. *Appetite, 78C,* 102–109.

Volkow, N., Wang, G., Fowler, J., Logan, J., Gatley, S., Hitzemann, R. et al., (1997). Decreased striatal dopaminergic responsiveness in detoxified cocaine-dependent subjects. *Nature, 386,* 830–833.

Volkow, N., Wang, G., Telang, F., Fowler, J., Logan, J., Hayne, M. et al., (2007). Profound decreases in dopamine release in striatum in detoxified alcoholics: Possible orbitofrontal involvement. *Journal of Neuroscience, 27,* 12700–12706.

Volkow, N., Wang, G., Telang, F., Fowler, J., Thanos, P. Logan, J., ... Pradhan, K. (2008). Low dopamine striatal D2 receptors are associated with prefrontal metabolism in obese subjects: Possible contributing factors. *NeuroImage, 42,* 1537–1543.

Wang, G. J., Volkow, N. D., & Fowler, J. S. (2002). The role of dopamine in motivation for food in humans: Implications for obesity. *Expert Opinion on Therapeutic Targets, 6,* 601–609.

Wang, G., Volkow, N., Logan, J., Pappas, N., Wong, C., Zhu, W. et al., (2001). Brain dopamine and obesity. *Lancet, 357,* 354–357.

Weller, R., Cook, E., Avsar, K., & Cox, J. (2008). Obese women show greater delay discounting than healthy-weight women. *Appetite, 51,* 563–569.

Werthmann, J., Field, M., Roefs, A., Nederkoorn, C., & Jansen, A. (2014). Attentional bias for chocolate increase chocolate consumption: An attention bias modification study. *Journal of Behavior Therapy and Experimental Psychiatry, 45,* 136–143.

Weygandt, M., Mai, K., Dommes, E., Leupelt, V., Hackmack, K., Kahnt, T., ... Haynes, J-D. (2013). The role of neural impulse control mechanisms for dietary success in obesity. *NeuroImage, 83,* 669–678.

Wilcox, C., Braskie, M., Kluth, J., & Jagust, W. (2010). Overeating behavior and striatal dopamine with 6-[F]-Fluoro-L-m-Tyrosine PET. *Journal of Obesity, 2010,* 909348.

Wise, R., & Rompre, P. (1989). Brain dopamine and reward. *Annual Review of Psychology, 40,* 191–225.

Yokum, S., Gearhardt, A., Harris, J., Brownell, K., & Stice, E. (2014). Individual differences in striatum activity to food commercials predicts weight gain in adolescence. *Obesity (Silver Spring), 22,* 2544–2551.

Yokum, S., Marti, C. N., Smolen, A., & Stice, E. (2015). Relation of the multilocus genetic composite reflecting high dopamine signaling capacity to future increases in BMI, *Appetite, 87,* 38–45.

Yokum, S., Ng, J., & Stice, E. (2011). Attentional bias for food images associated with elevated weight and future weight gain: An fMRI study. *International Journal of Obesity, 19,* 1775–1783.

Yokum, S., Ng, J., & Stice, E. (2012). Relation of regional gray and white matter volumes to current BMI and future increases in BMI: A prospective MRI study. *International Journal of Obesity, 36,* 656–664.

Zellner, M., & Ranaldi, R. (2010). How conditioned stimuli acquire the ability to activate VTA dopamine cells: A proposed neurobiological component of reward-related learning. *Neuroscience and Biobehavioral Reviews, 34,* 769–780.

Zhou, Q. Y., & Palmiter, R. D. (1995). Dopamine-deficient mice are severely hypoactive, adipsic, and aphagic. *Cell, 83,* 1197–1209.

4 Sugar Consumption
An Important Example Whereby Recognizing Food Addiction May Prove Important in Gaining Optimal Health

Harry G. Preuss
Georgetown University Medical Center
Washington, DC

Joan Ifland
Food Addiction Training, LLC
Cincinnati, OH

CONTENTS

4.1 INTRODUCTION

It is generally recognized that obesity, diabetes, and cardiovascular disorders are influenced greatly by nutrition and are among the most ubiquitous unhealthful conditions in the United States—for that matter over the entire globe [1,2]. Unfortunately, these particular disorders have become more prevalent during the past 20 years; and many think their occurrence rates and severity are continuing to escalate as a result of improper nutritional choices. Not only can bad nutritional habits diminish quality of life on an emotional level due to physical appearance, they also are associated with major risk factors for a variety of serious health situations including those mentioned above [1,2]. Although estimates are constantly changing, reasonable, current approximations for the incidences of the following disorders among the overall mature US population are 9.3% diabetic [3], 34.9% obese [4], 18%–32% hypertensive [5], and roughly 31% maintaining high circulating triglyceride levels [6]. The components providing these disturbing estimations occur so frequently in concert that they are commonly grouped together as the *metabolic syndrome* [2]. One popular theory is that previously mentioned improper nutritional choices cause insulin resistance and fat accumulation, which have been associated time and again with many of the elements of the metabolic syndrome [7].

Various nutritional elements affect health favorably as well as unfavorably. To give some examples on the favorable side, fiber consumption can lower blood pressure and ameliorate insulin resistance [8], while cruciferous vegetable such as broccoli, cauliflower, and brussels sprouts appear to have a favorable outcome regarding the development and progress of certain cancers [9]. It is generally accepted that high potassium consumption possesses the ability to lower blood pressure [10]. On the unfavorable side, salt (sodium), alone and in a variety of foods, has the potential to elevate blood pressure [10]. Also, high sugar intake correlates strongly with a multitude of chronic disturbances, including many elements of the metabolic syndrome [1,2].

A major question today concerns how the ubiquitous, serious health maladies making up the metabolic syndrome can be curbed. Obviously, sugar intake should be limited. However, this readily available knowledge has not seriously influenced the public's penchant for heavy sugar consumption. In this regard, an important question to ask is, "Does food addiction play a significant role in the continued widespread consumption of too much sucrose and high fructose corn syrup that many believe participate in the increasing development of many chronic health perturbations?" [11]. This point is important, because the presence of food addiction may explain, at least to some extent, not only prevalence but also failure to adequately manage numerous chronic health disorders emanating from unhealthful nutritional factors [12,13].

To clearly answer the questions concerning whether and, if necessary, how to curb serious harmful elements of the metabolic syndrome, various key points must be discussed in turn:

1. Previous evidence that sugar-associated maladies occur extensively
2. Knowledge that augmented sugar consumption corresponds with occurrence
3. Information concerning the role diagnosed diabetes plays in overall health
4. Link between sugar intake and glucose/insulin disorders (insulin resistance)
5. Influence of even mild levels of insulin resistance on general health
6. Means to prevent, ameliorate, and/or treat glucose-insulin perturbations—a role for addiction

4.2 HISTORICAL BACKGROUND CONCERNING WIDESPREAD HARM FROM DIETARY SUGAR

The years surrounding World War I were extremely important for those interested in preventing and treating a variety of chronic maladies [14–18]. During the war, disorders such as diabetes, obesity, and cardiovascular diseases like arteriosclerotic heart disease and elevated blood pressure decreased markedly in most involved countries where an accessible supply of nutritious food was deficient. Based upon this information, Paton [14] believed that the occurrence of obesity, diabetes, and arteriosclerosis declined to a great extent from a shortage of dietary sugar—sucrose, commonly referred to as *table sugar*, to be exact. This assumption was strengthened by knowledge from another nutritional happening—namely the enhanced prevalence of these chronic disorders prior to World War I, at which time a notable increase in sugar use had taken place [15]. Despite these factual correlations, other observers disagreed with the deduction. Aschoff put forth another theory [16]. He proffered that reduced fat consumption rather than that of sugar was the more logical reason behind the diminution of a number of metabolic disturbances. To support him, Himsworth, also aware of a less significant incidence of diabetes mellitus among the masses during World War I, linked the phenomenon to a lower consumption of dietary fats also common to those times [17].

The importance of the pathological changes occurring during wartime with food scarcities caused many interested parties to take sides as to what macronutrient was most responsible for the decreased presence of diabetes, obesity, and cardiovascular disorders. Was there a clear inciter when considering sugars and fats? Yudkin pointed out a thought-provoking dilemma when it came to deciding which—diminished intakes of both sugars and fats occurred to a similar extent during World War I [15]. However, it was not the usual case for health professionals to consider both to be equally involved. Whether sugars or fats were responsible became a key consideration. Unfortunately, data from World War II also lacked evidence to determine if sugars or fats were the more important cause of atherosclerotic heart disease and diabetes mellitus; because again both low sugar and fat intakes occurred simultaneously in the face of a falling incidence of these chronic maladies [18].

Following World War II, John Yudkin in a series of papers continued to defend the postulate that sucrose was largely responsible for the increasing incidence of diabetes mellitus (type 2) and coronary heart disease [19–21]. To strengthen his assertions, he pointed out that higher intake of sucrose was associated with elevated blood pressure in addition to higher circulating triglycerides and insulin levels. Based on his findings, Yudkin strongly supported a low carbohydrate diet for optimal health, a concept championed later by Atkins and others in their support for ketogenic diets [22]. More than four decades ago, Ahrens also supported the "sugar theory" as being behind the striking increase in cardiovascular disorders—"the most striking recent dietary change has been the sevenfold increase in consumption of sucrose" in the modern diet [18]. Ahrens especially noted an increased prevalence of hypertension in the Western world. Many of his concepts derived largely from the clinical reports provided earlier by John Yudkin [23].

While Yudkin received modest support for his postulates that metabolic disorders emanated to a large extent from too much sugar consumption, the opinion that fats, particularly saturated fats, are even more responsible for the increased prevalence of harmful medical situations gained considerably more favor from academics as well as the general community [24,25]. Ancel Keys supported and popularized the saturated fat–cholesterol theory. His epidemiologic findings favored the role of nutritional fats in cardiovascular diseases—the so-called seven-country study that promoted the commonly accepted belief that "fat causes heart disease" [26–31]. The "sugar hypothesis" continued to receive relatively poor acceptance over the ensuing years, even though the link of sucrose to these disorders was as strong as that from fats [23]. Nevertheless, several publications continued to report that sparse evidence existed to associate sugar consumption with any major cause of poor health, with the generally recognized exception of dental caries [32–34].

Even in the face of persistent opposition, Yudkin continued to favor sugar over fats as the major nutritional background cause of many chronic perturbations, especially cardiovascular and metabolic disorders such as diabetes mellitus. In the second half of the twentieth century, Yudkin mused in print that several settings contribute to the ubiquity of elevated blood pressure and ischemic heart disease, e.g., stress, smoking, physical inactivity, and poor dietary habits [19,23]. "We cannot therefore expect that any one isolated factor will show an exact association with the disease," because so many different entities could be involved. Still, Yudkin was unwavering in his conviction that excess sucrose consumption elevates circulating triglycerides and insulin and results in a diminished glucose tolerance [19–21,23].

In the face of the strong support for saturated fats being at the heart of many poor dietary outcomes, several different research groups continued to find that isocaloric consumption of sucrose (not more complex carbohydrates like starches) consistently perturbs glucose tolerance [35,36]. In 1978, a review paper by Yudkin published in the *Journal of the Royal Society of Medicine* gave his analysis behind the dissimilar responses between sucrose and starch: "Present evidence suggests that most of the effects of sucrose are due in small part to its ease of digestion and absorption compared with starch, also in small part to its being a disaccharide, but chiefly to the fructose released when sucrose is digested" [37]. Accordingly, Yudkin offered over four decades ago two important pathophysiological principles popular even today—damage from caloric sweeteners such as sucrose and high fructose corn syrup chiefly stems from their rapid absorption (high glycemic indices) and the presence of fructose [1,2,37,38].

The battle over the relative harm between sugars and fats in the diet has lasted for many years. This includes most of the twentieth century, where fats, especially saturated fats, largely won out as the most deleterious macronutrient to avoid. The suspected harm from fats was based on the theory that they caused damage mainly via increasing circulating cholesterol. However, diabetes and cardiovascular disorders like hypertension appeared to increase despite attempts to limit saturated fat intake. Accordingly, it seems likely that faith in the cholesterol theory was derived from imperfect information [39,40]. At present, avoiding consumption of rapidly absorbed sugars, particularly those containing fructose, is likely the most favored dietary means to prevent/treat cardiovascular disorders and diabetes [1,2]. Unfortunately, many individuals are not taking that sage advice.

Point 1: *There is a strong association between sugar consumption and a variety of chronic disease forms. This link has been under consideration for many years.*

4.3 US CARBOHYDRATE INTAKE OVER THE PRECEDING CENTURY AND BEYOND

It is safe to say that the public likes sugar. Despite awareness that obesity and type 2 diabetes mellitus are increasing at alarming rates, intake of sugar calories continues to remain high. A number of reports have stated such. For example, in 1986, Karanja and McCarron published a figure illustrating changes in the US food supply [41]. It showed that between 1909 and 1960, a significant decline in total carbohydrate intake had taken place, but this overall decrease occurred largely through reduced consumption of complex carbohydrates such as whole grains [41]. Important for the concept of a significant role for sugar in promoting chronic health disorders, a simultaneous increase in simple carbohydrate consumption like table sugar had simultaneously taken place. Another report reaffirmed that despite the fact that fiber consumption remained low, other carbohydrates in refined forms showed increased consumption [42]. In addition, a steady rise in sugar consumption also took place from 1983 to 1999—122 pounds per person in 1983 to 158 pounds in 1999 [43]. This represented a 30% increase over the 16-year period. Recent decreases in sucrose consumption have been balanced by higher intake of high fructose corn syrup.

Further examination of sugar intake reveals that in the twenty-first century (2005–2010) men took in more calories from sugar than women [44]. Men on an average consumed 335 kcal per day from added sugar compared with 239 kcal per day for women. Still, converting this to percent of total calories consumed daily from added sugar between men and women showed men at 12.7% compared to women at 13.2%. Interestingly, twice the calories from added sugar emanated from solid foods rather than beverages; and non-Hispanic black men and women consumed a larger percentage of sugar calories than non-Hispanic white and Mexican-American individuals according to this report. Presently, the unfortunate trend is to continue ingesting more sugar while consuming low amounts of fiber. Drinking sugar-containing sodas is an excellent example of this. This combination (high sugar, low fiber) has been shown in animal studies to greatly increase systolic blood pressure [45,46]. Although many factors are involved in the regulation of blood pressure, the augmented prevalence of hypertension in modern time may be caused, at least in part, by a greater upsurge in sugar consumption, especially that from sucrose and high fructose corn syrup [47,48].

Point 2: *The intake of common sugars such as sucrose, fructose, and high fructose corn syrup is substantial and widespread.*

4.4 BASIC KNOWLEDGE OF DIABETES MELLITUS: A DISTURBANCE OF GLUCOSE–INSULIN REGULATION

In Toronto, Canada, Frederick Banting and his team isolated insulin in the early twentieth century [49–52]. At that time, the major cause of diabetes was believed to be a deficit of production and release of insulin. Since the vital role of insulin in regulating glucose metabolism was widely recognized, replacement of the hormone was believed to be the final cure for diabetes mellitus, a condition in which circulating glucose levels are chronically elevated. Nevertheless, within a short time frame, the discovery was made that another even more omnipresent form of diabetes exists.

In this new form, circulating insulin is adequate or even elevated, at least initially. Accordingly, it soon became apparent that a poor response of peripheral tissue to insulin early on, commonly referred to as *insulin resistance*, was the primary basis for the diabetes [53,54]. The original form of diabetes ascribed to a lack of insulin production/release occurring generally in younger individuals and requiring treatment with insulin was referred to as *type 1* [55]. The other, more prevalent form, attributed to poor response to insulin primarily by muscle and fat, was labeled *type 2* [55].

Sadly, individuals with type 2 diabetes undergo a distressful assortment of microvascular complications (including retinopathy, nephropathy, and peripheral neuropathy) and macrovascular impediments (atherosclerosis, coronary vascular disease). These, in turn, are associated with increased morbidity, mortality, and premature aging [56–58]. The common course for type 2 diabetes mellitus is development of insulin resistance, followed by a compensatory rise in circulating insulin concentrations—an attempt to adapt to this situation. In due course, insulin production reaches a plateau and cannot compensate further for the rising circulating glucose levels. The final outcome is hyperglycemia, hyperinsulinemia, and further complications.

Point 3: ***Diagnosed type 2 diabetes is linked to retinopathy, nephropathy, peripheral neuropathy, coronary vascular disease, atherosclerosis, and premature aging.***

4.5 HIGH SUGAR INTAKE IS LINKED TO INSULIN RESISTANCE

Many medical experts believe that insulin resistance is the most important promoter of the metabolic syndrome—perhaps even the major cause [7,59]. The term *insulin resistance* connotes the inability of cells to react in a proper manner to insulin. This poor response, in turn, perturbs entry of glucose from the bloodstream into fat, muscle, and other tissues. An excellent review by DeFronzo and Ferranini clearly points out the close association of insulin resistance with many chronic medical disorders [59].

The status of insulin resistance is enhanced by isocaloric exchanges of dietary sucrose for starch. Such dietary exchanges have long been recognized to typically produce increases in circulating glucose and insulin in both humans [60,61] and rats [36], because responding to insulin resistance, circulating levels of glucose increase and bring about, at least initially, a compensatory increase in circulating insulin levels [62,63]. Consequently, elevated glucose and insulin concentrations can be harbingers of insulin resistance associated with sucrose intake [1,2,64,65]. So, we believe insulin resistance, even in relatively mild forms, can be approximated, at least to some extent, by examining circulating glucose and insulin levels [64,65].

Point 4: ***Clinical and laboratory studies have shown clearly that elevated consumption of sugars is associated with elevated circulating levels of glucose and insulin secondary to increased insulin resistance.***

4.6 MILD INSULIN RESISTANCE IN NONDIABETIC INDIVIDUALS PORTENDS A RISK TO GENERAL HEALTH

While the detriment to health of type 2 diabetes mellitus is universally accepted (cardiovascular disorders and premature aging come to mind), a valid question arises whether less recognized mild glucose-insulin disturbances contribute damage that may go unnoticed. A solid answer is necessary, since the Western diet provides heavy sugar intake that as outlined above has the possibility to upset glucose-insulin homeostasis, laying the basis for many ensuing health problems. While this postulate is popular among many nutritionists and physicians, definitive proof has been lacking. Recently, however, we scrutinized in nondiabetic subjects whether fasting circulating glucose levels representing the status of insulin sensitivity correlate with various health factors in an adverse manner.

Data from nearly 300 volunteers were obtained whose fasting glucose levels were in the nondiabetic range (<125 mg/dl) [64,65]. Significant alterations in health modalities were assessed via correlations and quartile measurements using fasting glucose as the independent factor. Several correlations between fasting glucose concentrations and various elements of the metabolic syndrome were deemed to be statistically significantly positive. These included HbA1C, circulating levels of insulin, body weight, body fat mass, systolic/diastolic BP, triglycerides, ALT, globulins, WBC/neutrophil count, and hsCRP. Reassuringly, HDL cholesterol correlated appropriately in a significantly negative fashion to stand true to diagnostic factors in the metabolic syndrome. Values derived from the highest and lowest quartiles based on glucose levels showed statistical significant differences consistent with the conclusions derived from the correlations. The findings also implied that higher glucose levels are linked to augmented inflammation and liver disturbances common in the metabolic syndrome. In a different manner, most risk factors showed improvement when total cholesterol became the independent variable. The findings imply that maintaining fasting glucose at the lowest safe levels suggesting a more sensitive insulin response allows for the most healthful outlook.

***Point 5:** Fasting blood glucose levels in the nondiabetic range, mirroring the status of insulin resistance, correlate appropriately with the various manifestations of the metabolic syndrome. Despite being in the "normal range," the higher the glucose reading, the more significant the association with factors composing the metabolic syndrome. In addition, evidence of liver perturbations and inflammation are significantly more prominent at the higher readings.*

4.7 MEANS TO PREVENT, AMELIORATE, AND/OR TREAT GLUCOSE-INSULIN PERTURBATIONS: A ROLE FOR ADDICTION

In light of the evidence that sugar and sweetener use is associated with severe consequences, it would seem curious that people continue to use it. It is especially curious that people use it in great enough quantities to be associated with substantial harm such as diabetes, leading to blindness and amputations. Developing elevated glucose requires repeated poor decisions to consume sugary products. This is unlike the consequences of a one-time poor decision such as driving in spite of sleepiness. As a researcher noted about the epidemic of obesity, "Despite the important progression in the study of obesity, prevalence rates continue to increase, suggesting that additional elements must be involved in the pathogenesis of this disease" [66]. We are proposing that food addiction could be such an element in the pathogenesis of consequences of repeated sugar intake.

Research into the addictive properties of sugar may help explain why people consume sugar in spite of knowledge of consequences. As described in Chapter 6 of this textbook, Criscitelli and Avena describe evidence that sweeteners in general, and sugar specifically, exhibit characteristic of addiction. Chapter 5 also describes evidence that fat has addictive characteristics. Consistent with polysubstance research in drug addiction, sugar/fat combinations appear to be more addictive than either food alone. Taking the evidence to the next step, researchers have also found similarities between more complex processed food combinations found in common grocery store snack foods and drugs of abuse [67].

This evidence could provide an answer to the otherwise puzzling question of why people eat so much sugar, fat, sugar/fat, and complex processed food combinations in spite of knowledge of consequences. Research is now showing that chronic consumption of processed foods is linked to the development of strong urges to consume these foods concomitant with diminished cognitive capabilities [68]. Neuroimaging research shows decreased activity in the prefrontal cortex during intense cravings for processed foods. In this paradigm, it could be argued that people simple cannot make a good decision because their cognitive functions are suppressed and they simply cannot remember why they are not supposed to be eating sugary processed foods.

The evidence for addictive properties in sugars and fat suggests a new approach to treating diet-related diseases. Although it may initially seem contrary, it may be easier for sufferers of the metabolic syndrome to give up processed foods altogether, rather than try to cut back. This proposal is derived from a drug addiction framework, in which abstinence from addictive substances and cue avoidance are often the keys to gaining control over harmful, compulsive use. Evidence to this affect is presented in Chapter 6, "Abstinent Food Plans for Processed Food Addiction." Abstinence from processed foods may hold the key to reducing cravings sufficiently to gain control over decisions to avoid addictive processed food in favor of a healthy diet.

The evidence suggests that practitioners in fields related to the metabolic syndrome might see improvement in outcomes by employing addiction recovery principles of abstinence from processed foods and avoidance of food cues implicated in triggering cravings. The intersection of food addiction with the metabolic syndrome may be seen to occur in the necessarily repetitious pattern of consumption of processed foods required to develop both the metabolic syndrome and food addiction.

Under the scenario of overlap in the etiology of food addiction and the metabolic syndrome, it is possible that health practitioners addressing aspects of the metabolic syndrome could *de facto* be a primary point of contact for food addicts. This suggests the benefit of guidelines calling for patients presenting for treatment for the metabolic syndrome to be routinely screened for food addiction. This is somewhat similar to the idea that often alcoholics' primary point of contact with the health system is hospital emergency departments (ED). Thus training ED staff to screen accident victims in emergency rooms for drug and alcohol use is productive in getting appropriate help to alcoholics.

Under the concept that both food addiction and diet-related diseases stem from repeat exposure to processed foods, training health practitioners in simple means for identifying food-addicted patients could develop effective screening for this condition. Adapted symptoms described in the substance use disorder (addiction) diagnostic criteria in the fifth edition of the *Diagnostic and Statistical Manual of Mental Disorders* include:

Failure to cut back on processed foods
Unintended use of processed foods
Use of processed foods in spite of knowledge of consequences

Practitioners in the treatment of the metabolic syndrome are well positioned to identify patients who are struggling with these behaviors. This is due to the routine prescription of special diets in treatment plans. If a patient is not able to implement a prescribed diet, the practitioner can reasonably suspect that processed food addiction might be a factor. Failure to implement a prescribed food plan could alert a practitioner that food addiction may have developed. In this case, practitioners can recommend an abstinent food plan as such described in Chapter 6, "Abstinent Food Plans for Processed Food Addiction."

Point 6: *The evidence suggests that dietary sugars and fats are implicated in symptoms of the metabolic syndrome, even at low levels of elevated blood glucose. It is puzzling that people would consume these foods in spite of recommendations to cut back. The processed food addiction model offers a plausible answer to the puzzle. It would appear that there is much to be gained from equipping health practitioners with knowledge of common signs of food addiction. This is especially the case for health practitioners treating patients suffering some aspect of the metabolic syndrome. Relief from noncompliance with diet recommendations is a potential benefit from advising clients use addiction recovery approaches such as abstinence from processed foods and cue avoidance. Improved outcomes could be a welcome result.*

REFERENCES

1. Preuss HG, Preuss JM. The global diabetes epidemic: Focus on the role of dietary sugars and refined carbohydrates in strategizing prevention. In: *Metabolic Medicine and Surgery*, (eds) MM Rothkopf, MJ Nusbaum, LP Haverstick, CRC Press, Boca Raton, FL, pp 183–206, 2014.
2. Preuss HG, Clouatre D. Potential of diet and dietary supplementation to ameliorate the chronic clinical perturbations of the metabolic syndrome. In: *Nutritional and Integrative Strategies in Cardiovascular Medicine*, (eds) S Sinatra and M Houston, CRC Press, Boca Raton, FL, pp 148–178, 2015.

3. Center for Disease Control and Prevention, National Diabetes Fact Sheet. http://www.cdc.gov/diabetes/pubs/estimates11.htm (Accessed 4-4-14).
4. Center for Disease Control and Prevention, National Diabetes Fact Sheet. http://www.cdc.gov/nchs/data/databriefs/db131.htm (Accessed 8-9-16).
5. Dreisbach AW, Batuman V. Epidemiology of hypertension (Updated Jul 11,2013) http://emedicine.medscape.com/article/1928048-overview#aw2aab6b3 (Accessed 8-9-16).
6. Miller M, Stone NJ, Ballantyne C, Bittner V, Criqui MH, Ginsberg HN, Goldberg AC, et al. Triglycerides and cardiovascular disease, A scientific statement from the American heart association. *Circulation* 123:2293–2294, 2011.
7. Reaven GM. The individual components of the metabolic syndrome: Is there a raison d'etre? *J Amer Coll Nutr.* 6:191–195, 2007.
8. Burke V, Hodgson JM, Beilin LJ, Giangiulioi N, Rogers P, Puddeya IB. Dietary protein and soluble fiber reduce ambulatory blood pressure in treated hypertensives. *Hypertension* 38:821–826, 2001.
9. Higdon JV, Delage B, Williams DE, Dashwood RH. Cruciferous vegetables and human cancer risk: Epidemiologic evidence and mechanistic basis. *Pharmacol Res.* 55: 224–236, 2007.
10. Preuss HG, Clouatre D. Sodium, chloride, and potassium. In: *Present Knowledge in Nutrition*, 10th edition, (ed) J Erdman, ILSI Press, Washington DC, pp 475–492, 2012.
11. Ifland JR, Sheppard K, Preuss HG, Marcus MT, Rourke KR, Taylor WC, Bureau K, Manso G. Refined food addiction: A classic substance use disorder. *Medical Hypotheses* 72:518–526, 2009.
12. Ifland J. Patterns of consumption and consequence. In: *Sugar and Flours*. First Book Library. Houston, TX, pp 37–44, 2003.
13. Yudkin J. Evolutionary and historical changes in dietary carbohydrates. *Amer J Clin Nutr.* 80:108–115, 1967.
14. Paton JHP. Relation of excessive carbohydrate ingestion to catarrhs and other diseases. *Br Med J.* 1:738, 1933.
15. Yudkin J. Patterns and trends in carbohydrate consumption and their relation to disease. *Proc Nutr Soc.* 23:149–162,1964.
16. Aschoff L. Observations concerning the relationship between cholesterol metabolism and vascular disease. *Br Med J.* 2:1131–1134, 1932.
17. Himsworth HP. Diet and the incidence of diabetes mellitus. *Clin Sci.* 2:117–148, 1935.
18. Ahrens RA. Sucrose, hypertension, and heart disease: An historical perspective. *Am J Clin Nutr.* 27:403–422, 1974.
19. Yudkin J. Sucrose and cardiovascular disease. *Proc Nutr Soc.* 31:331–337, 1972.
20. Yudkin J, Morland J. Sugar and myocardial infarction. *Am J Clin Nutr.* 20:503–506, 1964.
21. Yudkin J, Szanto SS. Hyperinsulinism and atherogenesis. *Br Med J.* 1:349, 1971.
22. Atkins R. *Dr Atkins' New Diet Revolution*, Revised Edition. Evans ISBN 978-1-59077-002-3, Harper Collins 2001.
23. Bruckdorfer KR, Khan IH, Yudkin J. Fatty acid synthetase activity in the liver and adipose tissue of rats fed with various carbohydrates. *Biochem J.* 129:439–446, 1972.
24. Grundy SM. Dietary therapy for different forms of hyperlipoproteinemia. *Circulation* 76:523–528, 1987.
25. Xu J, Eilat-Adar S, Loria C, Goldbourt U, Howard BV, Fabsitz RR, Zephier EM, Mattil C, Lee ET. Dietary fat intake and risk of coronary heart disease: The strong heart study. *Am J Clin Nutr.* 84:894–902, 2006.
26. Keys A, Blackburn H, Taylor HL. Relationship of blood pressure, serum cholesterol, smoking habit, relative weight and ECG abnormalities to incidence of major coronary events: Final report of the Pooling Project. *J Chronic Dis.* 31:201–306, 1978.
27. Keys A, Aravanis C, Blackburn, H, Buzina R, Djordjević BS, Dontas AS, Fidanza F, et al. *Seven Countries. Multivariate Analysis of Death and Coronary Heart Disease.* Harvard University Press, Cambridge, MA and London. pp 1–381, 1980.
28. Keys A, Menotti A, Karvonen MJ, Aravanis C, Blackburn H, Buzina R, Djordjevic BS, et al. The diet and 15-year death rate in the Seven Countries Study. *Am J Epidemiol.* 124:903–915, 1986.
29. Keys A, Aravanis C, Blackburn HW, Van Buchem FS, Buzina R, Djordjević BD, Dontas AS, et al. Epidemiologic studies related to coronary heart disease: Characteristics of men aged 40–59 in seven countries. *Acta Med Scand.* 460 (Suppl): 1–392, 1967.
30. No Authors listed. Coronary heart disease in seven countries. *Circulation* 41(Suppl 4):184–185, 1970.
31. Keys A. Coronary heart disease in seven countries. 1970. *Nutrition* 13:250–252, 1997.
32. Nuttall FQ, Gannon MC. Sucrose and disease. *Diabetes Care* 2:305–310, 1981.

33. Bierman EL. Carbohydrate, sucrose and human disease. *Am J Clin Nutr.* 32:2712–2722, 1979.
34. Walker ARP. Sucrose, hypertension, and heart disease. (Letter to Editor). *Amer J Clin Nutr.* 28:195–202, 1975.
35. Cohen AM, Teitelbaum A, Balogh M, Groen JJ. Effect of interchanging bread and sucrose as main source of carbohydrate in a low fat diet on the glucose tolerance curve of healthy volunteer subjects. *Am J Clin Nutr.* 19:59–62, 1966.
36. Hallfrisch J, Lazar D, Jorgensen C, Reiser S. Insulin and glucose responses in rats fed sucrose or starch. *Am J Clin Nutr.* 32:787–793, 1979.
37. Yudkin J. Carbohydrate confusion. *J Royal Soc Med.* 71:551–556, 1978.
38. Jenkins DJA, Srichaikul K, Mirrahimi A, Augustin LSA, Chiavarso L, Sievenpiper JL, Kendall CWC: Glycemic index. In: *Obesity. Epidemiology, Pathophysiology, and Prevention* (2nd ed.), (eds) D Bagchi, HG Preuss, CRC Press, Boca Raton, FL, pp 212–238, 2012.
39. Ravnskov U. Cholesterol lowering trials in coronary heart disease: Frequency of citation and outcome. *BMJ* 305:15–19,1992.
40. Stehbens WE. Coronary heart disease, hypercholesterolemia, and atherosclerosis 1. False premises. *Exper Mol Pathol.* 70:103–119, 2001.
41. Karanja N, McCarron DA. Effect of dietary CHO on blood pressure. *Prog Biochem Pharmacol.* 21:248–265, 1986.
42. Gross LS, Li l, Ford ES, Liu S. Increased consumption of refined carbohydrates and the epidemic of type 2 diabetes in the United States: An ecologic assessment. *Am J Clin Nutr.* 79:774–779, 2004.
43. CSPI. Sugar intake hit all-time high in 1999. http://cspinet.org/new/sugar_limit.html (Accessed 3-24-15).
44. Ervin RB, Ogden CL. *Consumption of added sugars among US adults 2005–2010.* NCHS Data Brief, No. 122, May 2013.
45. Preuss HG, Fournier RD. Effects of sucrose ingestion on blood pressure. *Life Sci.* 30:879–886, 1982.
46. Preuss MB, Preuss HG. Effects of sucrose on the blood pressure of various strains of Wistar rats. *Lab Invest.* 43:101–107, 1980.
47. Duffey KJ, Popkin BM. High-fructose corn syrup: Is this what's for dinner. *Am J Clin Nutr.* 88:1722S–1732S, 2008.
48. Bray GA, Nielsen SJ, Popkin BM. Consumption of high-fructose corn syrup in beverages may play a role in the epidemic of obesity. *Am J Clin Nutr.* 79:537–543, 2004.
49. No Author Listed. Frederick Grant Banting (1891–1941), co-discoverer of insulin. *JAMA* 198:660–661, 1966.
50. Rafuse J. Seventy-five years later, insulin remains Canada's major medical-research coup. *Canad Med Assoc J.* 155:1306–1308, 1996.
51. Preuss HG. The insulin system in health and disease (Editorial). 16:393–394, 1997.
52. Rosenfeld L. InsulIn: Discovery and controversy. *Clin Chem.* 48:2270–2288, 2002.
53. Himsworth H. Diabetes mellitus: A differentiation into insulin-sensitive and insulin-insensitive types. *Lancet* 1:127–130, 1936.
54. Ginsberg H, Kimmerling G, Olefsky JM, Reaven GM. Further evidence that insulin resistance exists in patients with chemical diabetes. 23:674–678, 1974.
55. Olefsky JM. Diabetes mellitus. In: *Cecil Textbook of Medicine* (19th ed), (eds) JB Wyngaarden, LH Jr Smith, JC Bennett, WB Saunders Co., Philadelphia, PA, pp 1291–1310, 1992.
56. Preuss HG, Zein M, Areas JL, Gao CY. Macronutrients in the diet: A possible association with age related hypertension. In: *Endocrine Function and Aging*, (eds). TJ Armbrecht, R Coe, N. Wongsurawat, Springer-Verlag, New York, NY, pp 161–174, 1990.
57. Preuss HG. Effects of glucose/insulin perturbations on aging and chronic disorders of aging: The evidence. *J Am Coll Nutr.* 16:397–403, 1997.
58. Preuss HG, Bagchi D, Clouatre D. Insulin resistance: A factor of aging. In: *The Advanced Guide to Longevity Medicine*, (eds) MJ Ghen, N Corso, H Joiner-Bey, R Klatz, A Dratz, Ghen, Landrum, SC pp 239–250, 2001.
59. DeFronzo RA, Ferrannini E. Insulin resistance. A multifaceted syndrome responsible for NIDDM, obesity, hypertension, dyslipidemia, and atherosclerotic cardiovascular disease. *Diabetes Care.* 14:173–194, 1991.
60. Reiser S. Effect of nutrient excess in animals and man: Carbohydrates. In: *Handbook Series in Nutrition and Food: Section E Nutritional Disorders*, Volume 1, (ed) M Rechcigl, Jr. CRC Press, West Palm Beach, FL, pp 409–436, 1978.
61. Reiser S, Handler HB, Gadner LB, Hallfrisch JG, Michaelis OE, Prather ES. Isocaloric exchanges of dietary starch and sucrose in humans. II. Effect on fasting blood insulin, glucose, and glucagon and on insulin and glucose response to a sucrose load. *Am J Clin Nutr.* 32:2206–2216, 1979.

62. Reaven GM. Role of insulin resistance in human disease (Banting Lecture 1988). *Diabetes* 37:1595–1607, 1988.
63. Yudkin J. Sucrose, coronary heart disease, diabetes and obesity. Do hormones provide a link? *Am Heart J.* 115:493–498, 1988.
64. Preuss HG, Mrvichin N, Bagchi D, Preuss J, Perricone N, Kaats GR. Importance of fasting blood glucose in screening/tracking over-all health. *Original Internist.* 23:13–20, 2016.
65. Preuss HG, Mrvichin N, Bagchi D, Preuss J, Perricone N, Kaats GR. Fasting circulating glucose levels in the non-diabetic range correlate appropriately with many components of the metabolic syndrome. *Original Internist.* 23:78–89, 2016.
66. Lerma-Cabrera JM, Carvajel F, Lopez-Legarrea P. Food addiction as a new piece of the obesity framework. *Nutr J.* 15:5, 2016. doi:10.1186/s12937-016-0124-6.
67. Morris MJ, Beilharz J, Maniam J, Reichelt A, Westbrook RF. Why is obesity such a problem in the 21st century? The intersection of palatable food cues and reward pathways, stress and cognition. *J Neurosci.* 58:36–45, 2014. doi:10.1523/jneurosci.
68. Val-Laillet D, Aarts E, Weber B, Ferrari M, Quaresima V, Stoeckel LE, Stice E. Neuroimaging and neuromodulation approaches to study eating behavior and prevent and treat eating disorders and obesity. *Neuroimage Clin.* 8:1–31, 2015.doi:10.1016/j.nicl.2015.03.016.

5 Sugar and Fat Addiction

Kristen Criscitelli and Nicole M. Avena
Icahn School of Medicine
Mount Sinai, New York

CONTENTS

5.1 INTRODUCTION

The rates of overweight and obesity have reached pandemic proportions over the last 30 years, with the United States having the greatest increase in BMI among all high-income countries (Finucane et al., 2011). Unfortunately, these rates are projected to continue to increase (Wang, Beydoun, Liang, Caballero, & Kumanyika, 2008). Although the development of obesity arises from multiple etiologies, including genetics and age, the primary contributor to weight gain is a misalignment of calories ingested and calories expended. A change in dietary patterns and a shift in the food environment have been cited as primary reasons that people exceed caloric limits, leading to long-term weight gain and obesity (Chaput, Klingenberg, Astrup, & Sjodin, 2011; Mozaffood addictionrian, Hao, Rimm, Willett, & Hu, 2011; Swinburn et al., 2011).

In most industrialized societies, the modern food environment is inundated with highly processed foods manipulated to contain exaggerated levels of sugar and fat. Hyperphagia of highly palatable foods perpetuates hedonic eating by overriding homeostatic mechanisms, which under normal circumstances regulate appetite and body mass (Arora & Anubhuti, 2006; Neary, Goldstone, & Bloom, 2004). Indeed, evidence taken from the preclinical and clinical literature support the addictive potential of certain foods due to their ability to alter reward circuitry within the brain. Chronic ingestion of highly palatable foods leads to excessive weight gain and adiposity, which further exacerbates the dysregulation within the reward related regions of the brain. Drugs of abuse and highly palatable foods are mediated by common neural mechanisms, which partially explains the addictive-like behaviors and neuroadaptations observed in response to exposure to highly palatable and obesogenic diets. These findings give rise to the concept of food addiction (food addiction). In this chapter we discuss how certain foods are capable of engendering addictive-like behaviors and how these responses parallel drugs of abuse. We also discuss how food addiction relates to obesity, as well as the implications for clinical practice. Lastly, we examine the controversies surrounding the food addiction construct as a clinical diagnosis, as well as future avenues of research.

5.2 HOW TO MEASURE FOOD ADDICTION

Currently, food addiction is not recognized as a clinical diagnosis within the fifth edition of the *Diagnostic and Statistical Manual of Mental Disorders* (DSM 5); however, it is often measured in the literature with the psychometrically validated Yale Food Addiction Scale (YFAS). Initially, this tool was based on the substance disorder criteria from the Diagnostic and Statistical Manual of Mental Disorders Fourth Edition, Text Revision as translated to the overconsumption of highly palatable foods. In order to meet the criteria for food addiction, three or more of the seven DSM-IV-TR substance-use disorder (SUD) criteria and evidence of clinically significant impairment must be met. In the DSM 5, significant changes were made to the diagnostic criteria for SUDs and addictive disorders. Substance dependence and abuse categories were collapsed into a single category of "substance related and addictive disorders." This category is divided into "substance related disorders" and "non-substance related disorders." Gambling addiction is the only behavioral, non–substance-related disorder added (APA, 2013).

In response to these changes, the YFAS 2.0 has been developed. In the first study to test this newly developed scale, 14.6% of the participants met the criteria for food addiction and a positive association between higher scores of food addiction, obesity, and pathological eating behaviors was found. Moreover, a stronger association between obesity and food addiction was found using the YFAS 2.0 than the YFAS (Gearhardt, Corbin, & Brownell, 2016). However, since most research conducted to date has been done utilizing the YFAS, the research discussed in this chapter is based on the original YFAS. The original YFAS has assessed food addiction in clinical (Pepino, Stein, Eagon, & Klein, 2014) and nonclinical samples (Davis et al., 2011), as well as children (Gearhardt, Roberto, Seamans, Corbin, & Brownell, 2013). It has been validated and used across many cultures (Brunault, Ballon, Gaillard, Reveillere, & Courtois, 2014; Chen, Tang, Guo, Liu, & Xiao, 2015). Before describing the clinical data, this chapter reviews the preclinical work that has laid the foundation supporting the food addiction construct to describe neuropsychological underpinnings of pathological eating manifesting as an addiction.

5.3 PRECLINICAL RESEARCH ON FOOD ADDICTION

The administration of a rewarding substance, whether a drug of abuse or highly palatable food, results in the release of dopamine (DA) within the mesolimbic pathway, the reward-related region of the brain. This leads to motivation of obtaining the rewarding substance as well as administering it. However, it is important to note that not all individuals who find these substances pleasurable end up becoming addicted, which suggests that several underlying genetic and behavioral traits contribute to the development and cycle of addiction. Studies conducted in laboratory animals have shown that food addiction and sugar, as well as highly palatable combinations of both, can elicit neurochemical and behavioral alterations akin to drugs of abuse (Murray, Tulloch, Gold, & Avena, 2014). These findings have strengthened the argument that certain foods are capable of causing addiction-like responses despite negative consequences associated with their compulsive consumption.

5.3.1 SUGAR

It has been shown that sugar bingeing in rats can be induced by maintaining the rats on a daily schedule of 12-hour food restriction, followed by 12-hours of access to standard chow in conjunction with 10% sucrose solution. While the immensity of food-induced DA release diminishes after repeated access to specific foods, DA release remains elevated after sugar ingestion (Rada, Avena, & Hoebel, 2005), mirroring the response seen to drugs of abuse (Di Chiara, 2002). In addition to the sugar bingeing behavior, cross sensitization (Avena & Hoebel, 2003), tolerance, and craving (Avena, Long, & Hoebel, 2005) also occur. Furthermore, rats intermittently exposed to high-sucrose pellets show resistance to punishment and compulsive-like behavior compared to rats only exposed to standard chow; these rats will continually respond for high sucrose pellets despite negative consequences (Velazquez-Sanchez et al., 2015). Indeed, short-term unlimited access to sweet palatable food increases future food consumption in mice, as well as increases synaptic density in regions associated with reward (Liu et al., 2016). When sugar is no longer available and rats are food deprived or given the opioid antagonist naloxone, a withdrawal syndrome has been observed. Moreover, an imbalance of DA and acetylcholine occurs, resembling the neurochemical changes that occur during withdrawal from drugs (Avena, Rada, & Hoebel, 2008). Taken together, the literature contains evidence that sugar is capable of inducing behavioral and neurochemical adaptations within the reward-related regions of the brain. However, it is important to note that sugar in and of itself does not induce obesity.

5.3.2 Fat

Similar to sugar, fat also evokes binge-like consumption in animals. Fat has been found to be a more effective reinforcer than cocaine in obese rats (Townsend, Beloate, Huskinson, Roma, & Freeman, 2015). Chronic exposure to fat decreases the reinforcing properties of cocaine (Wellman, Nation, & Davis, 2007), regardless of weight. Ad libitum access to a high-fat diet reduces DA turnover within the NAc and decreases the rewarding effect of sucrose (J. F. Davis et al., 2008). Exposure to a high-fat diet for 6 weeks was able to normalize the dysregulation of DA transmission within the nucleus accumbens and ventral tegmental area of mice genetically bred to have decreased DA transmission (Teegarden, Nestler, & Bale, 2008). Similar to sugar, intermittent access to a high-fat diet or hydrogenated shortening elicits a binge-like response in non–food-deprived animals. Although body composition changes did occur over prolonged access to these palatable diets, no significant difference in actual body weight was observed (J. F. Davis et al., 2007); however, this effect maybe partially mediated by the type of paradigm used (Bake, Morgan, & Mercer, 2014). Fat is also highly motivating, as rats given highly restricted access to shortening will work progressively harder to obtain it. Moreover, when rats where given baclofen, which is known to reduce self-drug administration, there was a significant reduction in responding for fat (Wojnicki, Roberts, & Corwin, 2006). A study conducted by Rada, Bocarsly, Barson, Hoebel, and Leibowitz (2010) showed that both obese-prone (OP) and obese-resistant (OR) rats had a significant increase of extracellular DA within the nucleus accumbens when given access to a high-fat challenge meal. However, it is important to note that OP rats had lower baseline levels of DA within the nucleus accumbens compared to OR rats. Although the high-fat challenge increased extracellular DA in both groups, levels were significantly lower when compared to the OR group. In summary, a diet high in fat is able to alter reward response within the mesolimbic pathway; however, baseline neural differences between those prone or resistant to weight gain may increase the risk for hedonic eating. However, unlike rats exposed to sugar, neither fasting nor administration of the opioid antagonist naloxone precipitated signs of withdrawal in rats previously exposed to high-fat diet (Bocarsly, Berner, Hoebel, & Avena, 2011). Therefore, unlike sugar, fat alone does not fully induce addictive-like behaviors.

5.3.3 High Sugar/High Fat

The combination of a high-sugar and high-fat (HSHF) diet is used as a model for "Western-style" diets. A HSHF diet is thought to be a more accurate depiction of what humans eat because commercial foods are typically comprised of multiple macronutrients. Hedonic ingestion of HSHF or a "cafeteria-style" diet leads to weight gain in susceptible animals and induces withdrawal and anxiety during forced abstinence (Pickering, Alsio, Hulting, & Schioth, 2009). The amount of time in which animals are granted access to a cafeteria-style diet will differentially affect weight. Although restricted access to a cafeteria-style diet tends to increase weight, the difference is not significant when compared to rats only fed chow, as total caloric intake is similar.

Conversely, chronic extended access leads to significant weight gain. Indeed, chronic extended access also induces hyperphagia, marked elevation in brain reward thresholds and a decrease in

DA receptor D2 striatal expression (Johnson & Kenny, 2010). A recent study conducted in satiated rats showed that potato chips and an isocaloric mixture with a similar macronutrient composition of mainly fat and carbohydrate (35% and 65%, respectively) are capable of triggering consumption despite lack of hunger, as well as more robustly activating regions within the brain associated with reward compared to standard chow (Hoch, Kreitz, Gaffling, Pischetsrieder, & Hess, 2015). Further, during forced abstinence, rats show greater resistance to punishment when previously exposed to highly palatable food than compared to methamphetamine (Krasnova et al., 2014). Taken together, obesogenic diets induce neuroadaptations similar to drugs of abuse.

5.4 CLINICAL RESEARCH IN FOOD ADDICTION

There is an inverse relationship between BMI and illicit drug use, suggesting addictive foods and drugs of abuse elicit their effects on the same areas of the brain (Bluml et al., 2012). Indeed, dysregulation of dopaminergic signaling occurs in people who meet the criteria for food addiction. When people who did not meet the criteria for food addiction were given the DA agonist, snack food consumption was suppressed. However, after those who met the criteria for food addiction received the DA agonist, snack food consumption was unchanged (C. Davis, Levitan, Kaplan, Kennedy, & Carter, 2014), supporting underlying neural differences between those who meet the criteria for food addiction and those who do not. The relationship between weight and a positive assessment for food addiction has also been demonstrated. Although many studies have found food addiction to be positively associated with BMI (Murphy, Stojek, & Mackillop, 2013; Pedram et al., 2013; Pursey, Stanwell, Gearhardt, Collins, & Burrows, 2014; Raymond & Lovell, 2015), others have found no association (Berenson, Laz, Pohlmeier, Rahman, & Cunningham, 2015; Gearhardt et al., 2011). The inconsistencies suggest that the relationship between obesity and food addiction is not linear (Meule, 2012). An exploratory study found that visceral adiposity, which is argued to be a better indicator of chronic disease and metabolic derangements than BMI, is associated with food addiction (Pursey, Gearhardt, & Burrows, 2016). Additional work on the relationship of food addiction to other chronic metabolic diseases, and not only weight, would be beneficial for both prevention and treatment.

In addition to the correlation between food addiction and weight status, it is also vital to consider the relationship between food addiction and other psychological impairments, particularly regarding the effect on weight loss outcomes. Those who meet the criteria for food addiction are more likely to have other maladaptive eating behaviors and have heightened hedonic responsiveness to food. This may hinder weight loss success as these people may be predisposed to compulsively overeat for pleasure (Davis & Loxton, 2014). Moreover, food addiction is associated with increased depressive symptomology, impulsivity, binge eating, and emotional eating (Burmeister, Hinman, Koball, Hoffmann, & Carels, 2013; Eichen, Lent, Goldbacher, & Foster, 2013; Pivarunas & Conner, 2015). Close to 20% of overweight and obese participants in a behavioral weight loss intervention met the criteria for food addiction, which was negatively associated with weight loss results. Similarly, Eichen et al. (2013) found that 15% of those who were seeking weight loss treatment met the criteria for food addiction, and this was positively correlated with depressive symptoms. Notably, those who endorsed three or more symptoms reported inability to stop eating, use in spite of knowledge of consequences, and tolerance. However, they denied feelings of distress or impairment, which is a prerequisite for a diagnosis of SUD. A disproportionate number of individuals seeking weight loss surgery meet the criteria for food addiction, with findings ranging from 40% to 53%. These participants report increased impulsivity, depression, and binge eating episodes (Clark & Saules, 2013; Meule, Heckel, Jurowich, Vogele, & Kubler, 2014).

The evidence suggests that it is important to evaluate the psychological health of the individual in conjunction with pathological eating behaviors, as both can ultimately impact weight loss success. Since heightened desire and craving increase the risk of relapse, it is also important to consider how cravings for fat and sugar differentially influence compulsive eating. It has been shown that cravings for sweets and carbohydrates are not related to elevated BMI; however, sweet cravings do mediate the relationship between binge episodes and pathological eating. Conversely, fat craving does play a role in the relationship between BMI and addictive-like eating but does not influence the relationship between binge episodes and addictive eating (Joyner, Gearhardt, & White, 2015). In summary, treatment plans should take into account the underlying psychopathological behaviors associated with food addiction in order to ameliorate poor weight loss outcomes in this population.

5.5 CONTROVERSIES

Although there has been a significant increase within the scientific literature on the topic of food addiction, it continues to be controversial. Some argue that this model has several inconsistencies when examined in the context of the neuroimaging research (Ziauddeen, Farooqi, & Fletcher, 2012). Although it is acknowledged that much of the evidence is convincing, some suggest it is still too premature to determine if food addiction is in fact a valid disorder and it may reflect an "eating addiction" (Hebebrand et al., 2014; Hone-Blanchet & Fecteau, 2014). The high overlap (ranging from 40% to 60%) between food addiction, obesity, and binge-eating disorder (BED) (Gearhardt, White, Masheb, & Grilo, 2013; Gearhardt et al., 2012) has also been a source of contention among the scientific community. However, it is necessary to distinguish between the two disorders, because not all people who meet the criteria for food addiction also have BED (C. Davis et al., 2011). Further, those with both BED and food addiction appear to have an increased severity of disease and related eating disorder pathology (Gearhardt, Boswell, & White, 2014; Gearhardt et al., 2012).

Another critique of the food addiction construct is determining *what* exactly is addictive. The literature supports highly processed foods as more problematic compared to foods found in the natural state. This may be partially related to the pace of digestion and absorption. Processed foods are manipulated to contain inordinate levels of sugar, salt, and fat. They contain very little insoluble and soluble fiber (Martinez Steele et al., 2016), which have been shown to slow the rate of digestion. Therefore, in general, these foods are metabolized more rapidly when compared to minimally processed foods such as fruits or vegetables. This is similar to abused substances, such as cocaine or heroin, which undergo multiple steps of processing from their natural state to an addictive state and once taken are quickly absorbed into the bloodstream (Schulte, Avena, & Gearhardt, 2015). However, it is argued that due to lack of solid evidence, there is no specific food or predetermined combination of macronutrients that can be labeled as "addictive." Further, there is not one standardized term used to describe these foods (e.g., highly palatable, highly processed, ultraprocessed food), and unlike drugs of abuse food is essential for survival. Therefore, it is both necessary and advantageous for future studies to determine *what* is addictive and agree on a standardized definition of *highly palatable* or *processed food*.

The way food addiction is measured is also quite controversial. Although the YFAS is a validated and reliable tool, because it is a self-reported scale, some individuals may have a distorted recollection of specific symptoms of addiction, such as "withdrawal" (Pressman, Clemens, & Rodriguez, 2015). Others argue that although tolerance and withdrawal occur in laboratory animals previously exposed to highly palatable foods, the evidence in humans is not as strong. It is unlikely that withdrawal from highly palatable foods would elicit a potentially severe biological or psychological response like many drugs of abuse, such as heroin (Ziauddeen et al., 2012). Lastly, although evidence suggests a genetic component mediating these aberrant behaviors related to altered DA signaling, food reward, and weight status (Stice, Burger, & Yokum, 2015; Yokum, Marti, Smolen, & Stice, 2015), a recent genome-wide association study questions the relationship between food addiction and drug addiction. While several loci associated with food addiction traits were discovered, there was little evidence of shared genetic variation between drug addiction and food addiction when using the modified YFAS (Cornelis et al., 2016). Additional genetic studies, including twin studies, would be of value to the field.

5.6 CONCLUSION

It is apparent that obesity is a heterogeneous disease, and of myriad treatments available many do not provide clinically significant results and are not without adverse reactions (Kakkar & Dahiya, 2015). However, the neurobehavioral commonalities between substance abuse and hedonic hyperphagia may pave the way for pharmacological and behavioral treatments to combat this growing epidemic. Treatment options mirroring current therapeutic modalities for SUD are an area worth exploring, as well as the possible overlap between food addiction and other psychiatric illnesses. The clinical relevancy, regardless of weight status, must also be further investigated. These future findings could ultimately lead to greater preventive and treatment strategies for both obesity and other pathological eating behaviors. Furthermore, if food addiction is accepted as a contributor of excessive weight gain, it will likely parlay into greater public acceptance of obesity, hopefully leading to more government support for obesity-related initiatives (Schulte, Tuttle, & Gearhardt, 2016). As evidence for addictive properties in processed foods is developed, it could impact food policy on a national level. If certain foods are deemed "addictive," taxes as well as changes in legislation would be supported. In summary, future neurobiological and behavioral findings from animal and human models can ultimately be used to mitigate the negative consequences associated with addictive-like eating behaviors and obesity. These findings can be used to develop different therapeutic strategies, which can then be added to the clinician's armamentarium for treating these chronic diseases.

REFERENCES

APA, A. P. A. (2013). *The Diagnostic and Statistical Manual of Mental Disorders*, Fifth Edition (Vol. 5), American Psychiatric Association, Washington DC..

Arora, S., & Anubhuti. (2006). Role of neuropeptides in appetite regulation and obesity--A review. *Neuropeptides*, *40*(6), 375–401. doi:10.1016/j.npep.2006.07.001.

Avena, N. M., Long, K. A., & Hoebel, B. G. (2005). Sugar-dependent rats show enhanced responding for sugar after abstinence: Evidence of a sugar deprivation effect. *Physiology and Behavior*, *84*(3), 359–362. doi:10.1016/j.physbeh.2004.12.016.

Avena, N. M., Rada, P., & Hoebel, B. G. (2008). Evidence for sugar addiction: Behavioral and neurochemical effects of intermittent, excessive sugar intake. *Neuroscience and Biobehavioral Reviews*, *32*(1), 20–39. doi:10.1016/j.neubiorev.2007.04.019.

Avena, N. M., & Hoebel, B. G. (2003). A diet promoting sugar dependency causes behavioral cross-sensitization to a low dose of amphetamine. *Neuroscience*, *122*(1), 17–20.

Bake, T., Morgan, D. G., & Mercer, J. G. (2014). Feeding and metabolic consequences of scheduled consumption of large, binge-type meals of high fat diet in the Sprague-Dawley rat. *Physiology and Behavior*, *128*, 70–79. doi:10.1016/j.physbeh.2014.01.018.

Berenson, A. B., Laz, T. H., Pohlmeier, A. M., Rahman, M., & Cunningham, K. A. (2015). Prevalence of food addiction among low-income reproductive-aged women. *Journal of Womens Health (Larchmt)*, *24*(9), 740–744. doi:10.1089/jwh.2014.5182.

Bluml, V., Kapusta, N., Vyssoki, B., Kogoj, D., Walter, H., & Lesch, O. M. (2012). Relationship between substance use and body mass index in young males. *American Journal on Addictions*, *21*(1), 72–77. doi:10.1111/j.1521-0391.2011.00192.x.

Bocarsly, M. E., Berner, L. A., Hoebel, B. G., & Avena, N. M. (2011). Rats that binge eat fat-rich food do not show somatic signs or anxiety associated with opiate-like withdrawal: Implications for nutrient-specific food addiction behaviors. *Physiology and Behavior*, *104*(5), 865–872. doi:10.1016/j.physbeh.2011.05.018.

Brunault, P., Ballon, N., Gaillard, P., Reveillere, C., & Courtois, R. (2014). Validation of the French version of the Yale Food Addiction Scale: An examination of its food addictionctor structure, reliability, and construct validity in a nonclinical sample. *Canadian Journal of Psychiatry. Revue Canadienne de Psychiatrie*, *59*(5), 276–284.

Burmeister, J. M., Hinman, N., Koball, A., Hoffmann, D. A., & Carels, R. A. (2013). Food addiction in adults seeking weight loss treatment. Implications for psychosocial health and weight loss. *Appetite*, *60*(1), 103–110. doi:10.1016/j.appet.2012.09.013.

Chaput, J. P., Klingenberg, L., Astrup, A., & Sjodin, A. M. (2011). Modern sedentary activities promote overconsumption of food in our current obesogenic environment. *Obesity Reviews*, *12*(5), e12–e20. doi:10.1111/j.1467-789X.2010.00772.x.

Chen, G., Tang, Z., Guo, G., Liu, X., & Xiao, S. (2015). The Chinese version of the Yale Food Addiction Scale: An examination of its validation in a sample of female adolescents. *Eating Behaviors*, *18*, 97–102. doi:10.1016/j.eatbeh.2015.05.002.

Clark, S. M., & Saules, K. K. (2013). Validation of the Yale Food Addiction Scale among a weight-loss surgery population. *Eating Behaviors*, *14*(2), 216–219. doi:10.1016/j.eatbeh.2013.01.002.

Cornelis, M. C., Flint, A., Field, A. E., Kraft, P., Han, J., Rimm, E. B., & van Dam, R. M. (2016). A enome-wide investigation of food addiction. *Obesity (Silver Spring)*, *24*(6), 1336–1341. doi:10.1002/oby.21476.

Davis, C., Curtis, C., Levitan, R. D., Carter, J. C., Kaplan, A. S., & Kennedy, J. L. (2011). Evidence that 'food addiction' is a valid phenotype of obesity. *Appetite*, *57*(3), 711–717. doi:10.1016/j.appet.2011.08.017.

Davis, C., Levitan, R. D., Kaplan, A. S., Kennedy, J. L., & Carter, J. C. (2014). Food cravings, appetite, and snack-food consumption in response to a psychomotor stimulant drug: The moderating effect of "food-addiction". *Frontiers in Psychology*, *5*, 403. doi:10.3389/fpsyg.2014.00403.

Davis, C., & Loxton, N. J. (2014). A psycho-genetic study of hedonic responsiveness in relation to "food addiction". *Nutrients*, *6*(10), 4338–4353. doi:10.3390/nu6104338.

Davis, J. F., Melhorn, S. J., Shurdak, J. D., Heiman, J. U., Tschop, M. H., Clegg, D. J., & Benoit, S. C. (2007). Comparison of hydrogenated vegetable shortening and nutritionally complete high-fat diet on limited access-binge behavior in rats. *Physiology and Behavior*, *92*(5), 924–930. doi:10.1016/j.physbeh.2007.06.024.

Davis, J. F., Tracy, A. L., Schurdak, J. D., Tschop, M. H., Lipton, J. W., Clegg, D. J., & Benoit, S. C. (2008). Exposure to elevated levels of dietary fat attenuates psychostimulant reward and mesolimbic dopamine turnover in the rat. *Behavioral Neuroscience*, *122*(6), 1257–1263. doi:10.1037/a0013111.

Di Chiara, G. (2002). Nucleus accumbens shell and core dopamine: Differential role in behavior and addiction. *Behavioural Brain Research*, *137*(1–2), 75–114.

Eichen, D. M., Lent, M. R., Goldbacher, E., & Foster, G. D. (2013). Exploration of "food addiction" in overweight and obese treatment-seeking adults. *Appetite*, *67*, 22–24. doi:10.1016/j.appet.2013.03.008.

Finucane, M. M., Stevens, G. A., Cowan, M. J., Danaei, G., Lin, J. K., Paciorek, C. J., . . . Ezzati, M. (2011). National, regional, and global trends in body-mass index since 1980: Systematic analysis of health examination surveys and epidemiological studies with 960 country-years and 9.1 million participants. *Lancet*, *377*(9765), 557–567. doi:10.1016/s0140-6736(10)62037-5.

Gearhardt, A. N., Boswell, R. G., & White, M. A. (2014). The association of "food addiction" with disordered eating and body mass index. *Eating Behaviors*, *15*(3), 427–433. doi:10.1016/j.eatbeh.2014.05.001.

Gearhardt, A. N., Corbin, W. R., & Brownell, K. D. (2016). Development of the Yale Food Addiction Scale Version 2.0. *Psychology of Addictive Behaviors*, *30*(1), 113–121. doi:10.1037/adb0000136.

Gearhardt, A. N., Roberto, C. A., Seamans, M. J., Corbin, W. R., & Brownell, K. D. (2013a). Preliminary validation of the Yale Food Addiction Scale for children. *Eating Behaviors*, *14*(4), 508–512. doi:10.1016/j.eatbeh.2013.07.002.

Gearhardt, A. N., White, M. A., Masheb, R. M., & Grilo, C. M. (2013b). An examination of food addiction in a racially diverse sample of obese patients with binge eating disorder in primary care settings. *Comprehensive Psychiatry*, *54*(5), 500–505. doi:10.1016/j.comppsych.2012.12.009.

Gearhardt, A. N., White, M. A., Masheb, R. M., Morgan, P. T., Crosby, R. D., & Grilo, C. M. (2012). An examination of the food addiction construct in obese patients with binge eating disorder. *International Journal of Eating Disorders*, *45*(5), 657–663. doi:10.1002/eat.20957.

Gearhardt, A. N., Yokum, S., Orr, P. T., Stice, E., Corbin, W. R., & Brownell, K. D. (2011). Neural correlates of food addiction. *Archives of General Psychiatry*, *68*(8), 808–816. doi:10.1001/archgenpsychiatry.2011.32.

Hebebrand, J., Albayrak, O., Adan, R., Antel, J., Dieguez, C., de Jong, J., . . . Dickson, S. L. (2014). "Eating addiction", rather than "food addiction", better captures addictive-like eating behavior. *Neuroscience and Biobehavioral Reviews*, *47*, 295–306. doi:10.1016/j.neubiorev.2014.08.016.

Hoch, T., Kreitz, S., Gaffling, S., Pischetsrieder, M., & Hess, A. (2015). Fat/carbohydrate ratio but not energy density determines snack food intake and activates brain reward areas. *Scientific Reports*, *5*, 10041. doi:10.1038/srep10041.

Hone-Blanchet, A., & Fecteau, S. (2014). Overlap of food addiction and substance use disorders definitions: Analysis of animal and human studies. *Neuropharmacology*, *85*, 81–90. doi:10.1016/j.neuropharm.2014.05.019.

Johnson, P. M., & Kenny, P. J. (2010). Dopamine D2 receptors in addiction-like reward dysfunction and compulsive eating in obese rats. *Nature Neuroscience*, *13*(5), 635–641. doi:10.1038/nn.2519.

Joyner, M. A., Gearhardt, A. N., & White, M. A. (2015). Food craving as a mediator between addictive-like eating and problematic eating outcomes. *Eating Behaviors*, *19*, 98–101. doi:10.1016/j.eatbeh.2015.07.005.

Kakkar, A. K., & Dahiya, N. (2015). Drug treatment of obesity: Current status and future prospects. *European Journal of Internal Medicine*, *26*(2), 89–94. doi:10.1016/j.ejim.2015.01.005.

Krasnova, I. N., Marchant, N. J., Ladenheim, B., McCoy, M. T., Panlilio, L. V., Bossert, J. M., Cadet, J. L. (2014). Incubation of methamphetamine and palatable food craving after punishment-induced abstinence. *Neuropsychopharmacology*, *39*(8), 2008–2016. doi:10.1038/npp.2014.50.

Liu, S., Globa, A. K., Mills, F., Naef, L., Qiao, M., Bamji, S. X., & Borgland, S. L. (2016). Consumption of palatable food primes food approach behavior by rapidly increasing synaptic density in the VTA. *Proceedings of the National Academy of Sciences of the United States of America*, *113*(9), 2520–2525. doi:10.1073/pnas.1515724113.

Martinez Steele, E., Baraldi, L. G., Louzada, M. L., Moubarac, J. C., Mozaffood addictionrian, D., & Monteiro, C. A. (2016). Ultra-processed foods and added sugars in the US diet: Evidence from a nationally representative cross-sectional study. *BMJ Open*, *6*(3), e009892. doi:10.1136/bmjopen-2015-009892.

Meule, A. (2012). Food addiction and body-mass-index: A non-linear relationship. *Medical Hypotheses*, *79*(4), 508–511. doi:10.1016/j.mehy.2012.07.005.

Meule, A., Heckel, D., Jurowich, C. F., Vogele, C., & Kubler, A. (2014). Correlates of food addiction in obese individuals seeking bariatric surgery. *Clin Obes*, *4*(4), 228–236. doi:10.1111/cob.12065.

Mozaffood addictionrian, D., Hao, T., Rimm, E. B., Willett, W. C., & Hu, F. B. (2011). Changes in diet and lifestyle and long-term weight gain in women and men. *New England Journal of Medicine*, *364*(25), 2392–2404. doi:10.1056/NEJMoa1014296.

Murphy, C. M., Stojek, M. K., & Mackillop, J. (2013). Interrelationships among impulsive personality traits, food addiction, and body mass index. *Appetite*, *73*, 45–50. doi:10.1016/j.appet.2013.10.008.

Murray, S., Tulloch, A., Gold, M. S., & Avena, N. M. (2014). Hormonal and neural mechanisms of food reward, eating behaviour and obesity. *Nature Reviews: Endocrinology*, *10*(9), 540–552. doi:10.1038/nrendo.2014.91.

Neary, N. M., Goldstone, A. P., & Bloom, S. R. (2004). Appetite regulation: From the gut to the hypothalamus. *Clinical Endocrinology*, *60*(2), 153–160. doi:10.1046/j.1365-2265.2003.01839.x.

Pedram, P., Wadden, D., Amini, P., Gulliver, W., Randell, E., Cahill, F., . . . Sun, G. (2013). Food addiction: Its prevalence and significant association with obesity in the general population. *PloS One*, *8*(9), e74832. doi:10.1371/journal.pone.0074832.

Pepino, M. Y., Stein, R. I., Eagon, J. C., & Klein, S. (2014). Bariatric surgery-induced weight loss causes remission of food addiction in extreme obesity. *Obesity (Silver Spring)*, *22*(8), 1792–1798. doi:10.1002/oby.20797.

Pickering, C., Alsio, J., Hulting, A. L., & Schioth, H. B. (2009). Withdrawal from free-choice high-fat high-sugar diet induces craving only in obesity-prone animals. *Psychopharmacology*, *204*(3), 431–443. doi:10.1007/s00213-009-1474-y.

Pivarunas, B., & Conner, B. T. (2015). Impulsivity and emotion dysregulation as predictors of food addiction. *Eating Behaviors*, *19*, 9–14. doi:10.1016/j.eatbeh.2015.06.007.

Pressman, P., Clemens, R. A., & Rodriguez, H. A. (2015). Food addiction: Clinical reality or mythology. *American Journal of Medicine*, *128*(11), 1165–1166. doi:10.1016/j.amjmed.2015.05.046.

Pursey, K. M., Gearhardt, A. N., & Burrows, T. L. (2016). The relationship between "food addiction" and visceral adiposity in young females. *Physiology and Behavior*, *157*, 9–12. doi:10.1016/j.physbeh.2016.01.018.

Pursey, K. M., Stanwell, P., Gearhardt, A. N., Collins, C. E., & Burrows, T. L. (2014). The prevalence of food addiction as assessed by the Yale Food Addiction Scale: A systematic review. *Nutrients*, *6*(10), 4552–4590. doi:10.3390/nu6104552.

Rada, P., Avena, N. M., & Hoebel, B. G. (2005). Daily bingeing on sugar repeatedly releases dopamine in the accumbens shell. *Neuroscience*, *134*(3), 737–744. doi:10.1016/j.neuroscience.2005.04.043.

Rada, P., Bocarsly, M. E., Barson, J. R., Hoebel, B. G., & Leibowitz, S. F. (2010). Reduced accumbens dopamine in Sprague-Dawley rats prone to overeating a fat-rich diet. *Physiology and Behavior*, *101*(3), 394–400. doi:10.1016/j.physbeh.2010.07.005.

Raymond, K. L., & Lovell, G. P. (2015). Food addiction symptomology, impulsivity, mood, and body mass index in people with type two diabetes. *Appetite*, *95*, 383–389. doi:10.1016/j.appet.2015.07.030.

Schulte, E. M., Avena, N. M., & Gearhardt, A. N. (2015). Which foods may be addictive? The roles of processing, fat content, and glycemic load. *PloS One*, *10*(2), e0117959. doi:10.1371/journal.pone.0117959.

Schulte, E. M., Tuttle, H. M., & Gearhardt, A. N. (2016). Belief in food addiction and obesity-related policy support. *PloS One*, *11*(1), e0147557. doi:10.1371/journal.pone.0147557.

Stice, E., Burger, K. S., & Yokum, S. (2015). Reward region responsivity predicts future weight gain and moderating effects of the TaqIA allele. *Journal of Neuroscience*, *35*(28), 10316–10324. doi:10.1523/JNEUROSCI.3607-14.2015.

Swinburn, B. A., Sacks, G., Hall, K. D., McPherson, K., Finegood, D. T., Moodie, M. L., & Gortmaker, S. L. (2011). The global obesity pandemic: Shaped by global drivers and local environments. *The Lancet*, *378*(9793), 804–814. doi:10.1016/s0140-6736(11)60813-1.

Teegarden, S. L., Nestler, E. J., & Bale, T. L. (2008). Delta FosB-mediated alterations in dopamine signaling are normalized by a palatable high-fat diet. *Biological Psychiatry*, *64*(11), 941–950. doi:10.1016/j.biopsych.2008.06.007.

Townsend, E. A., Beloate, L. N., Huskinson, S. L., Roma, P. G., & Freeman, K. B. (2015). Corn oil, but not cocaine, is a more effective reinforcer in obese than in lean Zucker rats. *Physiology and Behavior*, *143*, 136–141. doi:10.1016/j.physbeh.2015.03.002.

Velazquez-Sanchez, C., Santos, J. W., Smith, K. L., Ferragud, A., Sabino, V., & Cottone, P. (2015). Seeking behavior, place conditioning, and resistance to conditioned suppression of feeding in rats intermittently exposed to palatable food. *Behavioral Neuroscience*, *129*(2), 219–224. doi:10.1037/bne0000042.

Wang, Y., Beydoun, M. A., Liang, L., Caballero, B., & Kumanyika, S. K. (2008). Will all Americans become overweight or obese? Estimating the progression and cost of the US obesity epidemic. *Obesity (Silver Spring)*, *16*(10), 2323–2330. doi:10.1038/oby.2008.351.

Wellman, P. J., Nation, J. R., & Davis, K. W. (2007). Impairment of acquisition of cocaine self-administration in rats maintained on a high-fat diet. *Pharmacology, Biochemistry and Behavior*, *88*(1), 89–93. doi:10.1016/j.pbb.2007.07.008.

Wojnicki, F. H., Roberts, D. C., & Corwin, R. L. (2006). Effects of baclofen on operant performance for food pellets and vegetable shortening after a history of binge-type behavior in non-food deprived rats. *Pharmacology, Biochemistry and Behavior*, *84*(2), 197–206. doi:10.1016/j.pbb.2006.04.015.

Yokum, S., Marti, C. N., Smolen, A., & Stice, E. (2015). Relation of the multilocus genetic composite reflecting high dopamine signaling capacity to future increases in BMI. *Appetite*, *87*, 38–45. doi:10.1016/j.appet.2014.12.202.

Ziauddeen, H., Farooqi, I. S., & Fletcher, P. C. (2012). Obesity and the brain: How convincing is the addiction model? *Nature Reviews: Neuroscience*, *13*(4), 279–286. doi:10.1038/nrn3212.

6 Abstinent Food Plans for Processed Food Addiction

Joan Ifland
Food Addiction Training, LLC
Cincinnati, OH

Harry G. Preuss
Georgetown University Medical Center
Washington, DC

Marianne T. Marcus and Wendell C. Taylor
The University of Texas Health Science Center at Houston
Houston, TX

Kathleen M. Rourke
SUNY Polytechnic Institute
Utica, NY

H. Theresa Wright
Renaissance Nutrition
East Norriton, PA

Kathryn K. Sheppard
Private Practice
Palm Bay, FL

CONTENTS

6.1 INTRODUCTION

A common confusion regarding "abstinence" in the treatment of processed food addiction (PFA) is that food addicts, like all beings, must eat food to live. So how can someone become abstinent from food? The answer lies in the division of foods into processed addictive foods versus unprocessed nonaddictive foods. No one would argue that alcoholics cannot achieve abstinence because they must drink fluids to survive. The difference between alcoholic versus nonalcoholic fluids is well known.

Researchers are beginning to recognize the addictive properties of foods identified as processed, ultraprocessed, calorie-dense, energy-dense, hedonic, high-fat/high-sugar, palatable, refined, cafeteria, grocery, or junk foods. These are as opposed to bland, natural, or unprocessed foods. For this chapter, the term *processed foods* is used. This chapter describes the foundation for abstinent foods and food plans in the treatment of PFA.

In the history of research into obesity, much attention has been paid to the behaviors of obese and eating disordered populations. Patterns of eating, emotions around eating, and cue reactivity of chronic overeaters are examples of well-studied topics. By contrast, in drug addiction research, attention has been more focused on the properties of the substances being misused. Bodies of research exist for alcohol, cocaine, nicotine, cannabis, and heroin.

In recent years, these divergent approaches to research into disordered eating versus drug misuse have begun to converge. Researchers have come to focus on the properties of specific foods used in chronic overeating. Research has now emerged showing addictive properties for sugars/sweeteners, fats, sugar/fat combinations, and formulations resembling grocery store products. This has yielded important new evidence for the role of processed foods in obesity and eating disorders.

The wealth of new findings in addictive properties for specific foods has provided the foundation for a series of recent review articles on the topic. Lerma-Cabrera, Carvajal, and Lopez-Legarrea argued that because obesity is increasingly prevalent, additional elements such as food addiction must be involved in its pathogenesis (Lerma-Cabrera, Carvajal, & Lopez-Legarrea, 2016). Carter et al. and Kalon et al. both noted that chronic consumption of energy-dense foods causes changes in the brain's reward pathways and that overeating displays patterns of behaviors that are consistent with drug addiction (Carter et al., 2016; Kalon, Hong, Tobin, & Schulte, 2016). Carr et al. described excessive motivation combined with low impulse control in both overeating and drug abuse (Carr, Daniel, Lin, & Epstein, 2011). Small described the individual's propensity for neural encoding of food cues as the pathology that leads to overeating (Small, 2009). Wiss et al. added to these arguments by noting the increase in the prevalence of cues for processed foods in obesogenic environments in the context of cue-induced cravings (Wiss, Criscitelli, Gold, & Avena, 2016). Schulte et al. argued in favor of food addiction as a substance-use disorder rather than a behavioral addiction by noting the evidence for addictive properties in processed foods (Schulte, Potenza, & Gearhardt, 2016). Carlier et al. described the genetic similarities between substance addiction phenotypes and overeating compulsions (Carlier, Marshe, Cmorejova, Davis, & Muller, 2015). These review articles reflect a growing consensus that processed foods play a role in chronic overeating.

In spite of these findings, there are challenges to conceiving of processed foods as psychoactive substances capable of the types of brain disturbances that are found in addictive drugs. Substances with abuse liability are described as compounds with central nervous system (CNS) activity, by design or as a side effect, with abuse and dependence potential. This includes compounds designed for peripheral targets that may have the potential to enter the CNS, either as the parent compound or as a metabolite (Swedberg, 2016). As will be seen in the "Review of Evidence" section of this chapter, there is extensive evidence that processed foods are associated with CNS activity that resembles reactions to drugs of abuse. The purpose of this chapter is to describe how abstinence can be achieved in recovery from PFA.

6.1.1 Concepts of Abstinence

Abstinence from addictive substances is generally well understood in the treatment of drug and alcohol addictions. Either the addicted client is using, or is not using, or is attempting to reduce harmful use. In PFA, controversy exists about which foods are addictive and which must be avoided to achieve abstinence and relief from cravings. Evidence exists for addictive properties in sugar, flour, gluten, excessive salt, processed fats, dairy, and caffeine. There is also evidence for addictive neuroreactions to volume-eating. This chapter examines the evidence for each category of addictive food.

Practitioners may find that outcomes improve significantly when abstinence protocols are applied to overeaters. It is possible that the high rate of relapse into overeating (Foster, Makris, & Bailer, 2005) stems from the client's continued use of addictive processed foods that could maintain both cravings and suppression of impulse control (Boswell & Kober, 2016). At the onset of abstinence, clients are likely to experience a withdrawal. Withdrawal symptoms are a good indication that the client is following abstinence guidelines. If no withdrawal is experienced, the practitioner may review the list of excluded foods to see what the client has not yet eliminated.

Addiction is a complex brain disease characterized by craving, seeking, and compulsion that persists despite widespread consequences (Volkow, Koob, & McLellan, 2016). Replacing cravings, obsession, and loss of control with healthy food choices and rational thought patterns is a core goal of recovery. In a PFA model, addictive processed foods may be conceptualized as rekindling the addiction and preventing normal food use. The core concept of this chapter is that abstinence from addictive processed foods stops the provocation of reward pathways and supports reduction of cue reactivity in a manner similar to that of recovery from addictive drugs.

Both the discovery of abstinence from addictive substances for treatment and the founding of Alcoholics Anonymous are credited to Bill Wilson in the 1930s. Similarly, Overeaters Anonymous began advocating abstinence from some processed carbohydrates in the 1960s (Rozanne, 2005). The use of abstinent food plans for the treatment of overeating have now spread to other 12-step groups such as Food Addicts in Recovery Anonymous (FA) and Food Addicts Anonymous (FAA). The concept has been popularized by books such as *Food Addiction: The Body Knows* (Sheppard, 1993). There is consistent agreement about which foods should be included in definitions of abstinence including processed carbohydrates, fatty and salty foods, as well as personal binge foods. Dairy and soy remain controversial. These 12-step societies see abstinence as the key to stopping the cravings, obsession, and loss of control that are the hallmarks of addictions.

This chapter describes the argument that PFA is so easily reignited and the consequences are so severe that a conservative approach to abstinence is warranted. Clients who are more severely addicted may need to practice greater abstinence, which means eliminating more foods more consistently. Approaches to clients who are preaddicted, or mildly addicted, may be more difficult due to resistance and the inconvenience of eliminating processed foods. The best approach involves balancing concerns about cue reactivity, relapse, and progression against the inconvenience of avoiding a range of processed foods. Recovery that is imbedded in more comprehensive support, cue avoidance, and cognitive restoration may be able to accommodate occasional use of less addictive foods without risking relapse. However, painful consequences such as headache, depression, and fatigue may still ensue from even minimal use, even if full-blown relapse does not occur.

6.1.2 Names for Processed Foods

Researchers use various terms for addictive foods. It is important to use a word that accurately reflects the addictive properties of the food. Confusion as to what constitutes an addictive food is important to explain with simple concepts because clients may have cognitive impairment and be unable to sort through complex ideas. Accuracy and comprehension is confounded by the number of different substances used in addictive foods, as well as the broad range of processing methods used to produce them. Here are the strengths and limitations for each name.

6.1.2.1 Processed Foods

This term seems to capture the essential characteristic of addictive foods. It can be argued that by definition processed foods have been manipulated, which condenses and alters the benign properties of primarily plants. In the vast majority of cases, it is the processing that transforms a plant into an addictive substance. Removing fiber, powdering, crystalizing, distilling, and heating to high temperatures combine to accelerate absorption of naturally occurring endorphins and intensify the impact on the reward pathways of the brain to the point of engendering the neuroadaptations characteristic of addiction.

Processed is a comprehensive term. Further, the term embodies the essence of the problem insofar as processing can be thought of as the source of the problem. Thus associating the problem with the name of the product is valuable. The term *processed foods* can help clients develop the ability to discern properties of foods regardless of claims and advertising. This is important because addictive foods are marketed deceptively as healthy, fun, sexy, and promoting weight loss. Piercing the confusion is challenging. Clients who suffer from cognitive impairment could have difficulty in deciphering labels. Giving clients a descriptive yet simple name is helpful.

Use of this term could also help clients at home. The image of processing could help clients refrain from processing plants into liquids (smoothies) or powder (flour) in home food processors. It could also help clients avoid reducing fruits into syrups or frying foods at high temperatures.

There are three limitations to this term.

1. Nonaddictive foods such as meat and poultry have gone through processing plants without changing their fundamental biochemical nature. Cold-pressed and unrefined oils would also fall into this category, as would spices as well as plain frozen fruits and vegetables.
2. There is evidence that some unprocessed foods such as high-gluten grains, raw milk, and high-sugar fruits have addictive properties.
3. Unprocessed carbohydrates could elicit an addictive response if eaten without balancing it with protein, fat, and fibrous fruit or vegetable. Unprocessed fats are similar.

The practitioner is faced with explaining these exceptions to clients who suffer from cognitive impairment. Fortunately, the ideas are fairly straightforward and understandable. This textbook uses the term *processed foods*. The rationale for choosing this term versus other names follows.

6.1.2.2 Ultraprocessed Foods

Martinez Steele et al. defined these foods as industrial formulations that, besides salt, sugar, oils, and fats, include substances not used in culinary preparations, in particular additives used to imitate sensorial qualities of minimally processed foods and their culinary preparations (Martinez Steele et al., 2016). This definition leaves out less processed foods for which addictive properties have been demonstrated.

6.1.2.3 Calorie-Dense or Energy-Dense

Calorie-dense and *energy-dense* are terms that reflect high sugar and high fat foods. However, these terms miss the noncaloric but addictive substances of artificial sweeteners, salt, caffeine, and food additives.

6.1.2.4 Hedonic

Hedonic refers to foods that are eaten for pleasure as opposed to eaten to assuage hunger. Hedonic eating is thought to be driven by reward rather than metabolic need (Ziauddeen, Alonso-Alonso, Hill, Kelley, & Khan, 2015). Research now shows that addictive eating, like drug use, can shift from liking to wanting. This raises the question of whether someone who is eating in response to an urge but does not like it is having a hedonic experience. It is also a term that is not in common use and could leave clients confused. It wouldn't necessarily help a client decide whether or not a food were acceptable.

6.1.2.5 High Fat/High Sugar

The limitation of the term *high fat/high sugar* is that it leaves out addictive substances such as artificial sweeteners, salt, caffeine, and food additives. It also leaves out low-fat dairy, which contains casomorphine. It also seems to leave out gluten and flour.

6.1.2.6 Palatable

Palatable is defined as "pleasant to taste." Food addicts report that they might be compulsively eating something that they do not like. People may not like the taste of coffee, sugary foods, or salty products, although they are addictive. It can be argued that palatability is in the eye of the beholder and thus the term *palatable* is not sufficiently universal to describe addictive foods.

6.1.2.7 Cafeteria, Grocery, or Junk Foods

These terms effectively capture the range of addictive substances that might be used in addictive foods. However, some addictive foods are not consistent with the lowbrow image that these terms suggest. Processed foods can be *haute cuisine*, gourmet, expensive, or make aggressive claims for healthy properties. Use of the term *junk food* may not be consistent with the image of an expensive, artisan, "whole grain" bread or raw "natural" cheese sold in a farmer's market or gourmet setting.

6.1.2.8 Addictive Foods

This term is perhaps the most accurate but it is not in common use. It does not help clients decide which foods to consume. Even researchers disagree on what is an addictive food. It is helpful to give clients a term that includes a descriptor of the key property of the food, i.e., processed.

6.1.2.9 Other

Practitioners may read research that uses terms such as *snack foods*, which could include processed foods such as cookies and chips. *Refined* is not broad enough to include foods that have been condensed without being refined. It is also not a term that is in common use.

6.1.3 Origins of Processed Foods as Addictive Substances

This chapter proposes that the difference between addictive processed foods and nonaddictive, unprocessed foods is a key factor in the loss of control over eating. Like drugs of abuse, sugars and flours are substances found in nature, where they exist in much smaller concentrations than in processed foods and in combination with fiber, water, vitamins, and minerals. Like drugs, they are not addictive until extracted and concentrated by modern industrial processes. Examples from the world of drugs include cocaine extracted from cocoa leaves, opium extracted from poppies, nicotine smoked from dried tobacco, and ethanol distilled from grains, fruits, and potatoes. Addictiveness may also be increased by consuming processed foods without proteins, fats, and fiber, which would modulate absorption.

Importantly, there is good evidence that carbohydrate preference (and likely fat preference and salt preference) is "hard-wired" into humans because it plays a crucial role in attracting people to eat safe and nutritious foods such as fruits. Whereas small concentrations of these substances contained in natural foods also have significant amounts of fiber, vitamins, and trace minerals that serve the useful purpose of directing us to eat such foods, large concentrations of these substances contained in processed foods may subvert this adaptation and lead some people to compulsively seek and consume processed foods.

In addition, a factor in the development of PFA is the practice in industrial cultures of combining these substances in ways that are entirely unnatural but that may enhance their potentially addictive force (Moss, 2013). Examples of these artificial combinations include soft drinks, which contain sugar and caffeine; doughnuts, which contain flour, gluten, sugar or high fructose corn syrup, salt, fat, and possibly caffeine from chocolate; and french fries, which contain fat, salt, and possibly dextrose. The combinations are in concentrations much larger than those found in nature and are dissociated from foods with nutritional value such as meats, vegetables, and fruits (Ifland et al., 2009).

The use of addictive processed foods in combination with easy availability, cheap prices, lots of advertising, introduction at a young age, and reinforced addictive properties in the processed products may arguably be framed as an epidemic of polysubstance misuse, which manifests as chronic overeating.

6.2 REVIEW OF EVIDENCE

The goal of the review of evidence is to improve understanding of the elements of PFA in order to discern direction for the successful resolution of eating disorders and obesity. Abstinence or reduction in harmful use is one of the desired outcomes in treatment of substance use disorders. So this review will describe the evidence that abstinence or reduced use of processed foods can be efficacious in the treatment of chronic overeating. Research findings can be summarized into three broad categories.

1. Evidence that addiction symptomology is found in chronic overeaters
2. Evidence for addictive characteristics in specific processed foods
   a. Processed foods associated with addiction-like neuroadaptations
   b. Processed foods that were used increasingly during the rise of the obesity epidemic
   c. Processed foods that are described in loss of control in qualitative data taken from 12-step food addiction literature
3. Evidence that abstinence from addictive processed foods reduces cravings and improves satiation

As discussed in other chapters of Part I of this textbook, there is a body of literature that shows characteristics of neuroadaptations in overeating as sensitized craving and reward neuropathways that suppress cognitive functions, while activating stress pathways (Moore, Sabino, Koob, & Cottone, 2017; Stice & Yokum, 2016). There is evidence for addictive properties in processed foods including sweeteners, flour, gluten, salt, processed fats, dairy, and caffeine (Wright & Ifland, 2014). Research into diabetes, Mediterranean, and Paleo diets demonstrates that unprocessed foods, specifically proteins combined with unprocessed vegetables, fruits, and starches as well as cold-pressed oils, are effective at reducing the symptoms of the metabolic syndrome and promoting satiety (Jonsson, Granfeldt, Erlanson-Albertsson, Ahren, & Lindeberg, 2010; Jonsson et al., 2009; Lindeberg et al., 2007). These three bodies of evidence support the model that chronic overeating is an addiction to specific processed foods and that abstinence from those processed foods can aid in recovery from overeating. Protein, carbohydrate, and fat balance in the meal plan is also essential.

6.2.1 Addictive Neuroadaptations in Chronic Overeaters

A number of chapters in Part I, "Fundamentals," of this textbook describe addictive neurofunctioning in overeaters. What follows is a brief summary of this evidence. The findings of neuroadaptations in chronic overeaters that are similar to the neuroadaptations found in drug and alcohol addicts offers evidence for the addictive properties of processed foods.

Brain imaging technology introduced in the 1990s gave insight into the origins of addictive behaviors. With scanning technology such as magnetic resonance imaging (MRI) and positron emission topography, addictions could be defined as the presence of specific dysfunctions in the brain (Wang, Volkow, Thanos, & Fowler, 2004) These dysfunctions appear as hyperactivation of craving, reward, and instrument transfer pathways simultaneous with suppression of inhibition and decision-making centers that fail to curb drug- and processed food–taking (Stice & Yokum, 2016). Sensitized stress pathways are also evident (Cottone et al., 2009).

The literature describing neuroadaptations in chronic overeating is extensive. A number of review articles articulate these findings comprehensively (D'Addario et al., 2014; Kelley, Baldo, Pratt, & Will, 2005; Kringelbach & Stein, 2010; Moore et al., 2017; Stice, Figlewicz, Gosnell, Levine, & Pratt, 2013; Wang, Tomasi, Convit, et al., 2014). Criscitelli and Avena recently found overlaps in neurodysfunction between chronic overeaters and users of nicotine (Criscitelli & Avena, 2016). In this model, success in the application of abstinent food plans to overeating results from reconditioning and stabilizing sensitized craving and reward pathways while restoring impulse control functions and reducing sensitivities in stress pathways.

There is evidence that the neurodysfunction found in addictive overeating is the result of Pavlovian conditioning in response to repeated use of addictive foods as well as repeated exposure to processed food cues (Petrovich, 2013; Small, 2009; Stice & Yokum, 2016; Volkow, Wang, Fowler, Tomasi, & Baler, 2012). Pavlovian conditioning is a process by which neurons encode experiences to create a history and then react based on the history of memories (Kelley, 2004). Peptides influence the reactivity of the brain, including insulin (Jastreboff, Gaiser, Gu, & Sinha, 2014; Kroemer, Krebs, Kobiella, Grimm, Vollstadt-Klein, et al., 2013; Taguchi, Wartschow, & White, 2007), leptin (Grosshans et al., 2012), ghrelin (Folgueira, Seoane, & Casanueva, 2014; Kroemer, Krebs, Kobiella, Grimm, Pilhatsch, et al., 2013), and orexin (Ho & Berridge, 2013; Williams, 2014). Peptides have been shown to comprehensively influence dopamine activity (Liu & Borgland, 2015). In addition, other conditions such as stress and hunger can enhance cravings and reward sensitivity (Ventura, Santander, Torres, & Contreras, 2014). This evidence helps explain the compulsive eating behavior that leads to overweight.

6.2.1.1 Reward Functions

The craving pathways activated in addictions include dopamine, opiate, serotonin, endorphin, and endocannabinoid. Of all the craving pathways, the dopamine pathway in the nucleus accumbens is perhaps the best understood (Wang, Tomasi, Volkow, et al., 2014). Both dopamine surfeit and deficit have been proposed for the role of dopamine in addiction and overeating (Blum et al., 2015). Sugar more than fat has been implicated in excessive dopamine activation (van de Giessen et al., 2013). In a rat antagonist study, both sucrose and fructose cues and ingestion activated dopamine circuits including both D1 and D2 circuitry but differently (Pritchett & Hajnal, 2011).

However, excessive fat intake has been linked to downregulated dopamine receptors, which suggests the progression of tolerance (Tellez et al., 2013). Dopamine production in the striata has also shown tolerance in a functional MRI (fMRI) study as receptor activity decreased with repeat consumption of ice cream (Burger & Stice, 2012). Dopamine tolerance to sugar was also found in rats (Alsio et al., 2010). In a rat study, a diet of junk food during pregnancy and lactation was shown to alter the development of dopamine and opiate pathways in offspring and to leave an increased preference for junk foods in the offspring (Gugusheff, Ong, & Muhlhausler, 2015).

Three other craving pathways are also susceptible to Pavlovian conditioning in response to processed food cues. The opiate pathways encode positive responses to sugar and fat within ventral striatal medium spiny neurons (Kelley et al., 2002). Downregulated opioid pathways were found in a morbidly obese population (Karlsson et al., 2015). Davis and Loxton found heightened opiate responses to palatable foods (Davis & Loxton, 2014). Euphoric endorphins have been found to be released excessively in the nucleus accumbens in both people with alcoholism and in those with sweet preference as well as their children (Fortuna, 2010).

Evidence for the impact of sugar on serotonin was found in that "elevated blood glucose levels catalyze the absorption of tryptophan through the large neutral amino acid (LNAA) complex and its subsequent conversion into the mood-elevating chemical serotonin" (Fortuna, 2012).

Endocannabinoid functioning has been found to integrate many of the functions described above (Karatsoreos et al., 2013). Endocannabinoids impact 22 neuroprocesses (D'Addario et al., 2014). Recently, dietary fats have been shown to activate endocannabinoid pathways in the gut and that this was necessary for rats to develop a preference for fat (DiPatrizio, Joslin, Jung, & Piomelli, 2013). Recent research reinforces the finding of a key role for endocannabinoid activation in the use of processed foods (Cristino, Becker, & Di Marzo, 2014; O'Keefe, Simcocks, Hryciw, Mathai, & McAinch, 2014; Sharma, Murumkar, Kanhed, Giridhar, & Yadav, 2014; Watkins & Kim, 2014) The evidence shows a complex of craving neuropathways, conditioned to respond to processed food cues.

The reward-sensitive pathways stimulate food-seeking and are also vulnerable to Pavlovian conditioning. The pathways include long-recognized connections between the amygdala and the hypothalamus that play a crucial role in developing learning that drives addictive overeating. An associated cue can acquire strong motivational properties by being paired with food under conditions of hunger. Cues are powerful enough to override satiety and cause eating in sated rats that have eaten and are sated. Neuropathways through which cues control feeding behavior describe maladaptive, conditioned control of eating that contributes to eating disorders (Petrovich & Gallagher, 2003).

The instrument transfer pathways translate cravings and reward-seeking into action. These pathways are also susceptible to Pavlovian conditioning. They include two anatomically and functionally distinct processes. The first is a goal-directed process that is based in the prefrontal cortex and dorsomedial striatum and encodes the causal relationship between an action and the motivational value of the outcome. The second process is a dorsolateral striatum–based habit function that learns associations between actions and antecedent stimuli (Schwabe & Wolf, 2011).

6.2.1.2 Cognitive Impairment

At the same time that craving, reward-seeking, and instrument transfer pathways respond to processed food cues, a parallel reaction is seen in the suppression of "control" pathways including executive decision-making, memory, learning, and inhibition (Hege et al., 2014; Lopez, Hofmann, Wagner, Kelley, & Heatherton, 2014; Stice & Yokum, 2016; Volkow et al., 2012). The evidence suggests that even though cravings, reward-seeking, and instrument transfer can be conditioned to respond to processed food cues, this would not be enough to explain chronic overeating. The suppression of control pathways is needed for the addictive behavior to take place (Martin & Davidson, 2014; O'Doherty, Buchanan, Seymour, & Dolan, 2006; Stice & Yokum, 2016). Loss of inhibition has been shown to be a particularly prominent feature in loss of control over eating (Stice & Yokum, 2016). Repair of neurocontrol systems plays a key role in recovery.

6.2.1.3 Sensitization of Stress Functions

Evidence for the progressive sensitization of stress pathways is thought to support progression of use through an increasing desire to avoid the stress of withdrawal (Koob, 2013). Research suggests that increased stress is experienced as a result of reactions of corticotropin-releasing factor pathways to surges of dopamine (Volkow et al., 2016). The theory is that increased stress counteracts the dopamine surge in an attempt to keep the brain balanced. This phenomenon is found in drug addiction as well as resulting from repeated exposure to high-fat/high-sugar foods (Moore et al., 2017).

6.2.1.4 Other Factors

In addition to craving stimulation and suppression of "brakes," food-related peptides enhance reactions (Murray, Tulloch, Gold, & Avena, 2014). These include leptin (Grosshans et al., 2012), insulin (Jastreboff et al., 2013; Kroemer, Krebs, Kobiella, Grimm, Vollstadt-Klein, et al., 2013), orexin (Ho & Berridge, 2013), and ghrelin (Folgueira et al., 2014; Kroemer, Krebs, Kobiella, Grimm, Pilhatsch, et al., 2013). These peptides originate elsewhere in the body including adipose tissue, pancreas, gut, and liver. They travel to the brain and can contribute at multiple points to the excitation of the above-described pathways (Sobrino Crespo, Perianes Cachero, Puebla Jimenez, Barrios, & Arilla Ferreiro, 2014). Alcaraz-Iborra and Cubero suggested that drug/food binge-like consumption in vulnerable organisms increases orexin activity, which in turn elicits enhanced impulsivity and further impulsivity-driven binge consumption in a synergistically reinforcing manger (Alcaraz-Iborra & Cubero, 2015).

Other factors that can exacerbate sensitivity include external stress (Meye & Adan, 2014), prior drug use (Orsini et al., 2014), and hunger (Witt, Raggio, Butryn, & Lowe, 2014).

6.2.2 Evidence for Addictive Properties in Specific Processed Foods

The addictive neuroanomalies found in overeaters is not enough to determine that overeating is a substance use disorder (SUD) such as heroin, alcohol, nicotine, or cocaine addiction. This position is so because process addictions such as sex, shopping, and gambling also exhibit similar neuroanomalies (Frascella, Potenza, Brown, & Childress, 2010). In order to make the case for PFA as an SUD rather than a process addiction, addictive substances must be misused in the behavior. There is growing evidence for addictive properties in a number of processed foods.

It has been shown that processed foods and cues precipitate the cascade of neuroreactions described above while bland foods do not (Beaver et al., 2006; Ferreira, Tellez, Ren, Yeckel, & de Araujo, 2012; Guerrieri, Nederkoorn, & Jansen, 2008; Pelchat, Johnson, Chan, Valdez, & Ragland, 2004; Stice, Spoor, Bohon, Veldhuizen, & Small, 2008). This extensive evidence supports the argument that foods, like beverages, can be divided into addictive and nonaddictive categories. Knowledge of the addictive properties of foods is important as it has been shown to correlate with support for public policies to regulate their use (Moran et al., 2016).

Addictive foods fall into six general categories of sweeteners, flour/gluten, excessive salt, processed fat, dairy, caffeine, fat/sugar, and other combinations of processed foods. Different categories of foods affect different neuropathways.

6.2.2.1 Sweeteners

Sweeteners include sugar and any products that include the word *sugar*. Sweeteners also include any product with the word *syrup*, including high fructose corn syrup. Words ending in *-itol* such as *mannitol* and *sorbitol* are considered to be sweeteners. Words ending in *-ose* such as *sucrose* and *lactose* are also sweeteners as are stevia, and artificial sweeteners such as Equal and Splenda.

The research literature has found addictive properties for sugar in the form of tolerance and withdrawal in rats (Avena, Bocarsly, & Hoebel, 2012) and heightened cue responsivity in humans (Yau & Potenza, 2013). Addictive properties for sugar were further documented in a rat study conducted with fast-scan cyclic voltammetry. Cameron et al. found that sugar was associated with a more rapid and voluminous rise in dopamine than cocaine when administered similarly (Cameron, Wightman, & Carelli, 2014). Tunstall and Kearns showed that rats chose grain over cocaine, but they chose sugar over grain (Tunstall & Kearns, 2014). Rats have been shown to choose sugar and saccharine over heroin and cocaine (Ahmed, Guillem, & Vandaele, 2013). Wang et al. showed that sugar ingestion in the obese resulted in lower dopamine response than lean participants (Wang, Tomasi, Convit, et al., 2014), contributing to evidence for tolerance. Fowler et al. found that problematic use of sugar predicted the development of drug abuse in a population of weight-loss surgery patients (Fowler, Ivezaj, & Saules, 2014). This can be interpreted as a demonstration of transference. Fructose has also been found to have addictive properties similar to corn alcohol (Lustig, 2013). Sugar and fructose use have been found to correlate with heart disease (Preuss & Preuss, 2014; Yudkin, 1988). Fructose in breast milk was found to correlate with increased weight in infants while lactose and glucose did not (Goran, Martin, Alderete, Fujiwara, & Fields, 2017).

In a study of the US diet, Martinez Steele et al. found that ultraprocessed foods comprised 57.9% of energy intake. Ultraprocessed foods contributed 89.7% of energy intake of added sugars (Martinez Steele et al., 2016). Repeat ingestion of sugar has been found to cause neuroadaptations in rats after 7 days (Tukey et al., 2013). The volume of sugars ingested, combined with evidence that neuroadaptations are rapid in response to ingestion of sugar, suggest the possibility that sugar addiction may be widespread in the United States.

Counotte found that adult rats exhibited incubation of sucrose cravings in withdrawal, while adolescent had less cravings and young rats not at all (Counotte, Schiefer, Shaham, & O'Donnell, 2014). Noble found that early exposure to either high-fat or high-sugar diets can impair learning and memory regardless of weight status and that the effect can persist into adulthood (Noble & Kanoski, 2016). This is similar to the cognitive impairment found in drug misuse (Rezapour, DeVito, Sofuoglu, & Ekhtiari, 2016).

Tukey et al. found that sucrose in two different amounts as well as saccharine all resulted in the same increase in activity in a locomotion pathway in the nucleus accumbens following activation of dopamine pathways. The study proposed that this effect, regardless of amount or type of sweeteners, occurred because the process of activation of dopamine pathways was instigated by sweet taste receptors (Tukey et al., 2013). The study described sensitization of the locomotion pathways in 7 days compared to sensitization in 14 days for cocaine.

In a rat study of cross-over incentive salience, Wyvell & Berridge found that amphetamine sensitization resulted in increased cue reactivity for sucrose including increased cue-triggered pursuit behaviors (Wyvell & Berridge, 2001).

The evidence for neuroadaptations to sugar ingestion is varied and consistent.

6.2.2.2 Flour and Gluten

This category includes any carbohydrate that has been ground into a powder, including wheat, rye, kamut, spelt, barley, corn, bean, and lentil flours. A morphine peptide has been isolated from wheat and a gluteomorphine has been discovered in gluten (Fanciulli et al., 2005; Fukudome & Yoshikawa, 1992; Huebner, Lieberman, Rubino, & Wall, 1984; Takahashi, Fukunaga, Kaneto, Fukudome, & Yoshikawa, 2000). Peters et al. found gluten-induced depression in a small study of humans (Peters, Biesiekierski, Yelland, Muir, & Gibson, 2014). Lachance and McKenzie found that serum markers for gluten sensitivity were elevated in schizophrenics and that the response differed from that found in celiac disease (Lachance & McKenzie, 2014). In a rat study, Larsen et al. found that dietary gluten increased natural killer cell activity against pancreatic beta cells and could be a factor in the development of type 1 diabetes (Larsen et al., 2014). The evidence suggests addictive properties and consequences for gluten.

The acellular properties of ground carbohydrates contribute to rapid breakdown, absorption, and inflammation (Spreadbury, 2012). Corn is often eliminated from abstinent food plans, possibly because of sensitivities developed through overexposure to processed corn derivatives such as high fructose corn syrup and corn starch commonly found in processed foods. Corn also has a high sugar content.

6.2.2.3 Salt

Research shows that salt has addictive properties. Morphine addicts have been observed to consume excessive salt in withdrawal, suggesting transference (Cocores & Gold, 2009). Salt use has been seen to conform to the DSM 4 addiction diagnostic criteria (Tekol, 2006). It has also been shown to be associated with the metabolic syndrome (Preuss & Clouatre, 2012). Salt use, both in excess and in total elimination, was demonstrated to be associated with higher mortality in a population study (Graudal, Jurgens, Baslund, & Alderman, 2014). Rudelt et al. found an increase of 23.4% in salt content at eight leading fast food outlets between 1997–1998 and 2009–2010 (Rudelt, French, & Harnack, 2014). The evidence suggests addictive properties for salt as well as consequences for excessive use.

6.2.2.4 Fat

Fat consumption has been shown to trigger addictive activity in mu opioid receptors (Ziauddeen et al., 2013) and has shown a withdrawal syndrome (Sharma, Fernandes, & Fulton, 2013). It is tied to activity in the endocannabinoid pathways (Engeli et al., 2014). Kuhn et al. found a preference response and greater hyperactivity for amphetamines in second generation rats fed a diet high in soy oil or hydrogenated vegetable fat but not fish oil (Kuhn et al., 2014). Del Rio et al. found that a high-fat diet increased gene expression in the dopamine pathways (Del Rio et al., 2015). Feinle-Bisset found that high-fat, energy-dense diets compromise the satiating effects of gut hormones (Feinle-Bisset, 2014). Schwander et al. found that a high-fat meal resulted in inflammation in an obese population (Schwander et al., 2014). Martin et al. found that rat pups born to dams fed a high-fat diet during pregnancy had impaired memory (Martin, Jameson, Allan, & Lawrence, 2014). Sobesky et al. found that a high-fat diet impaired memory in rats but that the effect was reversed with a regular diet and that the effect occurred before excess fat was normalized (Sobesky et al., 2014). The research suggests addictive properties for processed fat and consequences for neurofunction.

Beaulieu et al. found that obese and nonobese participants, regardless of exercise levels, consumed more calories on a high-fat diet than a high-carb diet (Beaulieu, Hopkins, Blundell, & Finlayson, 2017).

In a rat study, Dingess et al. found that a high-fat diet was associated with a significant reduction in the density of thin spines on the apical and basal segments of dendrites within the infralimbic medial prefrontal cortex (Dingess, Darling, Kurt Dolence, Culver, & Brown, 2017). This suggests biological plausibility for associations between loss of executive function and poor diet. Noble found that early exposure to either high-fat or high-sugar diet can impair learning and memory regardless of weight status and that the effect can persist into adulthood (Noble & Kanoski, 2016). In a study of a high-fat diet in rats, Brown demonstrated synaptic plasticity similar to that found in drug addiction (Brown et al., 2015).

6.2.2.5 Dairy

Dairy includes milk, ice cream, cheese, cream, sour cream, cottage cheese, yogurt, kefir, and butter. The findings of addictive properties for fat shown above also apply here for high-fat dairy products. Dairy is composed of sugar (lactose), fat, bovine hormones, and opiates. Four types of opiates have been isolated from milk, of which beta-casomorphine has been shown to attach to opiate receptors (Teschemacher, Koch, & Brantl, 1997). Milk has been shown to have a numbing effect in rats (Blass & Shide, 1994). Sweetened condensed milk and cocaine show identical reinstatement of reward seeking after extinguishment (Matzeu, Cauvi, Kerr, Weiss, & Martin-Fardon, 2015). A casomorphine isolated from milk is the only peptide that when injected peripherally stimulates the craving neuropathways (Bray, 2000). The presence of opiates in milk suggests an effect from concentrating dairy into cheese somewhat like the opiates in poppies are concentrated into opium. A correlation between milk drinking, bone fractures, and mortality was found in a Swedish population (Michaelsson et al., 2014), which calls into question the need for dairy for bone health.

Dairy is also being implicated in development of the metabolic syndrome. In a review article, Melnik described the impact on gene transcription:

> In a retrovirus-like manner milk exosomes may transfer *dairy cow mammary epithelial cells* (DCMEC)-derived miRNA-29s and bovine *fat mass and obesity-associated* (FTO) mRNA to the milk consumer amplifying FTO expression. There is compelling evidence that obesity, T2DM, prostate and breast cancer, and neurodegenerative diseases are all associated with increased FTO expression. Maximization of lactation performance by veterinary medicine with enhanced miRNA-29s and FTO expression associated with increased exosomal miRNA-29 and FTO mRNA transfer to the milk consumer may represent key epigenetic mechanisms promoting FTO/mTORC1-mediated diseases of civilization 2015. (Melnik, 2015b)

In a second review article, Melnik pointed out that:

> In all mammals except Neolithic humans, postnatal activation of mTORC1 (rapamycin complex 1 (mTORC1), the pivotal regulator of translation) by milk intake is restricted to the postnatal lactation period. It is of critical concern that persistent hyperactivation of mTORC1 is associated with aging and the development of age-related disorders such as obesity, type 2 diabetes mellitus, cancer, and neurodegenerative diseases. Persistent mTORC1 activation promotes endoplasmic reticulum (ER) stress and drives an aimless quasi-program, which promotes aging and age-related diseases. (Melnik, 2015a)

Dairy can be seen to exacerbate the metabolic syndrome through the mechanism of regulation of expression of FTO mRNA.

6.2.2.6 Caffeine

There are several diagnoses in the DSM 5 for caffeine use (Addicott, 2014; Thomasius, Sack, Strittmatter, & Kaess, 2014). These include caffeine withdrawal, caffeine intoxication, caffeine-related anxiety, and caffeine-related disordered sleep. The research on the addictive properties of caffeine shows both tolerance and a withdrawal syndrome (Bernstein, Carroll, Thuras, Cosgrove, & Roth, 2002). A study of the soft drink Coke showed that it activates reward regions in adolescents (Burger & Stice, 2014b).

6.2.2.7 Fat and Sugar Combinations

The combination of fat and sugar was found to have addictive properties. In a demonstration of withdrawal, Morris et al. found that rats deprived of supermarket foods high in sugar and fat exhibited a stress-like response and that the stress was attenuated when the sugar/fat was reintroduced (Morris, Beilharz, Maniam, Reichelt, & Westbrook, 2014). In a demonstration of progression and tolerance, Burger and Stice found that repeated exposure to cues for milkshakes (fat and sugar) increased reward learning but that receipt of the milkshake diminished reward response *in vivo* in 35 females (Burger & Stice, 2014a). The increase in reward learning and the decrease in reward response did not occur simultaneously but each predicted weight gain after 2 years. Cleobury and Tapper found that 79% of snacks chosen by an overweight and obese population were high in sugar and fat (Cleobury & Tapper, 2014). Soto et al. found that rats fed a high fat diet also overconsumed sugar and vice versa (Soto et al., 2015).

6.2.2.8 Polysubstance Processed Foods

As seen above, there is evidence that different processed foods impact different reward neuropathways. This evidence suggests that processed food products can typically be characterized as polysubstance products because they are rarely sold or consumed singly. This is an aspect of processed foods as addictive substances that is dissimilar from drug addiction. Drugs are typically purchased individually and used in combination. For example, the drinker purchases alcohol and nicotine separately and uses them together (Shiffman et al., 2014). However, processed foods are already combined into packaged goods and fast food meals, i.e., *de facto* polysubstance products. Highly processed foods are identified with problematic eating more so than unprocessed foods (Schulte, Avena, & Gearhardt, 2015).

In drug addiction, polysubstance use has been shown to be associated with more severe neuroconsequences (Meyerhoff, 2017), poorer functioning (Kelly et al., 2017), psychosis and impulsivity (Martinotti et al., 2009), and emotional distress (Connor et al., 2013). Polysubstance users may be more resistant to treatment (Moss, Chen, & Yi, 2014).

Researchers involved in understanding disordered eating have begun to use polysubstance food formulations in their studies. In light of typical polysubstance formulation in processed foods, this would seem to replicate common conditions and perhaps yield more applicable results.

In a rat study, Oginsky examined the effect of a combination of Ruffles original potato chips (40 g), Chips Ahoy original chocolate chip cookies (130 g), Jif smooth peanut butter (130 g), Nesquik powdered chocolate flavoring (130 g), and powdered Lab Diet 5001. This formula increased CP-AMPARs in the nucleus accumbens, which is associated with increased cue reactivity and food seeking. This response is consistent with the role of CP-AMPARs in cue-triggered cocaine-seeking (Oginsky, Goforth, Nobile, Lopez-Santiago, & Ferrario, 2016). The study demonstrates that a blend of processed foods can elicit neuroadaptations similar to those elicited by cocaine.

The formulation of Ruffles, Chips Ahoy, peanut butter, powdered chocolate flavoring, and Lab Powder has been used in two other studies. In a rat study using real-time microdialysis and liquid chromatography–mass spectrometry, Vollbrecht et al. used this formulation to study dopamine transmission for responding to cocaine in rats that were either obesity-prone or obesity-resistant. Obesity-prone rats showed greater cocaine-induced locomotion before any diet alteration. After exposure to the junk-food formulation, obesity-prone rats became more sensitive. The obesity-resistant rats also became more sensitive but not as much (Vollbrecht, Mabrouk, Nelson, Kennedy, & Ferrario, 2016). This study suggests that repeat exposure to processed foods can sensitize dopamine reactivity even in the absence of predisposition.

Robinson et al. used the formulation of Ruffles, Chips Ahoy, peanut butter, powdered chocolate flavoring, and Lab Powder to demonstrate sensitization to sucrose cues. Before the diet alternation, obesity-prone rats showed greater response to cues for sucrose than obesity-resistant rats. After exposure to the processed food blend, rats that developed obesity showed heightened "wanting" in response to sucrose cues as compared to levels before the processed food exposure. The obese rats also showed reduced mu opioid receptor mRNA expression in regions involved in eating or hedonic activity. However, regardless of weight gain, all rats showed increased amphetamine-induced locomotion and downregulation of dopamine mRNA expression. This study shows the progression of cravings in response to repeated ingestion of a blend of processed foods.

Kendig et al. used a combination of Oreos, Pringles, and Jelly Snakes candy in a study of conditioning in rat behavior. Habit-driven compulsion was exhibited in seeking the processed foods but was not exhibited in responding for chow (laboratory food for rats). Similarly, cues for the processed foods elicited attention bias, which could be ameliorated by cues for the chow (Kendig, Cheung, Raymond, & Corbit, 2016).

In a rat study, Martin-Fardon et al. found that cues associated with cocaine and sweetened condensed milk equally reinstated seeking behavior but the cocaine cue persisted longer (Martin-Fardon, Cauvi, Kerr, & Weiss, 2016).

In two studies of adolescent girls, Stice et al. used fMRI data in response to a milkshake to test for incentive salience. Participants who showed elevated orbitofrontal cortex responding to cues had greater weight gain (Stice, Burger, & Yokum, 2015). In a successful evaluation of a cognitive reappraisal training, Stice et al. used cognitive reappraisal of a Snicker's bar to reduce reward region response and increase inhibitory region response (Stice, Yokum, et al., 2015). Snickers bars are composed of sugar, cocoa butter, chocolate, skim milk, lactose, milkfat, soy lecithin, artificial flavor, peanuts, corn syrup, sugar, palm oil, skim milk, partially hydrogenated soybean oil, salt, and egg whites.

Martinez Steele found that ultraprocessed foods comprised 57.9% of energy intake in a US population (Martinez Steele et al., 2016). The research demonstrating a variety of neuroadaptations to processed foods suggests that the impact of ultraprocessed foods could be widespread in Westernized cultures.

Temple et al. used crisps (potato chips) and cookies to demonstrate that repeat exposure to these foods reliably produces behavioral sensitization (willingness to work for the food) in a subset of obese people but not in lean people (Temple, 2016). Caprioli et al. found that rats chose a 67% carbohydrate pellet over methamphetamine even if the rats had free access to the high-carbohydrate pellets in their home cage (Caprioli, Zeric, Thorndike, & Venniro, 2015). In a rat study of responding to cues for bacon, Thanos et al. demonstrated that Roux-en-Y gastric bypass is associated with greater activation of subjective neural processes related to reward or expectation, gustatory processing, motivation, cognition, and addiction (Thanos et al., 2015).

Research shows that combinations of processed foods elicit adaptations that are similar to those of addictive drugs. The psychotropic properties of processed foods help clarify factors in the global development of chronic overeating.

6.2.2.9 Volume

There is a general caveat in food addiction recovery that any food that the client loses control over should be eliminated from the diet (Food Addicts Anonymous, 2010, 271). This is supported by research showing that gastric distension activates the craving pathways that are also sensitized in drug addiction (Wang et al., 2006). The possibility here is that repeated volume eating could sensitize craving pathways as has been demonstrated in repeated exposure to drugs or processed foods.

6.2.2.10 Summary of Food-Specific Evidence

In summary, there is evidence for addictive properties in various processed foods including drug-like neuroadaptations in reward (dopamine, opiate, serotonin, endocannabinoid), cognitive (learning, decision-making, memory, impulse control, satiation), and stress pathways. There is evidence for psychotropic properties for sugar, sweeteners, flour, gluten, excessive salt, dairy, and caffeine. This evidence supports the concept of PFA as a substance-based use disorder rather than a behavioral disorder. With this evidence, the use of abstinent food plans that eliminate these foods gains credibility.

6.2.2.11 Food Disappearance Data

There is corroborating macro evidence for the role of specific processed foods in the development of the obesity epidemic. Insofar as obesity can be used as a surrogate for PFA, these data support the notion that specific processed foods play a key role in the loss of control over eating. The USDA Economic Service food disappearance data shows how much food disappears into the US economy and thus includes consumption as well as waste. Between 1970 and 1997, the years of the development of the obesity epidemic in the United States, the data shows significant increases in the annual per capita consumption of foods with addictive properties as shown in Table 6.1 (Putnam & Allshouse, 1999).This dramatic increase in consumption indicates the possibility of the addictive properties of these foods and the need to eliminate them in a food plan addressing food addiction.

Research shows that processed foods continue to be consumed in large quantities. Through an analysis of data taken from the National Health and Nutrition Examination Survey (NHANES) 2009–2010, Martinez Steele et al. found that 57.9% of energy intake for a US population came from ultra-processed foods. Ultraprocessed foods provide 89.7% of sugar intake (Martinez Steele et al., 2016).

TABLE 6.1
Increase in the US Annual Per Capita Consumption of Addictive Foods from 1970 to 1997

Processed Food	Increase 1970–1997 (pounds per capita)	Total in 1997 (pounds per capita)
Corn and wheat flour	50.8	172.8
Sweeteners	31.8	154.1
High-fructose corn syrup	61.9	62.4
High-fat dairy	20.4	36.7
Frozen potatoes (french fries)	30.5	59.0

6.2.2.12 Qualitative Data from 12-Step Food Addiction Literature

The literature from two 12-step groups, FAA and FA, describes a classic substance addiction syndrome in terms of loss of control over processed foods, implementation of abstinent food plans, and recovery, particularly from obsession and cravings (Food Addicts Anonymous, 2010; Food Addicts in Recovery Anonymous, 2013).

6.2.2.12.1 Abstinent Food Plans

Both of the 12-step food addiction recovery fellowships advocate eliminating sugars, flours, and any foods that trigger volume eating. FA does not advocate specific abstinence beyond this (Food Addicts in Recovery Anonymous, 2013, 427). For FAA, in addition to sugars, flours, and trigger foods, it advocates eliminating caffeine and reducing salt, particularly for members with high blood pressure. Its food plan combines proteins with unprocessed vegetables, fruits, and starches as well as cold-pressed oils (Food Addicts Anonymous, 2010, 271–285).

Foods listed in the FAA food plan include the following (Food Addicts Anonymous, 2010, 276):

Protein: Beef, pork, goat, poultry, eggs, fish and shellfish, low- or normal-fat dairy, tofu, and tempeh.
Starch: Unprocessed starches including sweet potato, winter squash, beans, brown rice, quinoa, and buckwheat.
Vegetable: Any vegetable including asparagus, onion, broccoli, cauliflower, cabbage, carrots, celery, beets, lettuce, spinach, peppers, eggplant, tomato, cucumber, summer squash, zucchini, etc.

Fruit: Apples, pears, plums, peaches, apricots, nectarines, strawberries, blueberries, raspberries, oranges, grapefruit, tangerines, pineapple, melon.

Cold-pressed oils: Olive, avocado, flaxseed, coconut, sesame, sunflower, pumpkin seed, etc.

Foods eliminated from the FAA abstinent food plan include the following (Food Addicts Anonymous, 2010, 271–273):

Sweeteners: Any sugar or syrup. Words ending in *-itol* such as *mannitol* and *sorbitol*. Words ending in *-ose* such as *sucrose* and *dextrose*. Artificial sweeteners.

Flour: Any carbohydrate that has been ground into a powder including flours ground from grains, beans, quinoa, or buckwheat. This includes corn starch.

Wheat in any form, including close relatives such as kamut, spelt, and rye.

Excessive salt: Very salty foods including olives and excessive salting of otherwise abstinent foods.

Fats: Processed fats, fried foods, cheese, and cream.

Some foods may be categorized as either abstinent or nonabstinent depending on the addict's ability to each them normally, i.e., in measured quantities.

Nuts and seeds: Some practitioners exclude them because of their fat content and because nuts are a common allergic food.

6.2.2.12.2 Other Foods Eliminated from 12-Step Programs

These foods are not necessarily eliminated from all 12-step food plans. However, some practitioners and sponsors eliminate them.

Soy: May be excluded because it is a common allergic food and because its protein content is not high enough to offset carbohydrate servings.

Puffed grains found in puffed cereal and rice cakes may be eliminated if the client loses control over them..

Potato: May be eliminated because of cross cravings to commonly abused foods such as French fries, potato chips, and baked potatoes loaded with sour cream and cheese. Potatoes are also a low-nutrient food.

High-sugar fruits: These include tropical fruits such as guava, mango, papaya, bananas, and dates. Cherries and grapes are also problematic for food addicts.

Crunchy foods: Chips, potato chips, tortilla chips, popcorn, lentil chips, vegetable chips, etc.

6.2.2.13 Summary of Evidence for Addictive Properties for Specific Foods

In summary, the evidence for addictive properties in specific processed foods is varied but consistent. Addictive neuroadaptations occur in response to high-sugar/high-fat foods as well as concoctions of processed grocery products. Morphine-like elements are found in gluten as well as dairy. Behaviors found in relationship to processed foods such as salt conform to diagnostic criteria for drug addictions. Increased consumption of these processed foods was seen during the years of the rise of the obesity epidemic. Further, these are the foods that are eliminated in 12-step food addiction recovery societies because their elimination is associated with relief from cravings.

6.2.3 Evidence for the Efficacy of Unprocessed Food Plans

There is evidence that diets that eliminate some range of processed foods are associated with improvements in weight and satiation. These include diabetes, Mediterranean, and Paleo diets. Further, there is evidence that as the amount of processed foods in the food plan decreases, the results increase, supporting the idea of a dose-dependent response.

Jonsson et al. compared a diabetes diet with the paleo diet. The diabetes diet included, "vegetables, root vegetables, dietary fiber, whole-grain bread and other whole-grain cereal products, fruits and berries, and decreased intake of total fat with more unsaturated fat … Salt intake was recommended to be kept below 6 g per day" (Jonsson et al., 2009). By comparison, the Paleolithic diet included, "lean meat, fish, fruit, leafy and cruciferous vegetables, root vegetables, eggs and nuts, while excluding dairy products, cereal grains, beans, refined fats, sugar, candy, soft drinks, beer and extra addition of salt" (Jonsson et al., 2009). In the two meal plans, the Paleolithic diet had fewer addictive processed foods than did the diabetes diet.

Compared to the diabetes diet, the Paleolithic diet showed improved measures for diabetes, cholesterol, blood pressure, weight, BMI, and waist circumference. In a similar study, the Paleolithic diet was also found to be more satisfying than the diabetes diet (Jonsson, Granfeldt, Lindeberg, & Hallberg, 2013). Satiation and reduced cravings are important in the PFA model. Carbohydrate cravings are found more in diabetics with poor control than diabetics with good control (Yu et al., 2013).

Jonsson et al. also compared the Paleolithic diet with the Mediterranean diet. Similar to the Paleo vs. diabetic diet studies, the Paleolithic diet was based on lean meat, fish, fruit, vegetables, root vegetables, eggs, and nuts. The Mediterranean diet was based on whole grains, low-fat dairy products, vegetables, fruit, fish, and oils and margarines (Jonsson et al., 2010). The Paleolithic diet was as satiating as the Mediterranean group but consumed less energy per day. The primary differences between the two plans is whole grains and dairy. In yet another study, the Paleolithic diet controlled glucose better than the Mediterranean diet (Lindeberg et al., 2007).

As compared to either the diabetes or Mediterranean diet, the Paleolithic diet, which eliminated the most processed foods, showed improved efficacy in satiation, which is central to the treatment of PFA. The improved results in management of the metabolic syndrome in the Paleolithic diet are consistent with what is known about the effects of sugar and salt (Preuss & Clouatre, 2012; Preuss & Preuss, 2014).

6.2.3.1 Outcomes and Food Plans

In Table 6.2, food plans are ranked according to the number of addictive foods included in the plan. The "idealized" plan eliminates all foods for which there is evidence of addictive properties (Jonsson et al., 2009; Lindeberg et al., 2007; Putnam & Allshouse, 1999; Wright & Ifland, 2014).

In a PFA model, the progressive reduction in addictive foods leading to their elimination may be the most important change from the standard American diet to an ideal abstinent food plan. Although the standard deviations in the data are large, there is a meaningful reduction in addictive

TABLE 6.2
Progressive Reduction in Processed Foods

Food (g per day) Plan	Sweetened Drinks*	Cereals*	Dairy*	Results
Ideal abstinent	0	0	0	Cessation of overeating, cravings, and metabolic syndrome.
Paleolithic	56 ± 121 12 ± 35	18 ± 52 12 ± 20	45 ± 119 16 ± 32	Improved blood pressure, cholesterol, improved satiation.
Diabetes	48 ± 90	172 ± 96	183 ± 123	Less robust than Paleolithic. Diabetes epidemic persists.
Mediterranean	141 ± 231	268 ± 96	287 ± 193	Less robust than Paleolithic. Heart disease persists.
American	645	215	88.6	Epidemic of metabolic syndrome.

* Grams per day.

foods from the diabetes and Mediterranean diets to the Paleo and abstinent diets. Table 6.2 suggests that the ideal abstinent food plan could work best to relieve cravings because it eliminates all addictive foods such as sweetened beverages, processed cereals, and dairy. In the qualitative evidence taken from the food addiction 12-step literature, it is the elimination of craving foods that precedes control over overeating. It is significant to note that higher satiation was found in the Paleolithic diet, which eliminated more craving foods than the diabetes diet (Jonsson et al., 2009). As satiation can be related to cravings, this is evidence that reducing processed foods reduces cravings.

Of course, there are a number of other reasons for improvements in health beside reduction in cravings. Some of the eliminated foods, such as sugar, have been shown to remove minerals from the body in the process of digestion (Eaton & Eaton, 2000; Tsanzi, Light, & Tou, 2008). Some eliminated foods are considered to be inflammatory (Michaelsson et al., 2014; Schwander et al., 2014; Shriner, 2013; Spreadbury, 2012). Wheat and dairy may impede digestion and promote irritable bowel syndrome (Carroccio et al., 2011). Sweeteners and salt are associated with a broad range of disease (Preuss & Clouatre, 2012; Preuss & Preuss, 2014). However, in a PFA model, the cessation of cravings is valuable for gaining control of behaviors and reducing use of these harmful processed foods.

It can be argued that if the issue with the American diet were simply that people should know to eat healthier foods, there would not be an epidemic of overeating and its consequences. The PFA model may explain why people persist in eating processed foods in spite of knowledge of consequences. In an addiction model, cravings cessation and restoration of impulse control are the core goal. There is evidence that a food plan that abstains from processed foods could accomplish this objective.

6.3 APPLICATION

Through the lens of the PFA model, a number of points can be drawn together from the "Review of Evidence" section to understand how to use abstinent food plans in the treatment of PFA. Cravings cessation is the key result sought in recovery, as cravings could be considered as the core dysfunction of addiction. Bridging research to clinical practice is accomplished by describing challenges in implementation of abstinent food plans, especially in terms of the scope of abstinence and cue avoidance.

6.3.1 Issues in Implementing an Abstinent Food Plan

The key issue in designing treatment plans for addictions is to match severity of disease with scope of recovery program (McLellan, Luborsky, Woody, O'Brien, & Druley, 1983). In this regard, implementing an abstinent food plan in a Westernized food environment has important challenges. As in all addictions, successful treatment depends on a Pavlovian reconditioning of the cravings neuropathways (O'Brien et al., 1988). This is accomplished both by reducing cravings stimulation through elimination of substances of abuse and avoiding cues as well as engaging in activities that desensitize reward pathways while restoring cognitive functions in the brain. It is possible that people suffering from addiction to processed foods are broadly affected for the reasons described as follows.

6.3.1.1 PFA vs. Drug Addiction

Comparing food versus drug addiction illuminates the particular challenges of implementing an abstinent food plan. Basic guidelines in PFA parallel classic drug and alcohol addiction treatment insofar as the aim is to reduce cravings triggered by cues in order to maintain executive functions, especially impulse control. In recovery from PFA, the goal is to recondition reward pathways to disassociate cravings from loss of control over eating. Unprocessed foods that do not trigger cravings constitute an abstinent food plan and make disassociation possible. Avoidance of cued food environments is also critical. As will be seen in Part III, "Approaches to Recovery," abstinent food plans face the challenge of intense cuing, accidental reintroduction, neuroadaptations, impairments from comorbidities, common use in cultural rituals, PFA in children, and lack of awareness among health professionals.

These multiple barriers to recovery suggest that programs of recovery from PFA should be more comprehensive to compensate for increased risk of lapses. Part III of this textbook describes comprehensive approaches to recovery for food addicts.

6.3.1.2 Achieving Effective Abstinence from Addictive Foods

Adequate elimination of cravings foods from a Westernized diet is important to recondition neuropathways to reduce cue reactivity. However, achieving an adequate degree of abstinence can be challenging for a number of reasons.

1. Delusion is an element of the addiction syndrome (Ferrari, Groh, Rulka, Jason, & Davis, 2008). The broad range of addictive foods encourages denial. Many food addicts simply cannot believe that they need to eliminate so many foods (Food Addicts in Recovery Anonymous, 2013, 92).
2. Support groups are inconsistent about which foods to eliminate (Rozanne, 2005). Media and health professionals do not teach abstinent food plans. There is no central authority to create guidelines for abstinence.
3. In a society in which people consume on average of over 1 pound per person per day of processed foods (Ifland et al., 2009), abstaining from these foods sets recovering food addicts outside of mainstream culture. They may have less in common with friends, family, and colleagues. This may cause difficulties in family relationships. "Food pushers" around the addict may pressure the addict to consume addictive foods.
4. Food addicts who have achieved abstinence are generally healthy. They may be able to participate in activities that others of their age group cannot manage. They do not have the disease profiles commonly found in consumers of processed foods and thus have less in common with their friends, family, and colleagues.
5. Food addicts may have a history of weight cycling. The trauma of repeated failures of weight loss should be treated in order to support the client in a long-term, lifetime approach as opposed to a short-term diet framework. It is often difficult for the food addict to accept the goal of following a food plan for the long term.
6. Food addicts are likely to have a history of using fad diets. Diets have been shown to fail (Foster et al., 2005), but the framing of the problem as one of short-term weight loss versus a lifetime problem of recovery from substance abuse can be hard to convey to a food addict. A thorough diagnosis, assessment, and treatment plan using the approaches shown in Part II of this textbook can help reframe the problem for a food addict.

Given the likelihood of accidental relapses and cue exposures, a comprehensively abstinent client is likely to have more protective conditioning than a client who is occasionally using a food that has even minor addictive qualities. However, it may take years for clients to gain motivation to eliminate processed foods. Repeated painful consequences of use may be needed before effective aversion is developed.

Another important reason to advocate for comprehensive abstinence is the severity of the consequences of relapse. As seen in Part II of the textbook, "Assessment," PFA is a disease that when active can severely damage sufferers across many aspects of their lives. The grave consequences of relapse justify adopting comprehensive abstinence as a risk reduction strategy.

6.3.1.3 Achieving Reduced Harm in PFA

However, complete abstinence from harmful processed foods is unlikely, given the amount of cuing, availability, social norms, and the broad range of processed food substances used in PFA. Mirror neurons are a factor in Westernized cultures and clients are vulnerable to being persuaded by what the people around them are doing (Cohen, 2008). Preparing the client for a lapse is justified under the circumstances. Even drug and alcohol treatment considers reduction in harmful use to be a treatment success. Lapses in PFA carry heavy emotional associations because of their link to the trauma of weight loss failure and the attraction of stigma as a result.

Broadly speaking, regardless of guidance from a practitioner about the value of abstinence, clients are highly likely to lapse. Practitioners can prepare for this eventuality in several ways.

1. The practitioner can teach the client that lapsing is normal. This guidance is valuable to prevent the client from framing a lapse as failure, which could trigger self-loathing and even lead the client to quit a recovery program.
2. The practitioner can assure the client that it takes time and repetition to condition the brain to no longer react to food cues. It could take months, even years, to work with household members to reduce/eliminate cuing in the home.
3. The practitioner can help the client learn from a lapse by reviewing cue exposure, mood, fatigue, and stressors leading up to the lapse.
4. The practitioner can use a lapse to review the *Recover from a Craving* handout at www.foodaddictionresources.com. The lapse can be turned to good use as a motivator for adding more brain-healthy activities. The more brain-healing (reconditioning) activities, the faster cue reactivity is diminished.

It's vital that the practitioner avoid any appearance of judging the lapsing client.

There are two factors to consider when helping a client define abstinence as a means to prevent lapses.

The first factor in defining an abstinent regime for relapse prevention is the stability of the client. An unstable client needs more abstinence, more consistently. Stability can be evaluated by considering how many healthy-brain activities the client is using, how comprehensively food and stress cues are avoided, and how consistently meals are being prepared. If the client has a comprehensive routine of meditation, exercise, craft/arts, as well good cue avoidance and consistently well-prepared meals, it is likely that the client could take a bite of an addictive processed food without developing a full-blown relapse. However, some consequence in terms of mood or mental functioning can be expected.

On the other hand, the client may be at high risk of relapse, which supports encouraging the client to work toward a higher level of abstinence. If the client has had a recent lapse, is unavoidably exposed to food cues, and is struggling to get meals made reliably, then a bite of a processed food could be risky, even dangerous, in terms of provoking a long-term relapse. To help a high-risk client, the practitioner can encourage the client by describing the benefits of working toward consistent abstinence. Praise for progress made and celebration of results are valuable reinforcements.

The second factor preventing relapse is to consider the client's day-to-day environment, either physical or virtual. If the client lives in a household where abstinent eating is the norm, an occasional bite of a processed food is not likely to throw the client into a long-term relapse. If the client is well grounded in a daily environment of healthy people, either virtual or physical, who are eating an unprocessed food plan, the risk of a long-term relapse may be minimal, although distressing mental or emotional consequences could still occur. Guidelines about abstinence can be somewhat less stringent.

Reduction of the risk of long-term relapse and protection from devastating consequences is motivation for practitioners to create a virtual, online environment for their clients or to refer clients to a virtual, online recovery community as listed at www.foodaddictionresources.com.

Even if the client is at low risk of suffering a long-term devastating lapse, there are likely to be painful consequences to a lapse, even of just one bite. A commensurate degree of increased cravings, headache, nausea, depression, anxiety, fatigue, disturbed sleep, skin eruption, etc., could follow a lapse of even a small amount of a processed food. The client could go through a period of withdrawal. In this case, the practitioner can still use the experience to build motivation in the client to develop a more consistent abstinence. The point is that regardless of risk of severe relapse, bites of processed foods could make the client sick. By letting the client make the connection between bites and not feeling well, the practitioner can help the client develop a natural aversion to processed foods.

Consequences of a bite or several bites may not be apparent to the client. In this case, the practitioner runs the risk of losing credibility with the client if the practitioner insists that the bite was dangerous. This aspect of guiding clients requires skill and finesse. The best idea is to educate, plant ideas, share ideas about how to make decisions, create healthy "environments," and let the client experience the consequences of decisions.

If clients are discouraged by inability to avoid lapsing, the practitioner can help the client identify additional brain-restoration activities. Clients may also naturally develop more effective skills in terms of politely declining offers of addictive foods in business and social situations.

In summary, the recommendation to comprehensively eliminate addictive foods in abstinent food plans is supported by research, likelihood of cue exposure, and management of risk of relapse. Sweeteners, flour, gluten, excessive salt, processed fats, dairy, and caffeine are eliminated at a minimum. High-sugar fruits, nuts, olives, puffed cereals, and soy are also candidates for elimination. Any other food that the client eats excessively can be considered as a personal binge food and should be eliminated.

Employing classic addiction recovery techniques in the treatment of overeating provides a novel and valuable method for the obesity epidemic that has been resistant to improvement. The key issues in treatment are reducing the likelihood of exposure to cues and processed foods to an effective level of abstinence.

6.3.2 Discussing Neuroimpairment

As can be seen from the evidence, neuroimpairment in PFA can be extensive. Anomalies have been found in pleasure, cognitive, stress, locomotion, and emotion-processing functions. Neurofunctioning is the foundation for effective recovery, as it enables the client to execute complex tasks such as organizing meals, avoiding cues, and restructuring personal relationships. Clearly, restoration of a range of neurofunctioning is a priority, from reducing cue reactivity, to cognitive restoration and desensitization of stress pathways.

The neuroconsequences of PFA need to be explained to the food-addicted client. Clients have a right to information about their condition. After years of being subjected to distorted information about the problem as one of weight loss rather than addiction, the client should be educated about what has happened.

At the same time, clients may have internalized shame to a painful degree. Learning that their brains have been "injured" or "damaged" by chronic processed food use could overwhelm and devastate clients who have been unfairly blamed for their lack of control over processed foods.

The practitioner can employ compassionate education by emphasizing three points when advising clients about neuroimpairment.

1. It is important to emphasize that this is new information. The client could not have known that brain adaptations were occurring as a result of their food choices.
2. The food industry has the capability to condition brains to crave and be impulsive. This is not the fault of the client.
3. There are techniques for restoring brain functioning. The client is justified in having hope that healthy neurofunctioning can be achieved.

As the practitioner and client develop a relationship of trust based on compassion, ease of tasks, and celebrations of progress, the joy of recovery and the reclamation of neurofunction will be at the heart of the practice.

6.4 CONCLUSION

There is significant evidence that PFA is an SUD involving a number of processed foods. These include sweeteners, flour, gluten, excessive salt, processed fats, dairy, and caffeine. There is also evidence in the research and 12-step literature that abstaining from these foods results in reduced cravings in a pattern similar to that of abstinence from alcohol and drugs of abuse. The evidence also shows that reducing or eliminated processed foods is associated with improvements in the metabolic syndrome.

Although much is known in recovery circles about managing food addiction, research is needed to establish best practices in establishing and maintaining reliable abstinence. Because abstinence is inconvenient to maintain in Westernized cultures where processed foods proliferate, knowledge about matching degrees of abstinence to severity of addiction would be useful. Studies would be useful into treatment protocols, development of optimal food plans, and withdrawal management.

The evidence brings into focus a need to profoundly reconceptualize obesity in much the same way as drug addiction is presently being reframed. Findings into the nature of drug addiction as a lapsing disease of impaired neurofunction are replacing old concepts of addiction as a moral failure. Instead, lapses are now seen to be the result of the nature of the disease. As such, lapses should treated with compassion rather than judgment (Volkow et al., 2016). This is also the case with addiction to processed foods. As much as clients addicted to drugs have suffered from judgment, so have chronic overeaters. The obese attract severe stigmatization and suffer from internalizing blame and loathing (Ratcliffe & Ellison, 2015). Clients suffering from addiction to processed foods deserve profound compassion.

In the case of PFA, the role of the food industry in the creation of the condition can be questioned. The issue is illustrated by this quote, "The use of medical technology, such as functional magnetic resonance imaging, to quantitate hedonic responses to food, enhance taste, and effectively develop and market commercial food products has produced new areas of ethical concern and opportunities to better understand eating and satiety" (deShazo, Hall, & Skipworth, 2015).

Treating addictions in general is difficult, with recurring relapse a common feature. PFA presents special challenges in heavily cued cultures. Recognition of the need for a very comprehensive approach is the key to success.

REFERENCES

Addicott, M. A. (2014). Caffeine use disorder: A review of the evidence and future implications. *Curr Addict Rep, 1*(3), 186–192. doi:10.1007/s40429-014-0024-9.

Ahmed, S. H., Guillem, K., & Vandaele, Y. (2013). Sugar addiction: Pushing the drug-sugar analogy to the limit. *Curr Opin Clin Nutr Metab Care, 16*(4), 434–439. doi:10.1097/MCO.0b013e328361c8b8.

Alcaraz-Iborra, M., & Cubero, I. (2015). Do Orexins contribute to impulsivity-driven binge consumption of rewarding stimulus and transition to drug/food dependence? *Pharmacol Biochem Behav, 134*, 31–34. doi:10.1016/j.pbb.2015.04.012.

Alsio, J., Olszewski, P. K., Norback, A. H., Gunnarsson, Z. E., Levine, A. S., Pickering, C., & Schioth, H. B. (2010). Dopamine D1 receptor gene expression decreases in the nucleus accumbens upon long-term exposure to palatable food and differs depending on diet-induced obesity phenotype in rats. *Neuroscience, 3,* 779–787. doi:S0306-4522(10)01294-7 [pii] 10.1016/j.neuroscience.2010.09.046 [doi].

Avena, N. M., Bocarsly, M. E., & Hoebel, B. G. (2012). Animal models of sugar and fat bingeing: Relationship to food addiction and increased body weight. *Methods Mol Biol, 829*, 351–365. doi:10.1007/978-1-61779-458-2_23.

Beaulieu, K., Hopkins, M., Blundell, J., & Finlayson, G. (2017). Impact of physical activity level and dietary fat content on passive overconsumption of energy in non-obese adults. *Int J Behav Nutr Phys Act, 14*(1), 14. doi:10.1186/s12966-017-0473-3.

Beaver, J. D., Lawrence, A. D., van Ditzhuijzen, J., Davis, M. H., Woods, A., & Calder, A. J. (2006). Individual differences in reward drive predict neural responses to images of food. *J Neurosci, 26*(19), 5160–5166.

Bernstein, G. A., Carroll, M. E., Thuras, P. D., Cosgrove, K. P., & Roth, M. E. (2002). Caffeine dependence in teenagers. *Drug Alcohol Depend, 66*(1), 1–6.

Blass, E. M., & Shide, D. J. (1994). Some comparisons among the calming and pain-relieving effects of sucrose, glucose, fructose and lactose in infant rats. *Chem Senses, 19*(3), 239–249.

Blum, K., Thanos, P. K., Oscar-Berman, M., Febo, M., Baron, D., Badgaiyan, R. D., …Gold, M. S. (2015). Dopamine in the brain: Hypothesizing surfeit or deficit links to reward and addiction. *J Reward Defic Syndr, 1*(3), 95–104. doi:10.17756/jrds.2015-016.

Boswell, R. G., & Kober, H. (2016). Food cue reactivity and craving predict eating and weight gain: A meta-analytic review. *Obes Rev, 17*(2), 159–177. doi:10.1111/obr.12354.

Bray, G. A. (2000). Afferent signals regulating food intake. *Proc Nutr Soc, 59*(3), 373–384.

Brown, R. M., Kupchik, Y. M., Spencer, S., Garcia-Keller, C., Spanswick, D. C., Lawrence, A. J., …Kalivas, P. W. (2015). Addiction-like synaptic impairments in diet-induced obesity. *Biol Psychiatry*. doi:10.1016/j.biopsych.2015.11.019.

Burger, K. S., & Stice, E. (2012). Frequent ice cream consumption is associated with reduced striatal response to receipt of an ice cream-based milkshake. *Am J Clin Nutr, 95*(4), 810–817. doi:10.3945/ajcn.111.027003.

Burger, K. S., & Stice, E. (2014a). Greater striatopallidal adaptive coding during cue-reward learning and food reward habituation predict future weight gain. *NeuroImage, 99*, 122–128. doi:10.1016/j.neuroimage.2014.05.066.

Burger, K. S., & Stice, E. (2014b). Neural responsivity during soft drink intake, anticipation, and advertisement exposure in habitually consuming youth. *Obesity (Silver Spring), 22*(2), 441–450. doi:10.1002/oby.20563.

Cameron, C. M., Wightman, R. M., & Carelli, R. M. (2014). Dynamics of rapid dopamine release in the nucleus accumbens during goal-directed behaviors for cocaine versus natural rewards. *Neuropharmacology, 86*, 319–328. doi:10.1016/j.neuropharm.2014.08.006.

Caprioli, D., Zeric, T., Thorndike, E. B., & Venniro, M. (2015). Persistent palatable food preference in rats with a history of limited and extended access to methamphetamine self-administration. *Addict Biol.* doi:10.1111/adb.12220.

Carlier, N., Marshe, V. S., Cmorejova, J., Davis, C., & Muller, D. J. (2015). Genetic similarities between compulsive overeating and addiction phenotypes: A case for "Food Addiction"? *Curr Psychiatry Rep, 17*(12), 96. doi:10.1007/s11920-015-0634-5.

Carr, K. A., Daniel, T. O., Lin, H., & Epstein, L. H. (2011). Reinforcement pathology and obesity. *Curr Drug Abuse Rev, 4*(3), 190–196.

Carroccio, A., Brusca, I., Mansueto, P., Soresi, M., D'Alcamo, A., Ambrosiano, G., …Di Fede, G. (2011). Fecal assays detect hypersensitivity to cow's milk protein and gluten in adults with irritable bowel syndrome. *Clin Gastroenterol Hepatol, 9*(11), 965–971.e963. doi:10.1016/j.cgh.2011.07.030.

Carter, A., Hendrikse, J., Lee, N., Yucel, M., Verdejo-Garcia, A., Andrews, Z., & Hall, W. (2016). The neurobiology of "Food Addiction" and its implications for obesity treatment and policy. *Annu Rev Nutr, 36*, 105–128. doi:10.1146/annurev-nutr-071715-050909.

Cleobury, L., & Tapper, K. (2014). Reasons for eating 'unhealthy' snacks in overweight and obese males and females. *J Hum Nutr Diet, 27*(4), 333–341. doi:10.1111/jhn.12169.

Cocores, J. A., & Gold, M. S. (2009). The salted food addiction hypothesis may explain overeating and the obesity epidemic. *Med Hypotheses, 73*(6), 892–899. doi:S0306-9877(09)00484-8 [pii] 10.1016/j.mehy.2009.06.049 [doi].

Cohen, D. A. (2008). Neurophysiological pathways to obesity: Below awareness and beyond individual control. *Diabetes, 57*(7), 1768–1773. doi:10.2337/db08-0163.

Connor, J. P., Gullo, M. J., Chan, G., Young, R. M., Hall, W. D., & Feeney, G. F. (2013). Polysubstance use in cannabis users referred for treatment: Drug use profiles, psychiatric comorbidity and cannabis-related beliefs. *Front Psychiatry, 4*, 79. doi:10.3389/fpsyt.2013.00079.

Cottone, P., Sabino, V., Roberto, M., Bajo, M., Pockros, L., Frihauf, J. B., …Zorrilla, E. P. (2009). CRF system recruitment mediates dark side of compulsive eating. *Proc Natl Acad Sci U S A, 106*(47), 20016–20020. doi:10.1073/pnas.0908789106.

Counotte, D. S., Schiefer, C., Shaham, Y., & O'Donnell, P. (2014). Time-dependent decreases in nucleus accumbens AMPA/NMDA ratio and incubation of sucrose craving in adolescent and adult rats. *Psychopharmacology (Berl), 231*(8), 1675–1684. doi:10.1007/s00213-013-3294-3.

Criscitelli, K., & Avena, N. M. (2016). The neurobiological and behavioral overlaps of nicotine and food addiction. *Prev Med, 92*, 82–89. doi:http://dx.doi.org/10.1016/j.ypmed.2016.08.009.

Cristino, L., Becker, T., & Di Marzo, V. (2014). Endocannabinoids and energy homeostasis: An update. *Biofactors, 40*(4), 389–397. doi:10.1002/biof.1168.

D'Addario, C., Micioni Di Bonaventura, M. V., Pucci, M., Romano, A., Gaetani, S., Ciccocioppo, R., … Maccarrone, M. (2014). Endocannabinoid signaling and food addiction. *Neurosci Biobehav Rev.* doi:10.1016/j.neubiorev.2014.08.008.

Davis, C., & Loxton, N. J. (2014). A psycho-genetic study of hedonic responsiveness in relation to "food addiction". *Nutrients, 6*(10), 4338–4353. doi:10.3390/nu6104338.

Del Rio, D., Cano, V., Martin-Ramos, M., Gomez, M., Morales, L., Del Olmo, N., & Ruiz-Gayo, M. (2015). Involvement of the dorsomedial prefrontal cortex in high-fat food conditioning in adolescent mice. *Behav Brain Res.* doi:10.1016/j.bbr.2015.01.039.

deShazo, R. D., Hall, J. E., & Skipworth, L. B. (2015). Obesity bias, medical technology, and the hormonal hypothesis: Should we stop demonizing fat people? *Am J Med, 128*(5), 456–460. doi:10.1016/j.amjmed.2014.11.024.

Dingess, P. M., Darling, R. A., Kurt Dolence, E., Culver, B. W., & Brown, T. E. (2017). Exposure to a diet high in fat attenuates dendritic spine density in the medial prefrontal cortex. *Brain Struct Funct, 222*(2), 1077–1085. doi:10.1007/s00429-016-1208-y.

DiPatrizio, N. V., Joslin, A., Jung, K. M., & Piomelli, D. (2013). Endocannabinoid signaling in the gut mediates preference for dietary unsaturated fats. *Faseb J, 27*(6), 2513–2520. doi:10.1096/fj.13-227587.

Eaton, S. B., & Eaton, S. B., 3rd. (2000). Paleolithic vs. modern diets--selected pathophysiological implications. *Eur J Nutr, 39*(2), 67–70.

Engeli, S., Lehmann, A. C., Kaminski, J., Haas, V., Janke, J., Zoerner, A. A., …Jordan, J. (2014). Influence of dietary fat intake on the endocannabinoid system in lean and obese subjects. *Obesity (Silver Spring),* 22(5), E70–E76. doi:10.1002/oby.20728.

Fanciulli, G., Dettori, A., Demontis, M. P., Tomasi, P. A., Anania, V., & Delitala, G. (2005). Gluten exorphin B5 stimulates prolactin secretion through opioid receptors located outside the blood-brain barrier. *Life Sci, 76*(15), 1713–1719.

Feinle-Bisset, C. (2014). Modulation of hunger and satiety: Hormones and diet. *Curr Opin Clin Nutr Metab Care, 17*(5), 458–464. doi:10.1097/mco.0000000000000078.

Ferrari, J. R., Groh, D. R., Rulka, G., Jason, L. A., & Davis, M. I. (2008). Coming to terms with reality: Predictors of self-deception within substance abuse recovery. *Addict Disord Their Treat, 7*(4), 210–218. doi:10.1097/ADT.0b013e31815c2ded.

Ferreira, J. G., Tellez, L. A., Ren, X., Yeckel, C. W., & de Araujo, I. E. (2012). Regulation of fat intake in the absence of flavour signalling. *J Physiol, 590*(4), 953–972. doi:10.1113/jphysiol.2011.218289.

Folgueira, C., Seoane, L. M., & Casanueva, F. F. (2014). The brain-stomach connection. *Front Horm Res, 42,* 83–92. doi:10.1159/000358316.

Food Addicts Anonymous. (2010). *Food Addicts Anonymous.* Port St. Lucie, FL: Food Addicts Anonymous, Inc.

Food Addicts in Recovery Anonymous. (2013). *Food Addicts in Recovery Anonymous.* Woburn, MA: Food Addicts in Recovery Anonymous.

Fortuna, J. L. (2010). Sweet preference, sugar addiction and the familial history of alcohol dependence: Shared neural pathways and genes. *J Psychoactive Drugs, 42*(2), 147–151.

Fortuna, J. L. (2012). The obesity epidemic and food addiction: Clinical similarities to drug dependence. *J Psychoactive Drugs, 44*(1), 56–63. doi:10.1080/02791072.2012.662092.

Foster, G. D., Makris, A. P., & Bailer, B. A. (2005). Behavioral treatment of obesity. *Am J Clin Nutr, 82*(1 Suppl), 230s–235s.

Fowler, L., Ivezaj, V., & Saules, K. K. (2014). Problematic intake of high-sugar/low-fat and high glycemic index foods by bariatric patients is associated with development of post-surgical new onset substance use disorders. *Eat Behav, 15*(3), 505–508. doi:10.1016/j.eatbeh.2014.06.009.

Frascella, J., Potenza, M. N., Brown, L. L., & Childress, A. R. (2010). Shared brain vulnerabilities open the way for nonsubstance addictions: Carving addiction at a new joint? *Ann N Y Acad Sci, 1187*, 294–315. doi:NYAS5420 [pii] 10.1111/j.1749-6632.2009.05420.x.

Fukudome, S., & Yoshikawa, M. (1992). Opioid peptides derived from wheat gluten: Their isolation and characterization. *FEBS Lett, 296*(1), 107–111.

Goran, M. I., Martin, A. A., Alderete, T. L., Fujiwara, H., & Fields, D. A. (2017). Fructose in breast milk is positively associated with infant body composition at 6 months of age. *Nutrients, 9*(2). doi:10.3390/nu9020146.

Graudal, N., Jurgens, G., Baslund, B., & Alderman, M. H. (2014). Compared with usual sodium intake, low- and excessive-sodium diets are associated with increased mortality: A meta-analysis. *Am J Hypertens, 27*(9), 1129–1137. doi:10.1093/ajh/hpu028.

Grosshans, M., Vollmert, C., Vollstadt-Klein, S., Tost, H., Leber, S., Bach, P., …Kiefer, F. (2012). Association of leptin with food cue-induced activation in human reward pathways. *Arch Gen Psychiatry, 69*(5), 529–537. doi:10.1001/archgenpsychiatry.2011.1586.

Guerrieri, R., Nederkoorn, C., & Jansen, A. (2008). The interaction between impulsivity and a varied food environment: Its influence on food intake and overweight. *Int J Obes (Lond), 32*(4), 708–714.

Gugusheff, J. R., Ong, Z. Y., & Muhlhausler, B. S. (2015). The early origins of food preferences: Targeting the critical windows of development. *Faseb J, 29*(2), 365–373. doi:10.1096/fj.14-255976.

Hege, M. A., Stingl, K. T., Kullmann, S., Schag, K., Giel, K. E., Zipfel, S., & Preissl, H. (2014). Attentional impulsivity in binge eating disorder modulates response inhibition performance and frontal brain networks. *Int J Obes (Lond)*. doi:10.1038/ijo.2014.99.

Ho, C. Y., & Berridge, K. C. (2013). An orexin hotspot in ventral pallidum amplifies hedonic 'liking' for sweetness. *Neuropsychopharmacology, 38*(9), 1655–1664. doi:10.1038/npp.2013.62.

Huebner, F. R., Lieberman, K. W., Rubino, R. P., & Wall, J. S. (1984). Demonstration of high opioid-like activity in isolated peptides from wheat gluten hydrolysates. *Peptides, 5*(6), 1139–1147.

Ifland, J. R., Preuss, H. G., Marcus, M. T., Rourke, K. M., Taylor, W. C., Burau, K., …Manso, G. (2009). Refined food addiction: A classic substance use disorder. *Med Hypotheses, 72*(5), 518–526. doi:S0306-9877(08)00642-7 [pii] 10.1016/j.mehy.2008.11.035 [doi].

Jastreboff, A. M., Gaiser, E. C., Gu, P., & Sinha, R. (2014). Sex differences in the association between dietary restraint, insulin resistance and obesity. *Eat Behav, 15*(2), 286–290. doi:10.1016/j.eatbeh.2014.03.008.

Jastreboff, A. M., Sinha, R., Lacadie, C., Small, D. M., Sherwin, R. S., & Potenza, M. N. (2013). Neural correlates of stress- and food cue-induced food craving in obesity: Association with insulin levels. *Diabetes Care, 36*(2), 394–402. doi:10.1093/ntr/ntw088.

Jonsson, T., Granfeldt, Y., Ahren, B., Branell, U. C., Palsson, G., Hansson, A., …Lindeberg, S. (2009). Beneficial effects of a Paleolithic diet on cardiovascular risk factors in type 2 diabetes: A randomized cross-over pilot study. *Cardiovasc Diabetol, 8*, 35. doi:10.1186/1475-2840-8-35.

Jonsson, T., Granfeldt, Y., Erlanson-Albertsson, C., Ahren, B., & Lindeberg, S. (2010). A paleolithic diet is more satiating per calorie than a mediterranean-like diet in individuals with ischemic heart disease. *Nutr Metab (Lond)*, 7, 85. doi:10.1186/1743-7075-7-85.

Jonsson, T., Granfeldt, Y., Lindeberg, S., & Hallberg, A. C. (2013). Subjective satiety and other experiences of a Paleolithic diet compared to a diabetes diet in patients with type 2 diabetes. *Nutr J, 12*, 105. doi:10.1186/1475-2891-12-105.

Kalon, E., Hong, J. Y., Tobin, C., & Schulte, T. (2016). Psychological and neurobiological correlates of food addiction. *Int Rev Neurobiol, 129*, 85–110. doi:10.1016/bs.irn.2016.06.003.

Karatsoreos, I. N., Thaler, J. P., Borgland, S. L., Champagne, F. A., Hurd, Y. L., & Hill, M. N. (2013). Food for thought: Hormonal, experiential, and neural influences on feeding and obesity. *J Neurosci, 33*(45), 17610–17616. doi:10.1523/jneurosci.3452-13.2013.

Karlsson, H. K., Tuominen, L., Tuulari, J. J., Hirvonen, J., Parkkola, R., Helin, S., …Nummenmaa, L. (2015). Obesity is associated with decreased mu-opioid but unaltered dopamine D2 receptor availability in the brain. *J Neurosci, 35*(9), 3959–3965. doi:10.1523/jneurosci.4744-14.2015.

Kelley, A. E. (2004). Memory and addiction: Shared neural circuitry and molecular mechanisms. *Neuron, 44*(1), 161–179.

Kelley, A. E., Bakshi, V. P., Haber, S. N., Steininger, T. L., Will, M. J., & Zhang, M. (2002). Opioid modulation of taste hedonics within the ventral striatum. *Physiol Behav, 76*(3), 365–377.

Kelley, A. E., Baldo, B. A., Pratt, W. E., & Will, M. J. (2005). Corticostriatal-hypothalamic circuitry and food motivation: Integration of energy, action and reward. *Physiol Behav, 86*(5), 773–795. doi:10.1016/j.physbeh.2005.08.066.

Kelly, P. J., Robinson, L. D., Baker, A. L., Deane, F. P., McKetin, R., Hudson, S., & Keane, C. (2017). Polysubstance use in treatment seekers who inject amphetamine: Drug use profiles, injecting practices and quality of life. *Addict Behav, 71*, 25–30. doi:10.1016/j.addbeh.2017.02.006.

Kendig, M. D., Cheung, A. M., Raymond, J. S., & Corbit, L. H. (2016). Contexts paired with junk food impair goal-directed behavior in rats: Implications for decision making in obesogenic environments. *Front Behav Neurosci, 10*, 216. doi:10.3389/fnbeh.2016.00216.

Koob, G. F. (2013). Negative reinforcement in drug addiction: The darkness within. *Curr Opin Neurobiol, 23*(4), 559–563. doi:10.1016/j.conb.2013.03.011.

Kringelbach, M. L., & Stein, A. (2010). Cortical mechanisms of human eating. *Forum Nutr, 63*, 164–175. doi:10.1159/000264404.

Kroemer, N. B., Krebs, L., Kobiella, A., Grimm, O., Pilhatsch, M., Bidlingmaier, M., …Smolka, M. N. (2013). Fasting levels of ghrelin covary with the brain response to food pictures. *Addict Biol, 18*(5), 855–862. doi:10.1111/j.1369-1600.2012.00489.x.

Kroemer, N. B., Krebs, L., Kobiella, A., Grimm, O., Vollstadt-Klein, S., Wolfensteller, U., …Smolka, M. N. (2013). (Still) longing for food: Insulin reactivity modulates response to food pictures. *Hum Brain Mapp, 34*(10), 2367–2380. doi:10.1002/hbm.22071.

Kuhn, F. T., Trevizol, F., Dias, V. T., Barcelos, R. C., Pase, C. S., Roversi, K., …Burger, M. E. (2014). Toxicological aspects of trans fat consumption over two sequential generations of rats: Oxidative damage and preference for amphetamine. *Toxicol Lett, 232*(1), 58–67. doi:10.1016/j.toxlet.2014.10.001.

Lachance, L. R., & McKenzie, K. (2014). Biomarkers of gluten sensitivity in patients with non-affective psychosis: A meta-analysis. *Schizophr Res, 152*(2–3), 521–527. doi:10.1016/j.schres.2013.12.001.

Larsen, J., Dall, M., Antvorskov, J. C., Weile, C., Engkilde, K., Josefsen, K., & Buschard, K. (2014). Dietary gluten increases natural killer cell cytotoxicity and cytokine secretion. *Eur J Immunol, 44*(10), 3056–3067. doi:10.1002/eji.201344264.

Lerma-Cabrera, J. M., Carvajal, F., & Lopez-Legarrea, P. (2016). Food addiction as a new piece of the obesity framework. *Nutr J, 15*, 5. doi:10.1186/s12937-016-0124-6.

Lindeberg, S., Jonsson, T., Granfeldt, Y., Borgstrand, E., Soffman, J., Sjostrom, K., & Ahren, B. (2007). A Palaeolithic diet improves glucose tolerance more than a Mediterranean-like diet in individuals with ischaemic heart disease. *Diabetologia, 50*(9), 1795–1807. doi:10.1007/s00125-007-0716-y.

Liu, S., & Borgland, S. L. (2015). Regulation of the mesolimbic dopamine circuit by feeding peptides. *Neuroscience, 289c*, 19–42. doi:10.1016/j.neuroscience.2014.12.046.

Lopez, R. B., Hofmann, W., Wagner, D. D., Kelley, W. M., & Heatherton, T. F. (2014). Neural predictors of giving in to temptation in daily life. *Psychol Sci, 25*(7), 1337–1344. doi:10.1177/0956797614531492.

Lustig, R. H. (2013). Fructose: It's "alcohol without the buzz". *Adv Nutr, 4*(2), 226–235. doi:10.3945/an.112.002998.

Martin, A. A., & Davidson, T. L. (2014). Human cognitive function and the obesogenic environment. *Physiol Behav* doi:10.1016/j.physbeh.2014.02.062.

Martin, S. A., Jameson, C. H., Allan, S. M., & Lawrence, C. B. (2014). Maternal high-fat diet worsens memory deficits in the triple-transgenic (3xTgAD) mouse model of Alzheimer's disease. *PLoS One, 9*(6), e99226. doi:10.1371/journal.pone.0099226.

Martinez Steele, E., Baraldi, L. G., Louzada, M. L., Moubarac, J. C., Mozaffarian, D., & Monteiro, C. A. (2016). Ultra-processed foods and added sugars in the US diet: Evidence from a nationally representative cross-sectional study. *BMJ Open, 6*(3), e009892. doi:10.1136/bmjopen-2015-009892.

Martin-Fardon, R., Cauvi, G., Kerr, T. M., & Weiss, F. (2016). Differential role of hypothalamic orexin/hypocretin neurons in reward seeking motivated by cocaine versus palatable food. *Addict Biol*. doi:10.1111/adb.12441.

Martinotti, G., Carli, V., Tedeschi, D., Di Giannantonio, M., Roy, A., Janiri, L., & Sarchiapone, M. (2009). Mono- and polysubstance dependent subjects differ on social factors, childhood trauma, personality, suicidal behaviour, and comorbid Axis I diagnoses. *Addict Behav, 34*(9), 790–793. doi:10.1016/j.addbeh.2009.04.012.

Matzeu, A., Cauvi, G., Kerr, T. M., Weiss, F., & Martin-Fardon, R. (2015). The paraventricular nucleus of the thalamus is differentially recruited by stimuli conditioned to the availability of cocaine versus palatable food. *Addict Biol*. doi:10.1111/adb.12280.

McLellan, A. T., Luborsky, L., Woody, G. E., O'Brien, C. P., & Druley, K. A. (1983). Predicting response to alcohol and drug abuse treatments. Role of psychiatric severity. *Arch Gen Psychiatry, 40*(6), 620–625.

Melnik, B. C. (2015a). Milk--A nutrient system of mammalian evolution promoting mTORC1-dependent translation. *Int J Mol Sci, 16*(8), 17048–17087. doi:10.3390/ijms160817048.

Melnik, B. C. (2015b). Milk: An epigenetic amplifier of FTO-mediated transcription? Implications for western diseases. *J Transl Med, 13*, 385. doi:10.1186/s12967-015-0746-z.

Meye, F. J., & Adan, R. A. (2014). Feelings about food: The ventral tegmental area in food reward and emotional eating. *Trends Pharmacol Sci, 35*(1), 31–40. doi:10.1016/j.tips.2013.11.003.

Meyerhoff, D. J. (2017). Structural neuroimaging in polysubstance users. *Curr Opin Behav Sci, 13*, 13–18. doi:10.1016/j.cobeha.2016.07.006.

Michaelsson, K., Wolk, A., Langenskiold, S., Basu, S., Warensjo Lemming, E., Melhus, H., & Byberg, L. (2014). Milk intake and risk of mortality and fractures in women and men: Cohort studies. *BMJ, 349*, g6015. doi:10.1136/bmj.g6015.

Moore, C. F., Sabino, V., Koob, G. F., & Cottone, P. (2017). Pathological overeating: Emerging evidence for a compulsivity construct. *Neuropsychopharmacology*. doi:10.1038/npp.2016.269.

Moran, A., Musicus, A., Soo, J., Gearhardt, A. N., Gollust, S. E., & Roberto, C. A. (2016). Believing that certain foods are addictive is associated with support for obesity-related public policies. *Prev Med, 90*, 39–46. doi:10.1016/j.ypmed.2016.06.018.

Morris, M. J., Beilharz, J., Maniam, J., Reichelt, A., & Westbrook, R. F. (2014). Why is obesity such a problem in the 21st century? The intersection of palatable food, cues and reward pathways, stress, and cognition. *J Neurosci*. doi:10.1523/jneurosci.2013-14.2014 10.1016/j.neubiorev.2014.12.002.

Moss, H. B., Chen, C. M., & Yi, H. Y. (2014). Early adolescent patterns of alcohol, cigarettes, and marijuana polysubstance use and young adult substance use outcomes in a nationally representative sample. *Drug Alcohol Depend, 136*, 51–62. doi:10.1016/j.drugalcdep.2013.12.011.

Moss, M. (2013). *Salt, sugar*, fat: How the food giants hooked us, Random House, New York.

Murray, S., Tulloch, A., Gold, M. S., & Avena, N. M. (2014). Hormonal and neural mechanisms of food reward, eating behaviour and obesity. *Nat Rev Endocrinol, 10*(9), 540–552. doi:10.1038/nrendo.2014.91.

Noble, E. E., & Kanoski, S. E. (2016). Early life exposure to obesogenic diets and learning and memory dysfunction. *Curr Opin Behav Sci, 9*, 7–14. doi:10.1016/j.cobeha.2015.11.014.

O'Brien, C. P., Childress, A. R., Arndt, I. O., McLellan, A. T., Woody, G. E., & Maany, I. (1988). Pharmacological and behavioral treatments of cocaine dependence: Controlled studies. *J Clin Psychiatry, 49 Suppl*, 17–22.

O'Doherty, J. P., Buchanan, T. W., Seymour, B., & Dolan, R. J. (2006). Predictive neural coding of reward preference involves dissociable responses in human ventral midbrain and ventral striatum. *Neuron, 49*(1), 157–166.

Oginsky, M. F., Goforth, P. B., Nobile, C. W., Lopez-Santiago, L. F., & Ferrario, C. R. (2016). Eating 'Junk-Food' produces rapid and long-Lasting increases in NAc CP-AMPA receptors: Implications for enhanced cue-Induced motivation and food addiction. *Neuropsychopharmacology, 41*(13), 2977–2986. doi:10.1038/npp.2016.111.

O'Keefe, L., Simcocks, A. C., Hryciw, D. H., Mathai, M. L., & McAinch, A. J. (2014). The cannabinoid receptor 1 and its role in influencing peripheral metabolism. *Diabetes Obes Metab, 16*(4), 294–304. doi:10.1111/dom.12144.

Orsini, C. A., Ginton, G., Shimp, K. G., Avena, N. M., Gold, M. S., & Setlow, B. (2014). Food consumption and weight gain after cessation of chronic amphetamine administration. *Appetite, 78*, 76–80. doi:10.1016/j.appet.2014.03.013.

Pelchat, M. L., Johnson, A., Chan, R., Valdez, J., & Ragland, J. D. (2004). Images of desire: Food-craving activation during fMRI. *NeuroImage, 23*(4), 1486–1493.

Peters, S. L., Biesiekierski, J. R., Yelland, G. W., Muir, J. G., & Gibson, P. R. (2014). Randomised clinical trial: Gluten may cause depression in subjects with non-coeliac gluten sensitivity – an exploratory clinical study. *Aliment Pharmacol Ther, 39*(10), 1104–1112. doi:10.1111/apt.12730.

Petrovich, G. D. (2013). Forebrain networks and the control of feeding by environmental learned cues. *Physiol Behav, 121*, 10–18. doi:10.1016/j.neulet.2006.11.019.

Petrovich, G. D., & Gallagher, M. (2003). Amygdala subsystems and control of feeding behavior by learned cues. *Ann N Y Acad Sci, 985*, 251–262.

Preuss, H. G., & Clouatre, D. (2012). Sodium, chloride, and potassium. In J. Werman (Ed.), *Present Knowledge in Nutrition* (10 ed., pp. 475–492,). Washington, DC: ILSI Press.

Preuss, H. G., & Preuss, J. M. (2014). The global diabetes epidemic: Focus on the role of dietary sugars and refined carbohydrates in strategizing prevention. In M. Rothkopf (Ed.), *Metabolic Medicine and Surgery* (1 ed.), 183–206, Boca Raton FL: CRC Press.

Pritchett, C. E., & Hajnal, A. (2011). Obesogenic diets may differentially alter dopamine control of sucrose and fructose intake in rats. *Physiol Behav, 104*(1), 111–116. doi:10.1016/j.physbeh.2011.04.048.

Putnam, J., & Allshouse, J. (1999). Food consumption, prices and expenditures. *Economic Research Service Statistical Bulletin No. 965*, 1970–1997.

Ratcliffe, D., & Ellison, N. (2015). Obesity and internalized weight stigma: A formulation model for an emerging psychological problem. *Behav Cogn Psychother, 43*(2), 239–252. doi:10.1017/s1352465813000763

Rezapour, T., DeVito, E. E., Sofuoglu, M., & Ekhtiari, H. (2016). Perspectives on neurocognitive rehabilitation as an adjunct treatment for addictive disorders: From cognitive improvement to relapse prevention. *Prog Brain Res, 224*, 345–369. doi:10.1016/bs.pbr.2015.07.022.

Rudelt, A., French, S., & Harnack, L. (2014). Fourteen-year trends in sodium content of menu offerings at eight leading fast-food restaurants in the USA. *Public Health Nutr, 17*(8), 1682–1688. doi:10.1017/S136898001300236X.

Rozanne, S. (2005). *Beyond Our Wildest Dreams*. Rio Rancho, NM: Overeaters Anonymous.

Schulte, E. M., Avena, N. M., & Gearhardt, A. N. (2015). Which foods may be addictive? The roles of processing, fat content, and glycemic load. *PLoS One, 10*(2), e0117959. doi:10.1371/journal.pone.0117959.

Schulte, E. M., Potenza, M. N., & Gearhardt, A. N. (2016). A commentary on the "eating addiction" versus "food addiction" perspectives on addictive-like food consumption. *Appetite*. doi:10.1016/j.appet.2016.10.033.

Schwabe, L., & Wolf, O. T. (2011). Stress-induced modulation of instrumental behavior: From goal-directed to habitual control of action. *Behav Brain Res, 219*(2), 321–328. doi:10.1016/j.bbr.2010.12.038.

Schwander, F., Kopf-Bolanz, K. A., Buri, C., Portmann, R., Egger, L., Chollet, M., ...Vergeres, G. (2014). A dose-response strategy reveals differences between normal-weight and obese men in their metabolic and inflammatory responses to a high-fat meal. *J Nutr.* doi:10.3945/jn.114.193565.

Sharma, S., Fernandes, M. F., & Fulton, S. (2013). Adaptations in brain reward circuitry underlie palatable food cravings and anxiety induced by high-fat diet withdrawal. *Int J Obes (Lond), 37*(9), 1183–1191. doi:10.1038/ijo.2012.197.

Sharma, M. K., Murumkar, P. R., Kanhed, A. M., Giridhar, R., & Yadav, M. R. (2014). Prospective therapeutic agents for obesity: Molecular modification approaches of centrally and peripherally acting selective cannabinoid 1 receptor antagonists. *Eur J Med Chem, 79*, 298–339. doi:10.1016/j.ejmech.2014.04.011.

Sheppard, K. (1993). *Food Addiction: The Body Knows.* Deerfield Beach, FL: Health Communications.

Shiffman, S., Dunbar, M. S., Li, X., Scholl, S. M., Tindle, H. A., Anderson, S. J., & Ferguson, S. G. (2014). Smoking patterns and stimulus control in intermittent and daily smokers. *PLoS One, 9*(3), e89911. doi:10.1371/journal.pone.0089911.

Shriner, R. L. (2013). Food addiction: Detox and abstinence reinterpreted? *Exp Gerontol, 48*(10), 1068–1074. doi:10.1016/j.exger.2012.12.005.

Small, D. M. (2009). Individual differences in the neurophysiology of reward and the obesity epidemic. *Int J Obes (Lond), 33*(2), S44–48. doi:10.1038/ijo.2009.71.

Sobesky, J. L., Barrientos, R. M., De May, H. S., Thompson, B. M., Weber, M. D., Watkins, L. R., & Maier, S. F. (2014). High-fat diet consumption disrupts memory and primes elevations in hippocampal IL-1beta, an effect that can be prevented with dietary reversal or IL-1 receptor antagonism. *Brain Behav Immun, 42*, 22–32. doi:10.1016/j.bbi.2014.06.017.

Sobrino Crespo, C., Perianes Cachero, A., Puebla Jimenez, L., Barrios, V., & Arilla Ferreiro, E. (2014). Peptides and food intake. *Front Endocrinol (Lausanne), 5*, 58. doi:10.3389/fendo.2014.00058.

Soto, M., Chaumontet, C., Even, P. C., Nadkarni, N., Piedcoq, J., Darcel, N., ...Fromentin, G. (2015). Intermittent access to liquid sucrose differentially modulates energy intake and related central pathways in control or high-fat fed mice. *Physiol Behav, 140*, 44–53. doi:10.1016/j.physbeh.2014.12.008.

Spreadbury, I. (2012). Comparison with ancestral diets suggests dense acellular carbohydrates promote an inflammatory microbiota, and may be the primary dietary cause of leptin resistance and obesity. *Diabetes Metab Syndr Obes, 5*, 175–189. doi:10.2147/dmso.s33473.

Stice, E., Burger, K. S., & Yokum, S. (2015). Reward region responsivity predicts future weight gain and moderating effects of the TaqIA Allele. *J Neurosci, 35*(28), 10316–10324. doi:10.1523/jneurosci.3607-14.2015.

Stice, E., Figlewicz, D. P., Gosnell, B. A., Levine, A. S., & Pratt, W. E. (2013). The contribution of brain reward circuits to the obesity epidemic. *Neurosci Biobehav Rev, 37*(9 Pt A), 2047–2058. doi:10.1016/j.neubiorev.2012.12.001.

Stice, E., Spoor, S., Bohon, C., Veldhuizen, M. G., & Small, D. M. (2008). Relation of reward from food intake and anticipated food intake to obesity: A functional magnetic resonance imaging study. *J Abnorm Psychol, 117*(4), 924–935. doi:10.1126/science.1161550.

Stice, E., & Yokum, S. (2016). Neural vulnerability factors that increase risk for future weight gain. *Psychol Bull, 142*(5), 447–471. doi:10.1037/bul0000044.

Stice, E., Yokum, S., Burger, K., Rohde, P., Shaw, H., & Gau, J. M. (2015). A pilot randomized trial of a cognitive reappraisal obesity prevention program. *Physiol Behav, 138*, 124–132. doi:10.1016/j.physbeh.2014.10.022.

Swedberg, M. D. (2016). Drug discrimination: A versatile tool for characterization of CNS safety pharmacology and potential for drug abuse. *J Pharmacol Toxicol Methods, 81*, 295–305. doi:10.1016/j.vascn.2016.05.011.

Taguchi, A., Wartschow, L. M., & White, M. F. (2007). Brain IRS2 signaling coordinates life span and nutrient homeostasis. *Science, 317*(5836), 369–372. doi:10.1126/science.1142179.

Takahashi, M., Fukunaga, H., Kaneto, H., Fukudome, S., & Yoshikawa, M. (2000). Behavioral and pharmacological studies on gluten exorphin A5, a newly isolated bioactive food protein fragment, in mice. *Jpn J Pharmacol, 84*(3), 259–265.

Tekol, Y. (2006). Salt addiction: A different kind of drug addiction. *Med Hypotheses, 67*(5), 1233–1234.

Tellez, L. A., Medina, S., Han, W., Ferreira, J. G., Licona-Limon, P., Ren, X., ...de Araujo, I. E. (2013). A gut lipid messenger links excess dietary fat to dopamine deficiency. *Science, 341*(6147), 800–802. doi:10.1126/science.1239275.

Temple, J. L. (2016). Behavioral sensitization of the reinforcing value of food: What food and drugs have in common. *Prev Med, 92*, 90–99. doi:10.1016/j.ypmed.2016.06.022.

Teschemacher, H., Koch, G., & Brantl, V. (1997). Milk protein-derived opioid receptor ligands. *Biopolymers, 43*(2), 99–117. doi:10.1002/(sici)1097-0282(1997)43:2<99::aid-bip3>3.0.co;2-v.

Thanos, P. K., Michaelides, M., Subrize, M., Miller, M. L., Bellezza, R., Cooney, R. N., …Hajnal, A. (2015). Roux-en-Y gastric bypass alters brain activity in regions that underlie reward and taste perception. *PLoS One, 10*(6), e0125570. doi:10.1371/journal.pone.0125570.

Thomasius, R., Sack, P. M., Strittmatter, E., & Kaess, M. (2014). Substance-related and addictive disorders in the DSM-5. *Z Kinder Jugendpsychiatr Psychother, 42*(2), 115–120. doi:10.1024/1422-4917/a000278.

Tsanzi, E., Light, H. R., & Tou, J. C. (2008). The effect of feeding different sugar-sweetened beverages to growing female Sprague-Dawley rats on bone mass and strength. *Bone, 42*(5), 960–968.

Tukey, D. S., Ferreira, J. M., Antoine, S. O., D'Amour J, A., Ninan, I., Cabeza de Vaca, S., …Ziff, E. B. (2013). Sucrose ingestion induces rapid AMPA receptor trafficking. *J Neurosci, 33*(14), 6123–6132. doi:10.1523/jneurosci.4806-12.2013.

Tunstall, B. J., & Kearns, D. N. (2014). Cocaine can generate a stronger conditioned reinforcer than food despite being a weaker primary reinforcer. *Addict Biol.* doi:10.1111/adb.12195.

van de Giessen, E., la Fleur, S. E., Eggels, L., de Bruin, K., van den Brink, W., & Booij, J. (2013). High fat/carbohydrate ratio but not total energy intake induces lower striatal dopamine D2/3 receptor availability in diet-induced obesity. *Int J Obes (Lond), 37*(5), 754–757. doi:10.1038/ijo.2012.128.

Ventura, T., Santander, J., Torres, R., & Contreras, A. M. (2014). Neurobiologic basis of craving for carbohydrates. *Nutrition, 30*(3), 252–256. doi:10.1016/j.nut.2013.06.010.

Volkow, N. D., Koob, G. F., & McLellan, A. T. (2016). Neurobiologic advances from the brain disease model of addiction. *N Engl J Med, 374*(4), 363–371. doi:10.1056/NEJMra1511480.

Volkow, N. D., Wang, G. J., Fowler, J. S., Tomasi, D., & Baler, R. (2012). Food and drug reward: Overlapping circuits in human obesity and addiction. *Curr Top Behav Neurosci, 11*, 1–24. doi:10.1007/7854_2011_169

Vollbrecht, P. J., Mabrouk, O. S., Nelson, A. D., Kennedy, R. T., & Ferrario, C. R. (2016). Pre-existing differences and diet-induced alterations in striatal dopamine systems of obesity-prone rats. *Obesity (Silver Spring), 24*(3), 670–677. doi:10.1002/oby.21411.

Wang, G. J., Tomasi, D., Convit, A., Logan, J., Wong, C. T., Shumay, E., …Volkow, N. D. (2014). BMI modulates calorie-dependent dopamine changes in accumbens from glucose intake. *PLoS One, 9*(7), e101585. doi:10.1371/journal.pone.0101585.

Wang, G. J., Tomasi, D., Volkow, N. D., Wang, R., Telang, F., Caparelli, E. C., & Dunayevich, E. (2014). Effect of combined naltrexone and bupropion therapy on the brain's reactivity to food cues. *Int J Obes (Lond), 38*(5), 682–688. doi:10.1038/ijo.2013.145.

Wang, G. J., Volkow, N. D., Thanos, P. K., & Fowler, J. S. (2004). Similarity between obesity and drug addiction as assessed by neurofunctional imaging: A concept review. *J Addict Dis, 23*(3), 39–53. doi:10.1300/J069v23n03_04.

Wang, G. J., Yang, J., Volkow, N. D., Telang, F., Ma, Y., Zhu, W., …Fowler, J. S. (2006). Gastric stimulation in obese subjects activates the hippocampus and other regions involved in brain reward circuitry. *Proc Natl Acad Sci U S A, 103*(42), 15641–15645.

Watkins, B. A., & Kim, J. (2014). The endocannabinoid system: Directing eating behavior and macronutrient metabolism. *Front Psychol, 5*, 1506. doi:10.3389/fpsyg.2014.01506.

Williams, D. L. (2014). Neural integration of satiation and food reward: Role of GLP-1 and orexin pathways. *Physiol Behav.* doi:10.1016/j.physbeh.2014.03.013.

Wiss, D. A., Criscitelli, K., Gold, M., & Avena, N. (2016). Preclinical evidence for the addiction potential of highly palatable foods: Current developments related to maternal influence. *Appetite, 115*, 19–27. doi:10.1016/j.appet.2016.12.019.

Witt, A. A., Raggio, G. A., Butryn, M. L., & Lowe, M. R. (2014). Do hunger and exposure to food affect scores on a measure of hedonic hunger? An experimental study. *Appetite, 74*, 1–5. doi:10.1016/j.appet.2013.11.010.

Wright, H. T., & Ifland, J. R. (2014). Obesity epidemic: Understanding addiction in managing overeating. *Behavioral Health Nutrition Newsletter, Academy of Nutrition and Diet, 32*(2), 1 & 3–6.

Wyvell, C. L., & Berridge, K. C. (2001). Incentive sensitization by previous amphetamine exposure: Increased cue-triggered "wanting" for sucrose reward. *J Neurosci, 21*(19), 7831–7840.

Yau, Y. H., & Potenza, M. N. (2013). Stress and eating behaviors. *Minerva Endocrinol, 38*(3), 255–267.

Yu, J. H., Shin, M. S., Kim, D. J., Lee, J. R., Yoon, S. Y., Kim, S. G., …Kim, M. S. (2013). Enhanced carbohydrate craving in patients with poorly controlled Type 2 diabetes mellitus. *Diabet Med, 30*(9), 1080–1086. doi:10.1111/dme.12209.

Yudkin, J. (1988). Sucrose, coronary heart disease, diabetes, and obesity: Do hormones provide a link? *Am Heart J, 115*(2), 493–498.

Ziauddeen, H., Alonso-Alonso, M., Hill, J. O., Kelley, M., & Khan, N. A. (2015). Obesity and the neurocognitive basis of food reward and the control of intake. *Adv Nutr, 6*(4), 474–486. doi:10.3945/an.115.008268.

Ziauddeen, H., Chamberlain, S. R., Nathan, P. J., Koch, A., Maltby, K., Bush, M., …Bullmore, E. T. (2013). Effects of the mu-opioid receptor antagonist GSK1521498 on hedonic and consummatory eating behaviour: A proof of mechanism study in binge-eating obese subjects. *Mol Psychiatry, 18*(12), 1287–1293. doi:10.1038/mp.2012.154.

7 Mindfulness Therapies for Food Addiction

Marianne T. Marcus
University of Texas Health Science Center School of Nursing
Houston, TX

CONTENTS

7.1 INTRODUCTION

Mindfulness-based interventions (MBIs) have been used in the treatment of a growing number of clinical disorders in recent decades. The original mindfulness-based stress reduction (MBSR) program was created by Jon Kabat-Zinn in 1979, to help people with chronic pain (Kabat-Zinn, Lipworth, & Burney, 1986). MBIs have been adapted and are now offered around the world to support individuals with stress, anxiety, depression (Goyal et al., 2014), chronic pain (Cherkin et al., 2016; Maglione et al., 2016), and the stress related to medical conditions such as cancer (Carlson et al., 2013, 2016). The purpose of this chapter is to summarize current information concerning the role of mindfulness in the treatment of eating disorders, including food addiction. The content includes a discussion of the concept of mindfulness and descriptions of the underlying mechanisms. The use of MBIs for substance use disorders (SUDs) and the shared features of SUDs and food addiction will be presented to illustrate the potential utility of MBIs for treatment of food addiction. The chapter also includes selected empirical and theoretical evidence for mindfulness behavioral approaches to treatment of eating disorders in general, with examples of protocols.

7.2 MINDFULNESS

7.2.1 Basic Concepts

Mindfulness, a meditation technique with ancient Buddhist roots, is defined as "paying attention in a particular way: on purpose, in the present moment, and nonjudgmentally" (Kabat-Zinn, 1994, 4). Mindfulness training promotes awareness and acceptance of one's thoughts, feelings, and bodily sensations as they arise and recognizing their impermanence. Mindfulness fosters a change in one's present-moment experience, described as "reperceiving" or "attentional control," which may result in more mindful behavioral responses (Shapiro et al., 2006).

7.2.2 Mechanisms

The underlying mechanisms that promote therapeutic improvement in individuals receiving MBIs have been identified and expanded as the body of research has grown over the last two decades. According to Shapiro et al. (2006), those mechanisms are *attention*, or the deliberate aspect of mindfulness; *intention*, or focus on the present moment; and *attitude*, or nonjudgmental acceptance.

Holzel et al. (2011) conducted a theoretical review of mindfulness research that consolidated conceptual and psychological perspectives and integrated a neuroscientific perspective based on brain imaging. They proposed an array of distinct but interacting mechanisms, including (1) *attention regulation*, or sustaining attention on the chosen object; (2) *body awareness*, or focus on an internal experience such as breathing as the object of attention; (3) *emotion regulation*, or nonjudgmental and accepting reappraisal of experience; (4) *emotion regulation*, or exposing oneself to awareness of experience with nonreactivity; and (5) *change in perspective of self*, or detachment from identification with a static sense of self.

According to a recent review by Shonin and Van Gordon (2016), there are 10 evidence-based mechanisms of mindfulness. They include (1) *structural brain changes*, neuroplastic changes seen on brain imaging in areas associated with increased learning and memory, improved self-regulatory efficacy, and greater interoceptive awareness; (2) *reduced autonomic arousal*, increased vagus nerve response associated with increased relaxation response; (3) *perceptual shift*, "stepping back" or distancing and objectively observing distressing experiences; (4) *increase in spirituality*, growth in spiritual awareness, which may broaden life perspectives and promote reevaluation of life priorities; (5) *greater situational awareness*, effortless communication with the present moment that may improve decision-making, job performance, and ability to anticipate situational outcomes; (6) *values clarification*, identification of true values and finding meaning in life; (7) *increase in self-awareness*, ability to recognize and label negative moods and thinking; (8) *addiction substitution*, substituting mindfulness meditation for a negative addiction such as substance use; (9) *urge surfing*, observing but not reacting to mental urges such as craving; and (10) *letting go*, the ability to reduce attachments.

Common elements in the mechanisms include focusing on whatever is at hand, whether it is breathing, walking, or eating, and observing the activity carefully. The mindfulness practitioner is taught to bring the focus back to the target activity when the mind wanders, observing, and accepting the thoughts, sensations, or emotions that arise without judging or attempting to change them (Marcus, 2015). Factors that may influence the effectiveness of the intervention include the type of MBI being taught; the clinical disorder targeted; the educational, social, and spiritual history of the participant; and the preparation of the mindfulness teacher (Shonin & Van Gordon, 2016).

7.2.3 Mindfulness Interventions

Mindfulness-based behavioral interventions, incorporating the mechanisms described above, include MBSR (Kabat-Zinn, 1990), mindfulness-based cognitive therapy (MBCT) (Segal et al., 2002), dialectical behavior therapy (DBT) (Linehan, 1993), acceptance and commitment therapy (ACT) (Hayes et al., 1999), and mindful eating (Kristeller & Wolever, 2011). Descriptions of these intervention programs are presented next, followed by examples of how they have been used for specific eating disorders. Table 7.1 provides a summary of the interventions, their use for eating disorders, and outcomes measured.

TABLE 7.1
Mindfulness Approaches for Eating Disorders

Intervention	Protocol	Mindfulness Content	Outcome Measures
Mindfulness-based stress reduction	Eight weekly 2-hour classes, didactic information on stress, workbook Therapist qualifications: master's degree, mindfulness experience, retreat attendance Manual	Variety of mindfulness meditative exercises, experiential discussion Homework: 45 minutes of formal and 15 minutes of informal mindfulness practice daily guided by audiotape	Stress, binge eating, weight loss
Mindfulness-based cognitive therapy	Eight weekly 2-hour classes, didactic-cognitive therapy concepts without change concepts, relapse prevention action plans Therapist qualifications: training in counseling and cognitive therapy considered important Manual	Variety of meditative practices, 3-minute minimeditation	Decreased food cravings, stress Body image concerns, emotional eating, external eating
Dialectical behavior therapy	Individual and group psychotherapy Four skill modules: core mindfulness, interpersonal effectiveness, emotion regulation, distress tolerance central dialectic: acceptance and change Therapist qualifications: must understand mindfulness and plan and practice exercises Manual	Core mindfulness module	Treatment retention Binge eating, mindfulness Self-acceptance
Acceptance and commitment therapy	Behavioral and cognitive content to increase psychological flexibility, behaviors linked to values, varying length of sessions across studies Therapist qualifications: experience in treatment mindfulness-based interventions Manual	Mindfulness content directed at reducing experiential avoidance (emotional eating external eating)	Craving, negative affect, emotional reactivity, stress, positive affect, weight loss, physical activity, stigma, quality of life, distress tolerance, self-acceptance, psychological flexibility
MEAL	Two-hour group sessions for 6 weeks Lessons on hunger, satiety cues, craving and emotional and cognitive states associated with eating Home practice with tape (10-minute meditation)	Mindfulness meditation	Mindfulness, cognitive restraint around eating, decreased weight, eating disinhibition, binge eating, depression, stress, negative affect, C-reactive protein
Mindfulness-based awareness training	Ten group sessions Lessons on mindful eating, emotional tolerance, self-acceptance, hunger, satiety awareness	Mindfulness meditation	Binge eating Weight loss Stress

- *Mindfulness-Based Stress Reduction* The foundation of MBSR is mindfulness meditation. The program was developed by Kabat-Zinn in 1979 to teach patients with chronic illnesses to reduce stress. MBSR involves eight weekly class sessions of 2.5 or 3 hours each. The teaching of MBSR is guided by a manual and includes a variety of mindfulness meditative exercises including breathing, sitting, walking, and eating. Hatha yoga and the body scan, or sequential focus on bodily sensations, are taught to improve awareness. MBSR participants are given homework, including audiotapes to guide daily practice and workbooks in which to record experiences of stress and mindfulness practice. The sixth class day is an all-day experience of mindfulness, encompassing the various exercises, usually experienced in silence. The Center for Mindfulness at the University of Massachusetts recommends guidelines for MBSR teachers and offers teacher certification (Baer & Krietmeyer, 2006).
- *Mindfulness-Based Cognitive Therapy* Components of MBSR are combined with cognitive behavioral therapy (CBT) in MBCT, which was originally designed to focus on depression and depressive relapses (Segal et al., 2002). The intervention is also taught in 2-hour weekly group sessions over 8 weeks. Homework and group discussion are included but not the full day of mindfulness practice. MBCT practitioners are not taught to change thoughts, as in CBT, but to face them and work with them. Relapse prevention action plans are encouraged, as is the 3-minute minimeditation, or breathing space, during the day to discourage automatic reactive behavior. MBCT therapists should have training in counseling, psychotherapy, or cognitive therapy (Baer & Krietmeyer, 2006).
- *Dialectical Behavioral Therapy* Originally developed for borderline personality disorder (BPD) (Linehan, 1993), DBT has been adapted for eating disorders, depression, and BPD with SUDs (Dakwar & Levin, 2009). The central dialectic is between acceptance and change, accepting the self while acquiring skills to change. DBT requires an initial commitment of a year of individual and group psychotherapy and a cognitive behavioral component based on four skills modules: core mindfulness, interpersonal effectiveness, emotion regulation, and distress tolerance. DBT is guided by a manual. Therapist training does not require formal mindfulness practice but the therapist must be familiar with mindfulness and able to plan practice exercises accordingly.
- *Acceptance and Commitment Therapy* A goal of ACT is to decrease experiential avoidance of negative feelings, sensation, or urges and to take action to eliminate those experiences. ACT combines mindfulness and acceptance processes and links behavior change to the practitioner's values, encouraging redirection and commitment to behaviors that are in line with those values (Hayes et al., 2011). ACT is guided by a manual and taught in group format.
- *Mindful Eating* Clinicians are also introducing another strategy known as *mindful eating. Mindful eating* has been defined as "an experience that engages all parts of us, our bodies, our hearts, and our minds, in choosing, preparing, and eating food" (Bays, 2009). According to The Center for Mindful Eating (TCME), mindful eating is (1) allowing yourself to become aware of the positive and nurturing opportunities that are available through food selection and preparation by respecting your inner wisdom; (2) using your senses to eat food that is both satisfying to you and nourishing to your body; (3) acknowledging responses to food (likes, dislikes, or neutral) without judgment; and (4) becoming aware of physical hunger and satiety cues to guide your decisions to begin and end eating (The Center for Mindful Eating).

7.2.3.1 Mindfulness for SUDs

Treatment studies for SUDs, using the MBIs described above, inform the use of mindfulness to treat disordered eating. Empirical reports of MBIs for the treatment of SUDs began to appear in the literature in early 2000 (Black, 2012). There have been an increasing number of studies and two systematic reviews indicating the potential benefit of mindfulness in the treatment of SUDs since that time (Chiesa & Serretti, 2014; Zgierska et al., 2009). Zgierska et al. (2009) reviewed 22 studies, 13 of which were controlled, and concluded that there was preliminary evidence for the efficacy of mindfulness interventions but found significant methodological limitations in many of the studies. Methodological concerns were also noted in the 24 quantitative, controlled studies of mindfulness-based treatments reviewed by Chiesa and Serretti (2014). These authors indicated that the benefit of mindfulness to SUD treatment was related to the potential for mindfulness training to develop a nonjudgmental and accepting attitude toward distressing thoughts and feelings without attempting to suppress them by using substances of abuse. The study interventions reported in the review included MBSR, MBCT, DBT, ACT, and mindfulness-based relapse prevention (MBRP).

Marcus (2015) reviewed the literature on mindfulness-based approaches to SUDs, including MBSR, MBCT, DBT, ACT and recent modifications developed specifically for substance-abusing populations, MBRP (Witkiewitz et al., 2005), mindfulness-based therapeutic community treatment (Marcus et al., 2009), and mindfulness-oriented recovery enhancement (Garland et al., 2010). The various psychological constructs targeted in these studies included stress, craving, acceptance, thought suppression, acting with awareness, emotional reactivity, and negative affect, characteristics that are also associated with food addiction and other eating disorders. Overall, the results of the studies reviewed indicated that mindfulness is promising for the treatment of SUDs, but more rigorous research is needed.

7.2.3.2 Food Addiction and SUDs: Shared Features

A comprehensive white paper on food addiction from the National Center on Addiction and Substance Abuse (Richter, 2016) states that food addiction, binge eating disorder (BED), and obesity are distinct but related health problems that share the common behavior of excessive consumption of certain types of foods. Thus, the policy, practice, and research implications for these disorders may overlap and be informed by shared characteristics with each other and with those of SUDs. Food addiction, defined as a clinically significant physical and psychological dependence on high-fat, high-sugar, and highly palatable foods (Brownell & Gold, 2012), shares symptoms with other eating disorders and with SUDs. Those symptoms include loss of control (over eating or substance use), continued use (unhealthy eating or substance use) despite negative physical or psychological consequences, repeated attempts to stop the behavior, cravings, emotional dysregulation (difficulty with coping, negative moods and feelings), and impulsivity (Richter, 2016).

Hone-Blanchet and Fecteau (2014) noted that food addiction is characterized by food craving, risk of relapse, withdrawal symptoms, and tolerance, indicating further evidence of symptoms shared with SUDs. Moreover, food cravings, overeating, and tolerance show support for an addiction-like model through neurobiological data (Hone-Blanchet & Fecteau, 2014). Given the shared symptoms ascribed to food addiction and SUDs, Brewerton (2013) posits that treatment goals should be similar if not identical for changing associated deleterious behaviors. Those goals include elimination or control of harmful behaviors, reduction of anxiety, normalization of mood, and acceptance of self. How these treatment goals are achieved may be informed by the addiction field and research on MBIs for treatment of SUDs.

Wisniewski et al. (2014) reviewed the research on eating disorders and SUDs together and described how MBIs have been used to treat both entities. They considered studies of interventions where mindfulness is core, such as MBSR and MBCT, as well as interventions where mindfulness is a component, such as DBT and ACT. They concluded that MBIs may be useful to treat these disorders because of their potential to promote awareness and acceptance and reduce the need to avoid or escape by engaging in unhealthy behaviors. The skills acquired through mindfulness training may prevent relapse and result in a more sustained recovery. These authors also noted that mindfulness may be useful in treating eating disorders and SUDs because of its demonstrated influence on observable regions of the brain associated with selective attention, learning and memory, and self-referential processing. Two recent studies lend further empirical support for mindfulness in addressing constructs associated with food addiction, emotional eating (Levoy et al., 2017) and interoceptive awareness (Lattimore et al., 2017).

7.2.3.3 Mindfulness Approaches for Treating Eating Disorders

The utility of training in mindfulness as an adjunct to treatment of eating disorders, including obesity and binge eating, is particularly compelling. As an example, mindfulness promotes an accepting attitude of one's moment-to-moment thoughts and experiences, which may reduce the tendency to engage in excessive eating to avoid or suppress distressing thoughts or emotions. Various psychological constructs and features of disordered eating, including stress, craving, experiential avoidance, self-compassion, coping, impulsivity, loss of control, thought suppression, and risk of relapse, have been targeted for mindfulness interventions. Relevant research on mindfulness interventions for eating disorders follows.

7.2.3.4 Mindfulness Interventions for Obesity

A number of MBI studies have specifically targeted obesity or weight loss. Tapper et al. (2008) conducted an exploratory trial of a brief ACT-based group intervention for 62 women who were attempting to lose weight. ACT uses mindfulness strategies to target *experiential avoidance*, which involves both *emotional eating*, the tendency to overeat to avoid negative emotions, thoughts, or bodily sensations, and *external eating*, the tendency to overeat in response to the stimuli associated with hyperpalatable foods. ACT strategies link behavior change to the individual's values, encouraging redirection and commitment to actions that are in line with those values (Hayes et al., 2012). The intervention involved three weekly workshops, with a fourth session approximately 3 months later. Guided by a manual, the intervention used the participant's own weight loss plan rather than adding dietary advice. Study participants were randomized to the intervention or a control condition. At 6 months postintervention, participants showed significantly greater increases in physical activity but no significant differences in weight loss or mental health. When intervention participants who reported never applying ACT principles were excluded, results showed significantly greater increases in physical activity and decreases in weight compared to controls. Though brief, the intervention was successful in bringing about change.

Lillis et al. (2009) conducted a randomized control study of a 1-day ACT workshop addressing obesity-related stigma and psychological distress with 84 participants who had completed a 6-month weight-loss program. Compared to waitlist controls, the workshop participants showed greater improvement in stigma reduction, quality of life, psychological distress reduction, body mass, distress tolerance, weight-specific acceptance, and psychological flexibility.

Dalen et al. (2010) conducted a pilot study of a mindfulness-based training program (MEAL) designed specifically for overweight/obese individuals. The intervention is taught in 2-hour sessions over 6 weeks. The MEAL curriculum includes mindfulness meditation, group eating exercises, and group discussion. Participants are taught to examine hunger and satiety cues, craving, and emotional and cognitive states associated with eating. At-home practice includes a 10-minute meditation tape and instructions to engage in mindful eating as much as possible. Ten obese individuals participated in the study. Participants showed statistically significant increases in measures of mindfulness and cognitive restraint around eating, and statistically significant decreases in weight, eating disinhibition, binge eating, depression, perceived stress, negative affect, and C-reactive protein. Though small, the study provides preliminary evidence for the effectiveness of a mindfulness-focused intervention in changing eating behaviors.

A systematic review of mindfulness and weight loss reported on a total of 19 studies, 13 randomized controlled trials and 6 observational studies (Olson & Emery, 2015). Twelve of the studies were published in peer-reviewed journals and seven were unpublished dissertations. Most of the interventions were comprehensive and included components such as diet education, self-monitoring of eating behavior, and increase in physical activity in addition to mindfulness training, which varied across the studies. While significant weight loss was documented among participants in the mindfulness interventions for 13 of the 19 studies, none of the studies documented a relationship between weight loss and changes in mindfulness. The study authors concluded that measurement of mindfulness, and elucidating the relationship between changes in mindfulness and weight loss, are essential in overcoming this methodological limitation.

O'Reilly et al. (2014) conducted a literature review to examine the effectiveness of MBIs for reducing targeted obesity-related behaviors such as binge eating, emotional eating, and external eating. Interventions in the 21 studies identified for the review included combined mindfulness and CBTs, MBSR, acceptance-based therapies, mindful eating programs, and combinations of mindfulness exercises. Eighteen of the reviewed studies reported improvements in the targeted eating behaviors. The authors concluded that many different MBI exercises produce positive results, suggesting that mindfulness training can be accessible to meet the needs of a variety of obese individuals.

A recent meta-analysis evaluated the impact of MBIs on psychological and physical health outcomes in overweight and obese adults (Rogers et al., 2017). Posttreatment outcomes of MBIs in 560 individuals were identified in the 15 studies included in the meta-analysis. The study found that effect sizes were large for improving eating behaviors; medium for depression, anxiety, and eating attitudes; and small for body mass index (BMI) and metacognition. When higher quality randomized control trials ($n = 7$) were examined alone, the positive effects for BMI, anxiety, eating attitudes, and eating behaviors remained significant. The findings suggest that MBI may be both physically and psychologically beneficial for this population but the authors caution that future research should be rigorous and examine the specific mechanisms underlying therapeutic changes.

A systematic review provided evidence that eating attentively, as occurs in mindful eating, may influence food intake and increase weight loss without the need for calorie counting (Robinson et al., 2013). Studies of mindful-eating interventions have reported success in treating eating disorders; decreased BMI; weight loss; decreasing binge and emotional eating; reducing food cravings; and increasing self-efficacy (Beshara et al., 2013; Kidd et al., 2013).

7.2.3.5 Mindfulness Approaches for BED

BED is characterized by use of food to deal with emotional distress; dysregulation of interoceptive awareness, appetite, and satiety; and reactivity to food cues (Kristeller & Wolever, 2011). Mindfulness-based awareness training (MB-EAT) was developed to treat BED by re-regulating the balance between the physiological factors and non-nutritive factors that contribute to BED. MB-EAT is taught in 10 sessions, each of which include mindfulness meditation. Other concepts such as mindful eating, emotional balance, and self-acceptance are introduced over the course of the program. Participants are taught hunger and satiety awareness and they practice mindful eating. Self-acceptance is emphasized by encouraging participants to recognize and cultivate their "inner wisdom" (Kristeller & Wolever, 2011). The efficacy of MB-EAT for BED was compared to a psychoeducational/cognitive-behavioral (PECB) intervention and a waitlist control group in a large randomized clinical trial ($n = 150$). The PECB treatment contained education on obesity, BED, recognition of triggers for eating, and cultivation of alternative coping skills. Ninety-five percent of those individuals in the MB-EAT group no longer met BED criteria at 4 months postintervention, versus seventy-six percent in the PECB group. Decreased BED symptoms and weight loss were strongly predicted by the degree to which participants engaged in mindfulness practice (Kristeller et al., 2013).

Woolhouse et al. (2012) studied the effectiveness of a combined-CBT group therapy for women ($n = 30$) with BED. The intervention, Mindful Moderate Eating Group, incorporated CBT components such as planned meals and food monitoring and mindful eating and meditation. The program consisted of ten 3-hour sessions and a 3-month follow-up session. Pre-and postprogram assessments indicated significant changes in binge eating, dieting, and body image dissatisfaction. All of the reductions were maintained at the follow-up. Sixteen of the study participants indicated in qualitative interviews that mindfulness training increased their self-awareness.

Three systematic reviews provide further evidence for the efficacy of MBIs in the treatment of BED. Katterman et al. (2014) conducted a review of the effectiveness of interventions in which mindfulness was the primary intervention for BED. Studies were included in which mindfulness meditation was a part of each session such as occurs in MBSR. Results of this review of 14 studies suggest that MBIs effectively decrease binge eating and emotional eating in this population but the evidence on weight loss was mixed. Weight management strategies may be needed to supplement mindfulness in studies where weight loss is a goal.

In a systematic review of group or individual psychological interventions using DBT, ACT, MBSR, or an adapted intervention related to these therapies, Godfrey, Gallo, and Afari (2015) assessed binge eating as an outcome but not necessarily the primary outcome of treatment. Nineteen studies were included in the review, which found that mindfulness interventions can be considered effective in reducing binge eating, as was supported by large or medium-large effect sizes overall.

In a systematic review comprised of eight papers, Wanden-Berghe et al. (2011) found that MBIs may be effective in the treatment of eating disorders including bulimia nervosa, anorexia nervosa, and binge eating. The authors caution that study qualities were variable and sample sizes small, but all of the studies reported statistically positive outcomes. A variety of MBIs were used in the studies providing additional support for the versatility of these interventions in achieving the desired results.

7.2.3.6 Mindfulness Approaches to Psychological Constructs of Disordered Eating

In addition to research on MBIs targeting specific eating disorders, studies have been done to assess the effect of MBIs on associated psychological constructs such as craving and stress.

Craving Alberts et al. (2010) added an MBI, aimed at regulating craving by focusing on acceptance, to a dietary group treatment for overweight and obese individuals. Participants were randomly assigned to receive the dietary treatment either with or without the supplementary 7-week training on acceptance. Compared to the control group, participants in the acceptance group reported significantly lower food cravings. Acceptance was further found to reduce loss of control when participants in the experimental group were exposed to food cues.

Alberts et al. (2012) studied the efficacy of an adapted MBCT intervention with a nonclinical sample of 26 women with disordered eating. Participants were randomly assigned to the 8-week intervention. Compared to controls, participants in the mindfulness intervention not only showed greater decreases in food cravings but also in associated factors such as dichotomous thinking, body image concern, emotional eating, and external eating.

Stress The association between stress and eating patterns has been examined in a number of contexts that include stress, neurobiology, and obesity (Yau & Potenza, 2013) and emphasize the relationship between eating disorders and post-traumatic stress disorder (Brewerton et al., 2015; Mason et al., 2014; Tagay et al., 2014). The reported strength of this association has led researchers to call for improved assessment of the phenomenon by clinicians and greater emphasis on inclusion of evidence-based stress reduction interventions in treatment of eating disorders.

Daubenmier et al. (2011) specifically targeted stress eating in a study with overweight and obese women. Study participants were assessed on measures of mindfulness, psychological distress, eating behavior, weight, cortisol awakening response, and abdominal fat pre- and postintervention. Forty-seven overweight/obese women participated in the randomized control study to test a novel intervention that incorporated elements of MBSR, MBCT, and MB-EAT. The intervention consisted of nine, 2.5 hour classes and a day of silent retreat. Daily home assignments and meditation were encouraged. Participants in the mindfulness treatment group improved in mindfulness, anxiety, and external-based eating compared to the control group.

In a nonclinical population of college students, Masuda and Wendell (2010) found that disordered eating-related cognitions were inversely related to mindfulness and positively associated with general psychological ill-health and emotional distress. They concluded that mindfulness is a useful concept in promoting behavioral health in the treatment disordered eating-related cognitions.

Corsica et al. (2014) conducted a pilot study to compare three interventions targeting stress eating. The randomized control study had three arms, mindfulness-based treatment (MBSR), a tailored cognitive-behavioral intervention (stress-eating intervention, SEI), and a combination intervention (MBSR + SEI). They found that all three interventions resulted in significant improvement in perceived stress and stress eating, but the combination treatment resulted in greater reductions and a moderate effect on short-term weight loss. The beneficial effects were consistent at the 6-week follow-up. The authors concluded that interventions that address both perceived stress through mindfulness and disordered eating behaviors through exposure-based cognitive behavioral treatment have the greatest potential to change eating behaviors and increase weight loss.

7.3 CONCLUSION

In view of the shared symptoms of disordered eating, food addiction, and SUDs and the promising empirical support for mindfulness-based approaches for addressing these symptoms, mindfulness should be considered for the treatment of food addiction. Food addiction is a complex, multifaceted health problem that requires a combination of evidence-based approaches. Mindfulness may complement other treatment approaches such as education, by giving the client a tool with which to confront stress, craving, environmental cues, and other known facets of food addiction. MBIs may also be useful for preventing food disorders (Atkinson & Wade, 2015; Jayewardene et al., 2016).

Clinicians should be appropriately trained to offer MBIs for food addiction. Training is available in a number of places around the country including the original site where the first mindfulness intervention, MBSR, was developed, the Center for Mindfulness at the University of Massachusetts, Department of Medicine (www.umassmed.edu/cfml/). Information about mindful eating strategies is available for clinicians at TCME, established in 2006. TCME provides accessible information and opportunities to interact in various ways, including via the web. The mission of TCME includes training and encouraging professionals to foster mindful eating practices among clients. Teacher preparation is explicated on the website. Teacher supervision and assessment is critical to assure fidelity of MBIs and advance research in the field (Crane et al., 2013; Evans et al., 2015). Resources for the mindfulness teacher include websites from the American Mindfulness Research Association (AMRA) (http://goamra.org) and the Mindfulness Awareness Resource Center (MARC) (http://marc.ucla.edu/body/cfm) at the University of California and a guide for teachers (McCown et al., 2010). Although the evidence for MBIs in the treatment of food addiction is promising, more rigorous research is needed to clearly define the benefits of various MBIs and identify factors that contribute to success of these interventions with various populations.

REFERENCES

Alberts, H.J.E.M., Thewissen, R., & Raes, L. (2012) Dealing with problematic behaviour. The effects of a mindfulness-based intervention on eating behaviour, food cravings, dichotomous thinking and body image concern. *Appetite,* 58, 847–851. doi:10.1016/j.appet.2012.01.009

Alberts, H.J.E.M., Mulkens, S., Smeets, M., & Thewissen, R. (2010) Coping with food cravings. Investigating the potential of a mindfulness-based intervention. *Appetite,* 55, 160–163. doi:10.1016/j.appet.2010.05.044

Atkinson, M.J., & Wade, T.D. (2015) Mindfulness-based prevention for eating disorders: A school-based cluster randomized controlled study. *J Eat Disord,* 48 (7), 1024–1037. doi:10.1002/eat.22416

Baer, R.A., & Krietemeyer, J. (2006) Overview of mindfulness and acceptance based treatment approaches. In Baer R.A. (Ed) *Mindfulness-based treatment approaches: Clinicians guide to evidence-based treatment applications.* pp 3–27. New York: Academic.

Bays, J.C. (2009) *Mindful eating: A guide to rediscovering a healthy and joyful relationship with food.* Boston, MA: Shambala.

Beshara, M., Hutchinson, A.D., & Wilson, C. (2013) Does mindfulness matter? Everyday mindfulness, mindful eating and serving size of energy dense foods among a sample of South Australian adults. *Appetite,* 67, 25–29.

Black, D.S. (2012) Mindfulness and substance use intervention. *Subst Use Misuse,* 47(3), 199–201.

Brewerton, T.D. (2013) Are eating disorders addiction? In T.D. Brewerton and A.B. Dennis (Eds.) *Eating disorders, addictions and substance use disorders.* Berlin: Springer-Verlag, 267–299.

Brewerton, T., O'Neil, P.M., Dansky, B.S., & Kilpatrick, D.G. (2015) Extreme obesity and its associations with victimization, PTSD, major depression and eating disorders in a national sample of women. *J Obesity Eat Disord,* 1(2:6), 1–9.

Brownell, K.D., & Gold, M.S. (Eds.). (2012) *Food addiction: A comprehensive handbook*. New York: Oxford University Press.

Carlson, L.E., Doll, R., Stephen, J., Faris, P., Tamagawa, R., Drysdale, E., & Speca, M. (2013) Randomized controlled trial of a mindfulness-based cancer recovery versus supportive expressive group therapy for distressed survivors of breast cancer. *J Clin Oncol,* 32(32), 3686–3687. doi:10.1200/JCO.2012.47.5210

Carlson, L.E., Tamagawa, R., Stephen, J., Drysdale, E., Zhong, L., & Speca, M. (2016) Randomized-controlled trial of mindfulness-based cancer recovery versus supportive expressive group therapy among distressed breast cancer survivors (MINDSET); Long-term follow-up results. *Psychooncology,* 25(7), 750–759. doi. 10.1002/pon.4150

Cherkin, D., Sherman, K.J., Balderson, B.H., Cook, A.J., Anderson, M.S., Hawkes, B.S., Hansen, K.E., & Turner, J.A. (2016) Effect of mindfulness-based stress reduction vs cognitive behavioral therapy or usual care on back pain and functional limitations in adults with chronic low back pain: A randomized clinical trial. *JAMA*, 315(12), 1240–1249. doi:10.1001/jama.2016.2323

Chiesa, A., & Serretti, A., (2014) Are mindfulness-based interventions effective for substance use disorders? A systematic review of the evidence. *Subst Use Misuse,* 19, 492–512.

Corsica, J., Hood, M.M., Katterman, S., Kleinman, B., & Ivan, I. (2014) Development of a novel mindfulness and cognitive behavioral intervention for stress-eating: A comparative pilot study. *Eat Behav,* 15, 694–699. http://dx.doi.org/10.1016/j.eatbeh.2014.08.002

Crane, R.S., Eames, C., Kuyken, W., Hastings, R.P., Williams, J.M., Bartley, T., Evans, A., Silverton, S., Soulsby, J.G., & Surawy, C. (2013) Development and validation of the mindfulness-based interventions-teaching assessment criteria (MBI:TAC). *Assessment*, 20(6), 681–688. doi:10.1177/1073191113490790

Dalen, J., Smith, B.W., Shelley, B.M., Sloan, A.L., Leahigh, L., & Begay, D. (2010) Pilot study: Mindful eating and living (MEAL); Weight, eating behavior, psychological outcomes associated with a mindfulness-based intervention for people with obesity. *Compl Ther Med,* 18, 260–263. doi:10.1016/j.ctim.2010.09.008

Dakwar, E., & Levin, F.R. (2009). The emerging role of meditation in addressing psychiatric illness with a focus on substance use disorders. *Harv Rev Psychiatry*, 17(4), 254–267.

Daubenmier, J., Kristeller, J., Hecht, F.M., Maninger, N., Kuwata, M., Jhaveri, K. Lustig, R.H., Kemeny, M., Karan, L., & Epel, E. (2011) Mindfulness intervention for stress eating to reduce cortisol and abdominal fat among overweight and obese women: An exploratory randomized controlled study. *J Obes,* 1–13. doi:10.1155/2011/651936

Evans, A., Crane, R., Cooper, L., Mardula, J., Wilks, J., Surawy, C., Kenny, M., & Kuyken, W. (2015) A framework for supervision for mindfulness-based teachers: A space for embodied mutual inquiry. *Mindfulness,* 6(3), 572–582. doi:10.1007/s12671-014-0292-4

Garland, E.L., Gylord, S.A., Boettiger, C.A., & Howard, M.O. (2010) Mindfulness training modifies cognitive, affective, and physiological mechanisms implicated in alcohol dependence: Results of a randomized controlled pilot trial. *J Psychoactive Drugs,* 42(2), 177–192.

Godfrey, K.M., Gallo, L.C., Afari, N. (2015) Mindfulness-based interventions for binge eating: A systematic review. *J Behav Med,* 38, 348–362. doi:10.1007/s10865-014-9610-5

Goyal, M., Singh, S., Sibinga, E.M.S., Gould, N.F., Rowland-Seymor, A., Sharma, R., Berger, Z., et al. (2014) Meditation programs for psychological stress and well-being: A systematic review and meta-analysis. *JAMA Intern Med,* 174(3). 357–368. doi10.1001/jamainternmed.2013.13018

Hayes, S.C., Stroshal, K., & Wilson, K.G. (1999) *Acceptance and commitment therapy*. New York: Guildford Press.

Hayes, S.C., Levin, M.E., PlumbVilardaga, J., Villatte, J.L., & Pistorello, J. (2011) Acceptance and commitment therapy and contextual behavioral science: Examining the progress of a distinctive model of behavioral and cognitive science. *Behav Ther,* 44, 180–198.

Hayes, S.C., Pistorello, J., & Levin, M.E. (2012) Acceptance and commitment therapy as unified model of behavior change. *Couns Psychol,* 40(7), 976–1002.

Holzel, B.K., Lazar, S.W., Gard, T., Schuman-Olivier, Z., Vago, D.R., Ott, U. (2011) How does mindfulness work? Proposing mechanisms of action from a conceptual and neural perspective. *Perpect Psychol Sci,* 6(6), 537–559. doi:10.1177/1745691611419671

Hone-Blanchet, A., & Fecteau, S. (2014) Overlap of food addiction and substance use disorders: Analysis of animal and human studies. *Neuropharmacology,* 85, 81–90. http:dx.doi.org/10.1016/j.neuropharm.2014.05.019

Jayewardene, W.P., Lohrmann, D.K., Erbe, R.G., & Torabi, M.R. (2016) Effects of preventive online mindfulness interventions on stress and mindfulness: A meta-analysis of randomized control trials. *Preventive Medicine Reports*. doi:10.1016/j.pmedr.2016.11.013 Published online November 14, 2016.

Kabat-Zinn, J. (1990) *Full catastrophe living; using the wisdom of your body and mind to face stress, pain and illness*. New York: Dell Publishing.

Kabat-Zinn, J. (1994) *Wherever you go, there you are: Mindfulness, meditation in everyday life*. New York: Hyperion.

Kabat-Zinn, J., Lipworth, L., Burney, R., & Sellers, W. (1986) Four year follow-up of a meditation-based program for the self-regulation of chronic pan: Treatment outcomes and compliance. *Clin J Pain,* 2, 159–173.

Katterman, S.N., Kleinman, B.M., Hood, M.M., Nackers, L.M., & Corsica, J.A. (2014) Mindfulness meditation as an intervention for binge eating, emotional eating, and weight loss: A systematic review. *Eat Behav,* 15, 197–204. http://dx.doi.org/10.1016/jeatbeh.2014.01.005

Kidd, L.I., Heifner, G.C., & Murrock, C.J. (2013) A mindful eating group intervention for obese women: A mixed methods feasibility study. *Arch Psychiatr Nurs,* 27, 211–218.

Kristeller, J.L., & Wolever, R.Q. (2011) Mindfulness-based eating awareness training for treating binge eating disorder: The conceptual foundation. *Eat Disord,* 19, 49–61. doi:10.1080/10640266.2011.533605

Kristeller, J., Wolever, R.Q., & Sheets, V. (2013) Mindfulness-based eating awareness training (MB-EAT) for binge eating: A randomized clinical trial. *Mindfulness,* doi 10.1007/s12671-012-0179-1 Published online February 1, 2013.

Lattimore, P., Mead, B.R., Irwin, L., Grice, L. Carson, R., & Malinowski, P. (2017) 'I can't accept that feeling': Relationships between interoceptive awareness, mindfulness and eating disorder symptoms in females with, and at-risk of an eating disorder. *Psychiatr Res,* 247,163–171. http://dx.doi.org/10.1016/j.psychres.2016.11.022

Levoy, E., Lazaridou, A., Brewer, J., & Fulwiler, C. (2017) An exploratory study of mindfulness-based stress reduction for emotional eating. *Appetite,* 109, 124–130. http://dx.doi.org/10.1016/j.appet.2016.11.029

Lillis, J., Hayes, S.C., Bunting, M.A., & Masuda, A. (2009) Teaching acceptance to improve the lives of the obese: A preliminary test of a theoretical model. *Ann Behav Med,* 37, 58–69. doi 10.1007/s12160-009-9083-x

Linehan, M.M. (1993) *Cognitive-behavioral treatment of borderline personality disorder.* New York: Guildford Press.

Maglione, M.A., Hempel, S., Maher, A.R., Apaydin, E., Ewing, B., Hilton, L., Xenakis, L., et al. (2016) *Mindfulness meditation for chronic pain: A systematic review.* Santa Monica, CA: Rand Corporation http://www.rand.org/pubs/reserach_reports//RR1317.html

Marcus, M.T., Schmitz, J., Moeller, F.G., Liehr, P., Cron, S.G., Swank, P., Bankston, S., Carroll, D., & Granmayeh, L.K. (2009) Mindfulness-based stress reduction in therapeutic community treatment: A stage 1 trial. *Am J Drug Alcohol Abuse,* 35(2), 103–108.

Marcus, M.T., (2015) Mindfulness as behavioural approach in addiction treatment. In N. El-Guebaly, M. Galanter, G Carra (Eds.). *Textbook of addiction treatment: International perspectives,* Springer-Verlag Mailand. pp. 821–839.

McCown, D., Reibel, D.K., & Micozzi, M.S. (2010) *Teaching mindfulness: A practical guide for clinicians and educators.* New York: Springer.

Mason, S.M., Flint, A.J., Roberts, A.L., Agnew-Blais, J., Koenen, K.C., & Rich-Edwards, J.W. (2014) Posttraumatic stress disorder symptoms and food addiction in women by timing and type of trauma. *JAMA Psychiatry,* doi:10.10001/jamapsychiatry.2014.1208 Published online September 17, 2014.

Masuda, A., & Wendell, J.W. (2010) Mindfulness mediates the relation between disordered eating-related cognitions and psychological distress. *Eat Behav,* 11, 293–296. doi:10.1016/j.eatbeh.2010.07.001

Olson, K., & Emery, C.F. (2015) Mindfulness and weight loss: A systematic review. *Psychosom Med,* 77, 59–67.

O'Reilly, G.A., Cook, L., Spruijt-Metz, D., & Black, D.S. (2014) Mindfulness-based interventions for obesity-related eating behaviors: A literature review. *Obes Rev,* 15, 453–461.

Richter, L. (2016) *Understanding and addressing food addiction: A science-based approach to policy, practice and research,* The National Center on Addiction and Substance Abuse. Columbia University.

Robinson, E., Aveyard, P., Daley, A., Jolly, K., Lewis, A., Lycett, D., & Higgs, S. (2013) Eating attentively: A systematic review and meta-analysis of the effect of food intake memory and awareness on eating. *Am J Clin Nutr,* 97, 728–742. doi:10.3945/ajcn.122.045245

Rogers, J.M., Ferrari, M., Mosely, K., Lang, C.P., & Brennan, L. (2017) Mindfulness-based interventions for adults who are overweight or obese: A meta-analysis of physical and psychological health outcomes. *Obes Rev,* 18, 51–67. doi:10.1111/obr.12461

Segal, Z.V., Williams, J.M.G., & Teasdale, J.D. (2002) *Mindfulness-based cognitive therapy for depression: A new approach to preventing relapse.* New York: The Guildford Press.

Shapiro, S.L., Carlson, L.E., Astin, J.A., & Freedman, B. (2006) Mechanisms of mindfulness. *J Clin Psychol,* 62, 373–386.

Shonin, E., & Van Gordon, W. (2016) The mechanisms of mindfulness in the treatment of mental illness and addiction. *Int J Ment Health Addiction.* doi 10.1007/s11469-9653-7 Published online May 13, 2016.

Tapper, K., Shaw, C., Ilsley, J., Hill, A.J., Bond, F.W., & Moore, L. (2008) Exploratory randomized controlled trial of a mindfulness-based weight loss intervention for women. *Appetite,* 52, 396–404. doi:10.1016/j.appet.2008.11.012

Tagay, S., Schlottbohm, E., Reyes-Rodriquez, M.L., Repic, N., & Senf, W. (2014) Eating disorders, trauma, PTSD and psychosocial resources. *Eat Disord,* 22(1), 33–49. doi:10 .1080/10640266.2014.857517

The Center for Mindful Eating. www.the centerformindfuleating.org Accessed November 14, 2016.

Wanden-Berghe, R.G., Sanz-Valero, J., & Wanden-Berghe, C. (2011) The application of mindfulness to eating disorders treatment: A systematic review. *Eat Disord,* 19, 34–48. doi:10.1080/1064066.2011.533604

Wisniewski, L., Bishop, E.R., & Killeen, T.K., (2014) Mindfulness approaches in the treatment of eating disorders, substance use disorders, and addictions. In T.D. Brewerton and A.B. Dennis (Eds.). *Eating disorders, addictions and substance use disorders.* Berlin: Springer-Verlag.

Witkiewitz, K., Marlatt, G.A., & Walker, D. (2005) Mindfulness-based relapse prevention for alcohol and substance use disorders. *J Cognit Psychother,* 19(3), 211–228.

Woolhouse, H., Knowles, A., & Crafti, N. (2012) Adding mindfulness to CBT programs for binge eating: A mixed methods evaluation. *Eat Disord,* 20, 321–339. doi:10.1080/10640266.2012.691791

Yau, Y.H.C., & Potenza, M.N. (2013) Stress and eating behaviors. *Minerva Endocrinol,* 38(3), 255–267.

Zgierska, A., Rabago, D., Chawla, N., Kushner, K., Koehler, R., & Marlatt, A. (2009) Mindfulness meditation for substance use disorders: A systematic review. *Subst Abus,* 30(4), 266–294.

Section II

Diagnosis and Assessment

8 Diagnosing and Assessing Processed Food Addiction

Dennis M. Donovan
University of Washington
Seattle, WA

Joan Ifland
Food Addiction Training, LLC
Cincinnati, OH

CONTENTS

8.1 INTRODUCTION

It almost goes without saying that diagnosis and assessment are the keys to recovery from addictions. Without an adequate diagnosis and assessment, a health professional cannot develop a recovery treatment plan. Without an assessment, a client cannot perceive the need for and value of taking action. Accurate assessment is the key to getting appropriate help for the epidemic of overeating manifesting as processed food addiction (PFA).

For the purposes of diagnosing and assessing PFA, this textbook uses two gold standard instruments, the *Diagnostic and Statistical Manual of Mental Disorders, 5th edition* (DSM 5), Substance-Related Addiction Diagnostic Criteria (SUD) and the Addiction Severity Index (ASI). These are summarized as follows.

The DSM SUD for alcohol use disorder have been adapted for PFA as shown below (American Psychiatric Association, 2013, 490–491).

1. Processed foods are consumed in larger amounts or over a longer period than was intended.
2. There is a persistent desire or unsuccessful efforts to cut down or control processed food consumption.
3. A great deal of time is spent in activities necessary to obtain processed foods, consume processed foods, or recover from their effects.
4. Craving, or a strong desire or urge to consume processed foods.
5. Recurrent processed food consumption resulting in a failure to fulfill major role obligations at work, school, or home.
6. Continued processed food consumption despite having persistent or recurrent social or interpersonal problems caused or exacerbated by the effects of processed foods.
7. Important social, occupational, or recreational activities are given up or reduced because of processed food consumption.
8. Recurrent processed food consumption in situations in which it is physically hazardous.
9. Processed food consumption is continued despite knowledge of having a persistent or recurrent physical or psychological problem that is likely to have been caused or exacerbated by processed foods.
10. Tolerance, as defined by either of the following:
    a. A need for markedly increased amounts of processed foods to achieve intoxication or desired effect.
    b. A markedly diminished effect with continued consumption of the same amount of processed foods.
11. Withdrawal, as manifested by either of the following:
    a. The characteristic withdrawal syndrome for processed foods.
    b. Processed foods are consumed to relieve or avoid withdrawal symptoms.

The thresholds specified in the DSM for a use disorder are two to three symptoms for mild, four to five symptoms for moderate, and six or more for severe (American Psychiatric Association, 2013, 484).

The ASI is a semi-structured interview designed to address seven potential problem areas in substance-abusing clients: medical status, employment and support, drug use, alcohol use, legal status, family/social status, and psychiatric status. The severity ratings are the interviewer's estimates of the client's need for additional treatment in each area. The severity scale ranges from 0 (no treatment necessary) to 9 (treatment needed to intervene in life-threatening situation). Each rating is based upon the patient's history of problem symptoms, present condition, and subjective assessment of their treatment needs in a given area (Treatment Research Institute, 2017).

Information collected through the ASI informs the treatment plan. This information also helps the practitioner develop options for first steps. Allowing the client to choose from options can facilitate getting started. The ASI also yields information that can structure tracking progress toward goals. A copy of the ASI can be downloaded from http://www.tresearch.org/wp-content/uploads/2012/09/ASI_5th_Ed.pdf.

8.1.1 Challenges in Diagnosing PFA

In the field of PFA, the tasks of developing a diagnosis and assessment face numerous challenges. First, PFA assessment is in its infancy. Although various assessment tools have been proposed, they do not necessarily address PFA as a substance use disorder with many manifestations. They may underestimate use. As seen in Part I, "Fundamentals," there is evidence for the application of the

SUD model to overeating. This is as opposed to a behavioral or process model that would apply to gambling, shopping, Internet, or sex addiction. Addictive foods and cues have been shown to be at the heart of PFA. So, Part II, "Assessment," depends on established SUD diagnostic and assessment tools, i.e., the DSM 5 SUD criteria for diagnosing and the ASI for assessment as adapted for overeating of processed food.

Secondly, diagnosis and assessment for PFA need to cover a wide range of dysfunction across a range of functional areas. Dysfunction can extend from cognitive impairment and mood disorders, to extensive physical, relationship, financial, career, and family problems. In severe cases, the client may be experiencing cravings continuously and spending most days seeking, eating, and recovering from processed food use. The following chapters describing dysfunction under each of the DSM 5 SUD criteria demonstrate the breadth of the disorder. Although the extent and areas of impairment can be overwhelming, developing a complete picture is crucial to developing a sufficiently comprehensive treatment plan and motivating a client to see a need for treatment and to follow the plan.

Overlooking any comorbid impairment can lead to assignments that are beyond the abilities of the client. For example, failing to find memory loss may lead to the false assumption that a client can remember instructions. This in turn could lead to frustration over a lack of progress because the client cannot remember what to do. Patiently reviewing the extensive SUD diagnostic criteria as well as the results of the ASI will yield rewards in a well-matched treatment plan and good progress.

Another factor in the challenge of assessing PFA is that the addiction may have been diagnosed repeatedly as a weight-loss problem as opposed to a serious mental disorder. The client may have experienced multiple failures at "weight loss" as a result of the misdiagnoses. Thus the client may be fearful of failure in yet another "weight loss" program. Reframing the problem as an SUD may take some practice for the health care provider but could be the key to persuading the client to try again and to use different methods for putting the disorder into remission. The assessment can play an important role in diverting attention from weight loss to more serious impairments such as mobility, fatigue, symptoms of the metabolic syndrome, and loss of executive function. By describing the potential to recover from ailments well beyond the scope of weight loss, the practitioner may be able to motivate the client to begin and stay with recovery.

And finally, practitioners may find it hard to accept that PFA, as diagnosed by the DSM 5 SUD criteria, is quite common but does not necessarily correspond to weight status. Practitioners may benefit from the discipline of systematically developing a profile of behaviors that conform to the DSM 5 SUD criteria. With the detailed information provided in the following chapters, practitioners will be able to probe for instances of addictive behaviors that could otherwise escape notice and avoid being distracted by weight status.

Practitioners can self-monitor for the temptation to dismiss or downplay results at the minimal and mild end of the scale. Addictions are progressive and in the case of PFA, there are intense pressures in obesogenic environments that can accelerate the development of PFA. Aggressive treatment even in minimal or mild cases of preaddiction can be warranted.

8.1.2 Prevention Strategies

Selective prevention strategies can be applied to groups that are at risk for the development of PFA even if clients from these populations have not yet manifested clinically significant symptoms. These would include clients with a history of drug abuse (Odom et al., 2010; Yanos, Saules, Schuh, & Sogg, 2014), family history of eating disorders or metabolic syndrome (Franks & McCarthy, 2016; Lydecker & Grilo, 2016), childhood abuse or neglect (Brewer-Smyth, Cornelius, & Pohlig, 2016; Helton & Liechty, 2014; Williams, Canterford, Toumbourou, Patton, & Catalano, 2015; Zeller et al., 2015), a history of weight cycling (Martire, Westbrook, & Morris, 2015), mental or emotional illness (Henriksen, Mather, Mackenzie, Bienvenu, & Sareen, 2014; Sanders, Han, Baker, & Cobley, 2015; Yanos et al., 2014), availability of processed foods in the home (Schuz, Bower, & Ferguson 2015), interpersonal violence (Davies, Lehman, Perry, & McCall-Hosenfeld, 2015), and a profile of undereducation/poverty (Lee, Andrew, Gebremariam, Lumeng, & Lee, 2014; Veses et al., 2015; Wiers et al., 2016). In the United States, Hispanic, American Indian, and African-American populations are at greater risk of obesity (Ogden, Carroll, Kit, & Flegal, 2013).

Indicated prevention applies to clients who are eating processed foods routinely but are not yet manifesting behaviors that would justify a diagnosis of PFA. Clients who have been diagnosed with diet-related diseases but do not yet require medication could be considered for indicated prevention. Worsening metabolic symptoms such as prediabetes, rising hypertension, or elevated lipids could also be considered for indicated prevention. Even slender clients can benefit from indicated intervention if they are experiencing cravings or instances of loss of control (Odom et al., 2010).

Identifying prevention opportunities and overcoming barriers and undertaking to comprehensively look for symptoms of PFA in clients could yield significant rewards for the practitioner who has been frustrated by the failure of weight-loss protocols. Diagnosing PFA opens the door to the potential for improved outcomes. It is well worth learning about the manifestations of characteristics of SUD as they resemble addiction to processed foods. Practitioners will be pleased at how readily the SUD diagnostic criteria and ASI lend themselves to chronic overeating. With a positive diagnosis of PFA, practitioners will find themselves on firm ground in their recommendations to apply adapted substance use disorder treatment protocols.

In the diagnosis and assessment processes, practitioners will need to follow diagnostic descriptions presented in Part II to fully assess the consequences of PFA. Because Western cultures have framed the problem as one of weight loss for so long, practitioners are not necessarily accustomed to probe for the full extent of consequences beyond the accumulation of adipose tissue. Ironically, when the full force of PFA is recognized, excess adipose tissue becomes a secondary concern. Research has begun to consider whether excess fat tissue is the problem it was once thought to be. Weight may take a back seat to issues of cognitive impairment, depression, fatigue, strong cravings, distressing bingeing behavior, and mobility. This may be so because these nonweight issues such as cognitive impairment may present significant barriers to organizing unprocessed, nonaddictive meals. As such, nonweight issues may present insurmountable barriers to recovery if left unaddressed.

8.1.3 The PFA Diagnosis vs. Other Diagnoses

Practitioners may also be using eating disorder diagnoses and missing PFA as an SUD. These diagnoses may include binge eating disorder (BED), bulimia, and anorexia. In a PFA model, the BED diagnosis does not entirely fit for the reason that binge use of addictive substances is not a diagnosis in the DSM 5. No addictive substance includes a diagnosis for bingeing. However, BED has been shown to make PFA worse and so it is useful to establish whether the client is bingeing as opposed to grazing. Thus it remains an important construct to assess. Practitioners will want to discover whether the client is bingeing on processed foods or unprocessed foods. Bingeing on processed foods can be seen as an SUD while bingeing on unprocessed foods may be thought of as a separate disorder that could be treated more like a process disorder.

Bulimia may be thought of as an attempt to compensate for PFA. It is also associated with more difficult outcomes and should be described in the assessment. Likewise, anorexia may also be an attempt to overcome PFA. In any eating disorder, there is compelling evidence for the harmful properties of processed foods, particularly their role in the development of neuroanomalies. Thus, processed foods should be avoided in the treatment of eating disorders.

Although there is research on the validity of the Yale Food Addiction Scale (YFAS) (Brunault, Ballon, Gaillard, Reveillere, & Courtois, 2014; Carr, Catak, Pejsa-Reitz, Saules, & Gearhardt, 2016; Chen, Tang, Guo, Liu, & Xiao, 2015; Clark & Saules, 2013; Gearhardt, Corbin, & Brownell, 2016; Gearhardt, Roberto, Seamans, Corbin, & Brownell, 2013; Meule, Muller,

Gearhardt, & Blechert, 2016; Pursey, Stanwell, Gearhardt, Collins, & Burrows, 2014), there is some evidence that it is not measuring PFA as an SUD but rather as a behavioral disorder such as shopping, gambling, or sex. The scale operationalizes the DSM 5 SUD criteria. However, PFA is a disorder with many manifestations, some of which are missing from the YFAS. There are 35 items on the YFAS but PFA manifests in literally hundreds of ways.

For example, the YFAS identifies dangerous use as eating or thinking about food while crossing a street, operating equipment, or driving a car. However, food-addicted clients may also eat spoiled food and burn themselves eating foods that are too hot or still frozen. Clients may also run the danger of blacking out while driving. Research shows that they are prone to accidents due to balance issues related to joints, excess adipose tissue, and an inability to see their feet. The YFAS does not surface these possibilities. So it is possible that the YFAS is underdiagnosing for ion because it does not include enough of the range of manifestations of the pathology.

As another example, the YFAS asks about avoiding social events for fear of the foods that will be there or fear of loss of control. However, clients may also avoid social events due to fears related to weight and not fitting in. These possibilities are not included in the YFAS.

The YFAS appears to underdiagnose for PFA. A recent study evaluated the YFAS using an online general population provided through Amazon known as Amazon Mechanical Turks. Its prevalence rate in this population of was only 14% in spite of a study population that was 28.7% overweight and 31.1% obese (Schulte, 2015 #3582). It does not seem logical that the overweight and obese populations did not experience unintended use, failure to cut back, and/or use in spite of knowledge of consequences and distress as a result. This is not logical considering evidence that 46% of American women have been shown to be trying to lose weight and thusly meeting Criterion 1 (Bish et al., 2005). The failure rate for weight loss is measured at 95%, which would seem to demonstrate widespread unintended use (Turk et al., 2009). And research showing that diabetics are not diet-compliant with recommendations to manage diet and the prevalence of overweight and obesity would indicate widespread conformance with Criterion 9, use in spite of knowledge of consequences (Rivellese et al., 2008). Given that a pound per person per day of processed foods disappears into the US domestic economy (Ifland et al., 2009) and research shows that it takes only 16 ingestions of a milkshake before addictive neuroadaptations appear (Burger & Stice, 2014), it seems unlikely that only 14% of the population has developed PFA.

The YFAS also does not take into account that food-addicted people may be using a number of different substances in the addiction. Lumping all foods into a single category of processed foods may suppress endorsement rates. For example, a client may crave chocolate and endorse that criteria but may not even think of coffee as an addictive substance that should be considered in endorsing withdrawal (avoidance of fatigue). This seems to call into question the ability of the YFAS to assess the upper range of severity where strong recovery programs would be most needed.

This textbook recommends becoming familiar with the many facets of PFA as organized under the DSM 5 SUD criteria. These facets will become clearer in the following chapters.

The gaps in the YFAS illustrate a key point. It is easy to confuse PFA with eating behaviors. To maintain clarity, it is important for practitioners to remember that in PFA, eating is just a means for absorbing addictive substances. Eating for the food-addicted client is no different than drinking for the alcoholic, snorting for the cocaine addict, smoking for the nicotine/cannabis addict, or injecting for the heroin addict. This concept may help practitioners to focus on the addictive substances rather than being distracted or confused by the fact that the substances are being eaten rather than smoked or injected.

8.1.4 Probing for Subtleties and Severity

As practitioners read through descriptions of the DSM 5 SUD criteria as they manifest in chronic overeating, two thoughts may stand out. First, it is easy to miss the subtleties of PFA and therefore to miss its onset and understate its severity. Many addicts minimize use and its consequences. Food-addicted clients are no different, plus clients may be suffering from memory loss. Practitioners would benefit from probing and listening carefully for the nuances of food-addicted behavior. Asking about different foods that might have been used in each criterion also helps to jog memory.

Overeating is so common in obesogenic cultures that practitioners may be tempted to dismiss aberrant eating behaviors as normal. Recalling that cigarette smoking was "normal" at one time may help practitioners categorize food-related behaviors as pathological even though the behaviors may be very common. Taking into consideration the vast quantities of addictive foods that disappear into the US economy, practitioners may ascribe importance to behaviors that under other circumstances might be benign. A smoker in 1960 would not be identified as problematic; however, a smoker in 2010 would be. Similarly, instances of loss of control over eating in 1930 during the Great Depression could reflect anxiety about shortages of food. However, in the obesogenic environment of 2016, loss of control could indicate the beginning of an addictive relationship with processed foods. In short, practitioners would do well to consider the obesogenic culture in which the assessment is taking place.

The second point that may surface from reading the SUD criteria is that, in some cases, PFA could be a more serious addiction than drug addiction. The assessment for severity of PFA quickly surfaces comparisons with drug addiction. Food-addicted clients, e.g., may have experienced PFA as very young children, even toddlers. This is as opposed to drug and alcohol addicts, whose earliest experiences may be as adolescents. Drug addicts may be combining one or two addictive substances, whereas food-addicted clients are likely to be routinely combining all of the major categories of addictive foods. Food manufacturers may be formulating foods to be particularly addictive, using ingredients that are unknown to the public. Further, the cuing in terms of advertising and availability for processed foods is intense in Western cultures, far exceeding that of drugs of abuse. Assessments for severity may turn up a surprising number of very severe cases. If an unexpected number of severe cases turns up, practitioners can treat them as such rather than assuming that some of the criteria are not important.

Although it may seem uncomfortable to inform a client of a finding of severity, practitioners may be surprised that clients accept the diagnosis with relief. After grave suffering for decades, clients may be grateful to find a solution. They may already suspect that they have a serious problem. They may be glad that a practitioner is taking their problem seriously and helping them to devise a plan that is comprehensive enough to manage the problem.

8.1.5 Using the ASI

The ASI serves to formulate a list of options. This helps practitioner and client decide where to start in the development of a comprehensive recovery program. For example, the assessment takes into account the extent to which the client is required to be around addictive foods in order to fulfill life obligations. Processed foods and drinks are used throughout the day in many different social, business, school, and faith-based situations. If clients are exposed to extensive cuing, they may have to make lifestyle adjustments before attempting to produce clean food. In some cases, cue-avoidance strategies may need to be in place before the client can quell cravings enough to choose healthy foods. Clients may only need to avoid cuing for a few months while sensitivities in reward pathways are reduced.

The ASI also surfaces problems with frequency measures. PFA behaviors can be virtually continuous throughout the day for a client. As is shown in the chapters following this introduction, some of the DSM criteria may be experienced by clients simultaneously and frequently throughout the day. Practitioners can ask clients how often they experience SUD symptoms and give the client the option of answering continuously. This helps the practitioner see the degree of compulsion from which the client suffers.

Similarly, if the client is exposed to stressful family situations, it may be unrealistic to start trying to make clean foods. Stress, particularly relationship stress, is a known relapse trigger. If the stressful relationships are occurring inside the client's home, the client may need to learn and practice defensive relationship strategies before starting a food plan. This is especially the case if addicted children are present in the home. (See Chapter 30, "Strategies for Helping Food-Addicted Children," in Part III, "Treatment.") A client who is financially devastated may need budgeting skills in order to start a nonaddictive food plan. The ability to effectively prioritize approaches depends on a comprehensive, in-depth assessment.

The drug counselor and general health practitioner will hopefully feel at home with the similarities between assessing PFA and classic drug addiction assessment in terms of conformance with DSM 5 SUD diagnostic criteria as well as the ASI. Eating disorder professionals may be unfamiliar with these criteria themselves but familiar with the problems that eating-disordered clients face. ED counselors will be able to categorize known ED symptomology into the SUD diagnostic categories.

Counselors may find that some clients have such severe impairments of such a wide variety that if they were drug-addicted, residential treatment would be recommended. However, insurance coverage for PFA is nonexistent and eating-disorder clinics may be unwilling to support the abstinence and harm-reduction protocols that PFA calls for. Many clients will be unable to afford to go to residential facilities for lack of funds and obligations to jobs or families. Regardless of severity, some clients will not be able to develop abstinence from the full range of addictive foods. Accomplishing a reduction in harm through partial abstinence can be considered a treatment success, as is the case with drug and alcohol addiction. Nonetheless, a finding of severity based on the number of DSM 5 SUD criteria met could encourage the client to build a more comprehensive program at home than would be the case without a comprehensive diagnosis. A variety of treatment resources can be found at www.foodaddicitonresources.com.

Dissimilarities of PFA to drug addiction are found in terms of the young age of onset, prevalence of cues, easy availability, and polysubstance nature. Asking a client about their first memories of cravings or food obsession will quickly show practitioners that most clients meet this criteria for severity with age of onset starting as young as toddlerhood.

Practitioners may be uneasy with assessing for exposure to food cues because of the prevalence of cues and the feeling of the impossibility of avoiding processed food cues. However, cue management can be accomplished slowly and through education about the seriousness of exposure to food cues. Missing the extent of cuing in a client's daily routines could undermine an otherwise sound program.

The polysubstance nature of processed food abuse can be understood from a review of Chapter 6, "Abstinent Food Plans for Processed Food Addiction," in Part I of this textbook. Sweeteners, flour, gluten, salt, processed fats, dairy, and caffeine are consumed in great quantities in Westernized cultures and almost always in combinations. Fast food products can combine all of the addictive substances with flour and gluten in a bun, taco shell, or pizza crust. Sugar is found in sauces, French fry coatings, and drinks. Cheese and processed fats are added to virtually everything and caffeine is in the drinks. A quick question about what the client ate and drank for breakfast will surface these combinations. Addictions that use multiple substances are harder to treat. Practitioners can use this research to persuade clients to build sufficiently comprehensive programs of abstinence, cue avoidance, cognitive restoration, and group support.

Of course, even with an appropriate diagnosis and assessment, practitioners know that addictions are hard to treat. The conditioned vulnerabilities of an addict's brain lead to a lifelong risk of relapse. In environments where cues are rife, the risks run higher. Recovery from PFA suffers from this fact of life. Clients are comprehensively impaired, yet they need to learn how to make meals that are free from literally thousands of addictive ingredients. It is difficult to ask the client to consistently prepare abstinent meals without becoming overwhelmed. However, with a comprehensive assessment, the practitioner and client can work together to plan a "doable" course of action to yield a sufficiently comprehensive and focused program.

8.1.6 Strengths and Limitations

The strengths of diagnostic and assessment techniques lie in the body of research supporting the DSM 5 as the gold standard criteria for diagnosing SUD and in the ASI for assessment. There is a significant body of research showing that the characteristics of SUD as described in the DSM 5 exist in chronic overeaters. A second strength is the grave need for better approaches to assessment in the epidemic of disordered eating. The limitation of the processes is that the diagnostic and assessment tools have undergone limited testing for PFA.

8.2 WHY DIAGNOSE AND ASSESS: PURPOSES OF DIAGNOSIS AND ASSESSMENT

There are quite a few reasons to assess clients for PFA. The first is to avoid confusing the client's condition with weight loss and clarifying the condition of addiction. Secondly, an assessment identifies parameters and severity of the problem. This information can motivate a client to start undertaking the protocols associated with recovery. Next, an assessment defines the problem. It lets the client see the parameters of the problem, which can be relief for a client who has struggled with misdiagnoses. An assessment also yields the finding of severity, which can help clients stay with recovery until they have achieved adequate protection against painful lapses. Another reason for assessment is to educate the client about problems related to food abuse. People may not recognize the broad range of health problems associated with processed foods.

The assessment also helps both practitioner and client develop outcome expectancies that can offer hope to the client. The client can consider the cooking and coping skills that will support recovery and lead to self-efficacy. The assessment will also surface other disordered use of food such as anorexia, binge eating, and bulimia. These can make PFA even harder to treat.

8.2.1 Distinguishing Weight Loss from PFA

A central purpose of assessing for PFA is to avoid confusing PFA with weight issues. By carefully working through the DSM 5 SUD criteria, the practitioner avoids missing PFA in normally weighted clients. Addiction can be present before enough fat tissue accumulates to become a weight problem. As a corollary, the practitioner also avoids automatically diagnosing PFA in obese clients. It is possible for an obese client to be incidentally obese from eating the calorie-dense foods readily available in Westernized cultures without having developed dysfunctional consequences. This client may just need advice on foods to avoid and foods to consume.

By relying on the DSM 5 SUD criteria, the practitioner can uncover preaddiction. Even if the ASI assessment does not seem serious, given the consequences of progression, the practitioner can treat preaddiction aggressively. The data gathered from the diagnostic criteria can also be used to help inform an assessment of PFA in children. Those criteria are included in Chapter 30, "Strategies for Helping Food-Addicted Children," found in Part III of this textbook, "Treatment." It can be hard to disassociate the degree of overweight and obesity from PFA but dependence on the DSM 5 SUD criteria and the ASI are the keys.

8.2.2 Motivating the Client

The diagnostic and assessment processes will yield valuable data on failure to cut back. Clients are likely to present with a long history of failures to lose weight. They are likely to have developed a fear of failure and a reluctance to try again. Practitioners will recognize the discouragement from repeated failures to lose weight. The approach here is to emphasize the hope of a new protocol based on the addiction model. With this approach, the practitioner can allay fears of failure. It is also helpful to share examples of success by taking the program slowly. Encourage the client to buy into the idea that by going slowly and picking out easy tasks, a solid program can be built over time. Failure only comes from not meeting goals within a specified period of time. So assure the client that there are no deadlines and the client will have all the time they need to build a dependable program.

8.2.3 Defining the Scope of the Problem

A role for the assessment is defining the parameters of the target behavior and comorbidities. The assessment is the first stage of delineating benefits from recovery. The practitioner would do well to use both DSM 5 and ASI to develop a broad scope of the pathology in physical, mental, emotional, behavioral, financial, professional, and family management. PFA, like all addictions, can be associated with very broad impairment. While it is important not to overwhelm clients, it can be useful to give them hope for building a lifestyle that yields a broad range of important benefits.

As part of the problem assessment, it is important to ask about mobility and fatigue because they can be barriers to both meal preparation and exercise, and these are important elements of recovery. Asking about quality of sleep is helpful, as sleep can significantly impact cognitive functionality. If the practitioner is trained to assess cognitive functioning, it is important to do so, with and without the presence of food cues. This may help motivate the client to remove processed foods from the home and to avoid making decisions in the grocery store. Assessing impaired cognitive abilities will help create realistic expectations for early-stage skill acquisition.

Cuing is a leading problem in relapse avoidance. Assessing the client's unavoidable and elective exposure to cues in their daily and weekly routines can help determine how important developing strategies for cue avoidance in early recovery can be. Learning to avoid food cues may not be too difficult; however, developing the client's motivation to avoid cues can be a challenge. Clients may find it difficult to accept that it is dangerous for them to go into a grocery store, just as it would be dangerous for an alcoholic in early-stage recovery to go into a bar. The need to avoid the break room at work, the fast food outlets on the highway, and restaurants on friday night can all be hard for clients to accept.

If the client has minimal food preparation skills, the assessment will surface this important problem. Simple cooking methods such as filling a slow cooker will be best at first. Frying foods is also relatively easy. How to set up a baking tray or filling a soup pot are also easy to teach.

Cognitive impairment is a significant problem because of the need to acquire meal preparation and cue avoidance skills. Online brain training such as Lumosity and Brain Age may be effective for cognitive restoration (Hardy et al., 2015; Kesler et al., 2013; Mayas, Parmentier, Andres, & Ballesteros, 2014; Nouchi et al., 2012; Nouchi et al., 2013). At the same time, the burden of engaging in brain training games is light and flexible, so clients are generally willing to participate.

A surprisingly important problem to assess is the status of unavoidable stressful personal relationships for increased risk of relapse. If there is an unpleasant person in the client's life, it is possible that the attempt to work a clean food plan will attract ridicule and possibly sabotage. If addicted children are likely to endure emotional withdrawals, the client should be prepared for that. It is important to ask about these issues and offer strategies for setting boundaries.

Defining the scope of the problem is a crucial role for the assessment. This is especially true in assessing PFA because of the general focus on excess adipose tissue to the exclusion of the broad range of other dysfunctions associated with chronic abuse of processed foods.

8.2.4 Determining a Diagnosis

The DSM 5 SUD criteria provide a well-substantiated guide for developing a reliable diagnosis. Practitioners may find that PFA is common. The DSM specifies that meeting only two of the

SUD criteria and exhibiting distress within a year would indicate a problem with substance abuse. However, many people might meet at least four of the SUD criteria of failure to cut back, unintended use, cravings, and use in spite of knowledge of consequences. As practitioners gain experience with the 11 SUD criteria, they may be surprised at how many obese people meet all of them. At the other end of the spectrum, it may be hard to find anyone who doesn't meet at least one criteria, especially use in spite of knowledge of consequences.

Clients may be relieved to have an accurate diagnosis after years of failing to conform to weight-loss protocols. Sharing with a client a diagnosis and its severity may increase determination to put the disorder into remission. Practitioners can explain that severity of addiction translates into increased risk of relapse. Understanding these concepts is important in the development of treatment. Because of the prevalence of processed food cues, the common use of processed foods in Westernized cultures, as well as the stress of restructuring relationships, correctly assessing severity is important. Accurate assessment of severity is needed to determine the necessary extent of cue avoidance, abstinence, cognitive restoration, energy, relationship repair, physical recovery, etc. Underassessing severity can lead to a program that is too weak to keep the disease in remission. Overassessing can lead to unnecessary and unrewarding changes in lifestyle, which can erode confidence in the program. Accurate assessment of severity is vital.

Food-related conditions are also important to catalog during the assessment. The ASI helps practitioners identify:

1. Other psychiatric diagnoses and problematic psychological states including depression, anger, anxiety, and shame. The range of severity can run from mild to suicide ideation, rage, and panic.
2. Physical diagnoses including diabetes, heart disease, joint impairment, hypertension, excessive adipose tissue.
3. Mental diagnoses including ADD, ADHD, memory loss, poor decision-making, poor impulse control, and inability to achieve satiation.
4. Behavioral problems including hiding food, bingeing, starving, purging, disrupted sleep, night eating, and lethargy.

8.2.5 Developing Outcome Expectancies

Practitioners should outline outcome expectancies in the assessment. The emphasis should be on mental health over weight loss. Clients should be able to connect the full spectrum of diet-related diseases to processed foods. Practitioners should discuss the process of adjusting to a nonobese body in terms of sexuality and attractiveness. Heightened relapse risk should be clearly delineated and tied to number of DSM criteria met, young age of onset, prevalence of cues, polysubstance use (sugar, gluten, salt, processed fats, dairy, caffeine, additives), and ready availability of cheap, convenient fast foods. The practitioner should make explicit reference to meal preparation skills, either as not needing much attention in the case of skilled clients or needing to go slow and develop simple meal preparation routines in the case of inexperienced clients. The ability to shop for, cook, and assemble meals of nonaddictive, unprocessed foods is crucial to success. Planning ahead may be thought of as a separate skill that the practitioner can monitor. The ability to schedule on-time meals in the context of a busy life is also a skill that clients may not have. The practitioner can motivate the client to develop meal preparation skills by offering the expectancy of a range of valuable outcomes such as improvements in diet-related diseases, fatigue, depression, and cognitive abilities.

Self-efficacy is an arena that the practitioner will want to explore. Clients can build a belief in their own ability to succeed. In recovery from PFA, much depends on attracting the client to the addiction model and away from the "weight loss" model. It is helpful for the client to make a commitment to taking the process of recovery slowly to eliminate the possibility of failure.

8.2.6 Personal Assessment: Domains of Assessment

The personalities of food-addicted clients are similar to those of drug-addicted clients. They manifest depression, anxiety, and anger. These can be barriers to recovery and should be included in the assessment. PFA may be complicated by anorexia, bulimia, binge eating, and weight-loss surgery. If the client also has one of these conditions, specialized counseling may be needed. Treatment may be complicated by job or obligations to family care. While weight loss may be a powerful motivator, cognitive restoration is also generally a strong motivator.

8.2.7 Determining Readiness to Change and Readiness for Treatment

The stages of readiness for treatment of PFA are similar to those of drug addiction. The personalized feedback derived from the assessment process facilitates the motivation to change. Stages of readiness are covered in detail in Part III of the textbook, "Treatment," and include:

1. Reasons for change
2. Problem recognition
3. Optimism about change
4. Commitment to change
5. Action
6. Maintenance

The assessment plays a central role in identifying the reasons for change and the process of recognizing the problem. Based on the strategies that the assessment suggests, the practitioner can work through the client's concerns about making the change and build optimism and commitment. The treatment plan as developed from the assessment serves as a guide for the long, slow process of disengaging from cues, restoring cognitive function, developing a routine for meal preparation, setting boundaries in relationships, exercising and sleeping regularly, and becoming situated in a support system.

8.3 HOW AND WHEN TO ASSESS: PRACTICAL ASPECTS OF THE ASSESSMENT PROCESS

8.3.1 How Much Is Enough? Balancing Scope of Assessment with Cost and Utility

Although extensive assessment would yield valuable information, it is often not practical nor cost-effective to conduct full assessments. However, just developing the client's status according to the DSM 5 SUD criteria could yield enough information to accomplish the goals of persuading a client to the PFA model, of motivating a client to undertake recovery, and of laying out options to start recovery. Creating a baseline of problems organized by the DSM 5 SUD criteria would also be enough to track progress and encourage the client to keep building a recovery program.

If resources are available, it would be desirable to run a full physical to gather information about nutritional status, hidden needs for medication, and range of mobility. A full physical could impact treatment insofar as referrals to specialists may be needed. An assessment of mental capabilities could determine whether the client is capable of making decisions in a grocery store or needs to engage a shopping service. An assessment of mood would demonstrate the client's ability to manage difficult relationships as well as the ability to care for self. An in-depth review of the DSM 5 SUD criteria could take many visits. Each criteria could surface a long history of multiple dysfunctions. However, this textbook bears in mind that clients are likely to be of limited means, which points the practitioner in the direction of a single-visit data-collection effort based on the DSM 5.

In spite of limitations, getting the comprehensive information needed to develop a treatment plan would require more than just the DSM data. Information for a treatment plan would be collected in subsequent visits.

8.3.2 Timing and Sequence of Assessments

Periodically reassessing clients has significant benefits in terms of keeping the client on track. This is particularly true for PFA in an environment where competing nutritional and weight-loss ideas are often pressed on clients by media, health professionals, friends, and family. Clients can be motivated to stay on track by periodically reviewing progress. A periodic review reinforces the many connections between processed foods and diseases. Initially, it may be hard for clients to believe that so many problems could be associated with processed foods. These connections are not broadly disseminated by media, which is dependent on the food and medical industries for advertising revenues. Nor are medical personnel typically familiar with diet solutions to ailments, being versed rather in pharmaceutical and surgical solutions to health problems. So the PFA counselor may have the pleasure of sharing in the unexpected remission of a broad range of physical, mental, emotional, and behavioral problems.

It is important to remember that clients may be suffering from memory loss. So bringing benefits to mind enriches recovery and makes the recovery more valuable to the client. Also of importance is that recovery is taking place in an environment that is rife with friendly food-pushers. In short, the client can use a periodic rearming with reasons not to take other advice nor cave to a bite here and there. Information about the many benefits of recovery protects the client against the pressures of an obesogenic culture.

Clients who come into recovery with severe cases may need follow-up more often. Clients whose severity is demonstrated by a long history of attempts to lose weight may be challenged to let go of so much inappropriate information. Clients may still experience the urge to restrict calories; eliminate fats, protein, or carbs; fast; overexercise; expose the brain to heavy cueing; undertake harmful surgery; use sugary meal replacements; and process foods at home in food processors. Periodically touching back to the assessment can help clients remember that not only did these approaches fail, but they could possibly have worsened the PFA. Timing of reassessment can be based on severity of overeating, risk of relapse, and consequences.

8.3.3 Methods to Enhance Validity and Reliability of Assessments

Validity is an important challenge in assessment of PFA due to memory loss, denial, and shame issues in clients. Establishing an accurate assessment is quite important as a means to motivating the client to undertake the broad range of tasks necessary to protect against a complex obesogenic environment. It may not be advisable to use collateral informants, as the client may have hidden overeating from friends and family. A collateral informant may deepen shame and even contribute to distrust of the practitioner.

On the other hand, biological measures may be helpful. These include symptoms of the metabolic syndrome such as excess adipose tissue, diabetes, hypertension, inflammation markers, cardiovascular disease, and cancer. If a client is describing the consumption of only healthy foods, the practitioner may gently ask the client's opinion about what foods might have caused the weight gain or other metabolic disorder. This could elicit new information about patterns of consumption of addictive, calorie-dense foods.

Practitioners will want to be vigilant about not missing an early-stage diagnosis. In the absence of any metabolic disorders, including weight gain, clients may have still developed cravings, unintended use, failed attempts to cut back, or use in spite of knowledge of consequences. This information could be surfaced in a review of the DSM 5 SUD criteria. Meeting only two of the criteria along with distress indicates the presence of a problem. Information about the harmful properties of processed foods and cues could thwart the progression of the disease to a more severe case.

8.3.4 Interviewing Techniques and Styles

After practitioners have read through the following chapters describing the breadth and severity of the distress associated with PFA, it is hoped that they will develop a new depth of compassion for what clients have suffered. The evidence demonstrates that the consequences of chronic abuse of processed foods are painful on many levels including physical, mental, emotional, behavioral, and spiritual. Compounding the suffering are the judgmental, condescending attitudes of Westernized cultures to obese people. Unfortunately, condescension has been demonstrated in health professionals (Phelan et al., 2015). Through exposure to the difficulties that clients have suffered, health professionals can develop empathy with their plight and avoid ridicule, bullying, or criticism.

As with all addictions, motivational interviewing is appropriate for food-addicted clients. Motivational interviewing emphasizes empathy and supports client autonomy in a discussion of whether changes would be worth making. With this approach, practitioners can avoid power struggles and persuasion in favor of developing the client's own reasons for undertaking recovery. The style is to use the information collected in the diagnosis and assessment to explore the client's concerns rather than try to persuade the client that treatment is the only option (Moyers & Glynn, 2013, 381–382).

Practitioners will want to be respectful and patient throughout the diagnostic and assessment processes. Adopting a motivational style that is nonjudgmental and supportive will help. Practitioners will remember that clients suffer from memory loss and that recalling events, foods, and behaviors may be difficult. For the same reason, practitioners may need to repeat information. Handouts will help reinforce auditory information. Food-addicted clients also suffer from shame and may not be able to share about embarrassing situations, particularly around bingeing, perceived failures, and difficult relationships.

Practitioners may be helpful by reassuring clients that their situations are not their fault. Rather, an aggressive food industry has deliberately formulated and marketed products to be addictive. Explaining why weight-loss regimes could make PFA worse also helps clients reduce self-blame and move forward with confidence.

8.4 PUTTING IT ALL TOGETHER

8.4.1 Treatment Planning and Matching Clients to Treatment

The assessment will surface strategies for building a program of protection against relapse into the use of addictive processed foods. Programs have to accomplish many different complex objectives. These include meal preparation, cue avoidance, cognitive restoration, exercise, sleep, education, disease resolution, and especially relationship management. The initial stages of treatment can focus on the slow but steady development of skills to realize goals. The key challenge is how to sequence goals. The solution is to let the client pick from a list of options. The practitioner can develop the options based on the problems surfaced in the assessment. Options are described in Part III, "Treatment."

The practitioner can also point out the strengths of the client. The client can start with strengths in terms of comfort level with cooking skills, exercise, cognitive restoration, cue avoidance, etc. Advanced issues are similar to recovery from drug addiction and include relationship repair, financial stability, employment, and volunteer service activities.

8.4.2 Avoid Overwhelm with a Menu of Options of Small Steps

The menu could include starting with mental, physical, behavioral, or food issues. Because of limited cognitive abilities, clients are easily overwhelmed and prone to quitting if presented with too much information. Slow but steady wins the race. There are more suggestions in Part III, "Treatment."

8.5 SUMMARY

Relying on classic drug addiction diagnostic techniques furthers the field of PFA assessment. Use of the DSM 5 SUD diagnostic criteria gives both practitioners and clients a helpful orientation to overeating as a substance use disorder rather than only a behavioral disorder. Use of the DSM 5 also gives both practitioner and client the ability to see the broad range of pathology and dysfunction associated with chronic abuse of processed foods. This leads to the development of broad goals, recognition of broad results, and greater motivation to adhere to a recovery program. By widening the scope of benefits well beyond weight loss, clients can appreciate the program elements needed to adequately protect against relapse. They can also adopt a long-term view of recovery as opposed to a short-term weight-loss program.

By leaning on the DSM 5 SUD diagnostic criteria, practitioners can defend against the temptation to overlook, downplay, or minimize the seriousness of conformance to any of the criteria. By matching severity developed through the ASI to a comprehensive recovery program, the practitioner can look forward to improving outcomes.

Accurately identifying and quantifying the distress of PFA allows practitioners to help stem the epidemic of chronic overeating. Looking for PFA in a broad array of health-care settings can relieve the suffering associated with processed food use.

REFERENCES

American Psychiatric Association. (2013). *The Diagnostic and Statistical Manual of Mental Disorders, Fifth Edition* (Vol. 5), Washington DC.

Bish, C. L., Blanck, H. M., Serdula, M. K., Marcus, M., Kohl, H. W., 3rd, & Khan, L. K. (2005). Diet and physical activity behaviors among Americans trying to lose weight: 2000 Behavioral Risk Factor Surveillance System. *Obes Res*, *13*(3), 596–607. doi:10.1038/oby.2005.64.

Brewer-Smyth, K., Cornelius, M., & Pohlig, R. T. (2016). Childhood adversity and mental health correlates of obesity in a population at risk. *J Correct Health Care*, *22*(4), 367–382. doi:10.1177/1078345816670161.

Brunault, P., Ballon, N., Gaillard, P., Reveillere, C., & Courtois, R. (2014). Validation of the French version of the Yale Food Addiction Scale: An examination of its factor structure, reliability, and construct validity in a nonclinical sample. *Can J Psychiatry*, *59*(5), 276–284.

Burger, K. S., & Stice, E. (2014). Greater striatopallidal adaptive coding during cue-reward learning and food reward habituation predict future weight gain. *NeuroImage*, *99*, 122–128. doi:10.1016/j.neuroimage.2014.05.066.

Carr, M. M., Catak, P. D., Pejsa-Reitz, M. C., Saules, K. K., & Gearhardt, A. N. (2016). Measurement invariance of the Yale Food Addiction Scale 2.0 across gender and racial groups. *Psychol Assess*, *29*(8), 1044–1052. doi:10.1037/pas0000403.

Chen, G., Tang, Z., Guo, G., Liu, X., & Xiao, S. (2015). The Chinese version of the Yale Food Addiction Scale: An examination of its validation in a sample of female adolescents. *Eat Behav*, *18*, 97–102. doi:10.1016/j.eatbeh.2015.05.002.

Clark, S. M., & Saules, K. K. (2013). Validation of the Yale Food Addiction Scale among a weight-loss surgery population. *Eat Behav*, *14*(2), 216–219. doi:10.1016/j.eatbeh.2013.01.002.

Davies, R., Lehman, E., Perry, A., & McCall-Hosenfeld, J. S. (2015). Association of intimate partner violence and health-care provider-identified obesity. *Women Health*, *56*(5), 561–575. doi:10.1080/03630242.2015.1101741.

Franks, P. W., & McCarthy, M. I. (2016). Exposing the exposures responsible for type 2 diabetes and obesity. *Science*, *354*(6308), 69–73. doi:10.1126/science.aaf5094.

Gearhardt, A. N., Corbin, W. R., & Brownell, K. D. (2016). Development of the Yale Food Addiction Scale Version 2.0. *Psychol Addict Behav*, *30*(1), 113–121. doi:10.1037/adb0000136.

Gearhardt, A. N., Roberto, C. A., Seamans, M. J., Corbin, W. R., & Brownell, K. D. (2013). Preliminary validation of the Yale Food Addiction Scale for children. *Eat Behav*, *14*(4), 508–512. doi:10.1016/j.eatbeh.2013.07.002.

Hardy, J. L., Nelson, R. A., Thomason, M. E., Sternberg, D. A., Katovich, K., Farzin, F., & Scanlon, M. (2015). Enhancing cognitive abilities with comprehensive training: A large, online, randomized, active-controlled trial. *PLoS One*, *10*(9), e0134467. doi:10.1371/journal.pone.0134467.

Helton, J. J., & Liechty, J. M. (2014). Obesity prevalence among youth investigated for maltreatment in the United States. *Child Abuse Negl*, *38*(4), 768–775. doi:10.1016/j.chiabu.2013.08.011.

Henriksen, C. A., Mather, A. A., Mackenzie, C. S., Bienvenu, O. J., & Sareen, J. (2014). Longitudinal associations of obesity with affective disorders and suicidality in the Baltimore epidemiologic catchment area follow-up study. *J Nerv Ment Dis*, *202*(5), 379–385. doi:10.1097/nmd.0000000000000135.

Ifland, J. R., Preuss, H. G., Marcus, M. T., Rourke, K. M., Taylor, W. C., Burau, K., . . . Manso, G. (2009). Refined food addiction: A classic substance use disorder. *Med Hypotheses*, *72*(5), 518–526. doi:S0306-9877(08)00642-7 [pii] 10.1016/j.mehy.2008.11.035 [doi].

Kesler, S., Hadi Hosseini, S. M., Heckler, C., Janelsins, M., Palesh, O., Mustian, K., & Morrow, G. (2013). Cognitive training for improving executive function in chemotherapy-treated breast cancer survivors. *Clin Breast Canc*, *13*(4), 299–306. doi:10.1016/j.clbc.2013.02.004.

Lee, H., Andrew, M., Gebremariam, A., Lumeng, J. C., & Lee, J. M. (2014). Longitudinal associations between poverty and obesity from birth through adolescence. *Am J Public Health*, *104*(5), e70–e76. doi:10.2105/AJPH.2013.301806.

Lydecker, J. A., & Grilo, C. M. (2016). Children of parents with BED have more eating behavior disturbance than children of parents with obesity or healthy weight. *Int J Eat Disord*, *50*(6), 648–656. doi:10.1002/eat.22648.

Martire, S. I., Westbrook, R. F., & Morris, M. J. (2015). Effects of long-term cycling between palatable cafeteria diet and regular chow on intake, eating patterns, and response to saccharin and sucrose. *Physiol Behav*, *139*, 80–88. doi:10.1016/j.physbeh.2014.11.006.

Mayas, J., Parmentier, F. B., Andres, P., & Ballesteros, S. (2014). Plasticity of attentional functions in older adults after non-action video game training: A randomized controlled trial. *PLoS One*, *9*(3), e92269. doi:10.1371/journal.pone.0092269.

Meule, A., Muller, A., Gearhardt, A. N., & Blechert, J. (2016). German version of the Yale Food Addiction Scale 2.0: Prevalence and correlates of 'food addiction' in students and obese individuals. *Appetite*, *1*(115), 54–61. doi:10.1016/j.appet.2016.10.003.

Moyers, T. B., & Glynn, L. H. (2013). Enhancing motivation for treatment and change. In B. S. McCrady & E. E. Epstein (Eds.), *Addictions A Comprehensive Guidebook*, pp. 377–390, New York: Oxford University Press.

Nouchi, R., Taki, Y., Takeuchi, H., Hashizume, H., Akitsuki, Y., Shigemune, Y., . . . Kawashima, R. (2012). Brain training game improves executive functions and processing speed in the elderly: A randomized controlled trial. *PLoS One*, *7*(1), e29676. doi:10.1371/journal.pone.0029676.

Nouchi, R., Taki, Y., Takeuchi, H., Hashizume, H., Nozawa, T., Kambara, T., . . . Kawashima, R. (2013). Brain training game boosts executive functions, working memory and processing speed in the young adults: A randomized controlled trial. *PLoS One*, *8*(2), e55518. doi:10.1371/journal.pone.0055518.

Odom, J., Zalesin, K. C., Washington, T. L., Miller, W. W., Hakmeh, B., Zaremba, D. L., . . . McCullough, P. A. (2010). Behavioral predictors of weight regain after bariatric surgery. *Obes Surg*, *20*(3), 349–356. doi:10.1007/s11695-009-9895-6.

Ogden, C. L., Carroll, M. D., Kit, B. K., & Flegal, K. M. (2013). Prevalence of obesity among adults: United States, 2011–2012. *NCHS Data Brief*, (131), 1–8.

Phelan, S. M., Burgess, D. J., Yeazel, M. W., Hellerstedt, W. L., Griffin, J. M., & van Ryn, M. (2015). Impact of weight bias and stigma on quality of care and outcomes for patients with obesity. *Obes Rev*, *16*(4), 319–326. doi:10.1111/obr.12266.

Pursey, K. M., Stanwell, P., Gearhardt, A. N., Collins, C. E., & Burrows, T. L. (2014). The prevalence of food addiction as assessed by the Yale Food Addiction Scale: A systematic review. *Nutrients*, *6*(10), 4552–4590. doi:10.3390/nu6104552.

Rivellese, A. A., Boemi, M., Cavalot, F., Costagliola, L., De Feo, P., Miccoli, R., . . . Zavaroni, I. (2008). Dietary habits in type II diabetes mellitus: How is adherence to dietary recommendations? *Eur J Clin Nutr*, *62*(5), 660–664. doi:10.1038/sj.ejcn.1602755.

Sanders, R. H., Han, A., Baker, J. S., & Cobley, S. (2015). Childhood obesity and its physical and psychological co-morbidities: A systematic review of Australian children and adolescents. *Eur J Pediatr*, *174*(6), 715–746. doi:10.1007/s00431-015-2551-3.

Schuz, B., Bower, J., & Ferguson, S. G. (2015). Stimulus control and affect in dietary behaviours. An intensive longitudinal study. *Appetite, 87C*, 310–317. doi:10.1016/j.appet.2015.01.002.

Treatment Research Institute. (2017). *Addiction Severity Index 5th.* Accessed from http://www.tresearch.org/wp-content/uploads/2012/09/ASI_5th_Ed.pdf

Turk, M. W., Yang, K., Hravnak, M., Sereika, S. M., Ewing, L. J., & Burke, L. E. (2009). Randomized clinical trials of weight loss maintenance: A review. *J Cardiovasc Nurs, 24*(1), 58–80. doi:10.1097/01.jcn.0000317471.58048.32.

Veses, A. M., Gomez-Martinez, S., de Heredia, F. P., Esteban-Cornejo, I., Castillo, R., Estecha, S., . . . Marcos, A. (2015). Cognition and the risk of eating disorders in Spanish adolescents: The AVENA and AFINOS studies. *Eur J Pediatr, 174*(2), 229–236. doi:10.1007/s00431-014-2386-3.

Wiers, C. E., Shokri-Kojori, E., Cabrera, E., Cunningham, S., Wong, C., Tomasi, D., . . . Volkow, N. D. (2016). Socioeconomic status is associated with striatal dopamine D2/D3 receptors in healthy volunteers but not in cocaine abusers. *Neurosci Lett, 617*, 27–31. doi:10.1016/j.neulet.2016.01.056.

Williams, J. W., Canterford, L., Toumbourou, J. W., Patton, G. C., & Catalano, R. F. (2015). Social development measures associated with problem behaviours and weight status in Australian adolescents. *Prev Sci, 16*(6), 822–831. doi:10.1007/s11121-015-0559-6.

Yanos, B. R., Saules, K. K., Schuh, L. M., & Sogg, S. (2014). Predictors of lowest weight and long-term weight regain among Roux-en-Y gastric bypass patients. *Obes Surg, 55*(4), 792–798. doi:10.1007/s11695-014-1536-z.

Zeller, M. H., Noll, J. G., Sarwer, D. B., Reiter-Purtill, J., Rofey, D. L., Baughcum, A. E., . . . Becnel, J. N. (2015). Child maltreatment and the adolescent patient with severe obesity: Implications for clinical care. *J Pediatr Psychol, 40*(7), 640–648. doi:10.1093/jpepsy/jsv011.

9 Assessment of Food Cravings

Adrian Meule
University of Salzburg
Salzburg, Austria

CONTENTS

9.1 DEFINING FOOD CRAVING AND HUNGER

Craving refers to an intense desire to consume a substance. Frequent experiences of craving are a core feature of substance use disorders (Tiffany & Wray, 2012). However, the term *craving* not only refers to drug-related substances but also to other substances like food or nonalcoholic beverages (Hormes & Rozin, 2010). As *food craving* refers to an intense desire to consume a particular food, it is this specificity that differentiates food craving from feelings of hunger. A craving for a specific food can be typically only satisfied by consumption of that food, while hunger can be alleviated by consumption of any type of food. Moreover, food cravings can occur in the absence of hunger; i.e., food deprivation is not a necessary condition for the occurrence of food craving. In a study by Pelchat and Schaefer (2000), e.g., participants were instructed to adhere to a monotonous diet (vanilla-flavored, nutritionally complete drinks) for 5 days. In young adults, the number of food cravings were markedly increased during that period, indicating that sensory monotony without nutritional deprivation is sufficient to stimulate food cravings.

Just because hunger is not a prerequisite for experiencing food craving does not mean, however, that hunger and food craving do not co-occur. In fact, it is likely that in many instances hunger easily turns into a food craving: just imagine when you are feeling very hungry and you are then exposed to the smell of your favorite food—this will most likely induce craving for that exact same food. Nevertheless, even when hunger and craving co-occur, it seems that they can still be differentiated with regard to their physiological and behavioral correlates. In a recent study by Meule and Hormes (2015), participants underwent a chocolate exposure, during which current craving for chocolate increased. Unexpectedly, participants also reported an increase in current hunger. While this may be due to physiological reasons (chocolate exposure may induce a general preparatory response for food ingestion, thereby increasing feelings of hunger) or to methodological issues (it may be difficult for participants to differentiate between feelings of hunger and craving), several dissociations were found:

1. Longer food deprivation (hours since the last meal before the testing) was associated with higher current hunger but not with current chocolate craving.
2. Salivary flow was increased during chocolate exposure, and this increase was associated with increases in current chocolate craving but not with increases in current hunger.

3. Higher chocolate consumption in the laboratory was associated with higher current chocolate craving but not with current hunger.

To conclude, it appears that even when hunger and craving arise simultaneously, they can still be differentiated under certain circumstances, as food deprivation predicts current hunger but not current food craving, and current food craving, but not hunger, predicts food cue-elicited physiological responses and subsequent food intake.

9.2 CULTURAL ASPECTS

Although the concept of food craving exists in most cultures, it appears that the term *craving* does actually not lexicalize in most languages other than English; i.e., there is rarely a truly equivalent translation of the term. While individuals outside of English-speaking countries may well experience what native English speakers would designate as a *craving*, it appears that there is often not a specific word for this experience (Hormes & Rozin, 2010). Thus, the term *craving* (and its translation in other languages in particular) can be somewhat vague and, therefore, there is a need to assess food craving with standardized questionnaires instead of a single question.

Craved foods usually have high energy density brought about by a combination of high sugar and fat content. In North America, the most commonly craved food is chocolate. Other frequently craved foods include pizza, salty snacks, ice cream, other sweets and desserts, and meat and chicken (Weingarten & Elston, 1991). Studies from European countries are rare, but the types of craved foods are most likely very similar to North America. For example, chocolate-containing foods were the most frequently craved foods in a study with women from Germany and Austria (Richard, Meule, Reichenberger, & Blechert, 2017). However, it appears that there are indeed some cultural differences, even within Europe. In a study by Rodriguez et al. (2007), British women reported more frequent chocolate cravings than Spanish women. In other studies, gender differences were found in American participants such that chocolate was the most frequently craved food in women and savory foods were the most frequently craved foods in men. This gender difference was absent in Spanish participants, as chocolate was the most often craved food in both genders (Osman & Sobal, 2006; Zellner, Garriga-Trillo, Rohm, Centeno, & Parker, 1999). Other evidence for cultural differences comes from Arab and Asian countries. For example, it has been reported that savory rather than sweet foods were much more likely to be identified as craved foods in Egyptian adults (Parker, Kamel, & Zellner, 2003). In Japan, rice is the most frequently craved food (of note, however, is that chocolate is still the second most frequently craved food; Komatsu, 2008; Komatsu & Aoyama, 2014).

9.3 ASSESSMENT

As food craving is, by definition, a subjective, psychological experience, the most straightforward approach to measure it is self-report. Although several psychophysiological or behavioral variables have been found to correlate with subjectively reported craving (e.g., heart rate, blood pressure, salivation, attention allocation, consumption; Carter & Tiffany, 1999; Field, Munafò, & Franken, 2009; Nederkoorn, Smulders, & Jansen, 2000; Werthmann et al., 2011), they require technical equipment and usually lack specificity and reliability for indicating craving (Shiffman, 2000).

There are several questionnaires for the assessment of the frequency of food cravings, i.e., for measuring food craving as a trait (Table 9.1). These include questionnaires that measure the frequency of cravings in general or specify a particular type of food. One of the most often-used questionnaires for the assessment of trait food craving, the Food Cravings Questionnaire—Trait (FCQ-T), measures several dimensions of food cravings in general, but items can be easily modified

TABLE 9.1
Overview of Different Questionnaire Measures for the Assessment of Food Craving

Questionnaire	Reference	Number of Items	Time Frame	Description (subscale names in italics)	Translations	Modified versions
Attitudes to Chocolate Questionnaire	Benton, Greenfield, and Morgan (1998)	24	In general	Measures craving for chocolate and eating chocolate for emotional reasons (*craving*), negative feelings associated with eating chocolate (*guilt*), and eating chocolate for functional reasons (*functional*). However, subsequent studies revealed that a 22-item, two-factor solution representing *craving* and *guilt* ought to be preferred over the original factor structure (Cramer & Hartleib, 2001; Müller, Dettmer, & Macht, 2008; Van Gucht, Soetens, Raes, & Griffith, 2014).	Dutch (Van Gucht et al., 2014) German (Müller et al., 2008)	–
Cognitive Fusion Questionnaire—Food Craving	Duarte, Pinto-Gouveia, Ferreira, and Silva (2016)	7	In general	Measures cognitive fusion with undesirable and disturbing food-related thoughts and urges to eat.	Portuguese (Duarte et al., 2016)	–
Control of Eating Questionnaire	Dalton, Finlayson, Hill, and Blundell (2015)	21	In the past 7 days	Measures difficulties in resisting food cravings (*craving control*), affect (*positive mood*), intensity and frequency of craving for sweet foods (*craving for sweet*), and intensity and frequency of craving for savory foods (*craving for savory*).	–	–
Craving Experience Questionnaire—Strength form	May et al. (2014)	10	Right now/at that time	Measures intensity of the craving experience (*intensity*), vividness of the craving experience (*imagery*), and intrusiveness of the craving experience (*intrusiveness*). The substance or type of food needs to be specified by the investigator.	–	–

(Continued)

TABLE 9.1 ***(Continued)***
Overview of Different Questionnaire Measures for the Assessment of Food Craving

Questionnaire	Reference	Number of Items	Time Frame	Description (subscale names in italics)	Translations	Modified versions
Craving Experience Questionnaire—Frequency form	May et al. (2014)	10	To be specified by investigator	Measures frequency of urges (*intensity*), craving-related imaginations (*imagery*), and intrusive craving-related thoughts (*intrusiveness*). The substance or type of food needs to be specified by the investigator.	–	–
Food Cravings Questionnaire—Trait (FCQ-T)	Cepeda-Benito, Gleaves, Williams, and Erath (2000)	39	In general	Measures frequency of having plans to consume food (*plans*), anticipation of positive reinforcement that may result from eating (*positive reinforcement*), anticipation of relief from negative states and feelings as a result from eating (*negative reinforcement*), lack of control over eating (*lack of control*), thoughts or preoccupation with food (*thoughts*), craving as a physiological state (*hunger*), emotions that may be experienced before or during food cravings or eating (*emotions*), cues that may trigger food cravings (*environment*), and guilt from cravings and/or for giving into them (*guilt*).	German (Meule, Lutz, Vögele, & Kübler, 2012) Italian (Innamorati et al., 2014) Korean (Noh et al., 2008) Persian (Kachooei & Ashrafi, 2016) Portuguese (Queiroz de Medeiros, Campos Pedrosa, Hutz, & Yamamoto, 2016; Ulian, et al., 2017) Spanish (Cepeda-Benito, Gleaves, Fernández, et al., 2000)	Chocolate FCQ-T (Rodriguez et al., 2007) Chocolate FCQ-T reduced (Meule & Hormes, 2015) FCQ-T reduced (Meule, Hermann, & Kübler, 2014) General FCQ-T (Nijs, Franken, & Muris, 2007)
Food Cravings Questionnaire—State (FCQ-S)	Cepeda-Benito et al. (2000)	15	Right now, at this very moment	Measures an intense desire to eat (*desire*), anticipation of positive reinforcement that may result from eating (*positive reinforcement*), anticipation of relief from negative states and feelings as a result of eating (*negative reinforcement*), lack of control over eating (*lack of control*), and craving as a physiological state (*hunger*).	German (Meule, Lutz, et al., 2012) Italian (Lombardo, Iani, & Barbaranelli, 2016) Portuguese (Queiroz de Medeiros, Campos Pedrosa, Hutz, & Yamamoto, 2016; Ulian, et al., 2017) Spanish (Cepeda-Benito et al., 2000)	Chocolate FCQ-S (Meule & Hormes, 2015) General FCQ-S (Nijs et al., 2007)

(Continued)

TABLE 9.1 *(Continued)*
Overview of Different Questionnaire Measures for the Assessment of Food Craving

Questionnaire	Reference	Number of Items	Time Frame	Description (subscale names in italics)	Translations	Modified versions
Food Craving Inventory	White, Whisenhunt, Williamson, Greenway, and Netemeyer (2002)	28	In the past month	Measures frequency of cravings for high-fat foods (*high fats*), sweet foods (*sweets*), high-carbohydrate foods (*carbohydrates/starches*), and high-fat fast food (*fast-food fats*). As the questionnaire asks about specific foods, cultural adaptations appear to be necessary for countries outside of North America.	British (Nicholls & Hulbert-Williams, 2013) German (Tarragon, Stein, & Meyer, 2017) Japanese (Komatsu, 2008) Portuguese (Queiroz de Medeiros, Campos Pedrosa, & Yamamoto, 2017) Spanish (Jáuregui Lobera et al., 2010)	–
Questionnaire on Craving for Sweet or Rich Foods	Toll, Katulak, Williams-Piehota, and O'Malley (2008)	14	At this moment/ during the past week	Measures perceptions about the ability of sweet or rich foods to relieve negative affect and about self-control over eating (*relief/control*) and intensity of cravings (*intensity*).	–	–
Orientation to Chocolate Questionnaire	Cartwright and Stritzke (2008)	14	In general	Measures approach inclinations toward chocolate (*approach*), avoidance inclinations toward chocolate (*avoidance*), and feelings of guilt resulting from eating chocolate (*guilt*).	French (Rodgers, Stritzke, Bui, Franko, & Chabrol, 2011)	–

to refer to craving for a particular food (e.g., chocolate). As the FCQ-T is the food craving measure with the highest number of items (Table 9.1), a short version with a one-factorial structure, the FCQ-T-reduced, has been developed, items of which are displayed in Table 9.2. Validity of the FCQ-T and FCQ-T-reduced has been supported such that individuals with higher scores show higher reactivity in response to and approach tendencies towards high-calorie, palatable foods in experimental studies (Brockmeyer, Hahn, Reetz, Schmidt, & Friederich, 2015a; Meule, Skirde, Freund, Vögele, & Kübler, 2012; Ulrich, Steigleder, & Grön, 2016) and report more frequent and more intense food cravings in daily life as measured with ecological momentary assessment (Richard, Meule, Reichenberger, & Blechert, 2017). Furthermore, the scales have good test-retest reliability, suggesting that scores do indeed represent food craving as a stable trait (e.g., Meule, Beck Teran, et al., 2014). Yet, they are also sensitive to treatment changes as indicated by significant reductions of scores in interventional studies (e.g., Brockmeyer, Hahn, Reetz, Schmidt, & Friederich, 2015b; Meule, Freund, Skirde, Vögele, & Kübler, 2012; Schmidt & Martin, 2016). The Food Craving Inventory is another often used food craving measure and assesses craving for 28 foods (Table 9.1). Given the cultural differences outlined above, however, cultural adaptations of certain food items are necessary when using the scale in countries outside of North America (e.g., Jáuregui Lobera, Bolaños, Carbonero, & Valero Blanco, 2010; Komatsu, 2008; Nicholls & Hulbert-Williams, 2013).

Self-report questionnaires for the assessment of momentary food craving include the strength form of the Craving Experience Questionnaire and the Food Cravings Questionnaire—State (FCQ-S; Table 9.1). Similar to the FCQ-T, items of the FCQ-S can be easily modified to refer to a

TABLE 9.2
Items and Response Categories of the Food Cravings Questionnaire-Trait-reduced

	Never	Rarely	Sometimes	Often	Usually	Always
1. When I crave something, I know I won't be able to stop eating once I start.	1	2	3	4	5	6
2. If I eat what I am craving, I often lose control and eat too much.	1	2	3	4	5	6
3. Food cravings invariably make me think of ways to get what I want to eat.	1	2	3	4	5	6
4. I feel like I have food on my mind all the time.	1	2	3	4	5	6
5. I find myself preoccupied with food.	1	2	3	4	5	6
6. Whenever I have cravings, I find myself making plans to eat.	1	2	3	4	5	6
7. I crave foods when I feel bored, angry, or sad.	1	2	3	4	5	6
8. I have no willpower to resist my food crave.	1	2	3	4	5	6
9. Once I start eating, I have trouble stopping.	1	2	3	4	5	6
10. I can't stop thinking about eating no matter how hard I try.	1	2	3	4	5	6
11. If I give in to a food craving, all control is lost.	1	2	3	4	5	6
12. Whenever I have a food craving, I keep on thinking about eating until I actually eat the food.	1	2	3	4	5	6
13. If I am craving something, thoughts of eating it consume me.	1	2	3	4	5	6
14. My emotions often make me want to eat.	1	2	3	4	5	6
15. It is hard for me to resist the temptation to eat appetizing foods that are in my reach.	1	2	3	4	5	6

Note: Individuals are instructed to indicate how frequently each comment is true for them in general. Sum scores of 50 or higher may indicate pathologically elevated food craving levels (Meule, in press).

TABLE 9.3
Items and Response Categories of the Chocolate Version of Food Cravings Questionnaire—State

	Strongly Disagree	Disagree	Neutral	Agree	Strongly Agree
1. I have an intense desire to eat chocolate.	1	2	3	4	5
2. I'm craving chocolate.	1	2	3	4	5
3. I have an urge for chocolate.	1	2	3	4	5
4. Eating chocolate would make things seem just perfect.	1	2	3	4	5
5. If I were to eat chocolate, I am sure my mood would improve.	1	2	3	4	5
6. Eating chocolate would feel wonderful.	1	2	3	4	5
7. If I ate chocolate, I wouldn't feel so sluggish and lethargic.	1	2	3	4	5
8. Satisfying my chocolate craving would make me feel less grouchy and irritable.	1	2	3	4	5
9. I would feel more alert if I could satisfy my chocolate craving.	1	2	3	4	5
10. If I had chocolate, I could not stop eating it.	1	2	3	4	5
11. My desire to eat chocolate seems overpowering.	1	2	3	4	5
12. I know I'm going to keep on thinking about chocolate until I actually have it.	1	2	3	4	5
13. I am hungry.	1	2	3	4	5
14. If I ate right now, my stomach wouldn't feel as empty.	1	2	3	4	5
15. I feel weak because of not eating.	1	2	3	4	5

Note: Individuals are instructed to indicate the extent to which they agree with each statement "right now, at this very moment." Sum scores of Items 1–12 represent current chocolate craving, while sum scores of Items 13–15 represent current hunger.

specific food such as chocolate. As can be seen in Table 9.3, this chocolate version of the FCQ-S assesses both current chocolate craving and current hunger. Validity of the scale has been supported by differential relationships of the craving and the hunger subscale with current food deprivation, salivary flow, and chocolate consumption (see Section 9.1; Meule & Hormes, 2015).

9.4 CONCLUSION

Food craving is a multidimensional experience as it includes cognitive (e.g., thinking about food), emotional (e.g., desire to eat or changes in mood), behavioral (e.g., seeking and consuming food), and physiological (e.g., salivation) aspects (Rodríguez-Martín & Meule, 2015). Although some of these aspects can be measured objectively, subjective self-report appears to be the most viable method for the assessment of food craving. With these self-report measures, food craving can be assessed on a trait level (i.e., asking about the general frequency of food cravings) and as a transient state (i.e., asking about the intensity of momentary food craving). Several questionnaires have been developed for these purposes in the past two decades, with some of them having been well validated and further refined and some having been developed just recently (Table 9.1). While there is some conceptual overlap across measures, some questionnaires differ quite substantially, as they aim to assess different aspects of food craving or conceptualize food craving as unidimensional construct. Thus, researchers and practitioners have a pool of different food craving questionnaires available that allows for selection of the most suited measure, depending on the given research question, clinical purpose or cultural background.

REFERENCES

Benton, D., Greenfield, K., & Morgan, M. (1998). The development of the attitudes to chocolate questionnaire. *Personality and Individual Differences, 24*, 513–520.

Brockmeyer, T., Hahn, C., Reetz, C., Schmidt, U., & Friederich, H. C. (2015a). Approach bias and cue reactivity towards food in people with high versus low levels of food craving. *Appetite, 95*, 197–202.

Brockmeyer, T., Hahn, C., Reetz, C., Schmidt, U., & Friederich, H. C. (2015b). Approach Bias Modification in Food Craving—A Proof-of-Concept Study. *European Eating Disorders Review, 23*, 352–360.

Carter, B. L., & Tiffany, S. T. (1999). Meta-analysis of cue-reactivity in addiction research. *Addiction, 94*, 327–340.

Cartwright, F., & Stritzke, W. G. (2008). A multidimensional ambivalence model of chocolate craving: Construct validity and associations with chocolate consumption and disordered eating. *Eating Behaviors, 9*, 1–12.

Cepeda-Benito, A., Gleaves, D. H., Fernández, M. C., Vila, J., Williams, T. L., & Reynoso, J. (2000). The development and validation of Spanish versions of the state and trait food cravings questionnaires. *Behaviour Research and Therapy, 38*, 1125–1138.

Cepeda-Benito, A., Gleaves, D. H., Williams, T. L., & Erath, S. A. (2000). The development and validation of the state and trait Food-Cravings Questionnaires. *Behavior Therapy, 31*, 151–173.

Cramer, K. M., & Hartleib, M. (2001). The attitudes to chocolate questionnaire: A psychometric evaluation. *Personality and Individual Differences, 31*, 931–942.

Dalton, M., Finlayson, G., Hill, A., & Blundell, J. (2015). Preliminary validation and principal components analysis of the Control of Eating Questionnaire (CoEQ) for the experience of food craving. *European Journal of Clinical Nutrition, 69*, 1313–1317.

Duarte, C., Pinto-Gouveia, J., Ferreira, C., & Silva, B. (2016). Caught in the struggle with food craving: Development and validation of a new cognitive fusion measure. *Appetite, 101*, 146–155.

Field, M., Munafò, M. R., & Franken, I. H. A. (2009). A meta-analytic investigation of the relationship between attentional bias and subjective craving in substance abuse. *Psychological Bulletin, 135*, 589–607.

Hormes, J. M., & Rozin, P. (2010). Does "craving" carve nature at the joints? Absence of a synonym for craving in many languages. *Addictive Behaviors, 35*, 459–463.

Innamorati, M., Imperatori, C., Balsamo, M., Tamburello, S., Belvederi Murri, M., Contardi, A., ... Fabbricatore, M. (2014). Food Cravings Questionnaire-Trait (FCQ-T) discriminates between obese and overweight patients with and without binge eating tendencies: The Italian version of the FCQ-T. *Journal of Personality Assessment, 96*, 632–639.

Jáuregui Lobera, I., Bolaños, P., Carbonero, R., & Valero Blanco, E. (2010). Psychometric properties of the Spanish version of the Food Craving Inventory (FCI-SP). *Nutrición Hospitalaria, 25*, 984–992.

Kachooei, M., & Ashrafi, E. (2016). Exploring the Factor Structure, Reliability and Validity of the Food Craving Questionnaire-Trait in Iranian adults. *Journal of Kerman University of Medical Sciences, 23*, 631–648.

Komatsu, S. (2008). Rice and sushi cravings: A preliminary study of food craving among Japanese females. *Appetite, 50*, 353–358.

Komatsu, S., & Aoyama, K. (2014). Food craving and its relationship with restriction and liking in Japanese females. *Foods, 3*, 208–216.

Lombardo, C., Iani, L., & Barbaranelli, C. (2016). Validation of an Italian version of the Food Craving Questionnaire-State: Factor structure and sensitivity to manipulation. *Eating Behaviors, 22*, 182–187.

May, J., Andrade, J., Kavanagh, D. J., Feeney, G. F., Gullo, M. J., Statham, D. J., . . . Connor, J. P. (2014). The craving experience questionnaire: A brief, theory-based measure of consummatory desire and craving. *Addiction, 109*, 728–735.

Meule, A. (in press). Food cravings in food addiction: exploring a potential cut-off value of the Food Cravings Questionnaire-Trait-reduced. *Eating and Weight Disorders.*

Meule, A., Beck Teran, C., Berker, J., Gründel, T., Mayerhofer, M., & Platte, P. (2014). On the differentiation between trait and state food craving: Half-year retest-reliability of the *Food Cravings Questionnaire-Trait-reduced* (FCQ-T-r) and the *Food Cravings Questionnaire-State* (FCQ-S). *Journal of Eating Disorders, 2*(25), 1–3.

Meule, A., Freund, R., Skirde, A. K., Vögele, C., & Kübler, A. (2012). Heart rate variability biofeedback reduces food cravings in high food cravers. *Applied Psychophysiology and Biofeedback, 37*, 241–251.

Meule, A., Hermann, T., & Kübler, A. (2014). A short version of the *Food Cravings Questionnaire - Trait*: The FCQ-T-reduced. *Frontiers in Psychology, 5*(190), 1–10.

Meule, A., & Hormes, J. M. (2015). Chocolate versions of the *Food Cravings Questionnaires*. Associations with chocolate exposure-induced salivary flow and ad libitum chocolate consumption. *Appetite, 91*, 256–265.

Meule, A., Lutz, A., Vögele, C., & Kübler, A. (2012). Food cravings discriminate differentially between successful and unsuccessful dieters and non-dieters. Validation of the Food Craving Questionnaires in German. *Appetite, 58*, 88–97.

Meule, A., Skirde, A. K., Freund, R., Vögele, C., & Kübler, A. (2012). High-calorie food-cues impair working memory performance in high and low food cravers. *Appetite, 59*, 264–269.

Müller, J., Dettmer, D., & Macht, M. (2008). The attitudes to chocolate questionnaire: Psychometric properties and relationship to dimensions of eating. *Appetite, 50*, 499–505.

Nederkoorn, C., Smulders, F. T. Y., & Jansen, A. (2000). Cephalic phase responses, craving and food intake in normal subjects. *Appetite, 35*, 45–55.

Nicholls, W., & Hulbert-Williams, L. (2013). British English translation of the Food Craving Inventory (FCI-UK). *Appetite, 67*, 37–43.

Nijs, I. M. T., Franken, I. H. A., & Muris, P. (2007). The modified trait and state Food-Cravings Questionnaires: Development and validation of a general index of food craving. *Appetite, 49*, 38–46.

Noh, J., Kim, J. H., Nam, H., Lim, M., Lee, D., & Hong, K. (2008). Validation of the Korean version of the General Food Cravings Questionnaire-Trait (G-FCQ-T). *Korean Journal of Clinical Psychology, 27*, 1039–1051.

Osman, J. L., & Sobal, J. (2006). Chocolate cravings in American and Spanish individuals: Biological and cultural influences. *Appetite, 47*, 290–301.

Parker, S., Kamel, N., & Zellner, D. (2003). Food craving patterns in Egypt: Comparisons with North America and Spain. *Appetite, 40*, 193–195.

Pelchat, M. L., & Schaefer, S. (2000). Dietary monotony and food cravings in young and elderly adults. *Physiology & Behavior, 68*, 353–359.

Queiroz de Medeiros, A.C., Campos Pedrosa, L.d.F., & Yamamoto, M.E. (2017). Food cravings among Brazilian population. *Appetite, 108*, 212–218.

Queiroz de Medeiros, A.C., Campos Pedrosa, L.d.F., Hutz, C.S., & Yamamoto, M.E. (2016). Brazilian version of food cravings questionnaires: psychometric properties and sex differences. *Appetite, 105*, 328–333.

Richard, A., Meule, A., Reichenberger, J., & Blechert, J. (2017). Food cravings in everyday life: An EMA study on snack-related thoughts, cravings, and consumption. *Appetite, 113*, 215–223.

Rodgers, R. F., Stritzke, W. G. K., Bui, E., Franko, D. L., & Chabrol, H. (2011). Evaluation of the French version of the orientation towards chocolate questionnaire: Chocolate-related guilt and ambivalence are associated with overweight and disordered eating. *Eating Behaviors, 12*, 254–260.

Rodríguez-Martín, B. C., & Meule, A. (2015). Food craving: New contributions on its assessment, moderators, and consequences. *Frontiers in Psychology, 6*(21), 1–3.

Rodriguez, S., Warren, C. S., Moreno, S., Cepeda-Benito, A., Gleaves, D. H., Fernandez, M. D., & Vila, J. (2007). Adaptation of the Food-Craving Questionnaire Trait for the assessment of chocolate cravings: Validation across British and Spanish women. *Appetite, 49*, 245–250.

Schmidt, J., & Martin, A. (2016). Neurofeedback against binge eating: a randomized controlled trial in a female subclinical threshold sample. *European Eating Disorders Review, 24*, 406–416.

Shiffman, S. (2000). Comments on craving. *Addiction, 95*, S171–S175.

Tarragon, E., Stein, J., & Meyer, J. (2017). Psychometric properties of the German translated version and adaptation of the Food Craving Inventory. *Frontiers in Psychology, 8*(736), 1–7.

Tiffany, S. T., & Wray, J. M. (2012). The clinical significance of drug craving. *Annals of the New York Academy of Sciences, 1248*, 1–17.

Toll, B. A., Katulak, N. A., Williams-Piehota, P., & O'Malley, S. (2008). Validation of a scale for the assessment of food cravings among smokers. *Appetite, 50*, 25–32.

Ulian, M. D., Sato, P. D. M., Benatti, F. B., Campos-Ferraz, P. L. D., Roble, O. J., Unsain, R. F., ... & Scagliusi, F. B. (2017). Cross-cultural adaptation of the State and Trait Food Cravings Questionnaires (FCQ-S and FCQ-T) into Portuguese. *Ciência & Saúde Coletiva, 22*, 403–416.

Ulrich, M., Steigleder, L., & Grön, G. (2016). Neural signature of the Food Craving Questionnaire (FCQ)-Trait. *Appetite, 107*, 303–310.

Van Gucht, D., Soetens, B., Raes, F., & Griffith, J. W. (2014). The attitudes to chocolate questionnaire. Psychometric properties and relationship with consumption, dieting, disinhibition and thought suppression. *Appetite, 76*, 137–143.

Weingarten, H. P., & Elston, D. (1991). Food cravings in a college population. *Appetite, 17*, 167–175.

Werthmann, J., Roefs, A., Nederkoorn, C., Mogg, K., Bradley, B. P., & Jansen, A. (2011). Can(not) take my eyes off it: Attention bias for food in overweight participants. *Health Psychology, 30*, 561–569.

White, M. A., Whisenhunt, B. L., Williamson, D. A., Greenway, F. L., & Netemeyer, R. G. (2002). Development and validation of the food-craving inventory. *Obesity Research, 10*, 107–114.

Zellner, D., Garriga-Trillo, A., Rohm, E., Centeno, S., & Parker, S. (1999). Food liking and craving: A cross-cultural approach. *Appetite, 33*, 61–70.

10 Case Study
Severe Processed Food Addiction

Natalie Gold
Ryerson University
Gestalt Institute of Toronto
Toronto, ON

CONTENTS

10.1 INTRODUCTION

The weekly 1950s TV series, *This Is Your Life*, stands out in my memory because even as a young teen, I understood on a basic level that my confusing behavior with food was similar to the stories of some of the surprised guests, both celebrities and ordinary folks, honored for overcoming serious alcoholism or drug addiction. Today, I believe I have suffered from food addiction, which is increasingly demonstrated to be similar to drug and alcohol addiction (Tomasi et al. 2015; De Ridder et al. 2016). Throughout my life, I have unknowingly met the criteria for a substance use disorder (SUD) as described in the *Diagnostic and Statistical Manual of Mental Disorders* (DSM 5). This self-case study shows how I did so, starting at a young age and continuing well into my adult life.

In recent years, the scientific evidence for food addiction and its relationship to binge eating disorder has been accumulating (Stice and Yokum 2016; Moore et al. 2017). However, until I read the 11 DSM 5 SUD diagnostic criteria to prepare this chapter, I did not qualify myself as a full-fledged food addict. Now there's no doubt in my mind that I am, since my personal experiences meet all 11 conditions. As a registered psychotherapist in private practice since 2007, I present my story as a severe case of processed food addiction (PFA). As I grew older, many of the main symptoms progressed and intensified in form, essence, and impact, until I got the right kind of help.

DSM-5 SUD diagnostic criteria (described in detail in the next chapters of this textbook).

1. Unintended use
2. Failure to cut back
3. Time spent
4. Cravings
5. Failure to fulfill major roles
6. Interpersonal problems
7. Activities given up
8. Hazardous use

9. Knowledge of consequences
10. Tolerance
11. Withdrawal

10.2 BACKGROUND

I was born in 1945 in London, England, to parents who endured World War II. My mother was the second youngest of eight children born to Polish immigrants who settled in the poorer section of London's East End, and my father apparently had a similar beginning. They married shortly before the British army dispatched my father, a military policeman, to faraway places. During the war, their first child was stillborn. This left an unresolved grief mark on my mother, increased her anxiety and underscored her desperate need to be the perfect mother, and for me to be the perfect daughter.

Our little threesome emigrated to Canada in 1948, leaving behind my mother's large family and the austerity of food rationing. A year later, my sister came along, and the comparisons to me began. She was the "good girl"—obedient, calm, generous, and quiet—while I was the opposite. We quickly excelled at playing our respective roles; the worse I became, the more she stayed out of trouble. And trouble there was.

We moved several times, the last when my 40-something father decided to begin again in Niagara Falls, Canada, after his business partner betrayed him in what could have been a highly profitable business venture.

At our house, meals were especially hectic. My father devoured everything compulsively, finishing before my mother even sat down. My sister and I had to finish what was on our plates before we could leave the table. Conversation was sparse, except for interrogations about school. The stage was set.

10.3 ONSET

By age 10, my mother had decided I was a bit too fat and forbade me to eat sweets and desserts until I slimmed down, despite her routine of feeding me chocolate as an infant to soothe me to sleep in my crib. Chocolate has now been shown to be one of the most addictive foods (Asmaro and Liotti 2014). Refusing to deprive my sister on my account, my mother continued to buy the weekly chocolate cake, which probably intensified my PFA through the mechanism of cuing (Boswell and Kober 2016). Slowly I began to sneak slices of that cake whenever alone in the kitchen. Little slices at first, which was kind of fun. However, the sneaking became more frequent, the slices grew bigger, and I was surprised at how quickly the cake shrank. Within months, to my bafflement, entire cakes disappeared, which I cleverly replaced with new ones missing varying amounts. It began to bother me that I couldn't go into the kitchen without sneaking cake, even when I told myself I wouldn't. I couldn't stop. So at the age of 10, I manifested two SUD criteria: (1) unintended use of larger amounts and for longer periods than intended and (2) a persistent desire to cut back.

The cake increasingly led to other sweet foods, which seems to comply with DSM SUD 10: tolerance. Entire packages of cookies vanished. Poof! Did they ever exist? When my mother asked who ate them, no one replied. This pattern became the norm: me as the thief, my mother as the grand inquisitor. It drove her crazy and caused ugly scenes in our family, especially at the dinner table. So another criterion was met, number 6: continued use in spite of interpersonal problems.

By the time I was 11 or 12, I wanted to stop all the lying, stealing food, and sneaking around, but I couldn't. I didn't understand this at the time, and even more incomprehensible were legitimate urges and cravings to eat the "substance," which meets Criterion 4. When my parents were not home, I automatically raided cookie tins, drawers and cupboards, fridges and freezers in the kitchen and basement, in accordance with Criterion 3, time spent. My mother's hideaways were carefully devised to keep special treats for company only, with each container including a note specifying the exact number of goodies it held. I changed these after wolfing down what I could. Then, my cravings unsated, I shifted to other foods; whatever was available, sweet or not. This seems like another worsening of Criterion 10, tolerance. My eating pattern grew worse, my mother grew more vocal in her frustration over missing items, and my body expanded exponentially. At this point, I was also satisfying Criterion 9, use in spite of consequences.

Our home became an unpleasant place for everyone. While my father remained silent, his frequent glares at me for causing trouble spoke volumes. My mother, out of love and concern, relentlessly increased her efforts to help, goad, torment, bribe, and shame me into losing weight, which was actually an unrecognized symptom of my food addiction. This kind of teasing and bullying has been found to correlate with the development of binge eating (Saltzman and Liechty 2016), which progressed along with my food addiction. To the dismay of my mother and me, no matter how hard I tried, each dieting attempt ended with a greater weight gain—a perfect example of Criterion 2, failed attempts to cut back. Dieting meant my mother watched what I ate (at meals) like a hawk, which I unknowingly resented. I also wanted to lose weight, but my mental preoccupation with what I couldn't eat weighed heavily on my mind. I couldn't stop thinking about food. I escaped to the basement rec room to play piano and sing my pain away, but not enough to diminish what was becoming an increasing dependency on food.

Before entering high school, I now realize I was severely addicted to processed foods, and conformed to seven or eight of the criteria, including Criterion 1, unintended use; Criterion 2, failed attempts to cut back; Criterion 3, time spent; Criterion 4, cravings; Criterion 6, interpersonal problems; Criterion 9, use in spite of consequences; and Criterion 10, tolerance. I probably also met Criterion 5, failure to fulfill major roles, because I was not the daughter my mother and father wanted. Nor was I a good sister, since she got blamed for the food I stole.

When high school started, I wore a (Canadian) size 13–14 dress (no jeans/slacks allowed in the early 1960s) and earned a proficiency award at the end of ninth grade. By midterms in Grade 12, I barely squeezed into a size 18–20 and failed four subjects. So over the 4 high school years, I became the perfect example of Criterion 5: I was unable to do what I should at school or home (the inability to function at work would come later). Mental preoccupation with food, weight, and the ensuing emotional turmoil had grown into obsession, rendering me unable to focus on schoolwork. I lacked my previous ability to concentrate in class and certainly couldn't study in my home environment. Research has demonstrated cognitive difficulties in an adolescent obese population (Yau et al. 2014). I lived in my head, out of touch with my physical and emotional needs, obsessively performing mental math calculations, which involved matching hypothetical caloric intake with potential future weight-loss scenarios. For example, if I ate a certain number of calories per day or week, then I could lose a particular number of pounds by such-and-such a date, but if I cut the calories even more I might fit into a lower size sooner. And on it went.

I also incessantly tried to figure out why I couldn't stop eating and why I was such a horrible daughter and fantasized about a perfect life once I got thin. My mother encouraged this "thintasy," believing a girl stood no chance in this world if she was "fatandugly" (words perpetually fused together). By internalizing the stigmatization of my parents and the culture at large (Palmeira et al. 2017), my self-loathing blossomed.

I had developed compulsive behavior in relation to food, all part of the addictive process. Despite wanting to cut down or stop using the "substance," as described in Criterion 2, I couldn't stop myself from starting a binge and I couldn't stop binge eating once I started. What was wrong with me? No one knew.

My lies multiplied as I devised various schemes to sneak sugary and salty treats into the house and to destroy the evidence (packaging). For example, I would discard candy and chocolate bar wrappers on the way to school, and not in our own garbage bin, to avoid discovery by one of my parents. All of this plotting and behavior corresponds precisely with Criterion 3: spending a lot of time getting, using, or recovering from use of the substance. Irritation, frustration, self-hate, guilt, shame, and profound grief grew as I failed to keep promises to myself to stop. Self-trust disappeared. In addition, whatever I ate failed to last long enough, which indicates that by my early teens, I was continuing to meet Criterion 10, tolerance, for sugar-based foods, needing more to get the desired effect. I was also beginning to meet Criterion 11, withdrawal, since I always felt rotten afterwards.

The addictive process escalated during a summer visit to England at age 16. When a relative revealed some disturbing news about my father's past, my unacknowledged mistrust of him deepened, my addiction to chocolate skyrocketed, and I returned home several sizes larger. Stress has been shown to be a leading cause of relapse (Cottone et al. 2009; Sinha and Jastreboff 2013). Soon after, I overheard my father admit he hated how I looked, which meant he hated me, since I was suffering from fused thinking (Duarte et al. 2016). Despondent, I tried suicide, which certainly fits Criterion 8, dangerous or physically hazardous use. My failure even at that, due to the wrong type and dosage of pills, sent me into a deep depression. Driven by heightened urges and cravings, as set out in Criterion 4, I cared only about getting my next fix to numb the pain, despite the devastating consequences to my body and spirit. This epitomizes Criterion 9. I continued to use, despite knowing I had problems—both physical and psychological—that could have been caused or made worse by the substance.

Almost all my interactions with people were dysfunctional due to the humiliation of my secret life with food and binge eating. As indicated in Criterion 6, I continued to use (and abuse) food, even when it clearly caused problems in my relationships—the ones I had and the ones I avoided. For example, the obvious mutual resentment between my mother and me intensified from her initial frustration over missing goodies to her heartsick rages over my obesity and lies. More difficult to discern was the bitterness I felt toward my father for not protecting me from my mother's tirades, and my confusion about this troubled man. I ate over that, too, and over the guilt for letting my younger sister take the blame for food I stole. My once-flourishing friendships with girlfriends gradually shrank. Given my low self-esteem and shameful eating with its all-too-visible consequences, I couldn't be truly honest with anyone. Of course, there were no boyfriends: attendance at school dances and social functions had slowly eroded, as isolation and self-loathing expanded with my waistline. By this stage, I was conforming to Criterion 7, giving up important social, occupational, or recreational activities because of substance use.

Somehow, I squeaked through twelfth grade and started university in Buffalo, where my first self-designed diet (to impress a young man) was doomed to fail. For about a month I ate Jello, chewed gum, drank coffee, and smoked cigarettes, until I fainted in the bathtub. Once again, as set out in Criterion 2, I desperately wanted to cut down or stop my food binges, but I couldn't for any decent length of time. That particular failed attempt became license to go haywire with junk food. My cravings and urges became so strong (Criterion 4) that I had to steal money from my college roommate to raid the vending machines in the dormitory basement. And despite my success at many extracurricular university activities (theatre arts, student politics, and folk-singing gigs), I became unable to study or hand in papers on time and dropped out at the end of second year—evidence of a deep adherence to Criterion 5, failure to fulfill roles. I then decided to move back home with my parents. In retrospect, this was not the cleverest idea.

10.4 ADULTHOOD

Regardless of my fun job writing copy at a radio station and my first car, the difficult home situation created a strong desire for escape and more independence (i.e., my own apartment), which my father vehemently opposed. So early one morning I packed my car, set off for Toronto, quickly found a room, and landed a lowly junior clerk typist job in an ad agency. This newfound freedom shifted my addiction into an all-consuming pastime, where two criteria blossomed: Criterion 3, time spent getting, using, or recovering from use of the substance, and Criterion 4, cravings. I ate until I was full and then I ate even more. I didn't realize it at the time, but feeling full was actually a trigger to continue eating, which is now supported by new research (Kim et al. 2016).

Back then, all I could think about was my next food fix and how to get it. Binges were now planned, as I ensured my stock of treats did not run out. When not at work, I ate *en route* to the closest convenience store, takeout place, or supermarket and from there to the next food stop.

Voracious eating behind the wheel may not yet be equated with driving under the influence, but it should be, since a car can be a dangerous weapon. Eating while driving (EWD?) is a messy business—a frantic urge to devour as much food as quickly as possible, way beyond the need to satisfy hunger. From behind the wheel, I shoved the food down, all the while planning what to eat next and where to get it, even though I hadn't finished whatever I was consuming. I dropped food (on myself, the steering wheel, seat, and car floor) and retrieved it, mopping up spills, and driving one-handed as I opened packages with the other. Until I felt stoned and temporarily sated, straining to keep my eyes open. Until the next craving hit. My focus, it would be safe to say, was not on the road or the traffic. Such risky behavior behind the wheel again and again exemplifies Criterion 8, hazardous use.

At work, I ate throughout the day, carefully planning where to stock up unnoticed. Despite provisions in my desk drawer to munch on secretly and a lunch to consume at my desk publicly, I sometimes bought extra lunches at various underground venues. I strategized where to get enough for the commute home and for when I arrived. My mental preoccupation with acquiring and consuming a constant supply of food exemplifies several criteria: Criterion 1, I ate more than intended; Criterion 10, tolerance—I usually had to have more and more; Criterion 3, time spent; and Criterion 4, cravings. This behavior kept the ugly consequences of Criterion 11, withdrawal, at bay, along with the remorse, shame, and self-loathing about the whole sad experience. Many overeating episodes lasted from Friday nights to Monday mornings, sometimes longer, which easily conforms with Criterion 7, activities given up.

My second major diet (shots in the hip for 6 weeks and a daily 500-calorie limit) and significant weight loss (down to a Canadian size 16, or an American 14) rendered me almost unrecognizable to work colleagues. With this surge in uncomfortable and unfamiliar praise, I promptly ate my way up to a size 22–24, a failure which once again epitomized Criterion 2, failure to cut down or stop. As my dress size increased, so did my isolating behavior. As described in Criterion 7, activities given up, food addiction once again restricted my social life—but in a new way. I began to avoid making definite plans with friends, in case I had to back out due to a binge or its aftereffects.

I haven't explained the aftereffects before, but food addiction, like other SUDs, comes with its own set of withdrawal symptoms, which correspond with those described in Criterion 11, withdrawal. In my case, these symptoms had been going on in varying degrees since I was a child. As is common among addicts, that's one of the reasons why I felt compelled to keep eating—to relieve and stave off the consequences. On a physical level, my withdrawal could include thirst, insomnia, gas and bloating, diarrhea and/or constipation, headaches, sweating, feeling cold, sluggish, clammy, and drowsy. Emotionally, I'd be anxious, irritable, easily angered, easily given to tears, extremely sensitive to perceived slights, and full of remorse, shame, and guilt. Mentally, I'd be in a fog, unable to think coherently or concentrate for longer than a few seconds (Theoharides et al. 2015).

Usually, I functioned according to a four-phase cycle: binge eating, withdrawal, a tapering-off period that gradually morphed into extreme food restriction, and super control as typified by the diet/weight-loss math. Then boom! Back into binge mode to repeat the cycle yet again (Goldstone et al. 2009).

The 8-month period after losing so much weight so quickly and regaining it plus extra was an incredibly stress-filled time. First, by rendering me unable to work, my food addiction and the resulting do-nothing depression forced the ad agency to fire me, which conforms to Criterion 5, failure to fulfill roles. Eventually I found a great new car-dependent job involving travel, but after being sexually assaulted at night on my street I had to move apartments. When my car died, I lost that second job. After wallowing around in a binge-filled depression and fog for over a month, I applied to work at a children's mental health residence, where my somewhat bizarre behavior became clearly evident to the staff. After several interviews, meetings, and a tour of the facilities, I actually had to be physically escorted from the building since I refused to leave and sank to the floor when staff members tried to gently usher me out. To top that off, when accused by my mother of causing my father's heart attack, despite logic and common sense, I accepted the blame and holed up for weeks in my basement apartment in a food frenzy, once more typifying Criterion 7, foregoing social, occupational, or recreational activities because of substance use.

During this isolation, I also made pathetic phone calls to various people, including a man I obsessed over. My mental undoing led to a psychotic break at the end of March 1967, culminating in a visit to Toronto's brand new leading-edge mental hospital, where I became an inpatient for 10 months and an outpatient for another 15. Finally, I got some much-needed help. But in spite of good intentions, the approaches used were inappropriate for my condition.

In the mid-1960s, eating disorders were not recognized, and certainly no one diagnosed my issue as an addiction, especially to food. So the PFA went unaddressed. Based on memories and actual hospital records, I did benefit from a supportive treatment plan to help me separate emotionally from my family. The assumption was that with family issues resolved, my obesity would recede on its own. However, that is like telling a drug user that once she straightens out her life, she'll no longer need heroin. For most people, healing from addiction doesn't quite work that way. While my social worker's notes mention my binges, usually after an encounter with one or both parents, I was never honest about what, how much, or the manner in which I ate. The hospital staff lacked the knowledge, training, or skills to apply addiction diagnostic criteria and discover that I was suffering from PFA, along with binge eating disorder.

As an outpatient, the diet–binge roller-coaster persisted. I continued to use food to calm, reward, or punish myself, to express or suppress feelings, and to numb my considerable emotional and psychic pain. By this stage, I would say that I was meeting all 11 of the DSM-5 SUD criteria. I bemoaned the consequences of obesity and depression despite group therapy. Hospital staff helped me return to university as a "mature student" to study radio/TV arts. At that time, I tried another extreme diet (500 calories a day of specific protein sources plus all the water I could drink), which ended after 5 weeks when I demolished more than a pound of low-fat swiss cheese in a movie theatre (almost a week's worth), followed by a lengthy bender. At this point, Criterion 9, use in spite of consequences, was manifesting as I continued to use food, despite knowing that my physical problem of obesity and psychological problems of depression, anxiety, and being a former mental patient would be made worse.

Two years after reentering school, I had to drop out a second time, since I couldn't concentrate or focus on my studies, which again conforms with Criterion 5, failure to fulfill roles. Instead of schoolwork, I fixated on my usual obsession, weight, the visible manifestation of my addiction, which continued to be a persistent pattern for many years.

While temporary office work gave me the flexibility to pursue musical interests, it also accommodated my food habit. Several SUD criteria were at play here. For example, the hourly pay helped me maintain at least some integrity when I needed to take time off work, which exemplifies Criterion 7, occupational activities given up, and Criterion 3, time spent. I missed work during and after major binges as I tried to recover from eating so much food, which fits Criterion 11, withdrawal.

In 1971, with my meager savings I headed to London, England, to travel and pursue a singing career. While various Toronto venues had hired me as a folk singer, Toronto talent agents proffered a massive thumbs down because of my obesity (O'Brien et al. 2013). But in London I soon got gigs in between temp jobs and did travel, including a tour with a band entertaining US troops stationed in Germany. Even there, my food addiction did not abate, as I continued to sneak food whenever I could.

During this time, upon my return to London, I sincerely believed that once I became functional and happier, the need to use food would dissipate. Instead, my addiction grew stronger. I couldn't just get by on small amounts, which satisfies Criterion 1, unintended use, and Criterion 10, tolerance. One of anything was never enough. One of anything, particularly sugar, white flour, and junk food products, always triggered Criterion 4, cravings. In fact, over the years until I got help, the quantities of junk food and sugar products I'd consume in a binge or binge period increased, in line with Criterion 10, tolerance. It took more and more to get the effect I wanted. Sometimes I'd buy so much I'd throw what was left in the garbage, only to retrieve it later. Even after burying it under cigarette ashes, I'd still salvage it, clean it off, and shove it down the hatch. This is another way of meeting Criterion 8, hazardous use.

I ate so much that my body couldn't take it. After some binge benders preceded by highly restrictive and controlled dieting, I suffered simultaneous bouts of diarrhea and vomiting from having consumed so much sugar and junk. I call these appalling episodes "two-pailers" since that's exactly what I used when groveling on my hands and knees on the floor, my body wracked with uncontrollable eruptions. No less disgusting than a drug addict lying in their own filth in some dark alley.

The two-pailers happened first in London and continued as an occasional part of my pattern after returning to Toronto in 1976. I continued to abuse food despite the physical, emotional, and psychological problems it caused, exemplifying Criterion 9, use in spite of consequences. I really couldn't help it. My binge eating was far beyond my control.

Back in Toronto, I eked out my existence with temp work and various music gigs, and with group and individual therapy to help me get my life on track. Night eating episodes began around this time—the extreme version of several criteria: Criterion 2, failure to cut back; Criterion 9, consequences; and Criterion 10, tolerance. I'd awake in the morning to discover empty cartons and packaging on the kitchen counter, with no memory of having eaten it. This was blackout eating.

When an opportunity to learn computer programming on the job came along in 1980, I grabbed it and passed the probation period. However, 3 months later I was fired since I was mentally and emotionally not suited to the job. I commiserated, of course, with a month of continuous binge eating, with frequent two-pailers, rendering me helpless and desperate.

10.5 SOLUTION

On June 3, 1981, several weeks after seeing a chance TV spot (which I have never seen since), I attended my first 12-step meeting and the beginning of the rest of my life. There I met others who abused food like me but who had found a way to stop. They used the word "powerless," which washed over me as truth often does when heard the first time. There, people found a way to stop binge eating and lose weight through "abstinence"—a self-designed, structured plan of eating meals/snacks, minus specific binge foods. Binge foods were defined as foods that members craved, obsessed over, and couldn't limit to just one. In 1981, an individualized nondiet approach toward sustainable weight loss was far from mainstream.

The program asked people to take an honest look at how, what, when, where, and why they ate. For me, this became possible with personal, group, and spiritual support. While some struggled with the latter, I quickly developed a concept of a higher power (not the traditional "God") to rely on for help. This was easier for me than reaching out to people. And, after reading William Dufty's book *Sugar Blues* (citing Dr. John Yudkin's research), I soon understood how refined sugar and white flour created cravings (Dufty 1993). Ironically, John Yudkin's work on sugar (Yudkin 1964), in the 1970s, has recently been validated by neuroscientists and other medical professionals, such as Dr. Robert Lustig (Lustig 2013).

After going sugarless for a while, my brain cleared up. Imagine radio signals obscured by too much static, so that nothing can be heard. That would describe my brain on sugar. But off sugar, since the static is gone, individual thoughts are discernible, although many try to come in on the same station. This gave me a fighting chance to sort them out. And sorting out self-deception, confusion, negative thoughts, and beliefs is essentially the work of all 12-step programs, which seem to combine a cognitive, spiritual, and social approach to healing.

A year later, ecstatic over my 70–90 pound weight loss (I have no idea what I weighed at the start) and ability to concentrate, my career in qualitative market research began. It was to serve me for several decades. Food was "quiet," i.e., I had no cravings. However, anxiety, emotions, and unresolved issues began to surface, which I worked on using the 12 steps and individual psychotherapy.

However, after 2.5 years of solid abstinence, the pain of a failed romance led to relapse. This hit me like a ton of bricks. Sugar-laden binges rapidly escalated, the two-pailers returned with a vengeance, and I struggled for months to regain abstinence and stave off major weight gain. Even with 12-step and psychotherapy support, my efforts to get off and stay off sugar and junk food remained erratic. I was again manifesting most of the criteria, but especially Criterion 4, cravings and urges to use; Criterion 6, relationship problems; and Criterion 9, use in spite of consequences.

In the mid-80s, I added an important new component to my recovery. Gestalt therapy is a holistic, experiential approach to healing that focuses on emotions, the body, and cognitive restoration. It was exactly what I needed.

Since June 1981, most of my life has been spent abstinent. And while I can still wear clothes I've had for more than a decade, the path has been somewhat rocky. I've had several major relapses lasting weeks, a range of moderate setbacks lasting a day or two, minor lapses lasting an hour or so, and occasional "slips" of just having extra. These have occurred with multiple yearlong periods of peace in between. Each mistake has been a learning experience, and most have been predicated by unacknowledged emotions, beliefs, negative self-talk, or personal "research" into whether or not I am actually addicted to sugar. The results are consistent: I am a processed food addict. The latter has now been supported by a host of scientific research (Wiss et al. 2016; Burrows et al. 2017; Chao et al. 2017).

After the attack on New York's Twin Towers on September 11, 2001, I realized I wanted more meaning in my life. With sugar and junk food out of the picture, I was able to complete years of various academic and experiential training programs. I have earned an honors BA in psychology (my third kick at the higher learning can). I have also been awarded a postgraduate certificate in gestalt therapy (a 4-year training program at the time), and received a 1-year graduate certificate in addictions and mental health counseling. I became a registered psychotherapist, licensed in the province of Ontario, Canada. I work mainly with people who suffer from binge eating, bulimia, food, and other addictions—underneath which is a plethora of unresolved issues which might need to be addressed. I have also written a popular book about my experiences as a food addict and binge eater, *Binge Crazy: A Psychotherapist's Memoir of Food Addiction, Mental Illness, Obesity and Recovery* (Gold 2015). The absence of DSM 5 SUD-related behaviors in my life has allowed me to function at a high level of productivity.

With more than half my life in an ongoing recovery process from food addiction, I still celebrate every time relevant new information comes to light about this devastating and complex illness, no less soul-destroying than other SUDs.

10.6 APPLICATION

This case study demonstrates the depth to which PFA can alter a life. The environment in which the child is raised can foster PFA at an early age. The disease can derail education and result in financial upheaval and instability through adulthood. As this example illustrates, the application of well-intended but inappropriate mental health services can leave the patient in the throes of compulsive eating and extensive consequences. It also clearly shows the need to abstain from or reduce the use of processed foods to regain control of eating.

In addition, this case demonstrates the applicability of the DSM-5 SUD diagnostic criteria to overeating and binge eating, since these criteria manifest faithfully in chronic overconsumption of processed food products. From this example, practitioners can feel confident that by gently questioning clients about their behaviors based on the addiction diagnostic approaches, they can develop a picture of the depth of pathology endured by the client.

The next 11 chapters of this textbook delve into the research supporting the many addictive eating behaviors manifesting under the addiction diagnostic criteria. Practitioners may feel a newfound appreciation of the pathology of addiction in overeating and be supported in helping their clients understand and accept the diagnosis.

REFERENCES

Asmaro, D. and M. Liotti (2014). High-caloric and chocolate stimuli processing in healthy humans: An integration of functional imaging and electrophysiological findings. *Nutrients* **6**(1): 319–341.

Boswell, R. G. and H. Kober (2016). Food cue reactivity and craving predict eating and weight gain: A meta-analytic review. *Obes Rev* **17**(2): 159–177.

Burrows, T., J. Skinner, M. A. Joyner, J. Palmieri, K. Vaughan and A. N. Gearhardt (2017). Food addiction in children: Associations with obesity, parental food addiction and feeding practices. *Eat Behav* **26**: 114–120.

Chao, A. M., J. A. Shaw, R. L. Pearl, N. Alamuddin, C. M. Hopkins, Z. M. Bakizada, R. I. Berkowitz and T. A. Wadden (2017). Prevalence and psychosocial correlates of food addiction in persons with obesity seeking weight reduction. *Compr Psychiatry* **73**: 97–104.

Cottone, P., V. Sabino, M. Roberto, M. Bajo, L. Pockros, J. B. Frihauf, E. M. Fekete, et al. (2009). CRF system recruitment mediates dark side of compulsive eating. *Proc Natl Acad Sci U S A* **106**(47): 20016–20020.

De Ridder, D., P. Manning, S. L. Leong, S. Ross, W. Sutherland, C. Horwath and S. Vanneste (2016). The brain, obesity and addiction: An EEG neuroimaging study. *Sci Rep* **6**: 34122.

Duarte, C., J. Pinto-Gouveia, C. Ferreira and B. Silva (2016). Caught in the struggle with food craving: Development and validation of a new cognitive fusion measure. *Appetite* **101**: 146–155.

Dufty, W. (1993). *Sugar Blues*. New York, Warner Books.

Gold, N. (2015). *Binge Crazy: A Psychotherapist's Memoir of Food Addiction, Mental Illness, Obesity and Recovery*. Montgomery Village, MD, Arrow Publications.

Goldstone, A. P., C. G. Prechtl de Hernandez, J. D. Beaver, K. Muhammed, C. Croese, G. Bell, G. Durighel, E. Hughes, A. D. Waldman, G. Frost and J. D. Bell (2009). Fasting biases brain reward systems towards high-calorie foods. *Eur J Neurosci* **30**(8): 1625–1635.

Kim, G. W., J. E. Lin, A. E. Snook, A. S. Aing, D. J. Merlino, P. Li and S. A. Waldman (2016). Calorie-induced ER stress suppresses uroguanylin satiety signaling in diet-induced obesity. *Nutr Diabetes* **6**: e211.

Lustig, R. H. (2013). Fructose: It's "alcohol without the buzz". *Adv Nutr* **4**(2): 226–235.

Moore, C. F., V. Sabino, G. F. Koob and P. Cottone (2017). Pathological overeating: Emerging evidence for a compulsivity construct. *Neuropsychopharmacology* **42**(7): 1375–1389.

O'Brien, K. S., J. D. Latner, D. Ebneter and J. A. Hunter (2013). Obesity discrimination: The role of physical appearance, personal ideology, and anti-fat prejudice. *Int J Obes (Lond)* **37**(3): 455–460.

Palmeira, L., J. Pinto-Gouveia, M. Cunha and S. Carvalho (2017). Finding the link between internalized weight-stigma and binge eating behaviors in Portuguese adult women with overweight and obesity: The mediator role of self-criticism and self-reassurance. *Eat Behav* **26**: 50–54.

Saltzman, J. A. and J. M. Liechty (2016). Family correlates of childhood binge eating: A systematic review. *Eat Behav* **22**: 62–71.

Sinha, R. and A. M. Jastreboff (2013). Stress as a common risk factor for obesity and addiction. *Biol Psychiatry* **73**(9): 827–835.

Stice, E. and S. Yokum (2016). Neural vulnerability factors that increase risk for future weight gain. *Psychol Bull* **142**(5): 447–471.

Theoharides, T. C., J. M. Stewart, E. Hatziagelaki and G. Kolaitis (2015). Brain "fog," inflammation and obesity: Key aspects of neuropsychiatric disorders improved by luteolin. *Front Neurosci* **9**: 225.

Tomasi, D., G. J. Wang, R. Wang, E. C. Caparelli, J. Logan and N. D. Volkow (2015). Overlapping patterns of brain activation to food and cocaine cues in cocaine abusers: Association to striatal D2/D3 receptors. *Hum Brain Mapp* **36**(1): 120–136.

Wiss, D. A., K. Criscitelli, M. Gold and N. Avena (2016). Preclinical evidence for the addiction potential of highly palatable foods: Current developments related to maternal influence. *Appetite* **115**: 19–27.

Yau, P. L., E. H. Kang, D. C. Javier and A. Convit (2014). Preliminary evidence of cognitive and brain abnormalities in uncomplicated adolescent obesity. *Obesity (Silver Spring)* **22**(8): 1865–1871.

Yudkin, J. (1964). Patterns and trends in carbohydrate consumption and their relation to disease. *Proc Nutr Soc* **23**: 149–162.

11 DSM 5 SUD Criterion 1 *Unintended Use*

Joan Ifland
Food Addiction Training, LLC
Cincinnati, OH

H. Theresa Wright
Renaissance Nutrition
East Norriton, PA

CONTENTS

Processed foods are often eaten in larger amounts or over a longer period than was intended. (American Psychiatric Association, 2013, p. 490)

11.1 INTRODUCTION

Unintended use is a common occurrence in obesogenic cultures. So much processed food is available in so many home, work, school, and social environments (Lifshitz & Lifshitz, 2014) that it is easy to experience a cued craving, reach out, and consume a calorie-dense food without prior intention to do so (McLaren et al., 2014). At the relatively harmless end of the spectrum of severity, unintended use may just be a second sweet at a social function. However, unintended use may progress all the way to eating a week's worth of groceries in a single afternoon.

Incidents of unintended use may be minor initially, but as the addiction progresses the experience of unintended use can become deeply distressing to the client. Food-addicted clients report helplessly watching their hand reach out and repeatedly put food into their mouths, while not wanting this to be happening. The feeling of helplessness can be quite frightening. This behavior can produce the distress that is required for a diagnosis of processed food addiction (PFA) to be made according to the DSM 5 (American Psychiatric Association, 2013, p. 490). An example of this is found in the Food Addiction Manual for Food Addicts Anonymous (FAA):

> I was feeling scared as I recognized that I couldn't keep inappropriate foods out of my mouth for more than 2 or 3 days and that, no matter how much I didn't want to, I ate. (Food Addicts Anonymous, 2010, p. 199)

A subtle example of unintended use may occur in the use of calorie-dense fast foods. While the food addict may intend to order a meal, the nature of fast food may ensure that the addict is actually eating the caloric equivalent of several meals (Stender, Dyerberg, & Astrup, 2007). Some fast food meals have the caloric content of a full day of food. This is a situation that could be resolved just by educating the client about the caloric content prepared foods.

Although common, unintended use may not manifest in all food-addicted clients, the food addict may be planning the use of processed foods and eat what was planned. Even if progression has occurred, the food addict may not have acted out beyond the planned use. Unintended use may not manifest until the food addict tries to cut back and starts to experience Criterion 2, failure to cut back.

In the context of recovery, when abstinence from addictive foods has been established, unintended use is no longer a matter of excessive calorie consumption but rather an issue of relapse and the risk of kindling the addiction. One bite can serve to restart the addiction for a food addict in the same way that one sip of alcohol can do so for the alcoholic. Under all circumstances, gathering information about the frequency and severity of episodes of unintended use gives the practitioner a picture of how far PFA has progressed in the client. This quote illustrates the situation:

> I tried another Twelve Step program dealing with food, but I had a harder time there. Their definition of abstinence was unclear to me. They said I would pick a diet that was sane. If I could've done that, I wouldn't be obese. I never knew boundaries when it came to eating or my health. There was little or no recognition that this disease was biochemical and that sugar, flour and wheat were the culprits. (Food Addicts Anonymous, 2010, p. 140)

Binge eating may be an indication of unintended use. The DSM 5 has diagnostic criteria for binge eating. Research shows that the presence of binge eating correlates with deeper emotional distress and poorer treatment outcomes (Meany, Conceicao, & Mitchell, 2014; Yanovski, Nelson, Dubbert, & Spitzer, 1993). Where binge eating is present, the practitioner may use this information to help motivate the client to undertake a more comprehensive program. This quote illustrates the seriousness of unintended bingeing:

> On September 5th, I had the worst binge of my life. That day I knew I had to go to any length to make my life manageable. I finally admitted that I was powerless and needed help. I was killing myself. (Food-addicted clients Anonymous, 2010, p. 130)

Similarly, binge eating may be followed by purging and the development of bulimia:

> I had been going to a diet program where you gave them your money, they gave you a written diet, and you got weighed every week. My disease was so out of control that I couldn't stop eating. I was too ashamed to get weighed in, so I started throwing up. I couldn't bear the humiliation of letting someone see how out of control I was. I was convinced that I must be either weak-willed or stupid. Why couldn't I follow simple instructions? Why couldn't I eat like a normal human being? Why did I always make a pig of myself? (Food-addicted clients Anonymous, 2010, p. 137)

Again, neither bingeing nor purging are necessary to find conformance to Criterion 1 in diagnosing PFA. The volume and rapidity necessary for a finding of bingeing are not necessary for a finding of unintended use. An example would be the office worker who eats a sizable box of crackers daily and would like to stop but cannot. This is unintended use but not bingeing. Similarly, the client who eats a quart of ice cream throughout an evening may do so over 4–5 hours by helplessly traveling to the freezer again and again for a few spoonfuls each time. This pattern of grazing would not meet the criteria for bingeing but would meet the criteria for unintended use.

The syndrome of unintended use is well established in assessment of drug addiction. This chapter reviews the evidence for a syndrome of unintended use in PFA. Practitioners can gain the ability to incorporate information about unintended use into phases of recovery, including the definition of the problem, the process of motivating the client to undertake recovery, the list of options for starting, baseline pathology, and tracking of progress.

11.1.1 Importance

Assessing for unintended use will give the practitioner important information about the pattern and severity of loss of control over use of processed foods. Fear of an episode of unintended use is a factor in decisions by food addicts not to attend events and not to eat in front of other people. Thus the cessation of instances of unintended use could be instrumental in restoration of a full life for the addict.

Determining cues leading up to an episode of unintended use can be useful. Cue reactivity has been shown to gradually precede reward functions in the development of addictive neuroanomalies (Burger & Stice, 2014). Learning about the pattern of cuing can head off an episode of unintended use before it has a chance to develop into a distressing binge or prolonged graze. Information may be gathered about time of day, place, activities, type of food, size of package, encounters with people, and availability that precede unintended use. This cue inventory can serve as the basis of items in the initial list of options and encourage the client to stay with a program of cue avoidance.

One conundrum that is difficult to resolve is how to question the client about unintended use without triggering the addiction by recalling provocative images of addictive calorie-dense foods. Even associated cues can trigger cravings that lead to loss of cognitive function, including memory. The practitioner can use distraction to try to bring the client out of craving induced by remembering instances of loss of control.

Unintended use can dominate the consciousness of a food addict. Food addicted clients may wake up and make a plan not to eat processed foods. They may plan to not eat, or to eat less. This may manifest as the intention, "I'm going to be good today." The resolve may be overwhelmed by cravings within a few hours. This repeat failure to make good on a promise can be devastating to self-esteem. The addict may suffer for most of most days with the torment of unintended use as irrationally defined in the addict's mind. The addict may get to the point where every bite of food is subjected to self-recrimination as being indicative of loss of control (Duarte, Pinto-Gouveia, Ferreira, & Silva, 2016). Self-loathing about eating anything may become the genesis of anorexia. Rationalizing followed by self-blame may become virtually continuous. Examples include, "I'll just have one. Well, just this once. I think this time is different. I deserve it. It's a special occasion. Well, I have to eat something!" As such, it can also manifest in Criterion 2, failure to cut back, as the unintended termination of a weight-loss attempt. This quote from the FAA manual illustrates the rationalization and confusion of unintended use:

> I had always told myself I could stop eating anytime I wanted to, that I just didn't want to stop. (Food Addicts Anonymous, 2010, p. 119)

The internal confusion and sense of continuous failure associated with unintended use is a serious consequence of PFA. The ingestion of excessive harmful calorie-dense foods makes cessation of unintended use an important goal of recovery. Reestablishing a healthy dialog about the enjoyment of abstinent foods is a welcome benefit of recovery to a food addict who has suffered from unintended use.

11.1.2 Evidence for the Syndrome

Unintended use is a measure of impaired control. Two other criteria, failure to cut back and use in spite of consequences, are also indications that control is impaired. The behaviors involved in these three criteria share the characteristic of poor impulse control. The neurological basis for impaired control appears to emanate from dysfunction or downregulation in the restraint centers in the brain

(Lopez, Hofmann, Wagner, Kelley, & Heatherton, 2014). Impaired functioning in restraint centers has been shown in both drug addicts and in the obese (Weygandt et al., 2013). Research shows that impulse control can be compromised to the point that decisions are not coming to consciousness (Voon, 2015). Unintended use on a macro level can be seen in research showing weight regain after a weight-loss program (Kant, 2003; Turk et al., 2009).

11.1.3 Unintended Use in Motivating the Client

Information gathered about unintended use can be useful in helping the client develop motivation to undertake treatment for PFA. Episodes of unintended use are distressing to food-addicted clients. Because of the unpredictability of unintended use and the intensity of episodes, food-addicted clients may have removed themselves from social situations. The ability to resume a social life safe from fear of loss of control is a good incentive. Resolving the internal dialog about not wanting to eat but eating anyway can also be an important incentive to the food-addicted client. Reestablishing enjoyment of food is an attractive goal.

11.1.4 Resolving Unintended Use in Treatment

Tracking episodes of unintended use is valuable in developing strategies for avoiding the cues that lead to unintended use. Any episode of unintended use, however, major or minor, can be used to inventory exposures to cues. With knowledge of cue exposure, the practitioner can help the client shore up early defenses against a lapse. "Brain training" to restore impulse control can be highlighted in the program of an unintended eater. Functioning impulse control in the dorsolateral prefrontal cortex has been shown to be a factor in weight loss after 1 year (Weygandt 2015).

11.2 MANIFESTATIONS

Unintended use is a behavioral manifestation of PFA in the form of eating more than was planned. However, it is preceded by rationalizing thought patterns. It also manifests emotionally as fear of loss of control and shame over the loss of control. Physically, unintended use can result in being overfull. Food-addicted clients report fear of choking after severe episodes of unintended use and may sleep sitting up to avoid choking on food while sleeping.

11.2.1 Behaviors

There are three general categories of behaviors in unintended use: loss of control over eating itself, coping with loss of control, and hiding the loss of control over eating.

Loss of control over behaviors in unintended use can range from one bite in the case of breaking abstinence to the consumption of thousands of calories in an evening. One behavior that has been reported by food-addicted clients is the sensation of loss of control over foods that require repeated hand-to-mouth motion. This would include candies, chips, breakfast cereal, popcorn, nuts, olives, and high-sugar fruits such as grapes and cherries. Unintended use following a bite is illustrated in this quote:

> It took me a couple of attempts. I tried "sugar-free" yogurt and that sent me out into relapse. Later, I indulged in high-fat foods and questionable foods when my mother passed away, and that sent me out. After nine months of shaky abstinence, I picked up sugar and binged and purged non-stop for four days. I was having spontaneous nosebleeds, alarming my therapist and thinking constantly about suicide. I pray that four-day binge in December of 1995 was, God willing, my last. (Food Addicts Anonymous, 2010, p. 263)

Coping with loss of control can manifest as restricting calories or just not eating until evening. It can lead to the dieting behavior that is described under Criterion 2, failure to cut back. Reactions to unintended use can include purging, which can develop into bulimia. Anorexia could also be a reaction to unintended use. This is an example from the FAA Manual:

> I had isolated from my friends and family. I would eat before going out to be able to eat in small quantities while out. More than once I drove in a blackout after stopping at a drive-through restaurant. I stayed too busy to go home because I knew I would eat too much and flop on the couch or into bed in a comatose state. I was always exhausted. I had been relieved of the shame about my past, giving the shame to the people it belonged to. However, I was so ashamed of what and how I ate and the lying I did to enable my disease to flourish. I did not want to live. (Food Addicts Anonymous, 2010, p. 181)

Hiding can derive from a sense of profound embarrassment as the food addict completes episode after episode of overeating. Because of shame, the behavior may involve hiding or waiting until members of the household have gone to bed so the addict does not attract judgment. The addict may also hide and monitor the supply of foods. Avoidance of social events may develop due to fear of embarrassing loss of control. As unintended use progresses and the internal dialog of self-judgment intensifies, the addict may avoid eating in front of other people at all.

> Usually when I did heavy bingeing I was home alone on the couch in front of the television. (Food Addicts Anonymous, 2010, p. 139)

11.2.2 Mental

The mental anguish that occurs in unintended use is profound. Disassociating, obsessing, and loss of cognitive function can all be mental manifestations of unintended use. There is the distress of disassociating from the behavior, i.e., watching the behavior and being unable to stop it. The internal dialog about whether to eat and the self-shaming that follows eating can be virtually continuous in PFA.

Some eating may take place subconsciously. Memory loss may manifest. The addict may be surprised to find empty food containers with no memory of having eaten the contents. This is particularly so in cases of night eating. This quote illustrates the mental process in unintended use:

> As time evolved, I became less able to control either my starving or bingeing. The mental anguish that food addiction created for me was so painful that:
>
> I can't remember.
> My thought process stops midstream.
> My eyes are unable to focus.
> My body can't operate at its potential.
> I become numb and I create a fantasy world. (Food Addicts Anonymous, 2010, p. 166)

Being in a distracting situation can also lead to loss of decision-making (Kemps, Tiggemann, & Hollitt, 2014). People at a social event can be a distraction. The distraction may set up circumstances where the food addict is not consciously deciding to eat but rather is eating while distracted. This scenario can also play out in a restaurant, sports, or entertainment setting. It can occur while driving or at home in front of the television. The mental dysfunction associated with unintended use can be extensive.

11.2.3 Emotional

The distress of unintended eating is profound. If the food addict has been eating unconsciously, shock and dismay can occur upon discovering the quantity of food that has disappeared. This can be followed by deep and debilitating shame. Depression, anxiety, and self-loathing stemming from repeated episodes of loss of control may also result. Fear of discovery from eating in front of others may develop.

Unintended use can also feed the syndrome of shame from stigmatization. Unlike other addictions, unintended use can result in the accumulation of excess adipose tissue on the body of the food addict. As this progresses through overweight and into obesity, the addict may experience stigmatization, harsh judgment, and discrimination in the culture (Seacat, Dougal, & Roy, 2016). These can be sources of distressing shame. The food addict may fervently desire to stop the episodes of unintended use in order to stop the cultural oppression. The failure to control unintended use may be viewed as personal failure, lack of willpower, and even stupidity. Wearing the excess weight resulting from these failures in public and suffering the recriminations thereof is deeply shaming, as if forced to publicly admit being a failure over and over. The pain of the shame is stressful and can activate the disease.

For reasons of shame, the client may be unable to talk about unintended use early in the relationship with the practitioner. For reasons of avoiding triggering cravings in the client with detailed images of addictive foods, the practitioner can ask generally whether clients ever feel like they've lost control. Or whether they avoid social situations because they fear eating more than they'd like. Or even if they feel comfortable eating in front of other people at all.

11.2.4 Physical

The immediate physical manifestations of unintended use include bloating and being overfull. The addict may be afraid to go to sleep for fear of choking on food that travels back up the esophagus and into the windpipe. As unintended use occurs over many years, the addict may develop the full range of consequences of chronic processed food abuse. These are described in Criterion 9, use in spite of knowledge of consequences.

11.3 APPLICATION

Assessing for episodes of unintended use gives the practitioner the opportunity to begin the process of establishing trust with the client. As the client describes instances of unintended use, the practitioner can assure the client that such episodes are a normal expression of PFA and truly beyond the control of the client. The practitioner can frame such events as being of the nature of an allergic reaction such that exposure to cues sets off a chain reaction in the brain that suppresses decision-making and motor control. It can be described as a seizure or even an attack of the disease of PFA. Reassuring the client that recovery can curb unintended use can encourage the client to consider the value of a recovery program.

With a compassionate approach during the assessment and development of the scope of problem, the practitioner can begin the process of helping the client heal from the trauma of self-blame and even self-hatred stemming from unintended use. Education and understanding are the keys.

11.3.1 Care in Approach

The practitioner will want to take care not to judge the client's behavior. Remembering that food-addicted clients suffer from relationship sensitivity, practitioners would do well to go out of their way to avoid any appearance of disgust or impatience with clients as they share these episodes of shameful behavior. Reassurance about the possibility of remission of unintended use could be comforting to the client.

11.3.2 Developing Goals

Practitioners may find it helpful to sequence goals to address mental dysfunction before emotional and behavioral dysfunction. It may be useful to develop techniques to distract from thoughts of self-blame, restricting, obsessing about food, and self-criticism about eating at all. Substituting a calming activity such as a craft, exercise, reading recovery literature, or listening to a meditation can be helpful. These are described in the Part III of the textbook, "Recovery." As relief from the mental dysfunction progresses, emotions and behaviors can follow.

Agreeing on a food plan can also help the food addict give self-permission to enjoy the "safe" foods on the plan. The food addict may need time to develop the skills to execute an abstinent food plan, but just knowing that there are foods that the addict can enjoy without self-criticism can be a relief.

11.3.2.1 Tracking Progress

At baseline, the practitioner will have a description of the dysfunctional thought patterns, emotions, and behaviors associated with unintended use. Focusing on avoiding the cues that precede unintended use can be productive. Initially, tracking progress may cover instances where the client began to think dysfunctionally but employed distraction to switch to rational thoughts. Identifying instances of shame, fear, depression, and self-anger can create a platform from which to substitute positive thoughts. Setting boundaries with people on criticism about the addict's eating and weight can also reduce triggers to internalize stigma. With techniques to transform thoughts and emotions in place, the practitioner and client can track reductions in episodes of unintended use.

11.4 CONCLUSION

Unintended use may be found to be a crucial behavior in PFA insofar as it is at the core of important dysfunctions with behavioral, mental, emotional, and physical consequences. Impairment in restraint centers in the brain appear to underpin the syndrome of unintended use. Research shows that it is present in both drug addiction and obesity. Putting unintended use into remission takes a combination of cue avoidance as well as distraction from confusion about what to eat, self-blame, and cravings. A nonaddictive food plan gives the client the confidence to eat peacefully. The attitude of the practitioner should be compassionately reassuring and nonjudgmental. The remission of unintended eating can also open the door to the ability to eat in front of others and the resumption of a social life. Assessing carefully for unintended use yields returns in the development of the scope of problem, as well as the list of options to begin and tracking the progression of recovery.

REFERENCES

American Psychiatric Association. (2013). *The Diagnostic and Statistical Manual of Mental Disorders, Fifth Edition* (Vol. 5), American Psychiatric Association, Washington DC.

Burger, K. S., & Stice, E. (2014). Greater striatopallidal adaptive coding during cue-reward learning and food reward habituation predict future weight gain. *NeuroImage, 99*, 122–128. doi:10.1016/j.neuroimage.2014.05.066.

Duarte, C., Pinto-Gouveia, J., Ferreira, C., & Silva, B. (2016). Caught in the struggle with food craving: development and validation of a new cognitive fusion measure. *Appetite,* 101, 146–155.

Food Addicts Anonymous. (2010). *Food Addicts Anonymous.* Port St. Lucie, FL: Food Addicts Anonymous, Inc.

Kant, A. K. (2003). Interaction of body mass index and attempt to lose weight in a national sample of US adults: association with reported food and nutrient intake, and biomarkers. *Eur J Clin Nutr, 57*(2), 249–259. doi:10.1038/sj.ejcn.1601549.

Kemps, E., Tiggemann, M., & Hollitt, S. (2014). Biased attentional processing of food cues and modification in obese individuals. *Health Psychol, 33*(11), 1391–1401. doi:10.1037/hea0000069.

Lifshitz, F., & Lifshitz, J. Z. (2014). Globesity: the root causes of the obesity epidemic in the USA and now worldwide. *Pediatr Endocrinol Rev, 12*(1), 17–34.

Lopez, R. B., Hofmann, W., Wagner, D. D., Kelley, W. M., & Heatherton, T. F. (2014). Neural predictors of giving in to temptation in daily life. *Psychol Sci, 25*(7), 1337–1344. doi:10.1177/0956797614531492.

McLaren, I. P., Dunn, B. D., Lawrence, N. S., Milton, F. N., Verbruggen, F., Stevens, T., … Leknes, S. (2014). Why decision making may not require awareness state-dependent mu-opioid modulation of social motivation. *Behav Brain Sci, 37*(1), 35–36. doi:10.1037/xhp0000116.

Meany, G., Conceicao, E., & Mitchell, J. E. (2014). Binge eating, binge eating disorder and loss of control eating: effects on weight outcomes after bariatric surgery. *Eur Eat Disord Rev, 22*(2), 87–91. doi:10.1002/erv.2273.

Seacat, J. D., Dougal, S. C., & Roy, D. (2016). A daily diary assessment of female weight stigmatization. *J Health Psychol, 21*(2), 228–240. doi:10.1177/1359105314525067.

Stender, S., Dyerberg, J., & Astrup, A. (2007). Fast food: unfriendly and unhealthy. *Int J Obes (Lond), 31*(6), 887–890. doi:10.1038/sj.ijo.0803616.

Turk, M. W., Yang, K., Hravnak, M., Sereika, S. M., Ewing, L. J., & Burke, L. E. (2009). Randomized clinical trials of weight loss maintenance: a review. *J Cardiovasc Nurs, 24*(1), 58–80. doi:10.1097/01.jcn.0000317471.58048.32.

Voon, V. (2015). Cognitive biases in binge eating disorder: the hijacking of decision making. *CNS Spectr, 20*(6), 566–573. doi:10.1017/s1092852915000681.

Weygandt, M., Mai, K., Dommes, E., Leupelt, V., Hackmack, K., Kahnt, T., … Haynes, J. D. (2013). The role of neural impulse control mechanisms for dietary success in obesity. *NeuroImage, 83*, 669–678. doi: 10.1016/j.neuroimage.2013.07.028.

Yanovski, S. Z., Nelson, J. E., Dubbert, B. K., & Spitzer, R. L. (1993). Association of binge eating disorder and psychiatric comorbidity in obese subjects. *Am J Psychiatry, 150*(10), 1472–1479. doi:10.1176/ajp.150.10.1472.

12 DSM 5 SUD Criterion 2 *Failure to Cut Back*

Joan Ifland
Food Addiction Training, LLC
Cincinnati, OH

Diane Rohrbach
Fare Nutrition
Seattle, WA

CONTENTS

There is persistent desire or unsuccessful efforts to cut down or control processed food use. (American Psychiatric Association 2013, p. 490)

12.1 INTRODUCTION

Failure to cut back is perhaps the most common characteristic of processed food addiction (PFA) in obesogenic environments. Possibly due to an aggressive and ineffective diet industry in combination with stigmatization of the obese and ready availability of calorie-dense addictive foods, people are often motivated to reduce adipose tissue or "lose weight." Overweight and obese people are encouraged to attempt to cut back on their consumption of calories in order to achieve weight loss. Clients may also be faced with diet recommendations from their health professionals as treatment for diet-related diseases. However, research shows that these attempts are generally unsuccessful (Turk et al., 2009). Given that 36.9% of men and 38% of women worldwide are overweight (Ng et al., 2014) while the pressure to be thin is widespread, it is logical to assume that a majority of people have tried and failed to cut back on their caloric intake and achieve long-term weight loss.

However, failure to lose weight and to maintain the loss is not generally recognized as meeting the criteria for PFA.

For several reasons, assessing for failure to cut back in PFA might be more complicated than assessing for failure to cut back in drug addiction. From the standpoint of assessing an attempt to cut back on addictive substances, it is worthwhile to consider what happens to use of addictive foods in a weight-loss attempt. The attempt to cut back may not eliminate all addictive foods. It might fail because it was intentionally short term, so the addiction was rekindled upon reintroduction of addictive foods. The wrong foods may have been eliminated. And other addictive foods might have been substituted for the eliminated addictive foods.

Almost no weight-loss regimens completely eliminate addictive foods. Attempts to cut back for weight loss almost always involve only partial elimination of addictive substances at best. The wide range of different addictive food substances, their presentation as food, and claims for health properties confuses attempts to cut back considerably. The media encourages fads by focusing on one substance at a time, rotating sugar, fat, salt, gluten, red meat, and carbohydrates as the culprit *du jour*. This type of "partial" attempt to cut back can be seen to be sabotaged by the addictive foods remaining in the diet. These quotes from the Food Addicts Anonymous (FAA) manual illustrate the problem:

> Six times I failed in a national weight loss program, and two times in a self-help program. I did a stint in a weight reduction program at a gym. (Food Addicts Anonymous, 2010, 149)
>
> It seems that most of my life I was losing and gaining weight. I was obsessed about taking off the pounds, but once I reached the goal weight the old behavior took over. It was a constant yo-yo. (Food Addicts Anonymous, 2010, 172)
>
> My mother tried to help me lose weight. We would go on different diets, like the grapefruit and boiled egg diet. I didn't eat hard-boiled eggs for almost 20 years after that diet. I had little success at these diets and when I was twelve years old, my grandfather bought me a sewing machine because he thought if I had something else to do besides eat, I would lose weight. That didn't work, but enabled me to make my own clothes rather than face the mortification of shopping in the chubby department. I went on many weight-loss and exercise programs and was successful. But then once I started my relapse, the chains of food addiction pulled tighter around me and became like quicksand to my aching heart and soul. (Food Addicts Anonymous, 2010, 176)
>
> Food stayed my friend. It protected me. I am sure it saved me from insanity or worse. As with every food addict, the disease progressed in me. I was never honest on a diet and was still successful in losing weight. I would be "good" for the morning and adjust my intake by the end of the day. At 125 pounds, I thought I was so fat. I wasn't happy. Then, at 135 pounds, I was fat and wished I could weigh 125 pounds again. I tried every diet that came through friends and magazines. Eventually the diets just didn't work. I just kept getting fatter and fatter. (Food Addicts Anonymous, 2010, 181)
>
> I started stealing food from the store across the street from our house. I was totally out of control with my food, and at age fourteen I joined a weight-loss program. I did very well, so well I stopped going. Slowly, the weight came back, plus additional pounds. (Food Addicts Anonymous, 2010, 194)
>
> I was sixty years old when I reached my all-time high, 300-plus pounds. Since 1973, I had been in and out of another program and had lost 100 pounds two times. I never really "got it." I had worked only the physical aspect of the program. But I had always heard "keep coming back" and I'd kept it tucked in the back of my mind and, though I felt discouraged by my many weak attempts at recovery, I was finally brought back by my wonderful wife and my love for her. (Food Addicts Anonymous, 2010, 197)
>
> It is no longer normal for me to worry about weight, go on fifty or so fad diets a year or have ten different dress sizes in the closet. (Food Addicts Anonymous, 2010, 223)

Even if a weight-loss plan removes all addictive foods, the model of a weight-loss diet is that it ends when the weight-loss goal is achieved. In the PFA model, this is the equivalent of relapse, as illustrated by these quotes from the FAA manual:

> As the years went by, I got several sizes heavier. I joined a diet program and lost 50 pounds and kept off for several years. Through my first pregnancy, I didn't gain excessively. I discovered all those nice

> veggies and varieties of seafood that I had never bothered with before. So what went wrong this time? The maintenance program. All those toxic goodies that had been taken away during the weight loss period were given back in reasonable portions. Not knowing at the time that I'm a food addict who is unable to eat those toxic foods in reasonable amounts. (Food Addicts Anonymous, 2010, 96–96)
>
> As the years rolled by, I experienced the sadness and joy that is part of living, but where others could accept life on life's terms, more and more, I was losing my grasp on reality. A world of fantasy offered relief from the pain of everyday living. I panicked over minor situations; every decision was stress-filled. Fear and anxiety haunted me. My sedatives were sugar, cake, ice cream, candy, and rye bread. I couldn't stop with one serving. My family said, "You can have those things, just eat moderately." Maybe they could eat moderately, but for me it was impossible. (Food Addicts Anonymous, 2010, 111)

Reduced harm in drug addiction is considered a legitimate goal of recovery. However, due the prevalence of cuing found in PFA and the severity of PFA, trying to reduce as opposed to abstain from the range of addictive foods offers a possible explanation for the high rate of relapse from weight-loss efforts (Turk et al., 2009).

People may be exhorted to cut back on food substances that are not addictive such as red meat and unprocessed carbohydrates. In this example, there really is no attempt to cut back on addictive substances. Clients may have cut back on calories overall and have cut back on healthy foods while continuing the use of the addictive foods.

Another factor in relapse from weight-loss efforts is that other addictive foods may have been substituted for the eliminated addictive foods. An example is cutting out carbohydrates while increasing use of fats, as in an Atkins-style weight-loss scheme (Barnett, Barnard, & Radak, 2009). Addictive processed carbohydrates were replaced with addictive processed fats and high-fat dairy. The use of diet foods is another example. Diet foods can be loaded with addictive substances so if a dieter is using diet foods as a meal substitute or as snacks, an attempt to cut back on addictive foods has not actually occurred.

Fasting is an example of eliminating all addictive foods. However, because all nutritious foods have also been eliminated, PFA may have gotten worse due to intensified cravings (Stice, Davis, Miller, & Marti, 2008). Fasting has a built-in failure to cut back because it must end at some point, as illustrated by this quote from the FAA manual:

> Each day I would go as long as I could before I took the first bite of food, because I knew when I did, I wouldn't be able to stop until I passed out and went to bed. (Food Addicts Anonymous, 2010, 121)

Pharmaceuticals have also been shown to not just fail in weight loss but also to cause harmful side effects such as depression, heart damage, and memory loss (Merlo, Wandler, & Gold, 2014).

These weight-loss schemes can be considered as failed attempts to cut back, regardless of the underlying reason. Even though the addictive mechanism might have only been one of several factors, nonetheless the practitioner may count the event toward conformance with Criterion 2.

Nonconformance to Criterion 2 would be found in people who are overeating but have never tried to cut down. Nonconformance to failure to cut back may also occur in people who are overeating but may not be aware of it, as illustrated by this quote from the FAA manual:

> I can identify food as being a problem for me when I was as young as seven years old. I recall claiming that I was sick at school just so I could run home to Grandma's and eat. I couldn't get enough food. It was very hard for me to stop after the first bite. One serving turned into three. I recall the shame I would feel when told to put back a serving. I had no idea that I was overeating. I ate to calm my fears or to celebrate my joy. (Food Addicts Anonymous, 2010, 147)

Assessing for failure to cut back is also complicated by the goal of weight loss rather than recovery from an addiction. Using the DSM 5 substance use disorder (SUD) criteria to assess PFA helps clear the confusion between weight loss and recovery. Recovery from addiction focuses on putting specific behaviors into remission. These are the behaviors described in the DSM 5 SUD criteria. Weight gain is a factor in specific consequences of the addiction such as comorbidities, shame from stigmatization, and a motivator in failed attempts to cut back. In the assessment process, it is important to develop a full picture of dysfunctional addictive behaviors to help the client attach value to the recovery process. Weight loss may have been a powerful distraction from recovery goals such as control over a myriad of distressing behaviors.

It is important to develop a full history of failed attempts because the episodes of weight cycling can make PFA worse (Martire, Westbrook, & Morris, 2015). Throughout the process of developing the history of failed weight loss, it is important for the practitioner to repeatedly assure the client that the failure to cut back was a failure of the weight-loss scheme and not a failure on the part of the client. Because in public perception PFA is framed as a weight-loss issue rather than neurodysfunction, clients are likely to be frustrated with themselves over their failure to implement schemes that could never have worked no matter how carefully the client had followed the plan.

Another confounding factor is that failed attempts may not materialize for years. Bariatric surgery e.g., has been shown to fail gradually over years (Alvarez et al., 2016; Arapis et al., 2016). Bariatric surgery clients may also switch to alcohol or drugs (Bak, Seibold-Simpson, & Darling, 2016). However, the underlying syndrome may be addiction to processed foods. So the practitioner may count weight gain in the prior year as conformance to Criterion 2, even though the attempt may have started years before.

To avoid getting lost in the reasons for failure to cut back on addictive foods, practitioners can take a step back and remember why they're assessing for failure to cut back. It is to determine if the client conforms to the criterion. Conformance requires that the client have failed to cut back in the last year. Severity can be determined by how many times over the life of the client failures have occurred and how much weight was lost and regained.

12.1.1 Importance

Assessing Criterion 2 accurately is important for a number of reasons. Failure to cut back drives self-blame. Repeated episodes of dieting and weight cycling have been shown to make weight-loss more difficult (Petroni et al., 2007). There is evidence that weight-loss schemes may make PFA worse (Stice et al., 2008). And clinging to a weight-loss perspective can set clients up for relapse when a goal weight has been achieved. Practitioners will want to probe for all the different weight-loss methods that the client has endured, including the amount of weight lost and regained each time. Similar to drug addiction, a history of relapse can indicate the need for more extensive treatment (Turk et al., 2009). Understanding the history of failure to cut back can be used to develop a sense for the severity of the client's addiction to processed foods.

It is also important not to downplay the value of this criterion because "dieting" is so common. "Well, everyone has tried to lose weight" is not a reason to assume that it is not important. Rather, the broad prevalence of failed attempts in the general population could be interpreted as an indication that PFA may be widespread in obesogenic environments. This would be consistent with findings that severity of food addiction is loosely correlated with BMI (Gearhardt, Corbin, & Brownell, 2016).

It is also important to know how deeply attached the client is to "weight loss." Allowing a client to cling to the notion that diet-related problems will be solved by losing weight undermines recovery and sets the client up for relapse back into PFA when normal weight is attained. Addictive neuroconditioning has been shown to be permanent (Pavlov, 2015). Weight loss is a short-term effort that ceases when the weight has been lost. The conceptual framework of weight loss is not a fit for the treatment of PFA, which is a long-term condition. Understanding how attached the client is to weight loss can help the practitioner define the scope of the problem. Shifting the focus to cognitive restoration first with the understanding that weight loss will follow can be included in the options. Tracking a broad range of physical, mental, behavioral, and emotional improvements is the key to forestalling relapse upon attaining a particular goal weight.

In assessing for failure to cut back, the practitioner will want to listen carefully for the client's feelings about the experience of failure to cut back, particularly self-blame, self-loathing, and shame. Was weight loss the primary motivator in the attempts to cut back? Does the client believe that other health benefits proceed from weight loss or the elimination of processed foods? Is the client open to the idea that that it could be the processed foods and not adipose tissue that is causing the health problems? Is the client already aware that other benefits could ensue from eliminating processed foods? The answers to these questions can drive the formulation of the scope of problem, the list of options to start, as well as tracking the progression of treatment.

12.1.2 Evidence for the Syndrome

There is quite a bit of evidence that people fail to cut back in obesogenic environments. There is the research showing the failure of weight loss in general (Turk et al., 2009). There is also evidence that people are unable to conform to diet recommendations made by health professionals in the treatment of diet-related diseases (Pate et al., 1986; Zilli, Croci, Tufano, & Caviezel, 2000). The neurological basis for failure to cut back has several foundations. Cue-induced cravings have been shown to trigger the intense urge to eat addictive calorie-dense foods (Boswell & Kober, 2016), and food cues proliferate in obesogenic cultures (Lifshitz & Lifshitz, 2014). Loss of impulse control is another factor (Houben, Nederkoorn, & Jansen, 2014). Impaired decision-making and memory may play roles as well (Yesavage et al., 2014). Stress has also been shown to precede relapse into loss of control (Marks, 2016). Failure to cut back and a plausible basis in neurofunctioning have been demonstrated in the literature.

12.1.3 Use in Motivation

Using recovery from failed weight-loss attempts as motivation is a double-edged sword. The practitioner can motivate with the hope of fat loss but at the same time, it would be beneficial to the client to take the focus off weight loss and place it on the other benefits of recovery. The mental, behavioral, emotional, and physical benefits of abstaining from processed foods can be extensive. However, it may be a challenge to get the client to value other benefits enough to be motivated by them. Public awareness of the full range of the consequences of processed foods is limited. Many clients will not be aware of potential benefits such as recovery from chronic fatigue, depression, anxiety, and loss of cognitive functions. Information about other potential benefits of recovery will be gathered in Criterion 9, use in spite of consequences. The practitioner can help focus the client on the full range of results by periodically asking about results other than weight loss.

Another motivator might be the chance to stop dieting behaviors and to reframe the weight-loss failures as a failure of the weight-loss program and not the failure of the client. This idea could be very difficult for the client to accept, as self-blame for failure of weight loss may be a deeply ingrained belief that may have been reinforced by media and health professionals.

Another motivator could be the thought of pleasing a health professional. After years of failure to comply with a doctor's orders and concomitant shame, the client might look forward to proudly reviewing improved bloodwork numbers, for example.

The practitioner should try to persuade the client not to track success through a scale. People may be gaining muscle and bone mass, which could equal the loss of fat mass. A scale will report these two successes as lack of any progress.

12.1.4 Use in Treatment

Recovery from failure to cut back can be tracked by discussion of instances of cravings, loss of control, and days of abstinence. It is not recommended that continuous days of abstinence be counted. Many clients suffer from perfectionism and a slip with the concomitant shame of having to "start over" is stressful. As stress activates the addiction, it is to be avoided at all costs. Clients may be so shamed by having to start over that they give up.

Because of the intense prevalence of processed foods and cues, small lapses are much more likely in recovery from PFA than other SUDs. The 12-step model of rewarding and celebrating continuous days of abstinence is not appropriate in recovery from PFA for a number of reasons. The number of substances is much greater. Cuing is much more prevalent. Severity in general may be higher. Thus the chances of a slip are much higher. Added to the elevated probability of a slip is the devastating shame of yet another failure. This sensitivity to failure could have been developed at the hands of the diet and industries, which set food-addicted clients up for failure and shame. There are many other motivators in terms of the results that can be used more effectively and kindly than days of continuous abstinence.

12.2 MANIFESTATIONS

12.2.1 Behaviors

The types of weight-loss schemes are almost endless. An aggressive diet industry, along with a body-disordered glamor/media industry, and a misguided health industry have combined to create many heavily marketed weight-loss schemes. The pressure to maintain an idealized weight is intense, while the cuing to consume calorie-dense addictive foods is also quite intense. The weight-loss schemes do not work (Turk et al., 2009). The net result is that a sizeable portion of the general population is in the market for weight-loss products at any given moment (Kant, 2002).

12.2.2 Mental

The obsession with weight loss and the shame of failure may start as an occasional thought but increase to the point of being virtually continuous. The practitioner may ask a simple question about whether thoughts of weight loss mixed with thoughts of wanting to eat are somewhat continuous. Some clients will be able to identify with this. Some clients may be so afraid of weight gain that they think of it whenever they eat (Duarte, Pinto-Gouveia, Ferreira, & Silva, 2016). The point is that the mental dysfunction related to failure to cut back may be extensive. Practitioners can probe for its severity.

Weight cycling has been shown to correlate with intensity of cravings (Rodriguez-Martin, Gil-Perez, & Perez-Morales, 2014). In a rat study, Dore et al. simulated weight cycling in rats by alternating diets of regular chow with a high-sucrose palatable diet. Diet-cycled rats dramatically escalated the intake of the palatable diet during the first hour of renewed access. After withdrawal, the weight-cycling rats showed compulsive eating and heightened risk-taking behavior (Dore et al., 2014). The number of dieting attempts per year, BMI increase, and cumulative BMI loss since age 20 can be used as weight-cycling parameters (Petroni et al., 2007).

12.2.3 Emotional

The overriding emotional manifestation of failure to cut back is shame. There is shame of the failure itself, but in the case of PFA there is the additional shame of extra adipose tissue and the implicit admission of failure in the client's day-to-day activities. Weight cycling has been shown to be a risk factor for binge eating, depression, and interpersonal sensitivity (Petroni et al., 2007). The burden of repeated and public failure on such a crucial issue can lead to depression and anxiety (Phelan et al., 2015).

12.2.4 Physical

Repeated failure to cut back can be framed as weight cycling. Weight cycling has been shown to result in loss of lean mass (Beavers et al., 2011). Tragically, higher BMI correlated with more frequent weight cycling and efforts at weight loss (Delahanty, Meigs, Hayden, Williamson, & Nathan, 2002). The more the client has tried, the greater the weight gain.

12.3 APPLICATION

12.3.1 Care in Approach

Under all circumstances, practitioners will benefit from educating about lapses as a normal element of recovery. Getting ahead of the curve in this issue means assuring the client that lapses are a normal part of recovery. Every lapse is a valuable "discovery" experience. Understanding the cues and triggers leading up to the lapse is valuable. There can be no judgment about lapses. It may take the client months before developing the mental stability to remain clear-headed during a cue-induced craving. The ability to remember the painful consequences of a lapse in the face of cuing will come to each client at a very different pace as memory loss has been shown to occur in the obese (Manasse et al., 2014).

Circumstances leading up to a lapse can be dispassionately reviewed for ideas about how to prevent future lapses. A lapse may encourage adopting the goal of finding ways to ensure that clean food is readily available when needed. More comprehensive cue avoidance may be developed over time. Hopefully, the assessment of severity has motivated the client to build a program with sufficiently comprehensive abstinence, cue avoidance, and cognitive restoration programs, but this needs time. Minimizing what's needed for self-protection and consequences of use can be common in recovery.

Because lapses are generally associated with a painful reaction such as headache or grogginess, practitioners do not need to add to the pain by framing the lapse as a failure and increasing the humiliation by making the client "start over." The painful consequences of lapses can also prevent clients from giving themselves *cart blanche* to lapse whenever they feel like it. The strategy here is to let the headache serve as an associative cue to avoid lapses. The number of pairings of lapse to pain that occur before the consequence can be remembered in the face of a prolonged, compounded cue is going to be different for each client.

A warm, compassionate, approving attitude will let the process unfold as safely as possible. An easygoing, reassuring practitioner can help the client internalize self-acceptance and avoid the self-recrimination that can lead to further relapses. An unconditionally supportive environment with good education and a clear expectation that lapses are normal are the keys to helping a client get back to abstinence after a lapse.

12.3.2 Developing Goals

In an effort to focus the client on abstinent meals as opposed to weight loss, the practitioner can avoid setting weight-loss goals. In recovery from processed foods, healthy gain in muscle and bone can occur (Lee, Hong, Shin, & Lee, 2016). For this reason, it is wise to persuade the client to remove the scale from the house. A slogan such as "weigh your food not your body" might be helpful.

Education about the precursors to relapse would reduce risk of relapse. Precursors to relapse include cues to crave, stress, hunger, and sleep deprivation (Morris, Beilharz, Maniam, Reichelt, & Westbrook, 2014; Sample, Martin, Jones, Hargrave, & Davidson, 2015). Goals for cue avoidance could be removing processed foods from the house, reducing television time, throwing out the diet cookbooks, finding a cue-free route to work, avoiding the break room at work, and declining invitations to events centered on food. Stress reduction goals might include setting boundaries with food pushers and critics. Hunger reduction can be a process of eating on time and serving full portions. Setting and meeting a bedtime, as well as sleeping or meditating through the night (as opposed to getting out of bed), are great sleep goals.

These kinds of gentle and productive goals broken down into very small steps can accustom the client to success and heal the trauma of failure to cut back.

12.3.3 Tracking Progress

Tracking progress in recovery from failure to cut back should focus on behaviors. Tracking by weight-loss number derived from a scale is harmful. The scale itself is a powerful cue to shame from past failed attempts. The scale weighs muscle and bone, which on a successful recovery plan could be growing heavier. So, even though fat tissue may be reduced, the scale will not reflect this. Thus the scale may cue the client into a mindset of failure, shame, depression, and despair. Even stepping on a scale that measures percentage of fat versus other elements of the body could be a reminder of trauma.

Further if the client is exercising and muscles are getting bigger, clothes might not loosen. So using the method of how clothes are fitting may also lead to discouragement and trigger the fear of failure as well as the urge to quit.

A method that measures fat without measuring muscle or bone is by measuring a skin fold. Clients should be discouraged from even using this method as it encourages weight obsession, which is painful. Because of the attachment of pathological shame to fat, there may not be a safe nontriggering method for tracking fat loss. The best approach would be to emphasize progress in recovery from physical, emotional, behavioral, and mental distress. Celebrating these benefits can serve to reinforce the value of the program, as well as divert attention from the painful issue of fat.

Tracking progress toward goals should be done in very small steps. It should also be done at the client's discretion, depending on what is important to the client. In Chapter 22 of this textbook, the Addiction Severity Index helps in identifying the client's priorities. The practitioner should avoid setting time limits, as this is counterproductive to the goals of reducing stress, creating successes for the client, and avoiding the perception of failure. Whenever the client reports any movement toward a goal, the practitioner can express enthusiastic approval, compliments, and encouragement.

12.4 CONCLUSION

Although failure to cut back is common is obesogenic cultures, its seriousness should not be overlooked. A history of failed attempts to cut back can be a source of deep trauma for food-addicted clients because it could attract harsh judgment from media-driven cultures. Because attempts to cut back are generally focused on the limited goal of losing weight, the practitioner can beneficially educate clients about the broader range of results that could be attained from undertaking recovery from addiction to processed foods. As clients develop an understanding of the scope of possible benefits, results can be incorporated into the motivation phase of preparing for recovery. Small steps toward reducing the risk of relapse can be included in the list of options for starting. Relapse prevention strategies can form the basis for tracking progress toward a program of protection against relapse.

Healing from failure to cut back and laying down the burden of ineffective weight-loss schemes is a life-changing benefit for food-addicted clients.

REFERENCES

Alvarez, V., Carrasco, F., Cuevas, A., Valenzuela, B., Munoz, G., Ghiardo, D., . . . Maluenda, F. (2016). Mechanisms of long-term weight regain in patients undergoing sleeve gastrectomy. *Nutrition, 32*(3), 303–308. doi:10.1016/j.nut.2015.08.023.

American Psychiatric Association. (2013). *The Diagnostic and Statistical Manual of Mental Disorders, Fifth Edition* (Vol. 5), American Psychiatric Association, Washington DC.

Arapis, K., Tammaro, P., Parenti, L. R., Pelletier, A. L., Chosidow, D., Kousouri, M., . . . Marmuse, J. P. (2016). Long-term results after laparoscopic adjustable gastric banding for morbid obesity: 18-year follow-up in a single university unit. *Obes Surg, 27*(3), 630–640. doi:10.1007/s11695-016-2309-7.

Bak, M., Seibold-Simpson, S. M., & Darling, R. (2016). The potential for cross-addiction in post-bariatric surgery patients: Considerations for primary care nurse practitioners. *J Am Assoc Nurse Pract, 28*(12), 675–682. doi:10.1002/2327-6924.12390.

Barnett, T. D., Barnard, N. D., & Radak, T. L. (2009). Development of symptomatic cardiovascular disease after self-reported adherence to the Atkins diet. *J Am Diet Assoc, 109*(7), 1263–1265. doi:10.1016/j.jada.2009.04.003.

Beavers, K. M., Lyles, M. F., Davis, C. C., Wang, X., Beavers, D. P., & Nicklas, B. J. (2011). Is lost lean mass from intentional weight loss recovered during weight regain in postmenopausal women? *Am J Clin Nutr, 94*(3), 767–774. doi:10.3945/ajcn.110.004895.

Boswell, R. G., & Kober, H. (2016). Food cue reactivity and craving predict eating and weight gain: A meta-analytic review. *Obes Rev, 17*(2), 159–177. doi:10.1111/obr.12354.

Delahanty, L. M., Meigs, J. B., Hayden, D., Williamson, D. A., & Nathan, D. M. (2002). Psychological and behavioral correlates of baseline BMI in the diabetes prevention program (DPP). *Diabetes Care, 25*(11), 1992–1998.

Dore, R., Valenza, M., Wang, X., Rice, K. C., Sabino, V., & Cottone, P. (2014). The inverse agonist of CB1 receptor SR141716 blocks compulsive eating of palatable food. *Addict Biol, 19*(5), 849–861. doi:10.1111/adb.12056.

Duarte, C., Pinto-Gouveia, J., Ferreira, C., & Silva, B. (2016). Caught in the struggle with food craving: Development and validation of a new cognitive fusion measure. *Appetite, 101*, 146–155.

Food Addicts Anonymous. (2010). *Food Addicts Anonymous*. Port St. Lucie, FL: Food Addicts Anonymous, Inc.

Gearhardt, A. N., Corbin, W. R., & Brownell, K. D. (2016). Development of the Yale Food Addiction Scale Version 2.0. *Psychol Addict Behav, 30*(1), 113–121. doi:10.1037/adb0000136.

Houben, K., Nederkoorn, C., & Jansen, A. (2014). Eating on impulse: The relation between overweight and food-specific inhibitory control. *Obesity (Silver Spring)*, 22(5), E6–E8.

Kant, A. K. (2002). Weight-loss attempts and reporting of foods and nutrients, and biomarkers in a national cohort. *Int J Obes Relat Metab Disord, 26*(9), 1194–1204. doi:10.1038/sj.ijo.0802024.

Lee, J., Hong, Y. P., Shin, H. J., & Lee, W. (2016). Associations of sarcopenia and sarcopenic obesity with metabolic syndrome considering both muscle mass and muscle strength. *J Prev Med Public Health, 49*(1), 35–44. doi:10.3961/jpmph.15.055.

Lifshitz, F., & Lifshitz, J. Z. (2014). Globesity: The root causes of the obesity epidemic in the USA and now worldwide. *Pediatr Endocrinol Rev, 12*(1), 17–34.

Manasse, S. M., Juarascio, A. S., Forman, E. M., Berner, L. A., Butryn, M. L., & Ruocco, A. C. (2014). Executive functioning in overweight individuals with and without loss-of-control eating. *Eur Eat Disord Rev, 22*(5), 373–377. doi:10.1002/erv.2304.

Marks, D. F. (2016). Dyshomeostasis, obesity, addiction and chronic stress. *Health Psychol Open, 3*(1), 2055102916636907. doi:10.1177/2055102916636907.

Martire, S. I., Westbrook, R. F., & Morris, M. J. (2015). Effects of long-term cycling between palatable cafeteria diet and regular chow on intake, eating patterns, and response to saccharin and sucrose. *Physiol Behav, 139*, 80–88. doi:10.1016/j.physbeh.2014.11.006.

Merlo, L. J., Wandler, K., & Gold, M. S. (2014). Co-occurring addiction and eating disorders. In R. K. Ries, S. C. Miller, D. A. Fiellin, & R. Saitz (Eds.), *The ASAM Principles of Addiction Medicine*, pp. 529–534. Washington, DC: American Society of Addiction Medicine.

Morris, M. J., Beilharz, J., Maniam, J., Reichelt, A., & Westbrook, R. F. (2014). Why is obesity such a problem in the 21st century? The intersection of palatable food, cues and reward pathways, stress, and cognition. *J Neurosci*, 58: 36–45. doi:10.1523/jneurosci.2013-14.2014 10.1016/j.neubiorev.2014.12.002.

Ng, M., Fleming, T., Robinson, M., Thomson, B., Graetz, N., Margono, C., . . . Gakidou, E. (2014). Global, regional, and national prevalence of overweight and obesity in children and adults during 1980–2013: A systematic analysis for the Global Burden of Disease Study 2013. *Lancet, 384*(9945), 766–781. doi:10.1016/s0140-6736(14)60460-8.

Pate, C. A., Dorang, S. T., Keim, K. S., Stoecker, B. J., Fischer, J. L., Menendez, C. E., & Harden, M. (1986). Compliance of insulin-dependent diabetics with a low-fat diet. *J Am Diet Assoc, 86*(6), 796–798.

Pavlov, I. P. (2015). *Conditioned Relexes* (G. V. Anrep Ed.). Mansfield Centre, CT: Martino Publishing.

Petroni, M. L., Villanova, N., Avagnina, S., Fusco, M. A., Fatati, G., Compare, A., & Marchesini, G. (2007). Psychological distress in morbid obesity in relation to weight history. *Obes Surg, 17*(3), 391–399. doi:10.1007/s11695-007-9069-3.

Phelan, S. M., Burgess, D. J., Puhl, R., Dyrbye, L. N., Dovidio, J. F., Yeazel, M., . . . van Ryn, M. (2015). The adverse effect of weight stigma on the well-being of medical students with overweight or obesity: Findings from a national survey. *J Gen Intern Med, 30*(9), 1251–1258. doi:10.1007/s11606-015-3266-x.

Rodriguez-Martin, B. C., Gil-Perez, P., & Perez-Morales, I. (2014). Exploring the "weight" of food cravings and thought suppression among Cuban adults. *Eat Weight Disord, 20*(2), 249–256. doi:10.1007/s40519-014-0163-y.

Sample, C. H., Martin, A. A., Jones, S., Hargrave, S. L., & Davidson, T. L. (2015). Western-style diet impairs stimulus control by food deprivation state cues: Implications for obesogenic environments. *Appetite, 93*, 13–23. doi:10.1016/j.appet.2015.05.018.

Stice, E., Davis, K., Miller, N. P., & Marti, C. N. (2008). Fasting increases risk for onset of binge eating and bulimic pathology: A 5-year prospective study. *J Abnorm Psychol, 117*(4), 941–946. doi:2008-16252-019. 10.1037/a0013644.

Turk, M. W., Yang, K., Hravnak, M., Sereika, S. M., Ewing, L. J., & Burke, L. E. (2009). Randomized clinical trials of weight loss maintenance: A review. *J Cardiovasc Nurs, 24*(1), 58–80. doi:10.1097/01.jcn.0000317471.58048.32.

Yesavage, J. A., Kinoshita, L. M., Noda, A., Lazzeroni, L. C., Fairchild, J. K., Taylor, J., . . . O'Hara, R. (2014). Effects of body mass index-related disorders on cognition: Preliminary results. *Diabetes Metab Syndr Obes, 7*, 145–151. doi:10.2147/dmso.s60294.

Zilli, F., Croci, M., Tufano, A., & Caviezel, F. (2000). The compliance of hypocaloric diet in type 2 diabetic obese patients: A brief-term study. *Eat Weight Disord, 5*(4), 217–222.

13 DSM 5 SUD Criterion 3
Time Spent

Joan Ifland
Food Addiction Training, LLC
Cincinnati, OH

Elaine Epstein
Private Practice
Huntington Woods, MI

CONTENTS

A great deal of time is spent in activities necessary to obtain processed foods, eat processed foods, or recover from their effects. (American Psychiatric Association, 2013, 491)

13.1 INTRODUCTION

Time spent is a measure of salience of processed food addiction (PFA). It is a measure of how conspicuous or prominent the addiction has become in the life of the food-addicted client. Criterion 7, important activities given up, is another measure of the salience of PFA. In the early stages of addiction, the time lost may be just the occasional extra stop at a fast food restaurant. As the syndrome progresses in severity, the addiction may eventually consume the addict's life in terms of fatigue, sleepiness, brain fog, television, long hours at low-paying jobs, medical problems, visits to food outlets, and mental obsession. Attempts to compensate for overeating, such as attendance at weight-loss programs and exercising, can also absorb the addict's time. PFA can absorb the client's time almost continuously. Time spent can expand to virtually 24 hours per day if disrupted sleep and night eating are present.

A number of themes help explain how PFA may drive the ways in which food-addicted clients use time, including cognitive impairment, issues of immobility, and lower socioeconomic status. Chronic processed food abuse is associated with both fatigue and disrupted sleep. So food-addicted clients may spend time sleeping during the day (Patel, Spaeth, & Basner, 2016). Resulting obesity, shortness of breath, joint pain, and body shame may make it difficult to move, so time may be primarily spent in sedentary behaviors (Perez & Warren, 2012). Due to cognitive deficits and discrimination against obese people, the obese are more likely to spend time in low-paying jobs and shift work (Griep et al., 2014). Memory loss is associated with obesity so clients may not be able to remember how they spend time. A logbook can help collect data on how time is being spent (Igelstrom, Emtner, Lindberg, & Asenlof, 2013).

The findings in cognitive impairment suggest that food-addicted clients are unlikely to be engaged in intellectually challenging pursuits. Even reading may be an unrewarding pastime, possibly related to learning difficulties, attention deficit, and memory loss. Research shows that client's time is probably not spent in exercise, cooking, or socializing (Patel et al., 2016).

Although the food-addicted client may not remember or may be too ashamed to share, PFA can progress to the point that the client is spending time eating inordinate amounts of processed foods. Food obsession can start innocently with perusing cookbooks, making food, or studying gourmet techniques. The time spent can progress into hours spent going from one fast food outlet to the next. Entire weekends can be spent eating and sleeping (Patel et al., 2014). People can be so tired and brain-fogged (Theoharides, Stewart, Hatziagelaki, & Kolaitis, 2015) from consuming processed foods that they sleep, watch television, or surf the Internet whenever they're not at work or caring for family (Patel et al., 2016).

Another way in which PFA consumes time is obsession over food and body. PFA can literally consume every waking moment as the food addict thinks about what to eat constantly. Along with the obsession about what to eat, obsession with body image and weight loss can also occupy thoughts. This is not a quantifiable loss of time, but food-addicted clients may feel as if their life is slipping by because they cannot focus on anything but food and weight.

Because processed foods are not illegal, food-addicted clients will likely not exhibit one characteristic of recreational drug use, which is the time spent avoiding law enforcement personnel in order to obtain substances. In PFA, there is no need to contact a supplier or meet a pusher in an out-of-the way place. There is no need to find a secret place out of public view to indulge in illegal use. To the contrary, processed foods are pushed legally and enthusiastically in many venues (Lifshitz & Lifshitz, 2014). Indeed, the easy, cheap availability of processed foods may accelerate the development of severity of PFA. The food addict may be spending minimal time obtaining food but a significant amount of time recovering from its use in terms of sleepiness, fatigue, depression, and medical problems. Because the consequences of overuse are not illegal, food-addicted clients are less likely to have a history of legal problems as the result of drunk driving, for example. They also do not seem to engage in violent behavior that can generate legal problems.

13.1.1 Importance

Finding out how the client is spending time is vital to the effort to determine how far the disease has progressed. The information can provide valuable material for the development of the assessment, scope of problem, and options to begin recovery. It can also support the practitioner's efforts to motivate the client. It may be productive to go back in the history to a time before the client became "disabled" by fatigue, brain fog, sleep deprivation, and mobility issues. The practitioner can find out what activities the client used to enjoy. There may be hopes or dreams that the client gradually abandoned as the addiction consumed more and more time. Clients may not connect the loss of their dreams to fatigue and cognitive impairment from processed foods. Cataloging what has been lost and the value of being able to spend time on more rewarding activities is a valuable element of recovery and can be used to motivate the client to start a program of recovery.

13.1.2 Evidence for the Syndrome

Studies demonstrate that the obese spend more time in sedentary behaviors than lean people (Gupta et al., 2016). Research shows that the obese spend more time watching television and other screens than lean people. This is true for both older and younger populations (Patel et al., 2016). As would be expected from the findings on television viewing, the obese spend more time sitting than lean people do (Bond et al., 2011). Obese people do not exercise as much as lean people, but when they do they spend the same amount of time at it (Patel et al., 2016). Obese people are not spending time cooking, which is consistent with correlations of fast food visits to obesity (Patel et al., 2016). However, obese people attend sporting and entertainment events to the same extent as lean people (Song et al., 2012).

Regarding sleep, there is a finding of a U-shaped curve. Obese people who are holding down several jobs sleep less than average. Obese people who do not hold a job sleep more than obese people who do hold jobs (Basner, Spaeth, & Dinges, 2014). One study found that obese people are more likely to sleep during the day (Patel et al., 2016). The higher the BMI, the later the person goes to bed (Basner & Dinges, 2009).

Research also shows that the obese are more likely than lean populations to be holding down several jobs and to be working night shifts (Patel et al., 2016). These working patterns can be time-consuming and could also contribute to sleepiness during nonwork hours.

Igelstrom found that using recall to collect data about sleep, sedentary behaviors, and exercise was inaccurate, possibly because the obese population was sleep-deprived. Logbooks were found to be more accurate than recall for a questionnaire in terms of conformance to accelerometer data (Igelstrom et al., 2013).

Obese populations have been shown to suffer from mobility issues, which can limit options for spending time. These include joint pain, shortness of breath, and excess adipose tissue (McGregor, Cameron-Smith, & Poppitt, 2014). They also suffer from a myriad of chronic illnesses, which can absorb time from being sick in bed and from seeking medical treatment (Padula, Allen, & Nair, 2014).

For food addicted clients, the research shows a life of television, uneven sleep patterns, chronic illness, and the possibility of holding down several jobs. With this scenario in mind, practitioners can probe for information about how much the television and computer are turned on in the household. This can also be a time to ask about time spent cooking and the source of meals, including meals sourced from fast food restaurants.

13.1.3 Use in Motivation

Changing the way that time is spent may depend on improvements in health that make the changes possible. Improvements in mobility, cognition, and sleep may be thought of as primary motivators. The activities that then become possible as a result of improvements in health may be secondary motivators.

If the client is sedentary due to joint pain or fatigue, initially the motivation to change may come more from the prospect of resolving those issues than being able to exercise. Exploring the history of exercise is helpful. The client may have enjoyed exercise but been forced to give it up due to pain, body shame, or fear of failure. The ability to exercise might not be a great motivator, but other forms of physical activity could be. These might include being able to play with children, keep an orderly house, play a sport, or even get off a scooter and resume walking.

If cognitive impairment such as learning disabilities, memory loss, and attention deficit are interfering with activities, then the hope of improving cognition itself may be an effective motivator. The practitioner can reinforce this motivation by finding out about valued activities that could be resumed with improved cognition. Examples might be abandoned reading or writing projects. Clients may feel that they don't have the time to cook, when the underlying problem may be fear of learning how to prepare meals because they are suffering from learning disabilities.

Clients may have unfinished projects that were begun in impulsive moments but unfinished due to attention deficit. The practitioner may find that the food addict is valiantly attempting to go to school or work toward certifications and promotions in spite of brain fog. In these cases, the ability to work more efficiently and effectively could be an important motivator. Recovery of cognitive abilities may mean that the client can finish work more quickly and progress with more confidence.

A common motivator is the prospect of being able to sleep and wake up rested and alert. Sleep deprivation and being groggy and sleepy during the day are uncomfortable symptoms of PFA. Being energetic consistently could be an important benefit, even greater than weight loss. For some clients, a reduction in inflammation and excess adipose tissue that develops in recovery may mean that the client will be able to stop using a sleep machine. With healthy sleep, the food addict can spend time in interesting activities rather than sedentary activities such as watching television and surfing the Internet. These can be effective motivators as clients learn that the impairments are derived from processed foods.

Food-addicted clients may also confuse a lack of time with a lack of energy or mental focus. This can be a barrier to undertaking recovery so it's valuable to explore possible underlying reasons for a perception of "not enough time" to shop or cook. Resolving these perceptions may remove barriers to motivation.

Reviewing the lost opportunities suffered by the client due to PFA may provide important motivators to changing how clients use their time. Shifting from time spent in PFA to time spent in rewarding and pleasurable activities is a valuable benefit of recovery.

13.2 MANIFESTATIONS

Manifestations of how time is consumed by the addiction can be categorized into behavioral, mental, emotional, and physical.

13.2.1 Behavioral

The most prominent behaviors in time spent are watching television, sleeping, and working. Eating behavior does not appear in the research as time-consuming for obese people, possibly because study participants cannot remember it or because they're too ashamed to report it or because it doesn't take much time to obtain addictive convenience foods. However, the frantic pursuit of processed foods is reported in the manuals for the 12-step food addiction groups. Examples are provided below. As a corollary, there are also missing behaviors such as socializing, education, and the pursuit of career advancement, which will be covered in Criterion 7.

The relationship between television and PFA is complex and synergistic. Research shows that television contributes to the development of PFA through the way in which it stimulates brain activity (Yokum, Gearhardt, Harris, Brownell, & Stice, 2014). The impact of commercials has been shown to influence a toddler's choice after only five exposures (Borzekowski & Robinson, 2001). After the tobacco companies acquired major food corporations, the number of television commercials for refined foods shown on saturday mornings rose from 160 in 1987, to 264 in 1992, and 564 in 1994 (Nestle, 2002, 181). To support the role of television in the spread of obesity, 65 million households in the late 1990s watched Nickelodeon, which was a major broadcaster of commercials for processed food (Nestle, 2002, 181).

Television and the glamour industry may also promote PFA through the mechanism of dieting. Research shows that dieting contributes to weight cycling (Cottone, Sabino, Steardo, & Zorrilla, 2008), possibly through the mechanism of increased cravings. Episodes of weight cycling are found to correlate with severity of BMI (Cottone, Sabino, Steardo, & Zorrilla, 2009).

Once PFA has progressed to the point of fatigue and impaired cognition, the relationship between the addict and television may shift. Although television may continue to provoke cravings through commercials and body obsession through eating disordered actors and stressful programming, it may also take on a new role. It may provide a "cover" for the fact that the food addict is too compromised to do much of anything else (Ocon, 2013; Theoharides et al., 2015). As such, time spent watching television may be a good indicator of the severity of the disease.

The research shows that food-addicted clients spend time during the day sleeping (Patel et al., 2016). This might be the direct effect of eating processed foods, which may make people groggy, combined with the indirect effect of disordered sleep (Calhoun, 2011 #9156).

Working several jobs and working night shifts have been found to be prevalent among the obese (Patel et al., 2016). Due to the lack of education and discrimination, night-shift jobs and multiple low-paying jobs may be the only jobs available to the obese (Basner & Dinges, 2009). Fatigue and disrupted sleep as well as time spent at the job may all be considered as indirect manifestations of the time that the addiction consumes.

13.2.2 Mental

Time spent can manifest mentally as obsessive thought patterns. The addict may be thinking obsessively about food and experience intense cravings (Davis, Levitan, Kaplan, Kennedy, & Carter, 2014). Cravings are covered more extensively in Criterion 4, cravings. The client may also be thinking obsessively about weight and body image (Stice et al., 2001). Obsessive worry about food and body can then spread to chronic anxiety about life in general (Morris, Beilharz, Maniam, Reichelt, & Westbrook, 2014).

Loss of cognitive function plays a role in terms of encouraging food-addicted clients to avoid tasks that might require learning, decision-making, or memory (Noble & Kanoski, 2016; Yesavage et al., 2014). Because television does not require intellectual effort, it can be thought of as a default activity to pass time in food-addicted clients who are no longer capable of engaging in more demanding activities.

13.2.3 Emotional

In addition to cognitive impairment, negative affect can shape activity choices for the food addict. The food addict may be too stigmatized, depressed, or anxious to leave the house (Ratcliffe & Ellison, 2015; Vandewater, Park, Hebert, & Cummings, 2015). Unfavorable comparison to actors may encourage shame and depression from time spent with television and Internet (Do, Shin, Bautista, & Foo, 2013). The absence of exercise and healthy sleep can also contribute to negative affect (Katz et al., 2016).

13.2.4 Physical

Television and sleepiness can combine to keep the food addict from being active. The lack of physical activity can be associated with a myriad of physical problems, including circulation, cardiovascular disease, and diabetes (Goularte, Ferreira, & Sanvitto, 2012). Sedentary behavior may lead to sarcopenia and osteoporosis (Aggio et al., 2016; Zhang et al., 2014). All of these factors can contribute to the accumulation of excess adipose tissue. Time spent in sedentary behaviors has a significant impact on physical deterioration.

13.3 CASES OF TIME SPENT IN PFA

Here are examples of how food obsession can take up time by determining where the addict can access processed foods, by interfering with work, by seeking processed foods, by avoiding weight gain, by consuming thought patterns, and by interfering with sleep and relationships. Child food-addicted clients can also experience time spent in the addiction.

The addiction may drive clients to only spend time in venues where processed foods are available.

I think you can see the pattern of obsession with food. My life revolved around sports events, carnival type entertainment, movies and anywhere I could consume extra amounts of food. (Food Addicts Anonymous, 2010, 190)

His love for me was not enough, though, and I found other ways to be nurtured, usually through sweet foods. My father ran a movie theater and on the pretext of helping out the candy girls, I would work behind the candy counter and sell a few bars even as I ate several of them before, during and after the movies. They also sold ice cream cones and hot buttered popcorn, which I ate by the box full. It was impossible to go to the movies without these things. I was mainly responsible for making sure that the meals were ready for my brothers and sisters. I would make sure that they had dessert, so after school I always baked cookies, a cake, or something sweet. (Food Addicts Anonymous, 2010, 208–209)

The addiction can also divert the addict's time from work to the pursuit of processed foods and the management of consequences. Here are examples:

Instead of calling on customers for my work, I drove here and there, bingeing in my car. (Food Addicts in Recovery Anonymous, pp. 22–23)

Things had gotten so bad that I couldn't make it more than an hour or two at work without leaving the office to get something to eat. Some days, when things were really stressful, I would turn to the desk drawer full of sweets to help me cope. Sometimes it seemed like I ate non-stop. I looked forward to work for the chance to eat at my desk without anyone knowing about it and I looked forward to getting home to eat before, during, and after dinner. I looked forward to time spent at my in-laws house on the weekend where there was always food and alcohol galore. I looked forward to shopping by myself because I could get all kinds of sweets at the mall. (Food Addicts Anonymous, 2010, 225–226)

For the next 17 years my weight continued to increase until I weighed 270 pounds and suffered from severe pain in my back, legs and knees. Finally, in too much pain to continue working, I sought medical help. (Food Addicts Anonymous, 2010, 245)

Similar to drug addiction, the pursuit and consumption of food can be time-consuming:

I would walk around the supermarket and eat my way up and down the aisles. I ate burnt or frozen foods. Binge foods consumed my every thought and feeling. (Food Addicts Anonymous, 2010, 105)

I would heave my huge body out of my recliner chair, go and get food, go back to my chair and eat it and then be compelled to go back for more food, and so on, until bedtime. (Food Addicts Anonymous, 2010, 121)

I never wanted normal meals. I wanted junk foods. I could never eat one of anything. I would buy 6–8 donuts, a bag of cookies, or a box of crackers, and consume them all at once. My other habit was grazing. I ate from the time I woke up to the time I went to bed, vowing to behave differently tomorrow. I inhaled food and ate in secret. I would fix one sandwich after another, peanut butter and jelly, or cheese and mayonnaise. (Food Addicts Anonymous, 2010, 205)

My binges started with boxes of healthy Shredded Wheat with quarts of skim milk, along with boxes of Grapenuts and as many bagels as were in my house. Then I would move on to raw or cooked oatmeal. I would further lose control and eat a jar of jelly and/or peanut butter, frozen blintzes, and whatever else I could find. I ate until I blacked out. I would wake up on top of and surrounded by boxes and bags. (Food Addicts Anonymous, 2010, 130)

I found bingeing as a way to comfort the loneliness and stop the emotional "see-saw" which occupied my life. I binged daily in the living room, in the dark, with only the light of the television to guide my eating. After bingeing, I fell asleep. Some people call it a "blackout." When I woke up, I would continue bingeing on the leftover foods. (Food Addicts Anonymous, 2010, 91–92)

Attempts to avoid weight gain as a consequence of PFA also can take time:

From then on, I threw up after every binge, sometimes many times a day. Because of all I ate, I continued to gain weight, and though I was actively involved in the twelve-step food program, I was both bulimic and fat. (Food Addicts in Recovery Anonymous, p. 78)

I must have weighed myself sixty-two times a day. I'd get on the scale in the bathroom, but I didn't like what it read. The bathroom had a tile floor. It seemed best to take the scale out onto the smoother, wooden floor. That had seams in it, though, so I'd put the scale on top of a chair, which was just one plank of wood, and then I would climb up on top of the chair to see my weight. (Food Addicts in Recovery Anonymous, p. 90)

I was still taking amphetamines, even though the benefit of limiting what I ate had long worn off, because I was now dependent on them. I could not stay awake, nor could I function without them. (Food Addicts Anonymous, 2010, 96)

Along with the binge eating all day, I was stopping in stores and buying clothes to fit my new larger sizes. At one point I had four different sizes in my closet. (Food Addicts Anonymous, 2010, 103)

Because most of my waking hours were spent figuring how I would "get rid of" the calories I had ingested, managing my food and exercise became my primary purpose in college and gaining an education was secondary. (Food Addicts Anonymous, 2010, 134)

I was heavy into exercise, sometimes twice a day. Once wasn't enough. My mind wouldn't stop. I couldn't deal with my feelings, my emotions, or my thoughts. The only time I felt good was when I exercised. So that's all I wanted to do. Exercise and food were all I talked about. (Food Addicts Anonymous, 2010, 213)

After a rough pregnancy, I was obese for the first time in my life. I weighed in the 190s and was 5' 2" tall. I was humongous. It was hard to move in the aisle of a grocery store, and I couldn't touch my toes. I remember starting to jog and literally feeling like an elephant on my poor knees and feet. That was when my exercise addiction was born. I worked out four to five hours a day, rush-walked with the baby in the carriage, did high intensity aerobics at the spa, ran, and used my all-powerful Life Cycle at home. The scale became my close friend. The weight slid off. I was bingeing on sweets each day, but was burning the calories off. (Food Addicts Anonymous, 2010, 235)

I stayed too busy to go home because I knew I would eat too much and flop on the couch or into bed in a comatose state. (Food Addicts Anonymous, 2010, 181)

On weekends, I'd sleep three fourths of the day so I wouldn't be tempted to eat. (Food Addicts Anonymous, 2010, 234)

Shortly after my divorce I found the best, most successful diet in my life—crack cocaine and heroin. Within two years I lost 97 pounds. I also lost everything else I owned, but who cared? I was 200 pounds! I was also in major trouble, financial trouble, $300,000 in debt. I had legal problems, indictments and felony arrests. My life was in total shambles, but when I looked in the mirror, I looked marvelous, not just good, marvelous! (Food Addicts Anonymous, 2010, 257)

The obsession may take time in terms of what the food addict thinks about. Time-consuming thoughts can be present regardless of weight status.

My days were dominated by thoughts of food, and my puny allotment of toxic goodies was begging to be increased. (Food Addicts Anonymous, 2010, 97)

I was consumed by an obsession with weight and food so powerful that my every waking moment was devoted to my disease. I was never free from the craving for sugar in some form. (Food Addicts Anonymous, 2010, 112)

When I went away to college, I fought for my life. I knew that I would have to study harder than anyone else. I know today that was because of the sugar fog. I did work hard and eventually graduated with a degree in education. (Food Addicts Anonymous, 2010, 199)

There were times, though, that the weight did come off, but my thoughts about myself, other people, places, things and circumstances, stayed the same. The outside changed; the inside did not. My insanity, craving and obsession with food were always present, no matter what my outside looked like. (Food Addicts Anonymous, 2010, 259)

The addiction can also take time away from sleep during the night and cause sleepiness during the day.

I tried dieting, exercising, praying, reading books, reading my Bible and going to bed early only to wake up during the night for my donut binge. The compulsion inside me for food just escalated. (Food Addicts Anonymous, 2010, 213)

As I got older and needed more "fixes," I would sneak to the refrigerator and eat slices of raw butter or drink maple syrup out of the bottle. If there was ice cream in the freezer, I'd be there with a spoon. I began sneaking snacks and jars of peanut butter into my bedroom. I was actually hiding wrappers under my bed. Then I'd blame the missing food on one of my brothers. I didn't realize it then, but I was preoccupied with food. I remember being unable to concentrate in my classes because I was so tired from the sugar I had been eating. Then I would feel so irritable and shaky when my blood sugar would drop. (Food Addicts Anonymous, 2010, 229)

I never sat still much because, if I did, I would fall asleep as I did whenever I watched television or read a book. I fell asleep many times just riding home in the car. Two years after I was married, I went for a complete physical to find out why I was so tired all the time. It was interfering with my job. I would fall asleep at my desk in the afternoons and at computer classes, no matter how much caffeine I had consumed. I was drinking about 12 cans of caffeinated beverages per day. (Food Addicts Anonymous, 2010, 230)

Relationship problems that are associated with addictions can also consume time.

However, one day my frustrations and anger got the better of me and I walked off the job. Suddenly I was alone 12-16 hours a day while my husband worked. I started drinking more, and I began to eat almost constantly. As I gained weight, my self-esteem plummeted. In about a year, I went from 135 pounds to 198 pounds. I felt awful. I kept trying to diet and I would promise my husband that I would lose weight, yet I could not stick to a diet. My life was really falling apart. I was angry all the time. My husband and I had vicious fights that often resulted in physical abuse, initiated by either one of us. I was just as guilty as he was. (Food Addicts Anonymous, 2010, 242)

By sixteen, I was exercising three hours a day, destroying my body ... and still the roll [*note: of excess fat around the middle of his body*]. At eighteen, I was bingeing and purging two to three times a day. I was emaciated, and still the roll. At twenty-one I married. In one year I gained 117 pounds. The roll was finally gone. Now my whole body was one big roll. That's when the infidelity and promiscuity started, not by my wife, but by me. It was so sick. I was running and sleeping with women all over the place, as if all the conquests would negate the fact that I was a fat, disgusting pig. Obviously, my marriage ended and I was free to run amuck. I always had to do everything more and better than everyone else: more successful, more exciting, more dangerous. All this garbage was fueled by my food addiction and the way it made me see myself and feel about myself. (Food Addicts Anonymous, 2010, 257)

Children can also suffer from the issue of PFA and the consumption of time.

By the time I entered kindergarten I was on diet pills to curb my appetite. I remember having to take a pill around 11:00 a.m. each day, and that meant a trip out to the water cooler. It wasn't long before I started dropping the pill down the drain instead of swallowing it. My mother remarked to my father very often that she couldn't understand how come I was still eating so much. Finally the pills were stopped, and I was left to eat whatever and whenever I wanted to, which was nearly all the time.

During my grammar school years, I lived from one snack to the next. All I thought of was candy and cookies, and I always found ways to have them. My devoted grandfather, who lived with us for years, saw to it that I always had money in my pocket "for treats," as he would say. Every evening after supper he and I would go for a walk. He would get a cigar, and I would get a triple-decker ice cream cone. It was this beloved grandfather, who loved me dearly and whom I loved in return, who sustained me through all the abuse of living in a home of alcoholic parents.

By age ten I became preoccupied with food and began to seek the nurturing from food to replace the nurturing I had never received at home. (Food Addicts Anonymous, 2010, 133)

As far back as I can recall, food was my main focus in life. It was the only constant, dependable resource. A great majority of my time was focused on when, where and how much I was going to eat. It was the only thing a chubby five-year-old looked forward to when school got out at 3:00 pm. (Food Addicts Anonymous, 2010, 250)

These quotes from the 12-step food addiction manuals illustrate how comprehensively PFA can consume a life. Practitioners will want to delve into the many ways in which chronic use of processed foods can gradually impair the addict and absorb time.

13.4 APPLICATION

13.4.1 Care in Approach

Food-addicted clients may be somewhat embarrassed by the way in which they spend their time. The practitioner can assure clients that if they are tired, sleepy, sick, or in pain it would be natural for them to spend time resting, watching television, or sleeping during the day. It would be normal to spend time doing things that do not require movement or concentration. As clients accept the idea that they were given pseudofoods with addictive groggy-making properties without their knowledge, they can shrug off self-blame and shame. Through education and acceptance, practitioners can create an environment where food-addicted clients feel comfortable sharing about the realities of their lives.

13.4.2 Developing Goals

There are a number of beneficial goals in recovering from spending a great deal of time in PFA. The overall goal is to gradually shift from sedentary, passive activities to active, engaged behaviors that enhance mental and physical health. As with all recovery processes, the keys are to go slowly and to steer the client toward activities that they already enjoy. Work alongside the client to determine what activities would be easiest and most pleasurable to undertake. Celebrate with the client as the hours in front of the television diminish, alertness returns, and fun projects take the place of sitting.

Transitional steps can be helpful. For example, the client may be quite attached to particular television shows, as the characters might feel like friends. This can be the case if the client has been isolated due to fatigue and body shame. So, instead of just turning off the television, the client can engage in seated exercises while watching. Working with a resistance band or twisting and stretching can improve circulation, strength, and neurofunction. Each small step strengthens the client so they can take another step.

The client can be encouraged to gradually listen to the television instead of keeping eyes on the screen. Instead of watching, the client can assemble a puzzle, work on a craft, or fill in a coloring book. The impact of visual cuing related to eating-disordered actors is diminished. Exposure to food advertising or food-related programming are powerful compounded cues to relapse (Kemps, Tiggemann, & Hollitt, 2014).

The goal of disengaging from television can be implemented slowly over time. However, given the strength and consistency of the link between television and obesity, the total elimination of television and its removal from the home is a justifiable albeit distant goal.

Exercise goals can gradually be increased as the client is able. Delaying the start of television by 20 minutes can create the time for a 20-minute walking or sitting video, done in place. Very little space is needed, and no special equipment is required. Walking tapes that feature normally shaped people in decent clothing are produced by Leslie Sansone and shown for free at www.youtube.com. The videos start at 20 minutes and increase from there. There are also yoga and seated exercise videos at www.youtube.com.

Finding new things to do from home is a good reason for the practitioner to identify online support. Various groups are listed at www.foodaddictionresources.com. Online programs are often supplemented by phone calls, which are a reinforcing activity for the recovering food addict.

Of course, the client will spend time ordering, cooking, and packing clean food. As the client develops efficiencies around these tasks, the time required will be reduced. The client can spend a few minutes each day playing brain training exercises.

Curiously, food-addicted clients sometimes are energized to organize their homes. This seems to be a phase of recovery that can occur around the third week of abstinence from processed foods. Possibly with newfound mental clarity and energy, the client releases a pent-up desire to make their space orderly after years of lacking the energy and clarity to do so. This is a joyful activity for recovering food-addicted clients.

Activities that demand cognitive functions should be delayed for a few months until the client seems ready. This particularly pertains to reading. Although there is a plethora of books describing the harm of processed foods, it would be wise not to suggest them until clients have restored learning and memory functions. When the client is ready, books can be found at www.foodaddictionbooks.com.

In recovery from PFA, it is important to steer recovering addicts away from entertainment and sports venues that promote processed foods. Movie theaters with the smell of popcorn, the munching of theater-goers, provocative advertisements, and stressful movies featuring eating-disordered actors are perhaps the most heavily cued. Sporting events where vendors are walking up and down the aisles hawking processed foods are also heavily cued.

13.4.3 Tracking Progress

As with all aspects of recovery from PFA, the practitioner will want to go slowly. Progress can be seen in the undertaking of an exercise video or a jigsaw puzzle. It can be seen in the decision to work on a craft and listen to a book rather than turn on the television. Progress may manifest in the willingness to stay in bed and listen to a meditation rather than get up during a sleep-disturbed night. Activities with children are a mark of recovery. Parents may report joy and a sense of relief that they are alert and energetic enough to take their children on outings.

Here is an example of how one food addict developed new activities:

> I'm still learning what to do to occupy myself now that I'm not preoccupied with food. Physical activity is fun now that I no longer have a potbelly. Intellectual pursuits, learning a musical instrument or other art forms are intriguing. Shopping for clothes is actually fun, now that I am of a size that allows me to buy the fun clothes. I need to point out that finding activities to replace what was my greatest source of pleasure, eating, didn't just happen by itself. I had to put genuine effort into it. My new sources of enjoyment started out as just diversions; they were second best. In my mind at that time, there was a gulf between those new activities and the "fun" I used to have when eating was my diversion. Here's another miracle. As time goes on, my new diversions grow greater and the "eating diversion" lessens. (Food Addicts Anonymous, 2010, 100)

This is an area of recovery where patience will yield great rewards. Practitioners need to remember clearly that clients are devastated physically, mentally, and emotionally. Much healing may need to occur before time in front of the television can be curtailed and orderly sleep can be restored. Moving away from media will be an iterative process where, e.g., the cessation of joint pain may be needed before an exercise video becomes possible. Then perhaps the exercise video can take the place of 20 minutes of television. And then, the client feels better enough to go to bed on time and another 20 minutes of television is displaced. Little by little, the client finds rewarding activities in the real world that contribute to a sense of well-being.

13.5 CONCLUSION

Probing for how the client is spending time yields a trove of insight into the suffering of the food addict. Finding out how much time is spent watching television, sleeping, and working low-paying jobs will inform the scope of problem, the areas of motivation, the list of options to begin, and of course the tracking of progress. It is important for practitioners to bear in mind the depth of the mental, emotional, and physical barrios to changing habits about how time is spent. Small steps toward more rewarding use of time might seem like monumental progress to the client and should be celebrated as such.

REFERENCES

Aggio, D. A., Sartini, C., Papacosta, O., Lennon, L. T., Ash, S., Whincup, P. H., ... Jefferis, B. J. (2016). Cross-sectional associations of objectively measured physical activity and sedentary time with sarcopenia and sarcopenic obesity in older men. *Prev Med, 91*, 264–272. doi:10.1016/j.ypmed.2016.08.040.

American Psychiatric Association. (2013). *The Diagnostic and Statistical Manual of Mental Disorders, Fifth Edition* (Vol. 5), American Psychiatric Association, Washington DC.

Basner, M., & Dinges, D. F. (2009). Dubious bargain: Trading sleep for Leno and Letterman. *Sleep, 32*(6), 747–752.

Basner, M., Spaeth, A. M., & Dinges, D. F. (2014). Sociodemographic characteristics and waking activities and their role in the timing and duration of sleep. *Sleep, 37*(12), 1889–1906. doi:10.5665/sleep.4238.

Bond, D. S., Unick, J. L., Jakicic, J. M., Vithiananthan, S., Pohl, D., Roye, G. D., . . . Wing, R. R. (2011). Objective assessment of time spent being sedentary in bariatric surgery candidates. *Obes Surg, 21*(6), 811–814. doi:10.1007/s11695-010-0151-x.

Borzekowski, D. L., & Robinson, T. N. (2001). The 30-second effect: An experiment revealing the impact of television commercials on food preferences of preschoolers. *J Am Diet Assoc, 101*(1), 42–46. doi:S0002-8223(01)00012-8 [pii] 10.1016/S0002-8223(01)00012-8.

Cottone, P., Sabino, V., Steardo, L., & Zorrilla, E. P. (2008). Opioid-dependent anticipatory negative contrast and binge-like eating in rats with limited access to highly preferred food. *Neuropsychopharmacology, 33*(3), 524–535. doi:10.1038/sj.npp.1301430.

Cottone, P., Sabino, V., Steardo, L., & Zorrilla, E. P. (2009). Consummatory, anxiety-related and metabolic adaptations in female rats with alternating access to preferred food. *Psychoneuroendocrinology, 34*(1), 38–49. doi:10.1016/j.psyneuen.2008.08.010.

Davis, C., Levitan, R. D., Kaplan, A. S., Kennedy, J. L., & Carter, J. C. (2014). Food cravings, appetite, and snack-food consumption in response to a psychomotor stimulant drug: The moderating effect of "food-addiction". *Front Psychol, 5*, 403. doi:10.3389/fpsyg.2014.00403.

Do, Y. K., Shin, E., Bautista, M. A., & Foo, K. (2013). The associations between self-reported sleep duration and adolescent health outcomes: What is the role of time spent on Internet use? *Sleep Med, 14*(2), 195–200. doi:10.1016/j.sleep.2012.09.004.

Food Addicts Anonymous. (2010). *Food Addicts Anonymous*. Port St. Lucie, FL: Food Addicts Anonymous, Inc.

Goularte, J. F., Ferreira, M. B., & Sanvitto, G. L. (2012). Effects of food pattern change and physical exercise on cafeteria diet-induced obesity in female rats. *Br J Nutr, 108*(8), 1511–1518. doi:10.1017/s0007114511006933.

Griep, R. H., Bastos, L. S., Fonseca Mde, J., Silva-Costa, A., Portela, L. F., Toivanen, S., & Rotenberg, L. (2014). Years worked at night and body mass index among registered nurses from eighteen public hospitals in Rio de Janeiro, Brazil. *BMC Health Serv Res, 14*, 603. doi:10.1186/s12913-014-0603-4.

Gupta, N., Heiden, M., Aadahl, M., Korshoj, M., Jorgensen, M. B., & Holtermann, A. (2016). What is the effect on obesity indicators from replacing prolonged sedentary time with brief sedentary bouts, standing and different types of physical activity during working days? A cross-sectional accelerometer-based study among blue-collar workers. *PLoS One, 11*(5), e0154935. doi:10.1371/journal.pone.0154935.

Igelstrom, H., Emtner, M., Lindberg, E., & Asenlof, P. (2013). Level of agreement between methods for measuring moderate to vigorous physical activity and sedentary time in people with obstructive sleep apnea and obesity. *Phys Ther, 93*(1), 50–59. doi:10.2522/ptj.20120123.

Katz, P., Margaretten, M., Trupin, L., Schmajuk, G., Yazdany, J., & Yelin, E. (2016). Role of sleep disturbance, depression, obesity, and physical inactivity in fatigue in rheumatoid arthritis. *Arthritis Care Res (Hoboken), 68*(1), 81–90. doi:10.1002/acr.22577.

Kemps, E., Tiggemann, M., & Hollitt, S. (2014). Exposure to television food advertising primes food-related cognitions and triggers motivation to eat. *Psychol Health, 29*(10), 1192–1205. doi:10.1080/08870446.2014.918267.

Lifshitz, F., & Lifshitz, J. Z. (2014). Globesity: The root causes of the obesity epidemic in the USA and now worldwide. *Pediatr Endocrinol Rev, 12*(1), 17–34.

McGregor, R. A., Cameron-Smith, D., & Poppitt, S. D. (2014). It is not just muscle mass: A review of muscle quality, composition and metabolism during ageing as determinants of muscle function and mobility in later life. *Longev Healthspan, 3*(1), 9. doi:10.1186/2046-2395-3-9.

Morris, M. J., Beilharz, J., Maniam, J., Reichelt, A., & Westbrook, R. F. (2014). Why is obesity such a problem in the 21st century? The intersection of palatable food, cues and reward pathways, stress, and cognition. *J Neurosci, 58*, 36–45. doi:10.1523/jneurosci.2013-14.2014 10.1016/j.neubiorev.2014.12.002.

Nestle, M. (2002). *Food Politics.* Berkeley, CA: University of California Press.

Noble, E. E., & Kanoski, S. E. (2016). Early life exposure to obesogenic diets and learning and memory dysfunction. *Curr Opin Behav Sci, 9*, 7–14. doi:10.1016/j.cobeha.2015.11.014.

Ocon, A. J. (2013). Caught in the thickness of brain fog: Exploring the cognitive symptoms of Chronic Fatigue Syndrome. *Front Physiol, 4*, 63. doi:10.3389/fphys.2013.00063.

Padula, W. V., Allen, R. R., & Nair, K. V. (2014). Determining the cost of obesity and its common comorbidities from a commercial claims database. *Clin Obes, 4*(1), 53–58. doi:10.1111/cob.12041.

Patel, S. R., Hayes, A. L., Blackwell, T., Evans, D. S., Ancoli-Israel, S., Wing, Y. K., & Stone, K. L. (2014). The association between sleep patterns and obesity in older adults. *Int J Obes (Lond), 38*(9), 1159–1164. doi:10.1038/ijo.2014.13.

Patel, V. C., Spaeth, A. M., & Basner, M. (2016). Relationships between time use and obesity in a representative sample of Americans. *Obesity (Silver Spring), 24*(10), 2164–2175. doi:10.1002/oby.21596.

Perez, M., & Warren, C. S. (2012). The relationship between quality of life, binge-eating disorder, and obesity status in an ethnically diverse sample. *Obesity (Silver Spring), 20*(4), 879–885. doi:10.1038/oby.2011.89.

Ratcliffe, D., & Ellison, N. (2015). Obesity and internalized weight stigma: A formulation model for an emerging psychological problem. *Behav Cogn Psychother, 43*(2), 239–252. doi:10.1017/s1352465813000763.

Song, Y., Zhang, X., Ma, J., Zhang, B., Hu, P. J., & Dong, B. (2012). Behavioral risk factors for overweight and obesity among Chinese primary and middle school students in 2010. *Zhonghua Yu Fang Yi Xue Za Zhi, 46*(9), 789–795.

Stice, E., Agras, W. S., Telch, C. F., Halmi, K. A., Mitchell, J. E., & Wilson, T. (2001). Subtyping binge eating-disordered women along dieting and negative affect dimensions. *Int J Eat Disord, 30*(1), 11–27. doi:10.1002/eat.1050 [pii].

Theoharides, T. C., Stewart, J. M., Hatziagelaki, E., & Kolaitis, G. (2015). Brain "fog," inflammation and obesity: Key aspects of neuropsychiatric disorders improved by luteolin. *Front Neurosci, 9*, 225. doi:10.3389/fnins.2015.00225.

Vandewater, E. A., Park, S. E., Hebert, E. T., & Cummings, H. M. (2015). Time with friends and physical activity as mechanisms linking obesity and television viewing among youth. *Int J Behav Nutr Phys Act, 12 Suppl 1*, S6. doi:10.1186/1479-5868-12-s1-s6.

Yesavage, J. A., Kinoshita, L. M., Noda, A., Lazzeroni, L. C., Fairchild, J. K., Taylor, J., . . . O'Hara, R. (2014). Effects of body mass index-related disorders on cognition: Preliminary results. *Diabetes Metab Syndr Obes, 7*, 145–151. doi:10.2147/dmso.s60294.

Yokum, S., Gearhardt, A. N., Harris, J. L., Brownell, K. D., & Stice, E. (2014). Individual differences in striatum activity to food commercials predict weight gain in adolescents. *Obesity (Silver Spring), 22*(12), 2544–2551. doi:10.1002/oby.20882.

Zhang, Y., Liu, J., Yao, J., Ji, G., Qian, L., Wang, J., . . . Liu, Y. (2014). Obesity: Pathophysiology and intervention. *Nutrients, 6*(11), 5153–5183. doi:10.3390/nu6115153.

14 DSM 5 SUD Criterion 4 *Cravings*

Joan Ifland
Food Addiction Training, LLC
Cincinnati, OH

CONTENTS

Cravings, or a strong desire or urge to use processed foods. (American Psychiatric Association, 2013, 491)

14.1 INTRODUCTION

Cravings are a prominent feature of addictions and this is no less the case with processed food addiction (PFA) (Temple, 2016). When considering how to approach chronic overeating, it can be easy to miss the distress of cravings and obsession. While weight loss could be assumed to be the goal of dieting, for the food addict, the release from intense cravings and obsessive thinking about processed foods can also be an important outcome. There is evidence that processed food cravings may be worse than drug cravings (Oginsky, Goforth, Nobile, Lopez-Santiago, & Ferrario, 2016). Tracking desensitization of cue reactivity in the craving pathways is therefore a key measure of progress in recovery from PFA.

The American Society of Addiction Medicine includes cravings in its definition of addiction as follows:

> Addiction is a primary, chronic disease of brain reward, motivation, memory and related circuitry. Addiction affects neurotransmission and interactions within reward structures of the brain … such that motivational hierarchies are altered and addictive behaviors … supplant healthy, self-care related behaviors. Addiction also affects neurotransmission … such that the memory of previous exposures to rewards (such as food, sex, alcohol and other drugs) leads to a biological and behavioral response to external cues, in turn triggering craving and/or engagement in addictive behaviors. (American Society of Addiction Medicine, 2011)

Cravings are at the core of PFA. Their role can be missed in approaches focused only on weight loss. Cravings in overeating are well documented. Addressing cued cravings can reduce risk of relapse and improve outcomes.

Assessment of severity of cravings at intake and during the course of recovery helpful in structuring a program of recovery. Underestimating the power of cued cravings to induce relapse, and thereby undertreating cravings, may explain some part of the failure of weight-loss programs (Turk et al., 2009). A study of humans showed that that cravings measured by brain imaging during exposure to chocolate cues were greater than were cravings reported by subjects (Frankort et al., 2015). This suggests that it could be easy to underestimate cravings.

Cravings are also associated with loss of cognitive function (Meule, Skirde, Freund, Vogele, & Kubler, 2012). Because recovery from PFA may call for a comprehensive restructuring of the client's life, assessing the extent to which cravings coincide with cognitive impairment is crucial to success. The client who is still suffering from cravings may have trouble focusing on new tasks, such as organizing the food plan, avoiding food cues, and managing relationships to minimize stress. Inadequate assessment of cravings can lead to inadequate consideration of cue reactivity and cognitive impairment, which can lead to relapse.

For assessing severity, the Food Cravings Questionnaire (FCQ) is a well-validated assessment tool (Meule, Hermann, & Kubler, 2014). The FCQ is sensitive enough to measure the progression of cravings cessation during weight loss (Imperatori et al., 2013). It serves the practitioner as a guidepost to the progress of clients in restoring healthy thought patterns. See Chapter 9 for an in-depth description of the FCQ.

Sequencing craving desensitization early in recovery could help facilitate the restoration of cognitive functions needed to implement an abstinent food plan in heavily cued environments. Techniques to diminish cravings have been demonstrated (Brockmeyer, Hahn, Reetz, Schmidt, & Friederich, 2015b; Kemps & Tiggemann, 2014; Kemps, Tiggemann, & Bettany, 2012). These will be covered in the Treatment Section of this textbook. Explicitly assessing cravings can improve outcomes for PFA and overeating. Understanding the role of cravings in overeating and relapse is useful for the PFA practitioner.

14.1.1 Importance

Even though harm is apparent to the observer, the addict cannot perceive the harm sufficiently to stop using. Thus, the intense urges and longings that are characteristic of cravings can be considered as an important pathology that triggers chronic, addictive overeating. Without cravings, people would be better able to control overeating (Childress et al., 1993; de Bruijn, van den Brink, de Graaf, & Vollebergh, 2005; O'Brien, 2005).

14.1.2 Chapter Overview

This chapter is organized into two sections: "Evidence Review" and "Application." The "Evidence Review" section contains the subsection "Introduction to the Evidence," which discusses the centrality of cravings to the assessment and treatment of PFA especially as it impacts the acquisition of skills necessary to combat PFA. The "Evidence Review" section also describes factors in the development of cravings for processed foods. The evidence here helps practitioners understand how to focus recovery on key problems such as repeat exposure to processed foods and cues. The development discussion also covers the role of food cues as they provoke cravings. The next topic in development is "Factors That Intensify Reactivity to Cues." This topic helps practitioners prioritize goals for protecting against cue reactivity and cravings. The last topic under development is "Cravings, Reward, and Instrument Transfer." This describes neurological processes related to cravings. It helps practitioners understand otherwise puzzling behavior on the part of food addicts.

The next section, "Evidence Review," discusses the relative importance of cravings in PFA. The purpose of this discussion is to encourage practitioners to focus on cravings as a primary factor in relapse relative to other factors such as childhood problems, hunger, fatigue, etc. Secondly, the section covers evidence for the existence of intense cravings in obesity. The third section compares cravings in PFA with those in drug addiction. The information is included to help reinforce the idea that food cravings are severe and deserve center stage in the diagnosis, assessment, and treatment of PFA.

The last section of "Evidence Review" is "Assessment of Severity." Here is the evidence for an assessment tool, the FCQ.

The second section of this chapter ("Application") covers applications of the evidence. It compares the management of food cues to drug cues. It also helps practitioners teach clients about how cravings may have played a role in past failures to maintain weight loss. This section also suggests how to set goals for cravings cessation and how to track progress in this area.

14.2 EVIDENCE REVIEW

14.2.1 Introduction to the Evidence

Evidence that cravings pathology is a central issue in overeating has grown (Hone-Blanchet & Fecteau, 2014; Kelley, Schiltz, & Landry, 2005; Tomasi et al., 2015). The strength of this finding and its potential to improve outcomes in recovery from overeating has prompted a significant increase in the volume and rate of new research into cravings in recent years (Boswell & Kober, 2016; Rodriguez-Martin & Meule, 2015). Discoveries about the source and suppression of cravings are important because they can inform best practices in PFA recovery and improve outcomes.

Research demonstrates that cravings for processed foods are experienced during activation of reward pathways in the brain. In the case of processed foods, four major pathways are involved, including dopamine (Wang et al., 2014), serotonin (Carr et al., 2013; Wurtman & Wurtman, 1995), opiate (Davis et al., 2011), and endocannabinoid (Monteleone et al., 2015). The activation of cravings has been shown to suppress other key brain centers, including restraint/inhibition, learning, decision-making, memory, and satiation (Kendig, 2014; Noble et al., 2014; Zhang, Manson, Schiller, & Levy, 2014). Cravings can be seen as an indication of more widespread neurodysfunction.

Cravings have been shown to be provoked by cues for processed foods (Colagiuri & Lovibond, 2015). Cravings are worse in food addicts than nonfood addicts (Meule & Hormes, 2015). Cravings are for processed foods rather than unprocessed foods (Polk, Schulte, Furman, & Gearhardt, 2016).

Pavlovian conditioning of neuropathways in reaction to cueing has been shown to be a precursor for cravings (Petrovich & Gallagher, 2007). Cueing can include the sight, smell, touch, taste, or sound of processed foods. Importantly, the cravings can be activated by any suggestion or reminder associated with a food cue (Cole, Hobin, & Petrovich, 2015). Emotions are also associated with cues to crave (Rejeski et al., 2010). Craving activation is translated into action through conditioned instrument transfer (Petrovich & Gallagher, 2007). The importance of cues in sensitizing cravings reactions in addictive eating is well established.

Cravings in PFA may be a more serious issue than in drug addiction. In the process of obtaining abstinent food, recovering food addicts are exposed to intense cues for processed food in grocery stores, restaurants, and even home kitchens (Colagiuri & Lovibond, 2015). This unavoidable exposure to triggering cues early in recovery sets PFA apart from other substance-based addictions. In recovery from other addictions, avoiding cues for the substance of abuse is more feasible. Cravings in reaction to processed food cues require special attention in recovery from PFA.

14.2.1.1 The Importance of Cues in PFA

Another key distinction between PFA and drug addiction is that in recovery from PFA, the client will need to acquire skills in cued environments to assemble abstinent meals. Assembling abstinent meals can be quite a challenge to cognitive capabilities in light of the extensive impact of cue reactivity throughout the brain (Val-Laillet et al., 2015). Because most prepared foods contain addictive ingredients, they generally need to be eliminated in recovery from PFA. However, the prevalence of addictive ingredients in packaged and fast foods means that the food addict is left with the task of preparing meals from scratch in cued environments. The client will need to learn how to shop, organize, cook, assemble, and package meals using abstinent ingredients. These activities take place in food-cued environments, which can activate cravings and increase risk of relapse.

The evidence discussed in this chapter supports recommendations for strategies for avoiding cues. As will be seen in Part III, "Approaches to Recovery," strategies may include engaging a grocery shopping service and condensing food preparation into as short a time as possible. Research shows that cue-induced cravings precede extensive cognitive impairment (Rodriguez-Martin & Meule, 2015). So sequencing desensitization of craving pathways and the repair of cognitive abilities early in recovery is supported. With this approach, recovery should proceed in a stepwise fashion where improved meal preparation supports cognitive restoration, which supports better meal preparation, etc. (Logan & Jacka, 2014).

To explore the issues involved in pathological food cravings, the "Evidence Review" section covers three topics. The first topic covers factors in the development of cravings. The second topic is the importance of cued cravings in the perpetuation of overeating. The third topic addresses methods for the assessment of severity of cravings. Assessment of severity is critical to matching depth of need to depth of program. For purposes of illustration, the scientific findings are integrated with qualitative data taken from two manuals published by 12-step groups, Food Addicts Anonymous and Food Addicts in Recovery Anonymous (Food Addicts Anonymous, 2010; Food Addicts in Recovery Anonymous, 2013).

14.2.2 Development of Cravings for Processed Foods

Understanding the source of cravings guides practitioners in methods to prevent cravings flare-ups. There is evidence that the predominant cause of overeating is cues for processed foods that activate sensitized craving neuropathways while suppressing executive functions such as restraint, learning, decision-making, and memory (Kendig, 2014; Noble et al., 2014; Stice & Yokum, 2016; Zhang et al., 2014). The craving neuropathways activated by processed food cues include the dopamine (Tomasi et al., 2015), serotonin (Wurtman & Wurtman, 1995), opiate (Davis et al., 2011), and endocannabinoid (Monteleone et al., 2015; Watkins & Kim, 2014) pathways.

The evidence suggests that pathways are sensitized through Pavlovian conditioning in response to exposure to processed food cues. A number of recent review articles articulate these findings comprehensively (D'Addario et al., 2014; Kelley, Baldo, Pratt, & Will, 2005; Kringelbach & Stein, 2010; Petrovich, 2013; Stice, Figlewicz, Gosnell, Levine, & Pratt, 2013; Stice & Yokum, 2016; Wang et al., 2014). The instrument transfer pathways that translate cravings into action have also been shown to be susceptible to Pavlovian conditioning in response to processed food cues (Yin, Ostlund, & Balleine, 2008). Instrument transfer has been shown to activate eating even when the subject is sated (Colagiuri & Lovibond, 2015). The impact of processed food cues are greater when cue conditioning occurs during hunger (Zhang, Berridge, Tindell, Smith, & Aldridge, 2009). Conditioning can take place in a single training session of cueing for sucrose in rats (Tye, Stuber, de Ridder, Bonci, & Janak, 2008). The evidence demonstrates that reward and instrument transfer pathways are highly susceptible to conditioning in response to processed food cues.

It can be argued that the result of this conditioning process is increasingly intense cravings (incentive salience), cognitive impairment, and sensitized stress pathways. These can be thought of as the core dysfunctions in PFA. This progressive reactivity of craving pathways is reflected in the 12-step literature. The following quotes are from the manuals of two 12-step groups, Food Addicts in Recovery Anonymous (FA) and Food Addicts Anonymous (FAA). They describe cravings as the central issue in recovery from PFA.

We found a way to be free from food obsession and cravings … (Food Addicts in Recovery Anonymous, 2013, 4)

You look normal, or even thin. You've won this at a high cost. Perhaps your obsession with food and weight tortures you. Your mind no longer feels like it's your own. (Food Addicts in Recovery Anonymous, 2013, 4)

Either we can't stop ourselves from eating more or we're possessed by an unremitting obsession with food and weight. (Food Addicts in Recovery Anonymous, 2013, 10)

FA provides all that we need to obtain and sustain our recovery without struggling with obsession or food cravings. (Food Addicts in Recovery Anonymous, 2013, 11)

Now I say there are two days that I'll always consider the best days of my life. One was when my daughter was born healthy. The other was the day that I was finally willing to let go of my obsession with food. (Food Addicts in Recovery Anonymous, 2013, 70)

I know now that it doesn't matter how much I did those things [*diet and exercise*], it's the mental obsession that counts. (Food Addicts Anonymous, 2010, 214)

I think you can see the pattern of obsession with food. My life revolved around sports events, carnival type entertainment, movies and anywhere I could consume extra amounts of food. (Food Addicts Anonymous, 2010, 190)

About two and a half months later [*after achieving abstinence*], I was walking home from work when I realized that for the first time in my life, I had a moment when I felt no physical craving for any food and no wish to eat. (Food Addicts in Recovery Anonymous, 2013, 205)

I was stunned when one of them said she was free from food cravings. … I could never master my cravings. (Food Addicts in Recovery Anonymous, 2013, 236–237)

The cravings were terrible. It was storming outside and I didn't have a car, but Twinkies were dancing in my head, calling me and seducing me. (Food Addicts Anonymous, 2010, 236)

These quotes from the 12-step food addiction societies illustrate distressing cravings and mental obsession around processed foods. The quotes showing dysfunctional thought patterns help clarify why substance use disorders are classified as a mental illness in the DSM 5. Remission of cravings and obsession are primary goals of recovery and can serve practitioners as markers for a client's progress through recovery.

14.2.2.1 The Nature of Food Cues

Cravings can be associated with a variety of triggers. Understanding these associative cues can help practitioners prepare clients to withstand cue-induced triggers. For example, Ferrer-Garcia et al. found that cravings are most intense at particular times and places, including the afternoon/early evening; in the late evening/night; between meals; when alone; at the end of the week; and in the dining room, the kitchen, the bedroom, the bakery, and the supermarket (Ferrer-Garcia 2013). Silvers et al. found that cravings are more intense in young children than young adults (Silvers et al., 2014). Borgogna et al. found that television was associated with higher cravings in non-Hispanic adolescents. Phone messaging was associated with cravings in Hispanic youth. Video games were associated with cravings more in males than females (Borgogna et al., 2014). There is support in the evidence for including strategies in recovery programs for avoiding exposure to these associative cues.

14.2.2.2 Factors That Intensify Reactivity to Cues

Familiarity with conditions that can intensify cravings gives practitioners the ability to teach clients how to focus their lifestyle efforts to protect against cravings. Cravings have been found to be more intense in women (Becker & Koob, 2016; Hallam, Boswell, DeVito, & Kober, 2016). Not surprisingly, people with higher states of craving react to foods cues more strongly (Brockmeyer, Hahn, Reetz, Schmidt, & Friederich, 2015a).

One factor that can increase cue reactivity is sleep deprivation (St-Onge, Wolfe, Sy, Shechter, & Hirsch, 2014). Stress also increases reactivity through the release of glucocorticoids, as well as noradrenergic arousal in the corticostriatal circuits, which facilitate the formation of habits (Schwabe & Wolf, 2011). Stressed study participants chose sweets and fat over bland food (Oliver, Wardle, & Gibson, 2000). A study found that early stage withdrawal from a high-fat diet did not immediately attenuate dopamine and synapse signaling associated with conditioned cue responses (Fernandes, Sharma, Hryhorczuk, Auguste, & Fulton, 2013). The research suggests the value of focusing in healthy sleep and stress avoidance through early stage withdrawal.

Multiple types of simultaneous cues intensify responses (Kearns & Weiss, 2005), which suggests prioritizing avoidance of heavily cued commercial food environments. Repeated consumption of processed foods increases cravings (Temple, 2016), which supports use of an abstinent food plan. Prior drug-taking or smoking increases cue reactivity (Orsini et al., 2014). Imagining taste also increases reactivity (Frankort et al., 2012). Negative affect (bad mood) increases sensitivity (Wagner, Boswell, Kelley, & Heatherton, 2012). Impulsivity correlates with reactivity (Diekhof et al., 2012). Practitioners should assist clients to focus on avoiding cued environments, thoughts of food, and negative moods. Using an unprocessed food plan is essential.

Genetic variances also predict reactivity (Felsted, Ren, Chouinard-Decorte, & Small, 2010) and are associated with cravings, especially for fast food (Yeh et al., 2016). This is evidence that cravings and sensitivity to cues can be transmitted genetically.

14.2.2.3 Cravings, Reward, and Instrument Transfer

Cravings have been shown to initiate a cascade of reward and instrument transfer that tie food cues to the act of seeking addictive substances. Sensitivity to reward has been shown to correlate with cravings and BMI. The more sensitive a person is to cravings, the greater the reward sensitivity and the greater the BMI (Franken & Muris, 2005; Jastreboff et al., 2013). A questionnaire study (Burton, Smit, & Lightowler, 2007) and a genetic twin study (Keskitalo et al., 2007) both demonstrated that cravings modulate behavioral and neurotransmitter responses to cues and obesity. This means that cravings were present during the release of neurotransmitters and the action of overeating (Stice & Dagher, 2010). Sugar cravings have been shown to be a factor in mediating the relationship between addictive eating and bingeing (Joyner, Gearhardt, & White, 2015). Children overeat in response to processed food advertisements on television (Halford, Boyland, Hughes, Oliveira, & Dovey, 2007). Exposure to chocolate cues leads to more chocolate consumption (Werthmann, Field, Roefs, Nederkoorn, & Jansen, 2014). Chocolate cues increase salivation and consumption in high-craving students with high trait craving, but not low (Meule & Hormes, 2015). Hyperresponsivity and increased energy intake both occur in obese subjects in anticipation of processed foods (Burger & Stice, 2013; Tye et al., 2008). The evidence suggests that focusing on cravings cessation could be helpful in controlling eating.

This quote illustrates this condition.

> Inside my head, my brain said, “Stop, stop, stop. Don’t eat.” I keep hearing, “I don’t want to get fat,” but another part of my brain was controlling my fork and it would not stop my hand from moving to my mouth. (Food Addicts in Recovery Anonymous, 2013, 278)

14.2.3 The Relative Importance of Cravings in PFA

The research shows a central role for cued cravings in the development and perpetuation of addictive eating. In overeating, cues have been shown to be a more important factor than hunger (Hetherington, 2007) or mood (Hill, Weaver, & Blundell, 1991). Cues for processed foods were found to be a leading cause of overeating (Berthoud, 2004, 2011; Burton et al., 2007). In children, smell and taste cues were a greater factor in overeating than mood, body esteem, and a restrained eating style (Jansen et al., 2003). Three out of five factors cited for weight gain by bariatric patients related to cravings (Fallon, Shearman, Sershen, & Lajtha, 2007). Stress can be a cue to overeat (Gibson, 2006). Preoccupations with food (persistent cravings), emotional triggers, and environmental cues are the three primary factors that explain cravings in a questionnaire study (Crowley et al., 2014). Cravings are a central issue in overeating.

The intensity and relative importance of cravings in PFA is also illustrated in these quotes from the 12-step literature. Note comparisons of the mental distress to the distress of excess weight.

> There was no dreadful, terrible experience that made me hit a rock bottom with food, but I got so that I couldn't bear my obsession. Will I? Won't I? Can I? Can't I? How much? How little? When do I eat? What do I eat? How much should I eat? (Food Addicts in Recovery Anonymous, 2013, 213)
>
> I developed a mental obsession and a hopelessness that was frightening in its intensity. (Food Addicts Anonymous, 2010, 41)
>
> There were times, though, that the weight did come off, but my thoughts about myself, other people, places, things and circumstances stayed the same. The outside changed; the inside did not. My insanity, craving and obsession with food were always present, no matter what my outside looked like. (Food Addicts Anonymous, 2010, 259)
>
> There were times when I appeared to be doing very well, but in the end, I would always end up back into the sugar because I had not been freed of the cravings. So, when someone from FAA told me how she had been following the food plan for 15 months and that the cravings were gone, I felt a flicker of hope for the first time in years. (Food Addicts Anonymous, 2010, 252)
>
> We had plenty of food, but my desire for more was always there. I had a slim figure most of my life, but I had cravings. (Food Addicts Anonymous, 2010, 212)
>
> I can truthfully say that, from the age of fifteen until I found FAA, I was consumed by an obsession with weight and food so powerful that my every waking moment was devoted to my disease. I was never free from the craving for sugar in some form. (Food Addicts Anonymous, 2010, 112)
>
> It's wonderful to be the right weight, but the complete freedom I have from food is even more important to me. (Food Addicts in Recovery Anonymous, 2013, 174)

These quotes reveal that for these food addicts, cravings and obsession are core pathology. It is possible that this aspect of obesity has been overlooked because it's not physically visible as is excess adipose tissue. Indeed, the problem of overeating was initially defined by the consequences of weight gain (actually adipose tissue gain) in the obesity epidemic. While PubMed yields 8766 studies for the word *obesity*, only 30 of these also containing the word *cravings* in the abstract. The database yields only 148 studies for a search of *food cravings*. However, as can be seen in the above quotes, the mental illness can be more important than weight issues for the food addict.

14.2.3.1 Cravings and Cue Reactivity in Obesity

There is extensive evidence that elevated BMI is associated with heightened craving responsivity to cues. This may occur because of corresponding loss of inhibitory control (Batterink, Yokum, & Stice, 2010). Foods craved by obese people are found to be sweets, high fats, carbohydrates/starches, and fast-food fats (Chao, Grilo, White, & Sinha, 2014). Franken and Muris found that sensitivity to reward was significantly related to food craving and BMI and that sensitivity to reward correlated to BMI even when craving was removed as a factor (Franken & Muris, 2005). This may reinforce the importance of cue reactivity in cravings severity. Cravings for fats mediate the relationship between addictive-like eating and BMI (Joyner et al., 2015).

In a meta-analysis, Kennedy and Dimitropoulos found that obese people showed more active reward processing after a meal than lean (Kennedy & Dimitropoulos, 2014). In a PET scan study, Nummenmaa found that obese more so than lean subjects showed reward activation in response to pictures of processed foods (Nummenmaa et al., 2012). In a study of exposure to a pizza cue, Tetley, Brunstrom, and Griffiths found that individuals identified as overweight and participants who reported consuming the largest everyday portion sizes experienced a significantly greater change in their desired portion size of the cued food after the cue exposure (Tetley, Brunstrom, & Griffiths, 2009).

Obese children have also been shown to suffer from cravings more than lean children. Jansen et al. found that obese but not lean children overate in response to prolonged exposure to food cues (Jansen et al., 2003). Obese children show a tonic state of hyperactivity in reward circuitry (Black et al., 2014).

The evidence is significant in two respects. Explaining the role of involuntary craving responses to food addicts may help relieve them of the burden of self-judgment. It may help the obese food addict to understand that they do not lack control; rather, their craving and cognitive pathways have been conditioned to crave without restraint.

Secondly, although this evidence is significant, it does not negate the possibility that a person of normal weight could be suffering from cravings. Cravings have been shown to persist after bariatric surgery (Sudan, Sudan, Lyden, & Thompson, 2016). Some reward activity remains elevated in formerly obese people who have lost weight as opposed to people who have never been obese (DelParigi et al., 2004). Cravings assessment should be undertaken regardless of weight status.

14.2.3.2 Severity of Food vs. Drug Cravings

Research shows that food cravings may be more powerful than drug cravings. Oginsky found that addiction-related anomalies in the nucleus accumbens occur more quickly under high-fat/high-sugar ingestion than cocaine injection in rats (Oginsky et al., 2016).

Three factors may contribute to severity of food cravings as compared to cravings for addictive drugs: primal instincts, poly-food abuse, and peripheral signaling. Reinforcement of primal instincts means that PFA is complicated by the presence of strong survival instincts that encourage people to eat rapidly, eat in volume, and choose calorie-dense foods. These behaviors would have been valuable to primitive peoples as it would have helped them seek and consume vital calories (Cohen, 2008).

Food cravings may also be made more severe by their polysubstance nature (Schuckit et al., 2001). Almost all commercially prepared foods contain more than one addictive ingredient such as sugar, flour, fat, salt, dairy, gluten, and caffeine. For example, fast food meals tend to contain multiple addictive ingredients. Gluten (Huebner, Lieberman, Rubino, & Wall, 1984), flour (Spreadbury, 2012), processed fat (Trevizol et al., 2015), excessive salt (Cocores & Gold, 2009), and dairy (Bray, 2000) can be found in combinations of french fries, hamburgers, tacos, and pizza. Sweetener (Hone-Blanchet & Fecteau, 2014) and caffeine (Thomasius, Sack, Strittmatter, & Kaess, 2014) are contained in accompanying drinks. Recent research shows that polysubstance abuse is harder to treat than single substance use (Connor, Gullo, White, & Kelly, 2014; Moss, Chen, & Yi, 2014), which suggests that PFA based on poly-food abuse might be more difficult to treat than if the pattern is of single-food abuse.

Another factor that suggests that cravings in PFA may be worse than other addictions comes from studies of "peripheral signaling" (Bray, 2000; Hellstrom et al., 2004; Monteleone et al., 2013; Murray, Tulloch, Gold, & Avena, 2014). This means that systems throughout the body produce chemicals that reach the brain and impact the intensity of cravings by docking on craving-related neurotransmitters. Peptides that could enhance cravings reactivity include insulin (Jastreboff, Gaiser, Gu, & Sinha, 2014; Kroemer, Krebs, Kobiella, Grimm, Vollstadt-Klein, et al., 2013; Taguchi, Wartschow, & White, 2007), leptin (Grosshans et al., 2012), ghrelin (Folgueira, Seoane, & Casanueva, 2014; Kroemer, Krebs, Kobiella, Grimm, Pilhatsch, et al., 2013), and orexin (Ho & Berridge, 2013; Williams, 2014). Corticotropin-releasing factor produced in the nucleus accumbens has been shown to be vulnerable to conditioning and appears to enhance the motivation to seek food, possibly through increased stress (Cottone et al., 2009; Pecina, Schulkin, & Berridge, 2006).

More recent research is finding that the gut biome (bacteria) directly affect brain function. A range of transmitters and peptides travel to and from the brain. They can alter mood and impact behavior such as overeating (Borre, Moloney, Clarke, Dinan, & Cryan, 2014; Holzer & Farzi, 2014). This is especially true for fats as they activate the endocannabinoid pathway (Watkins & Kim, 2014).

Here are examples of the severity of food cravings in PFA.

> … years of struggle had kept landing me back in the same place: Can I, can't I, will I, won't I eat? It was a horrible way to live. (Food Addicts in Recovery Anonymous, 2013, 216)
>
> I also had food dreams, and my group assured me that it was not unusual for addicts of all kinds to crave their drug of choice. (Food Addicts Anonymous, 2010, 99)
>
> The unexpected miracle is not that I have lost 50 pounds and kept it off, but rather that my obsession and compulsion with food have been lifted. (Food Addicts in Recovery Anonymous, 2013, 25)

It is generally recognized that drug cravings are a serious mental condition but recognition that food cravings may be worse than drug cravings is not widespread. The evidence for cravings for processed foods illustrates the core pathology of overeating as a mental illness as opposed to an issue of lack of willpower.

14.2.4 Assessment of Severity

Assessment of severity of cravings generates data that is crucial for designing recovery programs and for tracking progress. The assessment helps guide development of strategies for cue avoidance in the more severely craving client. Assessment also identifies clients who are not suffering from cravings, rather perhaps from lack of information about eating. So assigning craving avoidance to a noncraving client would be misguided. The most common assessment method is the FCQ.

14.2.4.1 The Food Cravings Questionnaire

Assessment of cravings can be accomplished through the FCQ—Trait, which has been studied extensively. It was initially developed in Spain but has been validated for English, Italian, German, and Dutch populations (Franken & Muris, 2005; Innamorati, Imperatori, Balsamo, et al., 2014; Meule, Lutz, Vogele, & Kubler, 2012; Moreno, Rodriguez, Fernandez, Tamez, & Cepeda-Benito, 2008; Rodriguez et al., 2007). It been shown to be valid for specific foods but also food in general and for chocolate (Rodriguez et al., 2007). Originally a 39-item tool, a reduced version of 15 items has now been validated (Meule, Hermann, et al., 2014).

Items included in the reduced FCQ-Trait include lack of control over eating (five items), thoughts or preoccupation with food (five items), intentions and plans to consume food (two items), emotions before or during food craving (two items), and cues that may trigger food craving (one item). Respondents answer using a five-point scale ranging from *strongly agree* to *strongly disagree* (Meule, Hermann, et al., 2014). It has been shown to be associated with a measure of psychological pathology, BMI, impulsivity, lack of dieting success, and impaired cognitive ability during exposure to cues (Meule, Allison, & Platte, 2014; Meule & Kubler, 2014). It is sensitive enough to distinguish between a population that has started a diet and lost cravings and a population that has not yet begun to diet (Innamorati, Imperatori, Meule, et al., 2014).

A second 15-item scale, the FCQ—State measures changes in cravings from moment to moment and is used in research.

Through use of the validated FCQ, researchers and clinicians have found methods for measuring key brain functions in patients at intake and during the course of recovery.

14.2.5 Summary of the Evidence

This review of the literature provides evidence that cravings are the pathway from cues and life events to overeating. Cravings offer a possible explanation for overeating and are thus an area of potential to improve outcomes in recovery. Because craving pathways in the brain are so susceptible to learning or Pavlovian conditioning in response to cues and use, the research suggests that almost any association with a processed food could be remembered and could potentially serve as an associative trigger to overeat. The pathology develops from the ability of associated cues to trigger powerful cravings independently of hunger. Understanding how to reduce cravings is central to the cessation of addictive overeating.

There is a substantial body of literature demonstrating a primary role for cravings in addictive overeating. Cravings are found in the obese but not lean study subjects. Some aspects of cravings are seen to be more severe in PFA than in drug and alcohol addiction. A variety of research techniques demonstrate that cravings are associated chronic overeating. The distress of cravings and obsession is extensively described in the 12-step food addiction manuals and in some cases appears to be a more significant source of distress than excess weight. The evidence points to cravings as a hidden source of relapse. By evaluating cravings in clients and explicitly incorporating cravings desensitization into recovery, practitioners can look forward to more focused and successful recovery programs.

The research suggests a leading role for cue-induced cravings in the pathology of overeating. Key points are that (1) it is easy to trigger cravings; (2) during cravings, restraint, learning, memory, decision-making, and satiation are suppressed; and (3) symptoms of cravings are more prevalent in high BMI populations. It is possible that underestimating the role of cue-induced cravings could explain some part of the failure to stem the tide of obesity.

The evidence for food cravings is that cravings appear to be the factor that connects cues in the environment to chronic overeating. The findings suggest that overeating can be reduced or eliminated by focusing on strategies to avoid food cues and put cravings into remission.

14.3 APPLICATION

The research and practical experience of PFA point to the presence of a severe brain disease manifesting as obsessive cravings for processed foods, which translates into chronic overeating and a constellation of consequences. The cravings research is extensive, consistent across research techniques, strong in findings, and logical. It has intuitive appeal insofar as it demonstrates a neurophysical basis for overeating, which is more compelling than traditional explanations such as the loss of willpower or lack of moral fiber. As with drug addiction, the research reveals a brain that is so hyperactive in reward pathways that it overwhelms the ability to exercise restraint and make good decisions.

The qualitative data found in the quotes from the 12-step food addiction literature reveal the nature of the mental illness of PFA. The quotes illustrate the distress of cravings and obsession. Within the brains of food addicts, a storm rages of urges and longings for processed foods, while caring thoughts about family, education, career, and self-care are suppressed. The life of a food addict can be bleak when cravings are active.

The neuropathology discovered in the diagnostic criteria for cravings helps explain the pathological behavior found in the other 10 DSM 5 SUD criteria. In fact, the addictive behaviors can be seen as deriving from the all-consuming obsession with cravings, especially when the cognitive impairment that accompanies cravings is taken into consideration. Addicts are simply unable to surface rational thoughts, make good decisions, or engage in the behaviors needed to thrive.

14.3.1 Managing Drug vs. Food Cues

When compared to the requirements for managing cued cravings in drug and alcohol addiction, PFA presents more difficult challenges. Drug and alcohol cues are much less prevalent in obesogenic cultures than are processed food cues. While illegal recreational drugs are not commercially advertised, processed foods are heavily advertised on television, billboards, and magazines. There are restrictions on cigarette and alcohol availability and advertising. Recreational drugs are not found in grocery stores and restaurants, whereas processed foods proliferate. While sober friends may be made in drug and alcohol recovery, finding people who don't use processed foods is very difficult. So the risk of exposure to processed food cueing is much higher in recovery from PFA. This supports the idea that desensitization of cue reactivity in early stage recovery is a high priority.

14.3.2 Cravings in Weight-Loss Failure

The research and qualitative data reveal possibilities for why traditional weight-loss approaches to overeating have failed (Turk et al., 2009). Explaining inadequate treatment of cued cravings as the possible cause of failed weight-loss attempts may be very helpful to clients in terms of reducing shame, guilt, and self-judgment stemming from repeated loss of control over eating.

The "Evidence Review" section helps show why most diet plans would fail to curb cravings. Diet plans typically leave in processed ingredients that have been shown to ignite cravings. Popular plans such as Atkins contain high-fat foods (Atkins, 2009), which are now known to activate the endocannabinoid pathway (so-named because this pathway is also activated by cannabis) (Monteleone et al., 2015; Sharma, Fernandes, & Fulton, 2013). A current popular weight-loss cookbook, *Zero Belly Cookbook*, features a chocolate cake recipe (Zinczenko, 2015), while chocolate has perhaps the highest potential to activate cravings (Asmaro & Liotti, 2014). The cookbook for a popular weight loss program, Weight Watchers, suggests a sugary, bread-based dish (Weight-Watchers, 2014), while research shows sugar to be addictive (Avena, Rada, & Hoebel, 2008). In a PFA model, these programs would risk failure due to cue exposure. The cueing provocation of the recipes would activate the craving pathways in the brain and suppress executive functions, leaving the reader helplessly in the grip of intense cravings without the benefit of rational thought.

Further, cue avoidance would appear to be underemployed in approaches to weight loss. One example would be commonly given advice that weight-loss clients read labels and thereby prolong exposure to heavily cued grocery stores. Without desensitization, cooking in home kitchens could be triggering.

In short, traditional approaches to weight loss as opposed to recovery from PFA can be seen to fail because of a lack of consideration of neuropathology and inappropriate, even harmful, exposure to cueing. Sharing this insight with clients could reduce the barrier of fear of failure and allow clients to move forward into recovery.

14.3.3 Developing Goals

Food cue desensitization can occur naturally as the person eats nonaddictive, unprocessed foods in cue-free environments. The key study that demonstrated desensitization of a food cue was conducted by Pavlov (Pavlov, 2015). He taught dogs to associate a bell with food. Then he removed the food but rang the bell. He found that the bell could trigger the involuntary release of saliva through its association with food. However, he also found that continuing to ring the bell repeatedly without food eventually caused the release of saliva to cease. Thus Pavlov found that the cue could be disassociated from the involuntary reaction of saliva release.

In essence, this cue disassociation or desensitization is a key goal of recovery. The practitioner helps the client eat nonaddictive foods that avoid triggering the release of craving neurotransmitters. Instead of desensitizing the saliva gland in Pavlov's work with dogs, PFA practitioners seek to desensitize the craving pathways in the brain of food addicts. Instead of seeking to stop the release of saliva, practitioners seek to stop the release of craving neurotransmitters including dopamine, serotonin, opiates, and endocannabinoids. This is accomplished by abstaining from addictive, craving processed foods in the same way that alcoholics abstain from alcohol. Research shows that unprocessed foods do not trigger the release of craving neurotransmitters (Beaver et al., 2006;

Guerrieri, Nederkoorn, & Jansen, 2008; Passamonti et al., 2009). As the nontriggering foods fail to stimulate the release of neurotransmitters, the triggering effect of associated cues wanes and finally ceases to provoke cravings.

14.3.4 Tracking Progress

Even with substitution of nonaddictive foods for processed foods, "recovery" eating nonetheless exposes the client to many of the same cues that were present when "using." Drug paraphernalia is not needed to live, so drug addicts can shield themselves from these cues. However, food-cued utensils, equipment, and places are unavoidable when preparing unprocessed meals. This sets recovery from PFA apart from drug addiction and contributes to the difficulty of treating. Repeat assessment for cue reactivity of cravings is thus useful.

As seen in the quotes from the 12-step literature, the release from cravings can create valuable relief for a food addict. Cravings can start at a very young age, so many food addicts do not experience life without cravings until they start recovery. They may be well into adulthood, even old age. Abstinence protocols support a dramatic improvement in mental health for the food addict as the obsession ceases.

For cue desensitization, the challenge is to find methods for preparing abstinent meals that do not depend on decisions made by the craving brain of the client. The craving brain creates urgent and intense longings for processed foods, which somehow must be blocked out by the client wishing to shop for and prepare nontriggering meals. This is not easy and may explain by some clients are unable to start recovery. It is important that the practitioner match expectations of performance with a realistic assessment of the mental capabilities of the client.

The evidence suggests a need to find out how severely the client is craving and how much executive function has been lost. Fortunately, the FCQ has been validated for these evaluations. Assessment allows the practitioner to determine whether a client is capable of being in a cued environment without being triggered into cravings, which suppress the cognitive functions needed to execute a nonaddictive food plan. The practitioner can determine how likely it is that a client will be able to think clearly under the barrage of processed food cues found in typical food environments such as grocery stores and restaurants.

The assessment of severity of cravings occurs along a continuum of severity. As with all addictions, the practitioner is faced with developing a recovery program that matches the level of severity.

If the assessment of cravings indicates that the client will not be able to execute a food plan, then the practitioner can justify recommending residential treatment. If residential treatment is not an option, the practitioner can recommend that the client avoid shopping and meal preparation in favor of finding help with those tasks. This avoidance of cues could also be a good recommendation for lesser but still serious cravings. Through ongoing reassessment of cravings, the practitioner develops a justifiable basis for gradually reducing the amount of help needed for food preparation as cue reactivity is desensitized.

14.4 CONCLUSION

Assessing for cravings is important at the outset of recovery as it will impact key elements of the recovery program. Indeed, it can be argued that assessment of cravings could frame the recovery program, particularly in the early stages. The assessment allows the practitioner to evaluate meal-preparation alternatives such as the need for residential treatment, outpatient support for meal preparation, or client preparation of abstinent meals. Assessment of cravings gives the practitioner a solid basis for recommending residential versus supported outpatient treatment versus self-reliance by the client for meal preparation. Practitioners should periodically reassess for cravings to ascertain that clients are capable of other tasks associated with recovery such as rebuilding careers, relationships, and social activities.

Working directly on cravings desensitization relieves the practitioner of the frustration and distress of assigning tasks that are beyond the capability of the client. It gives clients confidence that they can recover as their capabilities are matched with the demands of their recovery. Taken altogether, addressing cravings can mean the difference between success and failure in recovery from PFA.

REFERENCES

American Psychiatric Association. (2013). *The Diagnostic and Statistical Manual of Mental Disorders, Fifth Edition* (Vol. 5), American Psychiatric Association, Washington DC.

American Society of Addiction Medicine. (2011). The Definition of Addiction. *Public Policy Statement.* Accessed from http://www.asam.org/advocacy/find-a-policy-statement/view-policy-statement/public-policy-statements/2011/12/15/the-definition-of-addiction

Asmaro, D., & Liotti, M. (2014). High-caloric and chocolate stimuli processing in healthy humans: An integration of functional imaging and electrophysiological findings. *Nutrients*, *6*(1), 319–341. doi:10.3390/nu6010319.

Atkins, R. C. (2009). *Dr. Atkins' New Diet Revolution.* New York: Harper.

Avena, N. M., Rada, P., & Hoebel, B. G. (2008). Evidence for sugar addiction: Behavioral and neurochemical effects of intermittent, excessive sugar intake. *Neurosci Biobehav Rev*, *32*(1), 20–39.

Batterink, L., Yokum, S., & Stice, E. (2010). Body mass correlates inversely with inhibitory control in response to food among adolescent girls: An fMRI study. *NeuroImage*, *52*(4), 1696–1703. doi:10.1016/j.neuroimage.2010.05.059.

Beaver, J. D., Lawrence, A. D., van Ditzhuijzen, J., Davis, M. H., Woods, A., & Calder, A. J. (2006). Individual differences in reward drive predict neural responses to images of food. *J Neurosci*, *26*(19), 5160–5166.

Becker, J. B., & Koob, G. F. (2016). Sex differences in animal models: Focus on addiction. *Pharmacol Rev*, *68*(2), 242–263. doi:10.1124/pr.115.011163.

Berthoud, H. R. (2004). Mind versus metabolism in the control of food intake and energy balance. *Physiol Behav*, *81*(5), 781–793.

Berthoud, H. R. (2011). Metabolic and hedonic drives in the neural control of appetite: Who is the boss? *Curr Opin Neurobiol*, *21*(6), 888–896. doi:10.1016/j.conb.2011.09.004.

Black, W. R., Lepping, R. J., Bruce, A. S., Powell, J. N., Bruce, J. M., Martin, L. E., . . . Simmons, W. K. (2014). Tonic hyper-connectivity of reward neurocircuitry in obese children. *Obesity (Silver Spring)*, *22*(7), 1590–1593. doi:10.1002/oby.20741.

Borgogna, N., Lockhart, G., Grenard, J. L., Barrett, T., Shiffman, S., & Reynolds, K. D. (2014). Ecological momentary assessment of urban adolescents' technology use and cravings for unhealthy snacks and drinks: Differences by ethnicity and sex. *J Acad Nutr Diet*, *115*(5), 759–766. doi:10.1016/j.jand.2014.10.015.

Borre, Y. E., Moloney, R. D., Clarke, G., Dinan, T. G., & Cryan, J. F. (2014). The impact of microbiota on brain and behavior: Mechanisms & therapeutic potential. *Adv Exp Med Biol*, *817*, 373–403. doi:10.1007/978-1-4939-0897-4_17.

Boswell, R. G., & Kober, H. (2016). Food cue reactivity and craving predict eating and weight gain: A meta-analytic review. *Obes Rev*, *17*(2), 159–177. doi:10.1111/obr.12354.

Bray, G. A. (2000). Afferent signals regulating food intake. *Proc Nutr Soc*, *59*(3), 373–384.

Brockmeyer, T., Hahn, C., Reetz, C., Schmidt, U., & Friederich, H. C. (2015a). Approach bias and cue reactivity towards food in people with high versus low levels of food craving. *Appetite*, *95*, 197–202.

Brockmeyer, T., Hahn, C., Reetz, C., Schmidt, U., & Friederich, H. C. (2015b). Approach bias modification in food craving-A Proof-of-Concept Study. *Eur Eat Disord Rev*, *23*(5), 352–360. doi:10.1002/erv.2382.

Burger, K. S., & Stice, E. (2013). Elevated energy intake is correlated with hyperresponsivity in attentional, gustatory, and reward brain regions while anticipating palatable food receipt. *Am J Clin Nutr*, *97*(6), 1188–1194. doi:10.3945/ajcn.112.055285.

Burton, P., Smit, H. J., & Lightowler, H. J. (2007). The influence of restrained and external eating patterns on overeating. *Appetite*, *49*(1), 191–197.

Carr, K. A., Lin, H., Fletcher, K. D., Sucheston, L., Singh, P. K., Salis, R. J., . . . Epstein, L. H. (2013). Two functional serotonin polymorphisms moderate the effect of food reinforcement on BMI. *Behav Neurosci*, *127*(3), 387–399. doi:10.1037/a0032026.

Chao, A., Grilo, C. M., White, M. A., & Sinha, R. (2014). Food cravings, food intake, and weight status in a community-based sample. *Eat Behav*, *15*(3), 478–482. doi:10.1016/j.eatbeh.2014.06.003.

Childress, A. R., Hole, A. V., Ehrman, R. N., Robbins, S. J., McLellan, A. T., & O'Brien, C. P. (1993). Cue reactivity and cue reactivity interventions in drug dependence. *NIDA Res Monogr*, *137*, 73–95.

Cocores, J. A., & Gold, M. S. (2009). The salted food addiction hypothesis may explain overeating and the obesity epidemic. *Med Hypotheses*, *73*(6), 892–899. doi:S0306-9877(09)00484-8 [pii] 10.1016/j.mehy.2009.06.049 [doi].

Cohen, D. A. (2008). Neurophysiological pathways to obesity: Below awareness and beyond individual control. *Diabetes*, *57*(7), 1768–1773. doi:10.2337/db08-0163.

Colagiuri, B., & Lovibond, P. F. (2015). How food cues can enhance and inhibit motivation to obtain and consume food. *Appetite*, *84*, 79–87. doi:10.1016/j.appet.2014.09.023.

Cole, S., Hobin, M. P., & Petrovich, G. D. (2015). Appetitive associative learning recruits a distinct network with cortical, striatal, and hypothalamic regions. *Neuroscience*, *286*, 187–202. doi:10.1016/j.neuroscience.2014.11.026.

Connor, J. P., Gullo, M. J., White, A., & Kelly, A. B. (2014). Polysubstance use: Diagnostic challenges, patterns of use and health. *Curr Opin Psychiatry*, *27*(4), 269–275. doi:10.1097/yco.0000000000000069.

Cottone, P., Sabino, V., Roberto, M., Bajo, M., Pockros, L., Frihauf, J. B., . . . Zorrilla, E. P. (2009). CRF system recruitment mediates dark side of compulsive eating. *Proc Natl Acad Sci U S A*, *106*(47), 20016–20020. doi:10.1073/pnas.0908789106.

Crowley, N., Madan, A., Wedin, S., Correll, J. A., Delustro, L. M., Borckardt, J. J., & Byrne, T. K. (2014). Food cravings among bariatric surgery candidates. *Eat Weight Disord*, *19*(3), 371–376. doi:10.1007/s40519-013-0095-y.

D'Addario, C., Micioni Di Bonaventura, M. V., Pucci, M., Romano, A., Gaetani, S., Ciccocioppo, R., . . . Maccarrone, M. (2014). Endocannabinoid signaling and food addiction. *Neurosci Biobehav Rev*, *47*, 203–224. doi:10.1016/j.neubiorev.2014.08.008.

Davis, C., Zai, C., Levitan, R. D., Kaplan, A. S., Carter, J. C., Reid-Westoby, C., . . . Kennedy, J. L. (2011). Opiates, overeating and obesity: A psychogenetic analysis. *Int J Obes (Lond)*, *35*(10), 1347–1354. doi:10.1038/ijo.2010.276.

de Bruijn, C., van den Brink, W., de Graaf, R., & Vollebergh, W. A. (2005). The craving withdrawal model for alcoholism: Towards the DSM-V. Improving the discriminant validity of alcohol use disorder diagnosis. *Alcohol Alcohol*, *40*(4), 314–322.

DelParigi, A., Chen, K., Salbe, A. D., Hill, J. O., Wing, R. R., Reiman, E. M., & Tataranni, P. A. (2004). Persistence of abnormal neural responses to a meal in postobese individuals. *Int J Obes Relat Metab Disord*, *28*(3), 370–377. doi:10.1038/sj.ijo.0802558.

Diekhof, E. K., Nerenberg, L., Falkai, P., Dechent, P., Baudewig, J., & Gruber, O. (2012). Impulsive personality and the ability to resist immediate reward: An fMRI study examining interindividual differences in the neural mechanisms underlying self-control. *Hum Brain Mapp*, *33*(12), 2768–2784. doi:10.1002/hbm.21398.

Fallon, S., Shearman, E., Sershen, H., & Lajtha, A. (2007). Food reward-induced neurotransmitter changes in cognitive brain regions. *Neurochem Res*, *32*(10), 1772–1782.

Felsted, J. A., Ren, X., Chouinard-Decorte, F., & Small, D. M. (2010). Genetically determined differences in brain response to a primary food reward. *J Neurosci*, *30*(7), 2428–2432. doi:10.1523/jneurosci.5483-09.2010.

Fernandes, M. F., Sharma, S., Hryhorczuk, C., Auguste, S., & Fulton, S. (2013). Nutritional controls of food reward. *Can J Diabetes*, *37*(4), 260–268. doi:10.1016/j.jcjd.2013.04.004.

Folgueira, C., Seoane, L. M., & Casanueva, F. F. (2014). The brain-stomach connection. *Front Horm Res*, *42*, 83–92. doi:10.1159/000358316.

Food Addicts Anonymous. (2010). *Food Addicts Anonymous*. Port St. Lucie, FL: Food Addicts Anonymous, Inc.

Food Addicts in Recovery Anonymous. (2013). *Food Addicts in Recovery Anonymous*. Woburn, MA: Food Addicts in Recovery Anonymous.

Franken, I. H., & Muris, P. (2005). Individual differences in reward sensitivity are related to food craving and relative body weight in healthy women. *Appetite*, *45*(2), 198–201.

Frankort, A., Roefs, A., Siep, N., Roebroeck, A., Havermans, R., & Jansen, A. (2012). Reward activity in satiated overweight women is decreased during unbiased viewing but increased when imagining taste: An event-related fMRI study. *Int J Obes (Lond)*, *36*(5), 627–637. doi:10.1038/ijo.2011.213.

Frankort, A., Roefs, A., Siep, N., Roebroeck, A., Havermans, R., & Jansen, A. (2015). Neural predictors of chocolate intake following chocolate exposure. *Appetite*, *87*, 98–107. doi:10.1016/j.appet.2014.12.204.

Gibson, E. L. (2006). Emotional influences on food choice: Sensory, physiological and psychological pathways. *Physiol Behav*, *89*(1), 53–61.

Grosshans, M., Vollmert, C., Vollstadt-Klein, S., Tost, H., Leber, S., Bach, P., . . . Kiefer, F. (2012). Association of leptin with food cue-induced activation in human reward pathways. *Arch Gen Psychiatry*, *69*(5), 529–537. doi:10.1001/archgenpsychiatry.2011.1586.

Guerrieri, R., Nederkoorn, C., & Jansen, A. (2008). The interaction between impulsivity and a varied food environment: Its influence on food intake and overweight. *Int J Obes (Lond)*, *32*(4), 708–714.

Halford, J. C., Boyland, E. J., Hughes, G., Oliveira, L. P., & Dovey, T. M. (2007). Beyond-brand effect of television (TV) food advertisements/commercials on caloric intake and food choice of 5-7-year-old children. *Appetite*, *49*(1), 263–267.

Hallam, J., Boswell, R. G., DeVito, E. E., & Kober, H. (2016). Gender-related differences in food craving and obesity. *Yale J Biol Med*, *89*(2), 161–173.

Hellstrom, P. M., Geliebter, A., Naslund, E., Schmidt, P. T., Yahav, E. K., Hashim, S. A., & Yeomans, M. R. (2004). Peripheral and central signals in the control of eating in normal, obese and binge-eating human subjects. *Br J Nutr*, *92 Suppl 1*, S47–S57.

Hetherington, M. M. (2007). Cues to overeat: Psychological factors influencing overconsumption. *Proc Nutr Soc*, *66*(1), 113–123.

Hill, A. J., Weaver, C. F., & Blundell, J. E. (1991). Food craving, dietary restraint and mood. *Appetite*, *17*(3), 187–197.

Ho, C. Y., & Berridge, K. C. (2013). An orexin hotspot in ventral pallidum amplifies hedonic 'liking' for sweetness. *Neuropsychopharmacology*, *38*(9), 1655–1664. doi:10.1038/npp.2013.62.

Holzer, P., & Farzi, A. (2014). Neuropeptides and the microbiota-gut-brain axis. *Adv Exp Med Biol*, *817*, 195–219. doi:10.1007/978-1-4939-0897-4_9.

Hone-Blanchet, A., & Fecteau, S. (2014). Overlap of food addiction and substance use disorders definitions: Analysis of animal and human studies. *Neuropharmacology*, *85*, 81–90. doi:10.1016/j.neuropharm.2014.05.019.

Huebner, F. R., Lieberman, K. W., Rubino, R. P., & Wall, J. S. (1984). Demonstration of high opioid-like activity in isolated peptides from wheat gluten hydrolysates. *Peptides*, *5*(6), 1139–1147.

Imperatori, C., Innamorati, M., Tamburello, S., Continisio, M., Contardi, A., Tamburello, A., & Fabbricatore, M. (2013). Gender differences in food craving among overweight and obese patients attending low energy diet therapy: A matched case-control study. *Eat Weight Disord*, *18*(3), 297–303. doi:10.1007/s40519-013-0054-7.

Innamorati, M., Imperatori, C., Balsamo, M., Tamburello, S., Belvederi Murri, M., Contardi, A., . . . Fabbricatore, M. (2014). Food Cravings Questionnaire Trait (FCQ-T) discriminates between obese and overweight patients with and without binge eating tendencies: The Italian version of the FCQ-T. *J Pers Assess*, *96*(6), 632–639. doi:10.1080/00223891.2014.909449.

Innamorati, M., Imperatori, C., Meule, A., Lamis, D. A., Contardi, A., Balsamo, M., . . . Fabbricatore, M. (2014). Psychometric properties of the Italian Food Cravings Questionnaire-Trait-reduced (FCQ-T-r). *Eat Weight Disord*, *20*(1), 129–135. doi:10.1007/s40519-014-0143-2.

Jansen, A., Theunissen, N., Slechten, K., Nederkoorn, C., Boon, B., Mulkens, S., & Roefs, A. (2003). Overweight children overeat after exposure to food cues. *Eat Behav*, *4*(2), 197–209.

Jastreboff, A. M., Gaiser, E. C., Gu, P., & Sinha, R. (2014). Sex differences in the association between dietary restraint, insulin resistance and obesity. *Eat Behav*, *15*(2), 286–290. doi:10.1016/j.eatbeh.2014.03.008.

Jastreboff, A. M., Sinha, R., Lacadie, C., Small, D. M., Sherwin, R. S., & Potenza, M. N. (2013). Neural correlates of stress- and food cue-induced food craving in obesity: Association with insulin levels. *Diabetes Care*, *36*(2), 394–402. doi:10.1093/ntr/ntw088.

Joyner, M. A., Gearhardt, A. N., & White, M. A. (2015). Food craving as a mediator between addictive-like eating and problematic eating outcomes. *Eat Behav*, *19*, 98–101. doi:10.1016/j.eatbeh.2015.07.005.

Kearns, D. N., & Weiss, S. J. (2005). Reinstatement of a food-maintained operant produced by compounding discriminative stimuli. *Behav Processes*, *70*(2), 194–202. doi:S0376-6357(05)00128-2 [pii] 10.1016/j.beproc.2005.04.007.

Kelley, A. E., Baldo, B. A., Pratt, W. E., & Will, M. J. (2005). Corticostriatal-hypothalamic circuitry and food motivation: Integration of energy, action and reward. *Physiol Behav*, *86*(5), 773–795. doi:10.1016/j.physbeh.2005.08.066.

Kelley, A. E., Schiltz, C. A., & Landry, C. F. (2005). Neural systems recruited by drug- and food-related cues: Studies of gene activation in corticolimbic regions. *Physiol Behav*, *86*(1–2), 11–14. doi:10.1016/j.physbeh.2005.06.018.

Kemps, E., & Tiggemann, M. (2014). A role for mental imagery in the experience and reduction of food cravings. *Front Psychiatry*, *5*, 193. doi:10.3389/fpsyt.2014.00193.

Kemps, E., Tiggemann, M., & Bettany, S. (2012). Non-food odorants reduce chocolate cravings. *Appetite, 58*(3), 1087–1090. doi:10.1016/j.appet.2012.03.002.

Kendig, M. D. (2014). Cognitive and behavioural effects of sugar consumption in rodents. A review. *Appetite, 80*, 41–54. doi:10.1016/j.appet.2014.04.028.

Kennedy, J., & Dimitropoulos, A. (2014). Influence of feeding state on neurofunctional differences between individuals who are obese and normal weight: A meta-analysis of neuroimaging studies. *Appetite, 75*, 103–109. doi:10.1016/j.appet.2013.12.017.

Keskitalo, K., Tuorila, H., Spector, T. D., Cherkas, L. F., Knaapila, A., Silventoinen, K., & Perola, M. (2007). Same genetic components underlie different measures of sweet taste preference. *Am J Clin Nutr, 86*(6), 1663–1669. doi:86/6/1663 [pii].

Kringelbach, M. L., & Stein, A. (2010). Cortical mechanisms of human eating. *Forum Nutr, 63*, 164–175. doi:10.1159/000264404.

Kroemer, N. B., Krebs, L., Kobiella, A., Grimm, O., Pilhatsch, M., Bidlingmaier, M., . . . Smolka, M. N. (2013). Fasting levels of ghrelin covary with the brain response to food pictures. *Addict Biol, 18*(5), 855–862. doi:10.1111/j.1369-1600.2012.00489.x.

Kroemer, N. B., Krebs, L., Kobiella, A., Grimm, O., Vollstadt-Klein, S., Wolfensteller, U., . . . Smolka, M. N. (2013). (Still) longing for food: Insulin reactivity modulates response to food pictures. *Hum Brain Mapp, 34*(10), 2367–2380. doi:10.1002/hbm.22071.

Logan, A. C., & Jacka, F. N. (2014). Nutritional psychiatry research: An emerging discipline and its intersection with global urbanization, environmental challenges and the evolutionary mismatch. *J Physiol Anthropol, 33*, 22. doi:10.1186/1880-6805-33-22.

Meule, A., Allison, K. C., & Platte, P. (2014). A German version of the Night Eating Questionnaire (NEQ): Psychometric properties and correlates in a student sample. *Eat Behav, 15*(4), 523–527. doi:10.1016/j.eatbeh.2014.07.002.

Meule, A., Hermann, T., & Kubler, A. (2014). A short version of the Food Cravings Questionnaire-Trait: The FCQ-T-reduced. *Front Psychol, 5*, 190. doi:10.3389/fpsyg.2014.00190.

Meule, A., & Hormes, J. M. (2015). Chocolate versions of the *Food Cravings Questionnaires*. Associations with chocolate exposure-induced salivary flow and ad libitum chocolate consumption. *Appetite, 91*, 256–265.

Meule, A., & Kubler, A. (2014). Double trouble. Trait food craving and impulsivity interactively predict food-cue affected behavioral inhibition. *Appetite, 79*, 174–182. doi:10.1016/j.appet.2014.04.014.

Meule, A., Lutz, A., Vogele, C., & Kubler, A. (2012). Food cravings discriminate differentially between successful and unsuccessful dieters and non-dieters. Validation of the Food Cravings Questionnaires in German. *Appetite, 58*(1), 88–97. doi:S0195-6663(11)00578-2 [pii] 10.1016/j.appet.2011.09.010.

Meule, A., Skirde, A. K., Freund, R., Vogele, C., & Kubler, A. (2012). High-calorie food-cues impair working memory performance in high and low food cravers. *Appetite.* doi:S0195-6663(12)00166-3 [pii] 10.1016/j.appet.2012.05.010.

Monteleone, A. M., Di Marzo, V., Aveta, T., Piscitelli, F., Dalle Grave, R., Scognamiglio, P., . . . Maj, M. (2015). Deranged endocannabinoid responses to hedonic eating in underweight and recently weight-restored patients with anorexia nervosa. *Am J Clin Nutr, 101*(2), 262–269. doi:10.3945/ajcn.114.096164.

Monteleone, P., Scognamiglio, P., Monteleone, A. M., Perillo, D., Canestrelli, B., & Maj, M. (2013). Gastroenteric hormone responses to hedonic eating in healthy humans. *Psychoneuroendocrinology, 38*(8), 1435–1441. doi:10.1016/j.psyneuen.2012.12.009.

Moreno, S., Rodriguez, S., Fernandez, M. C., Tamez, J., & Cepeda-Benito, A. (2008). Clinical validation of the trait and state versions of the Food Craving Questionnaire. *Assessment, 15*(3), 375–387. doi:10.1177/1073191107312651.

Moss, H. B., Chen, C. M., & Yi, H. Y. (2014). Early adolescent patterns of alcohol, cigarettes, and marijuana polysubstance use and young adult substance use outcomes in a nationally representative sample. *Drug Alcohol Depend, 136*, 51–62. doi:10.1016/j.drugalcdep.2013.12.011.

Murray, S., Tulloch, A., Gold, M. S., & Avena, N. M. (2014). Hormonal and neural mechanisms of food reward, eating behaviour and obesity. *Nat Rev Endocrinol, 10*(9), 540–552. doi:10.1038/nrendo.2014.91.

Noble, E. E., Mavanji, V., Little, M. R., Billington, C. J., Kotz, C. M., & Wang, C. (2014). Exercise reduces diet-induced cognitive decline and increases hippocampal brain-derived neurotrophic factor in CA3 neurons. *Neurobiol Learn Mem, 114*, 40–50. doi:10.1016/j.nlm.2014.04.006.

Nummenmaa, L., Hirvonen, J., Hannukainen, J. C., Immonen, H., Lindroos, M. M., Salminen, P., & Nuutila, P. (2012). Dorsal striatum and its limbic connectivity mediate abnormal anticipatory reward processing in obesity. *PLoS One, 7*(2), e31089. doi:10.1371/journal.pone.0031089.

O'Brien, C. P. (2005). Anticraving medications for relapse prevention: A possible new class of psychoactive medications. *Am J Psychiatry, 162*(8), 1423–1431.

Oginsky, M. F., Goforth, P. B., Nobile, C. W., Lopez-Santiago, L. F., & Ferrario, C. R. (2016). Eating 'Junk-Food' produces rapid and long-lasting increases in NAc CP-AMPA receptors: Implications for enhanced cue-induced motivation and food addiction. *Neuropsychopharmacology*, *41*(13), 2977–2986. doi:10.1038/npp.2016.111.

Oliver, G., Wardle, J., & Gibson, E. L. (2000). Stress and food choice: A laboratory study. *Psychosom Med*, *62*(6), 853–865.

Orsini, C. A., Ginton, G., Shimp, K. G., Avena, N. M., Gold, M. S., & Setlow, B. (2014). Food consumption and weight gain after cessation of chronic amphetamine administration. *Appetite*, *78*, 76–80. doi:10.1016/j.appet.2014.03.013.

Passamonti, L., Rowe, J. B., Schwarzbauer, C., Ewbank, M. P., von dem Hagen, E., & Calder, A. J. (2009). Personality predicts the brain's response to viewing appetizing foods: The neural basis of a risk factor for overeating. *J Neurosci*, *29*(1), 43–51. doi:29/1/43 [pii] 10.1523/JNEUROSCI.4966-08.2009 [doi].

Pavlov, I. P. (2015). *Conditioned Reflexes: An Investigation of the Physiological Activity of the Cerebral Cortex*. Eastford, CT: Martino Fine Books.

Pecina, S., Schulkin, J., & Berridge, K. C. (2006). Nucleus accumbens corticotropin-releasing factor increases cue-triggered motivation for sucrose reward: Paradoxical positive incentive effects in stress? *BMC Biol*, *4*, 8.

Petrovich, G. D. (2013). Forebrain networks and the control of feeding by environmental learned cues. *Physiol Behav*, *121*, 10–18. doi:10.1016/j.neulet.2006.11.019.

Petrovich, G. D., & Gallagher, M. (2007). Control of food consumption by learned cues: A forebrain-hypothalamic network. *Physiol Behav*, *91*(4), 397–403. doi:S0031-9384(07)00133-3 [pii] 10.1016/j.physbeh.2007.04.014.

Polk, S. E., Schulte, E. M., Furman, C. R., & Gearhardt, A. N. (2016). Wanting and liking: Separable components in problematic eating behavior? *Appetite*, *115*, 45–53. doi:10.1016/j.appet.2016.11.015.

Rejeski, W. J., Blumenthal, T. D., Miller, G. D., Lobe, M., Davis, C., & Brown, L. (2010). State craving, food availability, and reactivity to preferred snack foods. *Appetite*, *54*(1), 77–83. doi:S0195-6663(09)00625-4 [pii] 10.1016/j.appet.2009.09.009.

Rodriguez-Martin, B. C., & Meule, A. (2015). Food craving: New contributions on its assessment, moderators, and consequences. *Front Psychol*, *6*, 21. doi:10.3389/fpsyg.2015.00021.

Rodriguez, S., Warren, C. S., Moreno, S., Cepeda-Benito, A., Gleaves, D. H., Fernandez Mdel, C., & Vila, J. (2007). Adaptation of the food-craving questionnaire trait for the assessment of chocolate cravings: Validation across British and Spanish women. *Appetite*, *49*(1), 245–250.

Schuckit, M. A., Danko, G. P., Raimo, E. B., Smith, T. L., Eng, M. Y., Carpenter, K. K., & Hesselbrock, V. M. (2001). A preliminary evaluation of the potential usefulness of the diagnoses of polysubstance dependence. *J Stud Alcohol*, *62*(1), 54–61.

Schwabe, L., & Wolf, O. T. (2011). Stress-induced modulation of instrumental behavior: From goal-directed to habitual control of action. *Behav Brain Res*, *219*(2), 321–328. doi:10.1016/j.bbr.2010.12.038.

Sharma, S., Fernandes, M. F., & Fulton, S. (2013). Adaptations in brain reward circuitry underlie palatable food cravings and anxiety induced by high-fat diet withdrawal. *Int J Obes (Lond)*, *37*(9), 1183–1191. doi:10.1038/ijo.2012.197.

Silvers, J. A., Insel, C., Powers, A., Franz, P., Weber, J., Mischel, W., . . . Ochsner, K. N. (2014). Curbing craving: Behavioral and brain evidence that children regulate craving when instructed to do so but have higher baseline craving than adults. *Psychol Sci*, *25*(10), 1932–1942. doi:10.1177/0956797614546001.

Spreadbury, I. (2012). Comparison with ancestral diets suggests dense acellular carbohydrates promote an inflammatory microbiota, and may be the primary dietary cause of leptin resistance and obesity. *Diabetes Metab Syndr Obes*, *5*, 175–189. doi:10.2147/dmso.s33473.

Stice, E., & Dagher, A. (2010). Genetic variation in dopaminergic reward in humans. *Forum Nutr*, *63*, 176–185. doi:10.1159/000264405.

Stice, E., Figlewicz, D. P., Gosnell, B. A., Levine, A. S., & Pratt, W. E. (2013). The contribution of brain reward circuits to the obesity epidemic. *Neurosci Biobehav Rev*, *37*(9 Pt A), 2047–2058. doi:10.1016/j.neubiorev.2012.12.001.

Stice, E., & Yokum, S. (2016). Neural vulnerability factors that increase risk for future weight gain. *Psychol Bull*, *142*(5), 447–471. doi:10.1037/bul0000044.

St-Onge, M. P., Wolfe, S., Sy, M., Shechter, A., & Hirsch, J. (2014). Sleep restriction increases the neuronal response to unhealthy food in normal-weight individuals. *Int J Obes (Lond)*, *38*(3), 411–416. doi:10.1038/ijo.2013.114.

Sudan, R., Sudan, R., Lyden, E., & Thompson, J. S. (2016). Food cravings and food consumption after Roux-en-Y gastric bypass versus cholecystectomy. *Surg Obes Relat Dis*. doi:10.1016/j.soard.2016.09.001.

Taguchi, A., Wartschow, L. M., & White, M. F. (2007). Brain IRS2 signaling coordinates life span and nutrient homeostasis. *Science*, *317*(5836), 369–372. doi:10.1126/science.1142179.

Temple, J. L. (2016). Behavioral sensitization of the reinforcing value of food: What food and drugs have in common. *Prev Med*, *92*, 90–99. doi:10.1016/j.ypmed.2016.06.022.

Tetley, A., Brunstrom, J., & Griffiths, P. (2009). Individual differences in food-cue reactivity. The role of BMI and everyday portion-size selections. *Appetite*, *52*(3), 614–620. doi:S0195-6663(09)00034-8 [pii] 10.1016/j.appet.2009.02.005.

Thomasius, R., Sack, P. M., Strittmatter, E., & Kaess, M. (2014). Substance-related and addictive disorders in the DSM-5. *Z Kinder Jugendpsychiatr Psychother*, *42*(2), 115–120. doi:10.1024/1422-4917/a000278.

Tomasi, D., Wang, G. J., Wang, R., Caparelli, E. C., Logan, J., & Volkow, N. D. (2015). Overlapping patterns of brain activation to food and cocaine cues in cocaine abusers: Association to striatal D2/D3 receptors. *Hum Brain Mapp*, *36*(1), 120–136. doi:10.1002/hbm.22617.

Trevizol, F., Roversi, K., Dias, V. T., Roversi, K., Barcelos, R. C., Kuhn, F. T., . . . Burger, M. E. (2015). Cross-generational trans fat intake facilitates mania-like behavior: Oxidative and molecular markers in brain cortex. *Neuroscience*, *286*, 353–363. doi:10.1016/j.neuroscience.2014.11.059.

Turk, M. W., Yang, K., Hravnak, M., Sereika, S. M., Ewing, L. J., & Burke, L. E. (2009). Randomized clinical trials of weight loss maintenance: A review. *J Cardiovasc Nurs*, *24*(1), 58–80. doi:10.1097/01.jcn.0000317471.58048.32.

Tye, K. M., Stuber, G. D., de Ridder, B., Bonci, A., & Janak, P. H. (2008). Rapid strengthening of thalamo-amygdala synapses mediates cue-reward learning. *Nature*, *453*(7199), 1253–1257. doi:10.1038/nature06963.

Val-Laillet, D., Aarts, E., Weber, B., Ferrari, M., Quaresima, V., Stoeckel, L. E., . . . Stice, E. (2015). Neuroimaging and neuromodulation approaches to study eating behavior and prevent and treat eating disorders and obesity. *Neuroimage Clin*, *8*, 1–31. doi:10.1016/j.nicl.2015.03.016.

Wagner, D. D., Boswell, R. G., Kelley, W. M., & Heatherton, T. F. (2012). Inducing negative affect increases the reward value of appetizing foods in dieters. *J Cogn Neurosci*, *24*(7), 1625–1633. doi:10.1162/jocn_a_00238.

Wang, G. J., Tomasi, D., Volkow, N. D., Wang, R., Telang, F., Caparelli, E. C., & Dunayevich, E. (2014). Effect of combined naltrexone and bupropion therapy on the brain's reactivity to food cues. *Int J Obes (Lond)*, *38*(5), 682–688. doi:10.1038/ijo.2013.145.

Watkins, B. A., & Kim, J. (2014). The endocannabinoid system: Directing eating behavior and macronutrient metabolism. *Front Psychol*, *5*, 1506. doi:10.3389/fpsyg.2014.01506.

Weight-Watchers. (2014). *Weight Watchers New Complete Edition* (5th ed.). New York: Houghton Mifflin Harcourt.

Werthmann, J., Field, M., Roefs, A., Nederkoorn, C., & Jansen, A. (2014). Attention bias for chocolate increases chocolate consumption–an attention bias modification study. *J Behav Ther Exp Psychiatry*, *45*(1), 136–143. doi:10.1016/j.jbtep.2013.09.009.

Williams, D. L. (2014). Neural integration of satiation and food reward: Role of GLP-1 and orexin pathways. *Physiol Behav*, *136*: 194–199. doi:10.1016/j.physbeh.2014.03.013.

Wurtman, R. J., & Wurtman, J. J. (1995). Brain serotonin, carbohydrate-craving, obesity and depression. *Obes Res*, *3 Suppl 4*, 477S–480S.

Yeh, J., Trang, A., Henning, S. M., Wilhalme, H., Carpenter, C., Heber, D., & Li, Z. (2016). Food cravings, food addiction, and a dopamine-resistant (DRD2 A1) receptor polymorphism in Asian American college students. *Asia Pac J Clin Nutr*, *25*(2), 424–429. doi:10.6133/apjcn.102015.05.

Yin, H. H., Ostlund, S. B., & Balleine, B. W. (2008). Reward-guided learning beyond dopamine in the nucleus accumbens: The integrative functions of cortico-basal ganglia networks. *Eur J Neurosci*, *28*(8), 1437–1448. doi:10.1111/j.1460-9568.2008.06422.x.

Zhang, J., Berridge, K. C., Tindell, A. J., Smith, K. S., & Aldridge, J. W. (2009). A neural computational model of incentive salience. *PLoS Comput Biol*, *5*(7), e1000437. doi:10.1371/journal.pcbi.1000437.

Zhang, Z., Manson, K. F., Schiller, D., & Levy, I. (2014). Impaired associative learning with food rewards in obese women. *Curr Biol*, *24*(15), 1731–1736. doi:10.1016/j.cub.2014.05.075.

Zinczenko, D. (2015). *Zero Belly Cookbook.* New York: Ballentine.

15 DSM 5 SUD Criterion 5
Failure to Fulfill Roles

Joan Ifland
Food Addiction Training, LLC
Cincinnati, OH

Carrie L. Willey
Shades of Hope Treatment Center
Buffalo Gap, TX

CONTENTS

Recurrent processed food abuse resulting in a failure to fulfill major role obligations at work, school, or home. (American Psychiatric Association, 2013, p. 491)

15.1 INTRODUCTION

The failure to fulfill major role obligations at work, school, or home is a generally recognized characteristic of drug addiction. This criterion was included in the DSM IV SUD criteria and was retained in the DSM 5 SUD criteria. Like drug addicts, food-addicted clients may also suffer from the inability to fulfill role obligations. The etiology of the problem can be thought of as synergistic.

First, there is an initial preoccupation with obtaining the substance despite persistent physical or psychological consequences. Subsequent intoxication results in the failure to fulfill social, occupational, and recreational obligations. These failures often result in increased negative affect that is exacerbated by emerging withdrawal symptoms. A cycle of repeated failure to self-regulate follows, and each violation brings greater negative affect and results in greater tolerance than the last (Kassel, Veilleux, Heinz, Braun, & Conrad, 2013).

The development of this characteristic in processed food addiction (PFA) is gradual, with the preoccupation and consequences of processed food blocking out thoughts and activities necessary to fulfill role obligations at work, school, or home.

The desperation of this cycle is illustrated in these quotes from the 12-step food addiction manuals:

> I felt like I was being chased by a demon and the only way to keep it at bay was to do more and more—more food, more drugs. I finally had so many life experiences that filled me with such self-loathing that I quit doing the drugs. I was now alone with my primary addiction, food. My husband, children, job and other relationships all took a back seat to my disease of food addiction. The pain of who I was, the shame of who I had become, and the insanity caught up with me. I was forty-one years old and hated myself and almost everyone else. (Food Addicts Anonymous, 2010, p. 118)
>
> I weighed about 315 pounds and was still gaining. I was confused. I had been on Prozac, an anti-depressant, for [two and a half] years and I still could not hold down a full-time job. (Food Addicts Anonymous, 2010, p. 201)
>
> As time evolved, I became less able to control either my starving or bingeing. The mental anguish that food addiction created for me was so painful that:
>
> I can't remember.
> My thought process stops midstream.
> My eyes are unable to focus.
> My body can't operate at its potential.
> I become numb and I create a fantasy world.
>
> I promise myself recovery tomorrow, as if I have any control. I am not capable of decisions and forget any responsibilities. The time came when I was unable to care for anyone or anything, let alone myself. (Food Addicts Anonymous, 2010, p. 166)
>
> For a while, things looked good on the outside—the "white picket fence" syndrome. Then the devastation of this disease began to reveal itself as my children entered their teens. My emotional absence and immaturity had taken its toll. My life seemed like a painful nightmare from which I could not awake. Suicidal thoughts entered my mind on a frequent basis. (Food Addicts Anonymous, 2010, p. 217)

My disease progressed beyond my wildest imagination. Food became more important than my daughter, my husband, my integrity or anything else in my life. I would sneak food, hide food, leave the house at ungodly hours for it, stash it, and so on. I manipulated people, places and things so that I could be alone with my fix. One time, while my husband was paying our dinner check, I snuck back and ate the leftover food on his plate. My life consisted of bingeing, purging and exercising. It was nothing for me to do intense aerobic exercise for four hours a day. (Food Addicts Anonymous, 2010, pp. 235–236)

15.1.1 Importance

Failure to fulfill roles can create a stressful feedback loop in which the addiction is triggered by the anxiety of neglected situations at work, school, or home. PFA manifesting as obesity has been shown to be associated with failed educations, careers, and family management (Ali & Lindstrom, 2006; Feng & Wilson, 2015; Gonzalez-Casanova et al., 2014). Possible reasons for failed fulfillment of obligations could include cognitive impairment (Petrovich, 2013), fatigue (Patterson, Frank, Kristal, & White, 2004), general illness (Guh et al., 2009), depression (Goodman & Whitaker, 2002; Heo, Pietrobelli, Fontaine, Sirey, & Faith, 2006), and mental illness (Nguyen, Killcross, & Jenkins, 2014). These all help explain failure to fulfill obligations in chronic food abusers (Bray & Bellanger, 2006).

In the progression of the disease, it is possible that capabilities have declined while situations have become more demanding. In fact, the decline in capabilities and resulting neglect may be the cause of worsening situations. At some point, role obligations may become overwhelming. For example, as health deteriorates, side effects and expense of medications to address symptoms of the metabolic syndrome could further impair physical, mental, emotional, and financial capabilities (Christensen, Kristensen, Bartels, Bliddal, & Astrup, 2007). Each cycle of weight gain and loss could induce a deepening attitude of defeat, shame, and self-blame, which could erode the self-confidence needed to manage obligations (Foster, Makris, & Bailer, 2005). There may also be growing stress on the job as increasing daytime sleepiness makes performance more difficult (Jarosz et al., 2014). As PFA intensifies in the parents, it is possible that their underperforming, hyperactive, or ADD children could be acting out more and more (Mikolajczyk & Richter, 2008). It's important not to miss symptoms of PFA in children of clients as an indicator of demands on the parents. The synergistic relationship between the decreasing ability to meet role obligations and the growing demands of those obligations can be a symptom of PFA, as well as an indicator of its severity.

Here are illustrations of declining capabilities and increasing demands taken from the food addiction 12-step manuals.

> Comfort was sneaking back into my life and so did the weight. Single life was fun but expensive. The kids needed things, but child support was nil. There were bills and not enough money to pay them or to play. Food was then master, once again. (Food Addicts Anonymous, 2010, p. 146)
>
> I was trying to keep my family afloat, yet there wasn't money to buy food. The foods we got from the handouts were all sugary and high in carbohydrates—poison to me. My addiction was at an all-time low, and I started getting depressed and overwhelmed. (Food Addicts Anonymous, 2010, p. 178)
>
> As I threw back the sheets and lifted my obese legs off to one side of the bed, it was a struggle to move just a few inches. I knew I had responsibilities to face; pets to take care of and housework to do. I faced a 12-hour routine to keep my job in the federal government. But this day was different; I just couldn't do it anymore. The exhaustion was just too overwhelming. (Food Addicts Anonymous, 2010, p. 225)

As practitioners review the devastation of PFA through the assessment of SRAD Criterion 5, it may become apparent that it is unrealistic to expect a person with such a severe disease to be able to carry out obligations. It is especially important to assess the safety of children in the food addict's care. If children seem to be fed only nonnutritious processed foods, the practitioner may consider whether it's necessary to intervene and seek help for the household.

It is important to assess the extent of the failure to fulfill obligations across workplace, school, and home to support appropriate recovery strategies. It is very important to develop realistic strategies for managing obligations and to include them in the recovery program. It can be a significant relief to the client to have a plan. Reducing stress through proposing a plan of action can bring needed hope and a determination to take action.

15.1.2 Evidence for the Syndrome

There is quite a bit of evidence in the research suggesting that the obese can encounter barriers to fulfilling role obligations. Considering the comprehensive consequences of PFA, it is logical that PFA clients would not thrive in work, school, and home roles. Researchers have captured the distress and consequences in this area.

15.1.2.1 Work

In terms of fulfilling work roles, research shows that the obese tend to be economically disadvantaged with poor educations (An, 2015; Harper & Lynch, 2007; Stewart-Knox et al., 2012; Williams, Andrianopoulos, Cleland, Crawford, & Ball, 2013). A study in Washington State showed that jobs for the obese may be more readily available in lower-paying industries (Bonauto, Lu, & Fan, 2014; Gu et al., 2014).

PFA clients may suffer in work performance due to distraction of cravings (Meule & Kubler, 2014) and an inability to focus (Johnson et al., 2011). Research showing cognitive impairment in obese populations is extensive (Franken, Nijs, Toes, & van der Veen, 2016; Petrovich, 2013; Zhu et al., 2015).

PFA clients may also suffer from daytime sleepiness, which has been shown to impair memory (Igelstrom, Emtner, Lindberg, & Asenlof, 2013; Patel, Spaeth, & Basner, 2016).

It has also been shown that obese people suffer discrimination, which limits opportunities (Wang, Brownell, & Wadden, 2004). Excessive fat tissue, presentation in the workplace, and appropriate clothing are all issues in fulfilling roles at the workplace. Further, joint pain and bone deterioration can prevent standing for any length of time (Heo, Pietrobelli, Wang, Heymsfield, & Faith, 2010; Magnusson, Hagen, & Natvig, 2016; Wilkie, Blagojevic-Bucknall, Jordan, & Pransky, 2013). Depression could be a factor in finding a job as well as avoiding advancement (Olvera, Williamson, Fisher-Hoch, Vatcheva, & McCormick, 2015).

These quotes illustrate the researching findings.

> I had a hard time when I graduated from college. In an economy with double-digit unemployment and high interest rates, I couldn't find a job. I also couldn't find clothes that fit me. I weighed 175 pounds and had moved back in with my parents. (Food Addicts Anonymous, 2010, p. 21)
>
> Instead of calling on customers for my work, I drove here and there, bingeing in my car. How high is this scale going to go? I wondered. I could easily imagine it reading 200 pounds, but I knew it wouldn't stop there. Would it stop at 250? What would happen to me when none of my clothes fit and I could no longer buy the professional outfits required for my job? (Food Addicts Anonymous, 2010, p. 23)
>
> I went to bed with several bowls of cereal at night, trying to mask my unhappiness by eating. I had such anxiety attacks that I lasted only two or three days in a hospital job I found there. (Food Addicts in Recovery Anonymous, 2013, p. 101)
>
> I married a man who was morbidly obese. Before we divorced, I drove us into debt. I moved from job to job or didn't work at all. I wasn't actively suicidal, but I didn't want to live, and I was afraid I couldn't keep myself safe. (Food Addicts in Recovery Anonymous, 2013, p. 249)

In terms of understanding the phenomenon of barriers to fulfilling work roles in food-addicted populations, there may be synergy between the food industry targeting undereducated markets (Powell, Wada, & Kumanyika, 2014) and debilitating physical, mental, and emotional effects of the disease that combine to make it difficult for PFA clients to fulfill roles at work, particularly if the work is physically demanding and reduces sleep.

15.1.2.2 School

School can present a number of problems for the food addict. Dense cueing, stress, and negative interactions with classmates can combine to accelerate the disease and create barriers to success. College can accelerate the disease because of food availability (Kemps, Tiggemann, & Hollitt, 2014). The increased stress can provoke cravings and distraction (Nijs et al., 2010; Yau & Potenza, 2013). Furthermore, young adults may be away from home for the first time and be coping with unmonitored, unstructured time. Learning disabilities and cognitive impairment could also play an active role in preventing a food addict from fulfilling the role of student (Ells et al., 2006; Zamzow et al., 2014).

> By the time I was in high school, I was obese and had totally withdrawn. I had shut down. I hardly spoke to anyone. My appearance was poor, and I literally walked around in a sugar daze. In my second high school (we had moved again), I failed three courses. By then I had reached the weight of 160–180 pounds. I fought my way into college, but I still lived with my parents. I prolonged going home while attending college and often stayed up late to binge in the coffee shops to the point of blacking out. I knew no other way of life. I thought I was losing my mind, and I probably was. (Food Addicts Anonymous, 2010, p. 183)

15.1.2.3 Home

Research shows that obese parents may be challenged in the role of caring for children (Halliday, Palma, Mellor, Green, & Renzaho, 2014; Mogul, Irby, & Skelton, 2014). Problems of cognitive impairment may hamper parents from nurturing children intellectually (Levin et al., 2014). Parents may suffer from fatigue, which could interfere with child care (Maloney, Boneva, Lin, & Reeves, 2010). Parents who are experiencing loss of control in eating and restricting are more likely to have children who also suffer from these problems (Matheson et al., 2015). Poor impulse control and learning difficulties in obese children may make the demands of home greater in obese households (Schuchardt, Fischbach, Balke-Melcher, & Mahler, 2015). Limited mobility may also hamper abilities to care for children (Gerlach, Williams, & Coates, 2013; Vincent, Adams, Vincent, & Hurley, 2013).

Emotional instability can be a problem in obese populations and could interfere with the role of parent (Molyneaux, Poston, Ashurst-Williams, & Howard, 2014; Pasco, Williams, Jacka, Brennan, & Berk, 2013; Pasold, McCracken, & Ward-Begnoche, 2014; Raines, Boffa, Allan, Short, & Schmidt, 2015). In homes where food-addicted parents are distracted and tired, television watching by children may be higher, which could compound the likelihood of the development of pediatric PFA (Lioutas & Tzimitra-Kalogianni, 2015). Obesity in family systems could be interpreted as evidence of neglect of preparation of healthy foods (Kestila, Rahkonen, Martelin, Lahti-Koski, & Koskinen, 2009).

This quote illustrates how PFA can interfere with parenting.

> When my daughter asked me to read her a bedtime story, she interrupted my evening eating, and I begrudged her the time. (Food Addicts Anonymous, 2010, p. 22)

The evidence shows that PFA clients can suffer from failure to fulfill roles. In some ways, roles in the lives of the obese may be more demanding than roles in the lives of lean people. Although the manifestations may be different, the consequences of PFA can be as severe as those of drug addiction.

15.1.3 Use in Motivation

It is painful when a client feels that they're not meeting the demands of a job, school, or family and yet cannot improve the situation. The sense of shame around failing in roles can be reinforced by the failure to cut back as described in Criterion 2. This can be especially so if the client's children have developed weight problems (Dhingra, Brennan, & Walkley, 2011). The possibility of resolution of fear of losing a job, fear of being forced to abandon school, or shame over troubled children are all potential benefits from undertaking recovery. Gaining the mental, physical, and emotional capabilities to meet and even excel in roles is a powerful motivator. Assessment of abilities to fulfill roles will be an important element of the scope of problem. Gaining insight into the hopes and dreams lost can provide material to motivate clients to undertake recovery. Items from this assessment can help fill out the list of options to start recovery.

These quotes illustrate how motivating relief from despair could be.

> Eighteen years ago, when my father died suddenly and my world was crushed, I couldn't stop eating. I wanted to die. My life was unmanageable. I almost lost my job and I isolated from my support system. Luckily, a co-worker told me about Twelve-Step programs. That was the first time in my life I felt that there wasn't something wrong with me; I knew I had a disease. (Food Addicts Anonymous, 2010, p. 176)
>
> By the time the last baby was born and was about six months old, I'd decided it wasn't worth it to dress. I lived in nightgowns and housecoats, which fit over my fat. They were comfortable and convenient since I was always nursing one child or another. I was haunted by fears and was afraid to leave my house. I never answered the door or the phone. I thought if I left my home, someone would try to steal my children. If I drove, a car accident might kill them. I might run into someone and she would see that my clothes didn't fit me anymore. She'd notice that my hair was thin. So I stayed behind my door. (Food Addicts in Recovery Anonymous, 2013, p. 90)

Educating clients that recovery is healing from a specific disease with identifiable causes can be an effective motivator to start taking easy steps in a comprehensive program.

15.1.4 Use in Treatment

Like all aspects of symptoms of PFA, failure to fulfill roles can be healed in a stepwise fashion. The pace of recovery of the abilities to fulfill roles depends on the extent of cognitive impairment as well as the client's physical strength to keep up with demands. Fortunately, improvements in energy and mental clarity may occur even in the first week of abstinence. The ability of the client to prepare meals is key. The practitioner and client can work together to create an upward reinforcing spiral where, as abilities increase, demands decrease. As the client is able to finish tasks, performance reviews at work may improve or grades may come up at school. As abstinent foods are introduced to the home, the out-of-control behaviors of children may improve and the children may become less demanding. Recovery of ability to fulfill roles can be seen to converge from two directions, i.e., increasing competencies and decreasing problems.

15.2 APPLICATION

There are a number of ways in which gathering information about the client's ability to fulfill roles can be useful to the process of recovery. The results of assessing role fulfillment can help motivate clients. Clients may not have made the connection between their chronic food abuse and problems in their workplaces and homes. They may not have realized that their food use cut short an education. Holding out the promise of improvements in these areas through sobriety could be motivational.

Assessing role fulfillment could also generate valuable material for the recovery plan. As clients achieve sobriety, they may be interested in furthering their careers, resuming educations, and improving the lives of their household members. Steps to achieving progress in these areas can be included in the list of options that transition the client from contemplation to action.

15.2.1 Care in Approach

Although research has not yet progressed to consistent recommendations, a review article found that the most widely supported types of obesity treatment are family behavioral treatment and parent-only behavior treatment (Altman & Wilfley, 2015). Education about the link between food abuse and financial distress, abandoned educations, and neglected children could be helpful. The practitioner should check that possibly life-threatening conditions are under control in the children of clients. These include diabetes, obstructive sleep apnea, and fatty liver (Allen & Fost, 2012; Cheng, 2012; Garrahan & Eichner, 2012). Neglected children have higher rates of obesity in some cases (Helton & Liechty, 2014). Care neglect and supervisory neglect correlate with obesity in younger and older children, respectively (Knutson, Taber, Murray, Valles, & Koeppl, 2010). This is the case especially in single-child households (Chen & Escarce, 2014). Neglected children gain weight more quickly than non-neglected children (Shin & Miller, 2012). Practitioners can help clients prioritize the care of children in their recovery program.

Motivation needs to be sustained. Motivation at initiation did not produce weight loss in a family weight-loss intervention while sustained motivation did (Accurso, Norman, Crow, Rock, & Boutelle, 2014).

15.2.2 Developing Goals

After carefully listening to the client's routines, capabilities, and needs, the practitioner can develop easily attainable goals toward development of the capabilities needed to fulfill roles. It is important to establish goals that can be accomplished with certainty. Do not set deadlines to avoid setting clients up for failure. Giving clients permission to relax and take their time reduces stress, reduces fear of failure, reduces risk of relapse, and increases confidence.

Looking at the family as a whole has been shown to be key in the treatment of chronic overeating (Skelton, Buehler, Irby, & Grzywacz, 2012). In general, developing characteristics of resiliency in the family are good goals. These include routines, reduced stress, functioning, and structure (Sigman-Grant, Hayes, VanBrackle, & Fiese, 2015). Parents can work toward avoiding parenting styles that are associated with childhood obesity including uninvolved, indulgent, or highly protective parenting. Positive communication and an authoritative parenting style were found to be associated with a healthy BMI (Fiese, Hammons, & Grigsby-Toussaint, 2012; Shloim, Edelson,

Martin, & Hetherington, 2015). Responding to children's distress positively and without using food as a reward are also productive goals (Saltzman et al., 2016). New foods can be introduced in a positive environment that avoids pressuring. Pressuring can create avoidance of healthy foods later in life (Ventura & Worobey, 2013).

Other kinds of goals could be to establish meal times (Berge et al., 2015), set sleep times, limit screen time, and keep televisions out of bedrooms (Jones & Fiese, 2014). Signing up for a brain-training online program such as Lumosity is easy and fun (Hardy et al., 2015) and targets the important goal of cognitive restoration (Petrovich, 2013). More challenging goals might be to consolidate processed foods into one cabinet at home to reduce cuing (Boswell & Kober, 2016), as a step toward eventually clearing the home of processed foods (Werthmann, Jansen, & Roefs, 2014).

If the client has lost a job, or would like to prepare for a better job, the practitioner can put steps in that direction into the recovery program. Similarly, if the client wants to complete a degree or certification, the practitioner can describe the path needed to fulfill that role.

15.2.3 Tracking Progress

Goals related to fulfilling roles at work and school are likely to flow naturally from improvements in energy, mental clarity, alertness, weight loss, and confidence. In early stage recovery, rather than setting career or school goals, the practitioner can give clients benefits to watch for. Benefits that will enhance the ability to fulfill roles are reduction in sleepiness, fatigue, and joint pain. Improvements in cognitive function such as learning, decision-making, memory, and restraint will also naturally improve clients' abilities to fulfill roles. Similarly, reduced depression, anxiety, irritability, and shame that are derived from chemical imbalances will contribute naturally to clients' functionality and role fulfillment.

Practitioners can support clients as they take the lead in deciding how they will repair damage to careers and educations. It is likely that clients will surface lost dreams or will devise new hopes for goals that were submerged by the disease. Practitioners may need to be more involved in tracking improvements in childcare. Positive interactions, boundary setting, scheduling, and structuring children's time are all parenting skills that could benefit from devising scripts and rehearsing scenarios.

15.3 CONCLUSION

Practitioners will reap rewards from assessing clients for barriers to fulfilling major role obligations at work, school, or home. Determining conformance to Criterion 5 is important to fully assess and to treat.

Practitioners can reassure clients that they are not to blame by comparing PFA to any other serious illness or serious accident. With this perspective, the client can reduce shame about being unable to fulfill roles. In the scope of the problem, the practitioner will describe the extent of impairment that the client has suffered physically, emotionally, and mentally. Clients will be able to see that no one would expect an employee/student/parent to perform under these circumstances. Practitioners can watch for opportunities to provide immediate relief for children.

Clients and practitioners alike can remember that restoration is a long-term process for career or educations. The key is to emphasize recovery of abilities such as cognitive restoration as well as improvements in mood, alertness, and mobility. Restoring a client to the ability to fulfill important roles can be done with the right attention to attitudes and strategies.

REFERENCES

Accurso, E. C., Norman, G. J., Crow, S. J., Rock, C. L., & Boutelle, K. N. (2014). The role of motivation in family-based guided self-help treatment for pediatric obesity. *Child Obes, 10*(5), 392–399. doi:10.1089/chi.2014.0023.

Ali, S. M., & Lindstrom, M. (2006). Socioeconomic, psychosocial, behavioural, and psychological determinants of BMI among young women: Differing patterns for underweight and overweight/obesity. *Eur J Public Health, 16*(3), 325–331. doi:10.1093/eurpub/cki187.

Allen, D. B., & Fost, N. (2012). Obesity and neglect: It's about the child. *J Pediatr, 160*(6), 898–899. doi:10.1016/j.jpeds.2012.02.035.

Altman, M., & Wilfley, D. E. (2015). Evidence update on the treatment of overweight and obesity in children and adolescents. *J Clin Child Adolesc Psychol, 44*(4), 521–537. doi:10.1080/15374416.2014.963854.

American Psychiatric Association. (2013). *The Diagnostic and Statistical Manual of Mental Disorders, Fifth Edition* (Vol. 5).

An, R. (2015). Educational disparity in obesity among U.S. adults, 1984–2013. *Ann Epidemiol, 25*(9), 637–642.e635. doi:10.1016/j.annepidem.2015.06.004.

Berge, J. M., Wall, M., Hsueh, T. F., Fulkerson, J. A., Larson, N., & Neumark-Sztainer, D. (2015). The protective role of family meals for youth obesity: 10-year longitudinal associations. *J Pediatr, 166*(2), 296–301. doi:10.1016/j.jpeds.2014.08.030.

Bonauto, D. K., Lu, D., & Fan, Z. J. (2014). Obesity prevalence by occupation in Washington State, Behavioral Risk Factor Surveillance System. *Prev Chronic Dis, 11*, 130219. doi:10.5888/pcd11.130219.

Boswell, R. G., & Kober, H. (2016). Food cue reactivity and craving predict eating and weight gain: A meta-analytic review. *Obes Rev, 17*(2), 159–177. doi:10.1111/obr.12354.

Bray, G. A., & Bellanger, T. (2006). Epidemiology, trends, and morbidities of obesity and the metabolic syndrome. *Endocrine, 29*(1), 109–117. doi:10.1385/ENDO:29:1:109.

Chen, A. Y., & Escarce, J. J. (2014). Family structure and childhood obesity: an analysis through 8th grade. *Matern Child Health J, 18*(7), 1772–1777. doi:10.1007/s10995-013-1422-7.

Cheng, J. K. (2012). Confronting the social determinants of health—Obesity, neglect, and inequity. *N Engl J Med, 367*(21), 1976–1977. doi:10.1056/NEJMp1209420.

Christensen, R., Kristensen, P. K., Bartels, E. M., Bliddal, H., & Astrup, A. (2007). Efficacy and safety of the weight-loss drug rimonabant: A meta-analysis of randomised trials. *Lancet, 370*(9600), 1706–1713. doi:10.1016/s0140-6736(07)61721-8.

Dhingra, A., Brennan, L., & Walkley, J. (2011). Predicting treatment initiation in a family-based adolescent overweight and obesity intervention. *Obesity (Silver Spring), 19*(6), 1307–1310. doi:10.1038/oby.2010.289.

Ells, L. J., Lang, R., Shield, J. P., Wilkinson, J. R., Lidstone, J. S., Coulton, S., & Summerbell, C. D. (2006). Obesity and disability—A short review. *Obes Rev, 7*(4), 341–345. doi:10.1111/j.1467-789X.2006.00233.x.

Feng, X., & Wilson, A. (2015). Getting bigger, quicker? Gendered socioeconomic trajectories in body mass index across the adult lifecourse: A longitudinal study of 21,403 Australians. *PLoS One, 10*(10), e0141499. doi:10.1371/journal.pone.0141499.

Fiese, B. H., Hammons, A., & Grigsby-Toussaint, D. (2012). Family mealtimes: A contextual approach to understanding childhood obesity. *Econ Hum Biol, 10*(4), 365–374. doi:10.1016/j.ehb.2012.04.004.

Food Addicts Anonymous. (2010). *Food Addicts Anonymous*. Port St. Lucie, FL: Food Addicts Anonymous, Inc.

Food Addicts in Recovery Anonymous. (2013). *Food Addicts in Recovery Anonymous*. Woburn, MA: Food Addicts in Recovery Anonymous.

Foster, G. D., Makris, A. P., & Bailer, B. A. (2005). Behavioral treatment of obesity. *Am J Clin Nutr, 82*(1 Suppl), 230s–235s.

Franken, I. H., Nijs, I. M., Toes, A., & van der Veen, F. M. (2016). Food addiction is associated with impaired performance monitoring. *Biol Psychol*. doi:10.1016/j.biopsycho.2016.07.005.

Garrahan, S. M., & Eichner, A. W. (2012). Tipping the scale: A place for childhood obesity in the evolving legal framework of child abuse and neglect. *Yale J Health Policy Law Ethics, 12*(2), 336–370.

Gerlach, Y., Williams, M. T., & Coates, A. M. (2013). Weighing up the evidence—A systematic review of measures used for the sensation of breathlessness in obesity. *Int J Obes (Lond), 37*(3), 341–349. doi:10.1038/ijo.2012.49.

Gonzalez-Casanova, I., Sarmiento, O. L., Pratt, M., Gazmararian, J. A., Martorell, R., Cunningham, S. A., & Stein, A. (2014). Individual, family, and community predictors of overweight and obesity among Colombian children and adolescents. *Prev Chronic Dis, 11*, E134. doi:10.5888/pcd11.140065.

Goodman, E., & Whitaker, R. C. (2002). A prospective study of the role of depression in the development and persistence of adolescent obesity. *Pediatrics, 110*(3), 497–504.

Gu, J. K., Charles, L. E., Bang, K. M., Ma, C. C., Andrew, M. E., Violanti, J. M., & Burchfiel, C. M. (2014). Prevalence of obesity by occupation among US workers: The National Health Interview Survey 2004–2011. *J Occup Environ Med, 56*(5), 516–528. doi:10.1097/jom.0000000000000133.

Guh, D. P., Zhang, W., Bansback, N., Amarsi, Z., Birmingham, C. L., & Anis, A. H. (2009). The incidence of co-morbidities related to obesity and overweight: A systematic review and meta-analysis. *BMC Public Health, 9*, 88. doi:10.1186/1471-2458-9-88.

Halliday, J. A., Palma, C. L., Mellor, D., Green, J., & Renzaho, A. M. (2014). The relationship between family functioning and child and adolescent overweight and obesity: A systematic review. *Int J Obes (Lond), 38*(4), 480–493. doi:10.1038/ijo.2013.213.

Hardy, J. L., Nelson, R. A., Thomason, M. E., Sternberg, D. A., Katovich, K., Farzin, F., & Scanlon, M. (2015). Enhancing cognitive abilities with comprehensive training: A large, online, randomized, active-controlled trial. *PLoS One, 10*(9), e0134467. doi:10.1371/journal.pone.0134467.

Harper, S., & Lynch, J. (2007). Trends in socioeconomic inequalities in adult health behaviors among U.S. states, 1990–2004. *Public Health Rep, 122*(2), 177–189.

Helton, J. J., & Liechty, J. M. (2014). Obesity prevalence among youth investigated for maltreatment in the United States. *Child Abuse Negl, 38*(4), 768–775. doi:10.1016/j.chiabu.2013.08.011.

Heo, M., Pietrobelli, A., Fontaine, K. R., Sirey, J. A., & Faith, M. S. (2006). Depressive mood and obesity in US adults: Comparison and moderation by sex, age, and race. *Int J Obes (Lond), 30*(3), 513–519. doi:10.1038/sj.ijo.0803122.

Heo, M., Pietrobelli, A., Wang, D., Heymsfield, S. B., & Faith, M. S. (2010). Obesity and functional impairment: Influence of comorbidity, joint pain, and mental health. *Obesity (Silver Spring), 18*(10), 2030–2038. doi:10.1038/oby.2009.400.

Igelstrom, H., Emtner, M., Lindberg, E., & Asenlof, P. (2013). Level of agreement between methods for measuring moderate to vigorous physical activity and sedentary time in people with obstructive sleep apnea and obesity. *Phys Ther, 93*(1), 50–59. doi:10.2522/ptj.20120123.

Jarosz, P. A., Davis, J. E., Yarandi, H. N., Farkas, R., Feingold, E., Shippings, S. H., . . . Williams, D. (2014). Obesity in urban women: Associations with sleep and sleepiness, fatigue and activity. *Womens Health Issues, 24*(4), e447–e454. doi:10.1016/j.whi.2014.04.005.

Johnson, R. J., Gold, M. S., Johnson, D. R., Ishimoto, T., Lanaspa, M. A., Zahniser, N. R., & Avena, N. M. (2011). Attention-deficit/hyperactivity disorder: Is it time to reappraise the role of sugar consumption? *Postgrad Med, 123*(5), 39–49. doi:10.3810/pgm.2011.09.2458.

Jones, B. L., & Fiese, B. H. (2014). Parent routines, child routines, and family demographics associated with obesity in parents and preschool-aged children. *Front Psychol, 5*, 374. doi:10.3389/fpsyg.2014.00374.

Kassel, J. D., Veilleux, J. C., Heinz, A., Braun, A. R., & Conrad, M. (2013). Emotions and addictive processes. In P. M. Miller (Ed.), *Principles of Addiction: Comprehensive Addictive Behaviors and Disorders* (Vol. 1), pp. 213–222. New York: Elsevier.

Kemps, E., Tiggemann, M., & Hollitt, S. (2014). Biased attentional processing of food cues and modification in obese individuals. *Health Psychol, 33*(11), 1391–1401. doi:10.1037/hea0000069.

Kestila, L., Rahkonen, O., Martelin, T., Lahti-Koski, M., & Koskinen, S. (2009). Do childhood social circumstances affect overweight and obesity in early adulthood? *Scand J Public Health, 37*(2), 206–219. doi:10.1177/1403494808100827.

Knutson, J. F., Taber, S. M., Murray, A. J., Valles, N. L., & Koeppl, G. (2010). The role of care neglect and supervisory neglect in childhood obesity in a disadvantaged sample. *J Pediatr Psychol, 35*(5), 523–532. doi:10.1093/jpepsy/jsp115.

Levin, B. E., Llabre, M. M., Dong, C., Elkind, M. S., Stern, Y., Rundek, T., . . . Wright, C. B. (2014). Modeling metabolic syndrome and its association with cognition: The northern Manhattan study. *J Int Neuropsychol Soc, 20*(10), 951–960. doi:10.1017/s1355617714000861.

Lioutas, E. D., & Tzimitra-Kalogianni, I. (2015). "I saw Santa drinking soda!" Advertising and children's food preferences. *Child Care Health Dev, 41*(3), 424–433. doi:10.1111/cch.12189.

Magnusson, K., Hagen, K. B., & Natvig, B. (2016). Individual and joint effects of risk factors for onset widespread pain and obesity—A population-based prospective cohort study. *Eur J Pain, 20*(7), 1102–1110. doi:10.1002/ejp.834.

Maloney, E. M., Boneva, R. S., Lin, J. M., & Reeves, W. C. (2010). Chronic fatigue syndrome is associated with metabolic syndrome: Results from a case-control study in Georgia. *Metabolism, 59*(9), 1351–1357. doi:10.1016/j.metabol.2009.12.019.

Matheson, B. E., Camacho, C., Peterson, C. B., Rhee, K. E., Rydell, S. A., Zucker, N. L., & Boutelle, K. N. (2015). The relationship between parent feeding styles and general parenting with loss of control eating in treatment-seeking overweight and obese children. *Int J Eat Disord, 48*(7), 1047–1055. doi:10.1002/eat.22440.

Meule, A., & Kubler, A. (2014). Double trouble. Trait food craving and impulsivity interactively predict food-cue affected behavioral inhibition. *Appetite, 79*, 174–182. doi:10.1016/j.appet.2014.04.014.

Mikolajczyk, R. T., & Richter, M. (2008). Associations of behavioural, psychosocial and socioeconomic factors with over- and underweight among German adolescents. *Int J Public Health, 53*(4), 214–220. doi:10.1007/s00038-008-7123-0.

Mogul, A., Irby, M. B., & Skelton, J. A. (2014). A systematic review of pediatric obesity and family communication through the lens of addiction literature. *Child Obes, 10*(3), 197–206. doi:10.1089/chi.2013.0157.

Molyneaux, E., Poston, L., Ashurst-Williams, S., & Howard, L. M. (2014). Obesity and mental disorders during pregnancy and postpartum: A systematic review and meta-analysis. *Obstet Gynecol, 123*(4), 857–867. doi:10.1097/aog.0000000000000170.

Nguyen, J. C., Killcross, A. S., & Jenkins, T. A. (2014). Obesity and cognitive decline: Role of inflammation and vascular changes. *Front Neurosci, 8*, 375. doi:10.3389/fnins.2014.00375.

Nijs, I. M., Muris, P., Euser, A. S., Franken, I. H.,. (2010). Differences in attention to food and food intake between overweight/obese and normal-weight females under conditions of hunger and satiety. *Appetite, 54*(2), 243–254. doi:10.1016/j.appet.2009.11.004.

Effect of hedonic tone on event-related potential measures of cognitive processing. doi:10.1016/j.psychres.2005.08.013.

Olvera, R. L., Williamson, D. E., Fisher-Hoch, S. P., Vatcheva, K. P., & McCormick, J. B. (2015). Depression, obesity, and metabolic syndrome: Prevalence and risks of comorbidity in a population-based representative sample of Mexican Americans. *J Clin Psychiatry, 76*(10), e1300–e1305. doi:10.4088/JCP.14m09118.

Pasco, J. A., Williams, L. J., Jacka, F. N., Brennan, S. L., & Berk, M. (2013). Obesity and the relationship with positive and negative affect. *Aust N Z J Psychiatry, 47*(5), 477–482. doi:10.1177/0004867413483371.

Pasold, T. L., McCracken, A., & Ward-Begnoche, W. L. (2014). Binge eating in obese adolescents: Emotional and behavioral characteristics and impact on health-related quality of life. *Clin Child Psychol Psychiatry, 19*(2), 299–312. doi:10.1177/1359104513488605.

Patel, V. C., Spaeth, A. M., & Basner, M. (2016). Relationships between time use and obesity in a representative sample of Americans. *Obesity (Silver Spring), 24*(10), 2164–2175. doi:10.1002/oby.21596.

Patterson, R. E., Frank, L. L., Kristal, A. R., & White, E. (2004). A comprehensive examination of health conditions associated with obesity in older adults. *Am J Prev Med, 27*(5), 385–390. doi:10.1016/j.amepre.2004.08.001.

Petrovich, G. D. (2013). Forebrain networks and the control of feeding by environmental learned cues. *Physiol Behav, 121*, 10–18. doi:10.1016/j.neulet.2006.11.019.

Powell, L. M., Wada, R., & Kumanyika, S. K. (2014). Racial/ethnic and income disparities in child and adolescent exposure to food and beverage television ads across the U.S. media markets. *Health Place, 29*, 124–131. doi:10.1016/j.healthplace.2014.06.006.

Raines, A. M., Boffa, J. W., Allan, N. P., Short, N. A., & Schmidt, N. B. (2015). Hoarding and eating pathology: The mediating role of emotion regulation. *Compr Psychiatry, 57*, 29–35. doi:10.1016/j.comppsych.2014.11.005.

Saltzman, J. A., Pineros-Leano, M., Liechty, J. M., Bost, K. K., Fiese, B. H., & Team, S. K. (2016). Eating, feeding, and feeling: Emotional responsiveness mediates longitudinal associations between maternal binge eating, feeding practices, and child weight. *Int J Behav Nutr Phys Act, 13*, 89. doi:10.1186/s12966-016-0415-5.

Schuchardt, K., Fischbach, A., Balke-Melcher, C., & Mahler, C. (2015). The comorbidity of learning difficulties and ADHD symptoms in primary-school-age children. *Z Kinder Jugendpsychiatr Psychother, 43*(3), 185–193. doi:10.1024/1422-4917/a000352.

Shin, S. H., & Miller, D. P. (2012). A longitudinal examination of childhood maltreatment and adolescent obesity: Results from the National Longitudinal Study of Adolescent Health (AddHealth) Study. *Child Abuse Negl, 36*(2), 84–94. doi:10.1016/j.chiabu.2011.08.007.

Shloim, N., Edelson, L. R., Martin, N., & Hetherington, M. M. (2015). Parenting styles, feeding styles, feeding practices, and weight status in 4–12 year-old children: A systematic review of the literature. *Front Psychol, 6*, 1849. doi:10.3389/fpsyg.2015.01849.

Sigman-Grant, M., Hayes, J., VanBrackle, A., & Fiese, B. (2015). Family resiliency: A neglected perspective in addressing obesity in young children. *Child Obes, 11*(6), 664–673. doi:10.1089/chi.2014.0107.

Skelton, J. A., Buehler, C., Irby, M. B., & Grzywacz, J. G. (2012). Where are family theories in family-based obesity treatment? Conceptualizing the study of families in pediatric weight management. *Int J Obes (Lond), 36*(7), 891–900. doi:10.1038/ijo.2012.56.

Stewart-Knox, B., Duffy, M. E., Bunting, B., Parr, H., Vas de Almeida, M. D., & Gibney, M. (2012). Associations between obesity (BMI and waist circumference) and socio-demographic factors, physical activity, dietary habits, life events, resilience, mood, perceived stress and hopelessness in healthy older Europeans. *BMC Public Health, 12*, 424. doi:10.1186/1471-2458-12-424.

Ventura, A. K., & Worobey, J. (2013). Early influences on the development of food preferences. *Curr Biol, 23*(9), R401–R408. doi:10.1016/j.cub.2013.02.037.

Vincent, H. K., Adams, M. C., Vincent, K. R., & Hurley, R. W. (2013). Musculoskeletal pain, fear avoidance behaviors, and functional decline in obesity: Potential interventions to manage pain and maintain function. *Reg Anesth Pain Med, 38*(6), 481–491. doi:10.1097/aap.0000000000000013.

Wang, S. S., Brownell, K. D., & Wadden, T. A. (2004). The influence of the stigma of obesity on overweight individuals. *Int J Obes Relat Metab Disord, 28*(10), 1333–1337. doi:10.1038/sj.ijo.0802730.

Werthmann, J., Jansen, A., & Roefs, A. (2014). Worry or craving? A selective review of evidence for food-related attention biases in obese individuals, eating-disorder patients, restrained eaters and healthy samples. *Proc Nutr Soc, 74*(2), 99–114. doi:10.1017/s0029665114001451.

Wilkie, R., Blagojevic-Bucknall, M., Jordan, K. P., & Pransky, G. (2013). Onset of work restriction in employed adults with lower limb joint pain: Individual factors and area-level socioeconomic conditions. *J Occup Rehabil, 23*(2), 180–188. doi:10.1007/s10926-013-9443-z.

Williams, L. K., Andrianopoulos, N., Cleland, V., Crawford, D., & Ball, K. (2013). Associations between education and personal income with body mass index among Australian women residing in disadvantaged neighborhoods. *Am J Health Promot, 28*(1), 59–65. doi:10.4278/ajhp.120316-QUAN-143.

Yau, Y. H., & Potenza, M. N. (2013). Stress and eating behaviors. *Minerva Endocrinol, 38*(3), 255–267.

Zamzow, J., Culnan, E., Spiers, M., Calkins, M., Satterthwaite, T., Ruparel, K., . . . Gur, R. (2014). B-37 the relationship between body mass index and executive function from late childhood through adolescence. *Arch Clin Neuropsychol, 29*(6), 550. doi:10.1093/arclin/acu038.125.

Zhu, N., Jacobs, D. R., Meyer, K. A., He, K., Launer, L., Reis, J. P., . . . Steffen, L. M. (2015). Cognitive function in a middle aged cohort is related to higher quality dietary pattern 5 and 25 years earlier: The CARDIA study. *J Nutr Health Aging, 19*(1), 33–38. doi:10.1007/s12603-014-0491-7.

16 DSM 5 SUD Criterion 6 *Interpersonal Problems*

Joan Ifland
Food Addiction Training, LLC
Cincinnati, OH

Robin Piper
Turning Point of Tampa
Tampa, FL

CONTENTS

> Continued processed food use despite having persistent or recurrent social or interpersonal problems caused by or exacerbated by the effects of addictive foods. (American Psychiatric Association, 2013, p. 491)

16.1 INTRODUCTION

Like all addicts, processed food addiction (PFA) clients may use addictive substances in spite of social and interpersonal problems. However, due to the factor of weight gain in PFA, food-addicted clients may have more serious barriers to healthy interpersonal relationships than other drug addicts. A synergism can develop where eating, weight gain, neuroimpairment, and relationships reinforce one another negatively. Problems in interpersonal relationships can occur early in the development of drug addictions. "The morbidity moves from the intrapersonal sense of self (self-image, self-respect, self-concept, sense of self-efficacy, and even psychiatric symptomatology are often the earliest evidence of disease) to interpersonal relationships (family and close friends and then social relationships suffer)" (Parran, McCormick, & Delos Reyes, 2014, p. 342). Neurological impairments, childhood trauma, and weight-based stigmatization from the culture work together to create significant barriers within the food addict to engaging in healthy relationships.

16.1.1 Importance

In addition to probing for information for a diagnosis, information gathered under Criterion 6 can be used in treatment to reduce risk of relapse and to improve quality of life. Drug addicts with high trait rejection sensitivity and a critical interpersonal environment are vulnerable to relapse (Leach & Kranzler, 2013). It appears that the same is true for PFA clients (Carr, Friedman, & Jaffe, 2007). A Swedish study found that 26% of non–eating-disordered women experienced dysfunctional relationships while 55% of eating-disordered women did so (Broberg, Hjalmers, & Nevonen, 2001). Higher levels of interpersonal support were significantly associated with higher levels of health-promoting behaviors in a population of women with abdominal obesity (Cho, Jae, Choo, & Choo, 2014). Assessing the state of interpersonal relationships can inform the treatment plan in crucial areas and reduce risk of relapse.

For the food addict, social and interpersonal problems can emanate from dysfunctional emotions and behaviors. Developing a profile of active relationships could yield valuable insights into the client's distress. Long-term loneliness may be uncovered. The loneliness could be imbedded in isolation, but it could also be present in spite of active personal relationships. Addicts may be distancing themselves from friends and family because of shame and the distractions of disordered eating. Violence in relationships may be present as is the case in other addictions (Midei & Matthews, 2011; Parran et al., 2014). In a population of extremely obese people seeking bariatric surgery, the reported rate of interpersonal abuse was 30.5% (Salwen, Hymowitz, Vivian, & O'Leary, 2014). There are a myriad of reasons that the food addict could be experiencing dysfunctional relationships.

Assessing for relationship stress will provide items for the list of options to begin recovery and may be a major factor in a recovery treatment plan. Relationships may heal in the later stages of recovery, after stable emotions and thought patterns are established. However, relationship management skills could also be essential to early stage tasks such as reducing criticism and teasing at home, social events, and the workplace. Stress has been shown to lead to overeating and, in a feedback loop, the chronic overeating can lead to anomalies in the brain that are experienced as stress (Cottone et al., 2009; Gibson, 2006; Sinha, 2007). A significant body of research has demonstrated that interpersonal problems moderate the relationship between negative affect and binge eating (Ambwani, Roche, Minnick, & Pincus, 2015; Ansell, Grilo, & White, 2012; Ivanova et al., 2015). The ability to be in healthy relationships and reduce stress could be a crucial factor in reducing the risk of relapse.

Assessing for relationship status will also help the practitioner determine how to proceed with a crucial issue, i.e., will the client be able to reduce food cues in the home? Cuing and interpersonal stress are two leading causes of relapse (Grilo, Shiffman, & Wing, 1989). If relationships with household members are chaotic and the client is suffering from low self-esteem, achieving protection from processed food cues could be difficult. Household members may be vehemently attached to keeping cuing foods in the house. They may insist on eating processed foods in front of the food addict and on keeping processed foods out in sight in the kitchen. In this situation, early stage support for educating household members could be useful. Education could cover addictive foods, diseases associated with processed foods, the impact on cravings of availability of addictive foods, cost–benefit for each household member, etc. Handouts on these topics are available at www.foodaddictionresources.com.

The "Application" section of this chapter delves into the role of relationship problems in recovery from PFA. It reviews evidence suggesting how to manage relationship problems to improve outcomes in recovery. Assessing clients for the status of their social and interpersonal relationships will be fruitful in the effort to stabilize clients, develop a treatment plan, and work with clients to develop a sense of well-being.

16.1.2 Evidence for the Syndrome

As discussed in the introduction to assessment, PFA is a comprehensive disease. It can interfere with social and interpersonal relationships in a number of different ways. For the purposes of organizing this extensive syndrome, this section covers evidence for the character of relationship problems in the obese, then looks at the mechanisms of interpersonal problems including depression, anger, shame, self-hate, and family systems. Factors that are particular to PFA such as hiding and physical limitations are also described.

16.2 MANIFESTATIONS

Obese people exhibit a range of personalities and interpersonal relationships. Not all obese people are experiencing relationship problems. Obese people can be characterized as friendly and outgoing (Lo Coco, Gullo, Scrima, & Bruno, 2012). Lo Coco et al. used the Inventory of Interpersonal Problems to categorize the obese into four clusters of personality types that could have an impact on the nature of their interpersonal relationships. One cluster exhibited dominant characteristics, a second was less dominant but also more needy. A third cluster did not exhibit interpersonal problems, and the fourth showed a need to please other people (Lo Coco et al., 2012). None of the personality clusters were found in the cold or distant quadrants. This was an Italian population, which seems to be less stressed by obesity than US populations (Luppino et al., 2010). Each of these types suggests a different route to recovery. The dominant personalities may need to let go of controlling others, while the needy personality may need to work on self-sufficiency, and the approval-seeking obese person may need help with boundary setting. The Inventory of Interpersonal Problems can be used to surface and catalog the addict's situation.

The research suggests a prominent role for interpersonal relationships in the development of obesity. A review article found that difficulties in childhood interpersonal relationships, such as caregiver physical and sexual abuse and peer bullying, were associated with adult obesity (Midei & Matthews, 2011). Adverse childhood experiences are associated with obesity in adulthood (Van Niel, Pachter, Wade, Felitti, & Stein, 2014). In a prospective 9-year study, men's obesity was found to be influenced by a lack of emotional support while women's weight was reduced by becoming single after being married (Oliveira, Rostila, de Leon, & Lopes, 2013). Dysfunctions in adult relationships found in traumatized children include "expectancy of betrayal; expectancy of victimization; physical boundary diffusion; emotional boundary diffusion; expectancy of irresolvable attachment loss" (Courtois & Ford, 2013).

A review article found that social networks have an impact on obesity through social contagion, social capital (sense of belonging), and social selection where people join networks based on weight (Oliveira et al., 2013). People who were obese in childhood were more sensitive to interpersonal relationships and had more psychotic symptoms (Mills, 1995). Petroni et al. found that weight cycling and physical comorbidities influenced psychological health in a population of treatment-seeking, morbidly obese people (Petroni et al., 2007). Having more casual friends who were overweight at baseline and being part of a social network with stronger social norms for unhealthy eating predicted poorer weight loss (Leahey, Doyle, Xu, Bihuniak, & Wing, 2015). The research supports listening for childhood problems of obesity, abuse, and bullying to provide a basis for understanding adult problems of weight cycling, physical comorbidities, and social networks.

16.2.1 Mechanisms of Relationship Problems in Chronic Food Abusers

Research shows that neuroanomalies may explain the behavioral problems that characterize interpersonal problems in PFA clients. The mechanisms of relationship problems have been demonstrated in the brain. Impairments in control and emotion pathways can be conceptualized as manifesting as depression, anger, shame, and self-hate. These negative affects can form barriers to healthy relationships. Family systems then can be seen to foster PFA through the absence of healthy, warm relationships. There is a logical pattern of neuroimpairment leading to unhealthy behavior and dysfunctional relationships.

16.2.1.1 Neuroanomalies

Two paths of disordered behavior have been described in the brain. The first is loss of emotional control in the frontal lobe. The second is loss of functionality in the reward pathways, particularly serotonin and dopamine. A possible framework for understanding the link between processed foods and use in spite of interpersonal problems is that depression, anger, and shame originating in downregulated serotonin and dopamine pathways propel unhealthy relationship behaviors, and the control mechanisms that would otherwise mitigate negative behaviors, are not functioning.

> Alcohol, sedatives, and opioids reduce the contributions of the frontal lobes that facilitate recall, executive decision-making, interpersonal sensitivity, judgment, and morality. … Damage of particular areas of the brain can aid clinicians in recognizing certain stereotypic conditions associated with addiction. For example … damage to the frontal lobes can foster disinhibited, intrusive speech and behavior. (Westermeyer, 2013, p. 8)

A compromised frontal lobe has also been seen in fMRI research in the obese (Burger & Stice, 2014). The lack of behavioral control in the frontal lobes is a possible neurological underpinning of inability to control behaviors in relationships.

Serotonin has been shown to be an important factor in neuroanomalies found in addictions. Obesity and depression share pathological pathways such as hyperactivity of the hypothalamic–pituitary–adrenal axis, dysregulation of oxidant/antioxidant system balance, higher levels of inflammatory cytokines, leptin resistance, alternated plasma glucose, insulin resistance, reduced neuronal brain-derived neurotrophic factor (BDNF), and decreased serotonergic neurotransmission in various regions of the brain. Serotonin regulates diet intake, leptin, corticosterone, inflammatory mechanism, altered plasma glucose, insulin resistance, and BDNF concentration in the brain (Kurhe & Mahesh, 2015). Carbohydrates have been shown to stimulate serotonin production, which may be the beginning of the process of downregulation (Wurtman & Wurtman, 1986). Genetic polymorphisms in the serotonin systems have been correlated with obesity (Carr et al., 2013), as well as emotionality and risk for affective disorders (Firk, Siep, & Markus, 2013). In a rat study, it was shown that 16 weeks of a high-fat diet abolished the effect of serotonin on mood regulation. Replacing the high-fat diet with regular chow reestablished the functionality of serotonin in 6 weeks (Papazoglou, Jean, Gertler, Taouis, & Vacher, 2015). The impact of serotonin irregularities may explain depression in chronic processed food abusers.

Other mood-regulating pathways, including dopamine, opiate, and endocannabinoid, have been shown to be downregulated in obese people (Wang et al., 2014) and rats (Alsio et al., 2010). Opiate and dopamine systems share regulation of pleasure, but the interaction of opiate pathways with dopamine pathways has been shown to be abolished in the obese (Tuominen et al., 2015). There is also evidence for downregulation in endocannabinoid pathways in the brains of rats (Harrold, Elliott, King, Widdowson, & Williams, 2002) and downregulation of an endocannabinoid precursor in the guts of rats fed a high-fat diet (Diep et al., 2011). Significant dysregulation of mood-regulating pathways in chronic food abusers points to mood disorders as a compounding factor in relationship problems.

Quotes from the food addiction 12-step manuals illustrate the pathology.

> I had no friends. I began to wonder, "Who would know if anything happened to me?" Eating impaired my thinking. I had no access to good judgment about people. When I wanted something, I was determined to get it, come hell or high water. I didn't care who I hurt or how I affected others. I wanted what I wanted, and I steamrolled over anything necessary to get it. (Food Addicts in Recovery Anonymous, 2013, p. 140)
>
> I stole money from my dad's change drawer to buy sweets. I got in big trouble with a boy from my class when I was eight or nine. He suggested I steal a bottle of soft drink from the school canteen so we could drink it on the way home. I took one, and when we didn't have a bottle opener, we were so determined to have some that we smashed the top and tried to drink through the jagged glass. I felt a profound shame when we were caught. You might think that would have been enough for me, but I kept stealing—more from the canteen, sweets from the school staff room, and food and alcohol from stores. The consequences of my actions never deterred me. (Food Addicts in Recovery Anonymous, 2013, p. 211)

> Food affected my personality, as any drug does. (Food Addicts in Recovery Anonymous, 2013, p. 21)
>
> I was haunted by fears and was afraid to leave my house. I never answered the door or the phone. I thought if I left my home, someone would try to steal my children. If I drove, a car accident might kill them. I might run into someone and she would see that my clothes didn't fit me anymore. She'd notice that my hair was thin. So I stayed behind my door and watched everything that I ate. (Food Addicts in Recovery Anonymous, 2013, p. 90)
>
> I didn't recognize myself. I lost a lot of my ability to function. I'd always been a very high-functioning addict, but I almost got fired from my job. I had to quit before they let me go. (Food Addicts in Recovery Anonymous, 2013, p. 289)
>
> As my food addiction progressed, I didn't recognize myself. I didn't know that I was enough—that my own skills and assets were fine. I felt like I was breaking. (Food Addicts in Recovery Anonymous, 2013, p. 339)
>
> I'd lost a lot of my ability to function professionally by the time I reached the program. I'd been working as an operating room nurse and had helped prepare women for childbirth, but I was at the point where I could only handle one patient. (Food Addicts in Recovery Anonymous, 2013, pp. 103–104)
>
> Every experience I had in college was colored by my bingeing and purging. (Food Addicts in Recovery Anonymous, 2013, p. 279)
>
> I ate if I was lonely, if I was happy, if I was sad, and if I had a minute to spare. I ate especially when I didn't know where to turn or when I had the uncomfortable feeling of not knowing who I was. I had wonderful friends, and yet I couldn't talk with them as I needed to. I don't think I could have even identified what I wanted to say. (Food Addicts in Recovery Anonymous, 2013, p. 269)

As can be seen from the research and from the quotes, neuroimpairment in chronic food abusers is extensive and manifests in a variety of dysfunctional behaviors. It is to be expected that practitioners will find conformance to DSM 5 SUD Criterion 6 as they assess clients presenting for assessment for PFA.

16.2.1.2 Depression

Depression can be a significant barrier to healthy relationships. Depression is a well-established characteristic of obesity (Abou Abbas, Salameh, Nasser, Nasser, & Godin, 2015). Pratt and Brody found a higher rate of obesity in people with moderate to severe depressive symptoms whether or not they were taking an antidepressant (Pratt & Brody, 2014). Mediating factors between obesity and depression were found to be educational attainment, body image, binge eating, physical health, psychological characteristics, and interpersonal effectiveness (Preiss, Brennan, & Clarke, 2013).

The mechanisms of depression may be reinforced by stigma as well as feeling judged, social network changes, psychosocial stress, and the structural effects of discrimination, such as poor neighborhoods and low-paying jobs (Brewis, 2014). Combined obesity/depression in children can be affected by the role of the family, school, health care practitioners, and access to health care (Mihalopoulos & Spigarelli, 2015). Olvera et al. found that female gender, low education, and obesity were associated with depression and that severe obesity was associated with severe depression (Olvera, Williamson, Fisher-Hoch, Vatcheva, & McCormick, 2015). Roberts and Duong found a role for body image in the association of obesity with depression (Roberts & Duong, 2015). Even in a population of nondepressed obese women, Geil et al. found that they had reduced emotional intensity scores compared to lean participants in response to emotional stimuli (Giel et al., 2016). Arthritis, depression, and obesity are related to fatigue, which can also hamper interpersonal relationships (Giel et al., 2016). A review article found that obesity at baseline increased the odds of developing depression at follow-up, and the association was greater in Americans than Europeans and more so in people aged over 20 years (Luppino et al., 2010). Obesity can precede depression and vice versa (Marmorstein, Iacono, & Legrand, 2014). There is extensive evidence for the association of depression with chronic abuse of processed foods. This is consistent with the research showing impairment in pathways regulating emotions.

These quotes from the food addiction 12-step manuals illustrate depression in PFA clients.

> Life got more difficult as I continued high school. I was obsessed with food and was competing at high levels in academics, dance, and track. To get relief from the constant pressure and stress, I sometimes cried for hours, lying in bed by myself at night. (Food Addicts in Recovery Anonymous, 2013, p. 279)
>
> When I ate, I felt better. This caused a bad cycle. My feelings of inadequacy made me eat, but the eating made me fat. Fatness made me feel more inadequate, which increased my drive to eat. (Food Addicts in Recovery Anonymous, 2013, pp. 20–21)
>
> By the time I was forty, as I said, I no longer wanted to live. I had no hope. (Food Addicts in Recovery Anonymous, 2013, p. 54)

16.2.1.3 Anger

Anger has been shown to attenuate the relationship between childhood abuse and weight in a population of women in midlife (Midei, Matthews, & Bromberger, 2010). Pasco et al. found that, in general, women's BMI correlated with negative affect, including distress, anger, disgust, fear, and shame. Positive affect did not correlate with BMI (Pasco, Williams, Jacka, Brennan, & Berk, 2013). Applehans et al. found that distraction could reduce food intake in response to anger in an obese population (Appelhans, Whited, Schneider, Oleski, & Pagoto, 2011). In a study comparing dysfunction in obese men versus obese women, Iliceto et al. found that both men and women turn anger in toward themselves. Women had lower scores on self-empathy. Both men and women had lower scores on empathy for others (Iliceto et al., 2012). Surprisingly, anger does not seem to be as important an issue as depression and shame. Schneider at al. found that anxiety prompted more overeating than anger in an obese populations as compared to a lean population (Schneider, Appelhans, Whited, Oleski, & Pagoto, 2010).

Examples from the food addiction 12-step manuals illustrate how anger creates distress in interpersonal relationships.

> I was a big kid, so other kids made fun of me. I hated it and tried to be nice, tried to make friends with everyone, but at home I teased my sister and made my parents' lives difficult. (Food Addicts in Recovery Anonymous, 2013, p. 256)
>
> My fury came from nowhere. I never thought that I would be capable of abusing one of my children, but whatever made child abusers harm their children lived in me. (Food Addicts in Recovery Anonymous, 2013, p. 94)
>
> My addiction progressed to an even more deadly level, and I gained 40 pounds in three months. I had the personality to match. At 220 pounds, I was with my father in the hospital one day when I got frustrated. I was screaming like a maniac when the security officers came. (Food Addicts in Recovery Anonymous, 2013, p. 151)
>
> I was afraid to leave the house and used to have to call my mother to talk about my anxiety before I'd have the strength to walk out my front door. When my husband later decided to go to the United States, I didn't want to leave, and I made it as hard on him as I could. I spent lots of money to punish him. (Food Addicts in Recovery Anonymous, 2013, p. 297)

16.2.1.4 Shame

Shame has been shown to have a profound effect on self-esteem in chronic food abusers. Because PFA, unlike other drug addictions, often results in significant weight gain, shame is a pronounced issue in PFA. Inappropriate weight-loss regimens that result in repeat failure are also a source of shame that manifests in PFA. One study showed that when excluded from social situations, the obese experience more shame than normally weighted people (Westermann, Rief, Euteneuer, & Kohlmann, 2015). Another study found that shame, parental employment, and parental separation explained the relationship between depression and obesity (Sjoberg, Nilsson, & Leppert, 2005). Several studies showed that shame explained the relationship between obesity and low self-esteem (Albohn-Kuhne & Rief, 2011; Pila, Sabiston, Brunet, Castonguay, & O'Loughlin, 2015). Shame was also found to mediate the relationships between low self-esteem and risk of eating disorders

(Iannaccone, D'Olimpio, Cella, & Cotrufo, 2016). A long record of failed weight-loss attempts exacerbates shame in the obese (Kirk et al., 2014). High expectations for success from bariatric surgery were associated with shame (Homer, Tod, Thompson, Allmark, & Goyder, 2016). Shame, social anxiety, and depression (but not guilt) have been shown to be highly related to feeling inferior and to submissive behavior, which could inhibit the PFA client's ability to flourish in relationships (Gilbert, 2000). Shame has been shown to be a driver of how chronic food abusers view relationships.

These quotes illustrate how profoundly shame can interfere with interpersonal relationships.

> I withdrew because of my weight, too ashamed to let people see how I looked. We received a wedding invitation from my husband's cousin, and I never even sent a reply. Years later they spoke of how we'd missed their wedding. I missed my husband's grandfather's funeral for the same reason. (Food Addicts in Recovery Anonymous, 2013, pp. 295–296)
>
> By the time I entered first grade, I was self-conscious about my attachment to food and ashamed of my weight. (Food Addicts in Recovery Anonymous, 2013, p. 338; Kindle Locations 3778–3779).

16.2.1.5 Self-Hatred

Although not well covered in the literature (Weiss, 2004), self-loathing can contribute to depression, anger, and shame, which can then become barriers to healthy participation in interpersonal relationships. Internalized stigmatization is described in the research (Palmeira, Pinto-Gouveia, Cunha, & Carvalho, 2017). Self-hatred was found in eating-disordered female athletes when they broke an eating rule (Beals & Manore, 2000). These quotes illustrate the anguish of self-hatred.

> My illness got worse. I ate larger and larger quantities of baked goods and candies, but they no longer blunted my terrible feelings. Sometimes I bit and scratched myself because I couldn't stand the pressure of my self-hate. (Food Addicts in Recovery Anonymous, 2013, p. 77)
>
> I began to believe that I was a bad person. I'd begun babysitting, and I took food from people's cabinets and denied it later. I couldn't understand myself. My mother impressed upon me that I was a liar and a sneak. Obviously, my behavior was affecting my family, but I didn't know how to stop. (Food Addicts in Recovery Anonymous, 2013, p. 179)

16.2.1.6 Family Systems

There is a significant body of evidence showing that the nature of relationships within families can have an impact on the development of obesity. Assessing for problems in relationships within family systems is productive in this respect. The research demonstrates that households with warm, positive parenting styles are less likely to have obese children (Berge et al., 2014; Rhee et al., 2015). Households were more likely to have obese children if they exhibited poor family functioning including poor communication, poor behavior control, high levels of family conflict, and low family hierarchy values (Halliday, Palma, Mellor, Green, & Renzaho, 2014). Households where weight-teasing is taking place and parents are not attentive to children's negative affect are more likely to have obese children. Teasing and inattention were more influential in the development of obesity than the parents' weight status, race/ethnicity, or socioeconomic status (Saltzman & Liechty, 2016). Lack of response to negative emotions in the children as well as nonresponsive feeding patterns also predicted obesity in children (Saltzman et al., 2016). In a study of 24 countries, Al Sabbah et al. found that girls with body weight dissatisfaction had difficulties in talking to their mothers (Al Sabbah et al., 2009). This research is consistent with the findings of impaired emotional neuropathways and negative affect.

The inability to function in families is shown in these quotes.

> My sponsor was in intensive care for a month, in danger of dying. She lived five minutes away from me, and when she got home from the hospital, she needed my help, but I was so deep into eating, I couldn't reach out. I couldn't show up when she needed me most. (Food Addicts in Recovery Anonymous, 2013, p. 228)

> Looking back, I see no difference between myself and an alcoholic. I remember sitting on a park bench, cradling a brown bag of food at 2:00 in the morning when my wife was home struggling alone with a colicky baby. (Food Addicts in Recovery Anonymous, 2013, p. 235)
>
> By age sixteen, I was a full-blown food addict. I had no sense of my irresponsibility and immaturity, no awareness of the burdens I placed on my parents because of my eating. (Food Addicts in Recovery Anonymous, 2013, p. 356)

16.2.1.7 Unattractive Behaviors

There is no readily discernible research on the topic of behaviors in PFA that could be stressors in relationships. However, the food addiction 12-step manuals offer a number of examples that illustrate some of the behavioral difficulties a food addict might have in maintaining interpersonal relationships.

> I remember standing among the trees eating pies with my hands before I went home to throw up. I started running and taking laxatives again, which caused me to lose control of my bowels. (Food Addicts in Recovery Anonymous, 2013, p. 138)
>
> I was dating a man I'd met who was six years older than I. He came to my apartment one day when I had just finished eating a dozen doughnuts. I had flour all over my face and was sitting on the kitchen floor, curled up in a ball. I loved this man, but I wanted him to go away. He was banging on the door and looking in the window, thinking I was cheating on him, so I finally had to let him in. I was a mess, but I said, "I'll be with you in just a minute." I went into the bathroom, threw up, and took a shower. When I came out, I had my makeup all done, and I was dressed up—the girl he knew. "Okay," I said, "I'm ready." He was horrified, but we never spoke of it. (Food Addicts in Recovery Anonymous, 2013, p. 138)
>
> I was stealing desserts from the bags of food my agency bought for clients and purging as many as twenty-five times a day. (Food Addicts in Recovery Anonymous, 2013, p. 248)
>
> I couldn't brush my teeth or comb my hair. I wore dirty clothes and slept in dirty sheets. I disdained makeup and never learned how to buy nice shoes or match a skirt to a blouse. I felt unable to talk with my classmates and teachers, so I stayed silent most of the time. Worst of all, I began hearing a voice in my head that repeated over and over, "I hate myself. I wish I were dead." (Food Addicts in Recovery Anonymous, 2013, p. 76)

To summarize the evidence, chronic food-abusers have been shown to suffer from impairments in the neuropathways that regulate emotions and behaviors. These dopamine, opiate, serotonin, and endocannabinoid pathways have been shown to be downregulated and noncommunicative. This appears to contribute to emotional dysfunction, which in turn negatively affects interpersonal relationships. The situation is exacerbated by histories of failed weight loss and harsh judgment from the culture. Depression, anger, and shame are found in eating disorder research. The evidence is consistent and logical in creating a picture of personal misery and limitations that manifest in distressed relationships.

16.3 APPLICATION

The review of the evidence reveals extensive suffering and risk of relapse by PFA clients from their interpersonal relationships. To repeat the quote from the first paragraph of this chapter, "Drug addicts with high trait rejection sensitivity and a critical interpersonal environment are vulnerable to relapse" (Leach & Kranzler, 2013). PFA clients suffer from relationship sensitivity to a significant degree (Carr et al., 2007). And they are subject to high levels of criticism inside and outside the home (Seacat, Dougal, & Roy, 2016). Negative affect from interpersonal relationships is a core risk for relapse in PFA clients. Probing for severity of relationship problems is a key element of assessing PFA clients for conformance to Criterion 6, continued use despite having persistent or recurrent social or interpersonal problems caused by or exacerbated by the effects of processed foods (page 491; American Psychiatric Association, 2013).

The evidence suggests the value of developing a comprehensive picture of the client's relationship status. Reviewing relationships will show the practitioner how much the client is suffering from depression, fear, anger, and shame about relationships in general. The evaluation will also surface whether people in the client's life are triggering negative emotions. Both internally and externally derived relationship stressors are candidates for inclusion in the treatment plan. And setting boundaries on abusive behavior in current relationships could be an early item on the list of options for starting recovery. Improvements in self-esteem may need to precede the ability to set boundaries with family, colleagues, and friends on issues such as comments about food, weight, appearance, etc. Boundaries around being offered processed foods also may follow improvements in self-perception. Comprehensive probing will reveal both internal and external relationship stressors.

Practitioners can mine a rich vein of recovery by methodically reviewing the sources of distress about relationships and the etiology of negative affect associated with relationships. Fears and shame can originate in very young childhood as parents criticize children for weight issues (Kakinami, Barnett, Seguin, & Paradis, 2015). The client's parents are likely to have eaten processed foods, which could have diminished their ability to feel good about themselves and express positive thoughts to their family members. Education about these factors can bring relief to the client. Relief can translate into less self-blame and shame, which can in turn reduce stress and reduce risk of relapse.

Mending current relationships is a stepwise process. People in the client's life have likely witnessed a long series of failed attempts to control eating and weight. Collateral people could be derisive and critical of the client's "latest diet." People around the addict can be modeling a range of triggering behaviors from food abuse to jumping on the latest fad diet. Education and patience are the keys here. If collateral people are abusing processed foods, lessons about detaching may be borrowed from Al-Anon. Codependency training will also be useful here. As the clients becomes more stable emotionally, relationships may become less chaotic. These topics are covered more extensively in Part III of this textbook, "Treatment."

It is possible that clients may withhold information about relationship problems until they have established a relationship of trust with the practitioner. Clients may not be willing to admit the extent of problems. They may have been denying to themselves that problems exist, possibly because they feel helpless to do anything about dysfunctional interpersonal relationships. The practitioner can continue to monitor for new information about relationships even after the formal assessment has been developed.

The parent–child relationship is a special category. Recommendations for parents include (1) role modeling healthful behaviors, (2) providing an environment that makes it easy for their children to make healthful choices, (3) focusing less on weight and more on behaviors and overall health, and (4) providing a supportive environment for their children to enhance communication. The culture works against the development of a healthy weight and a positive body image in children and adolescents. Families may need support outside the home (Neumark-Sztainer, 2005).

As described in Part III, "Treatment," practitioners can take relationships' sensitivity into consideration in group functions by limiting criticism and replacing it with consistent positive feedback. Reworking negativity into optimism is a rewarding activity in recovery from PFA.

16.4 CONCLUSION

Assessing for relationship problems may take the practitioner and the client into painful aspects of the client's current and past situations. However, it is rewarding in terms of easing stressors that have been shown to lead to relapse. Practitioners can bring relief and hope to clients by reviewing the reasons that relationships may have failed or have been dysfunctional. Practitioners can assure clients that they did not cause the abuse, attract dysfunction, or fail to deserve healthy relationships. Healing current and past relationships can be a joyful aspect of recovery from processed foods.

REFERENCES

Abou Abbas, L., Salameh, P., Nasser, W., Nasser, Z., & Godin, I. (2015). Obesity and symptoms of depression among adults in selected countries of the Middle East: A systematic review and meta-analysis. *Clin Obes, 5*(1), 2–11. doi:10.1111/cob.12082.

Al Sabbah, H., Vereecken, C. A., Elgar, F. J., Nansel, T., Aasvee, K., Abdeen, Z., … Maes, L. (2009). Body weight dissatisfaction and communication with parents among adolescents in 24 countries: International cross-sectional survey. *BMC Public Health, 9*, 52. doi:10.1186/1471-2458-9-52.

Albohn-Kuhne, C., & Rief, W. (2011). Shame, guilt and social anxiety in obesity with binge-eating disorder. *Psychother Psychosom Med Psychol, 61*(9–10), 412–417. doi:10.1055/s-0031-1284334.

Alsio, J., Olszewski, P. K., Norback, A. H., Gunnarsson, Z. E., Levine, A. S., Pickering, C., & Schioth, H. B. (2010). Dopamine D1 receptor gene expression decreases in the nucleus accumbens upon long-term exposure to palatable food and differs depending on diet-induced obesity phenotype in rats. *Neuroscience, 171*(3), 779–787. doi:10.1016/j.neuroscience.2010.09.046.

Ambwani, S., Roche, M. J., Minnick, A. M., & Pincus, A. L. (2015). Negative affect, interpersonal perception, and binge eating behavior: An experience sampling study. *Int J Eat Disord, 48*(6), 715–726. doi:10.1002/eat.22410.

American Psychiatric Association. (2013). *The Diagnostic and Statistical Manual of Mental Disorders, Fifth Edition* (Vol. 5).

Ansell, E. B., Grilo, C. M., & White, M. A. (2012). Examining the interpersonal model of binge eating and loss of control over eating in women. *Int J Eat Disord, 45*(1), 43–50. doi:10.1002/eat.20897.

Appelhans, B. M., Whited, M. C., Schneider, K. L., Oleski, J., & Pagoto, S. L. (2011). Response style and vulnerability to anger-induced eating in obese adults. *Eat Behav, 12*(1), 9–14. doi:10.1016/j.eatbeh.2010.08.009

Beals, K. A., & Manore, M. M. (2000). Behavioral, psychological, and physical characteristics of female athletes with subclinical eating disorders. *Int J Sport Nutr Exerc Metab, 10*(2), 128–143.

Berge, J. M., Rowley, S., Trofholz, A., Hanson, C., Rueter, M., MacLehose, R. F., & Neumark-Sztainer, D. (2014). Childhood obesity and interpersonal dynamics during family meals. *Pediatrics, 134*(5), 923–932. doi:10.1542/peds.2014-1936.

Brewis, A. A. (2014). Stigma and the perpetuation of obesity. *Soc Sci Med, 118*, 152–158. doi:10.1016/j.socscimed.2014.08.003.

Broberg, A. G., Hjalmers, I., & Nevonen, L. (2001). Eating disorders, attachment and interpersonal difficulties: A comparison between 18- to 24-year-old patients and normal controls. *Eur Eat Disord Rev, 9*(6), 381–396. doi:10.1002/ERV.421.

Burger, K. S., & Stice, E. (2014). Greater striatopallidal adaptive coding during cue-reward learning and food reward habituation predict future weight gain. *NeuroImage, 99*, 122–128. doi:10.1016/j.neuroimage.2014.05.066.

Carr, D., Friedman, M. A., & Jaffe, K. (2007). Understanding the relationship between obesity and positive and negative affect: The role of psychosocial mechanisms. *Body Image, 4*(2), 165–177. doi:10.1016/j.bodyim.2007.02.004.

Carr, K. A., Lin, H., Fletcher, K. D., Sucheston, L., Singh, P. K., Salis, R. J., … Epstein, L. H. (2013). Two functional serotonin polymorphisms moderate the effect of food reinforcement on BMI. *Behav Neurosci, 127*(3), 387–399. doi:10.1037/a0032026.

Cho, J. H., Jae, S. Y., Choo, I. L., & Choo, J. (2014). Health-promoting behaviour among women with abdominal obesity: A conceptual link to social support and perceived stress. *J Adv Nurs, 70*(6), 1381–1390. doi:10.1111/jan.12300.

Cottone, P., Sabino, V., Roberto, M., Bajo, M., Pockros, L., Frihauf, J. B., … Zorrilla, E. P. (2009). CRF system recruitment mediates dark side of compulsive eating. *Proc Natl Acad Sci U S A, 106*(47), 20016–20020. doi:10.1073/pnas.0908789106.

Courtois, C. A., & Ford, A. D. (2013). *Treatment of complex trauma: A sequenced, relationship-based approach*, p. 49, New York: The Guilford Press.

Diep, T. A., Madsen, A. N., Holst, B., Kristiansen, M. M., Wellner, N., Hansen, S. H., & Hansen, H. S. (2011). Dietary fat decreases intestinal levels of the anorectic lipids through a fat sensor. *Faseb J, 25*(2), 765–774. doi:10.1096/fj.10-166595.

Firk, C., Siep, N., & Markus, C. R. (2013). Serotonin transporter genotype modulates cognitive reappraisal of negative emotions: A functional magnetic resonance imaging study. *Soc Cogn Affect Neurosci, 8*(3), 247–258. doi:10.1093/scan/nsr091.

Food Addicts in Recovery Anonymous. (2013). *Food Addicts in Recovery Anonymous*. Woburn, MA: Food Addicts in Recovery Anonymous.

Gibson, E. L. (2006). Emotional influences on food choice: Sensory, physiological and psychological pathways. *Physiol Behav, 89*(1), 53–61.

Giel, K. E., Hartmann, A., Zeeck, A., Jux, A., Vuck, A., Gierthmuehlen, P. C., … Joos, A. (2016). Decreased emotional perception in obesity. *Eur Eat Disord Rev, 24*(4), 341–346. doi:10.1002/erv.2444.

Gilbert, P. (2000). The relationship of shame, social anxiety and depression: The role of the evaluation of social rank. *Clin Psychol Pychother, 7*, 174–189.

Grilo, C. M., Shiffman, S., & Wing, R. R. (1989). Relapse crises and coping among dieters. *J Consult Clin Psychol, 57*(4), 488–495.

Halliday, J. A., Palma, C. L., Mellor, D., Green, J., & Renzaho, A. M. (2014). The relationship between family functioning and child and adolescent overweight and obesity: A systematic review. *Int J Obes (Lond), 38*(4), 480–493. doi:10.1038/ijo.2013.213.

Harrold, J. A., Elliott, J. C., King, P. J., Widdowson, P. S., & Williams, G. (2002). Down-regulation of cannabinoid-1 (CB-1) receptors in specific extrahypothalamic regions of rats with dietary obesity: A role for endogenous cannabinoids in driving appetite for palatable food? *Brain Res, 952*(2), 232–238.

Homer, C. V., Tod, A. M., Thompson, A. R., Allmark, P., & Goyder, E. (2016). Expectations and patients' experiences of obesity prior to bariatric surgery: A qualitative study. *BMJ Open, 6*(2), e009389. doi:10.1136/bmjopen-2015-009389.

Iannaccone, M., D'Olimpio, F., Cella, S., & Cotrufo, P. (2016). Self-esteem, body shame and eating disorder risk in obese and normal weight adolescents: A mediation model. *Eat Behav, 21*, 80–83. doi:10.1016/j.eatbeh.2015.12.010.

Iliceto, P., Pompili, M., Candilera, G., Natali, M. A., Stefani, H., Lester, D., … Girardi, P. (2012). Gender-related differences concerning anger expression and interpersonal relationships in a sample of overweight/obese subjects. *Clin Ter, 163*(5), e279–e285.

Ivanova, I. V., Tasca, G. A., Hammond, N., Balfour, L., Ritchie, K., Koszycki, D., & Bissada, H. (2015). Negative affect mediates the relationship between interpersonal problems and binge-eating disorder symptoms and psychopathology in a clinical sample: A test of the interpersonal model. *Eur Eat Disord Rev, 23*(2), 133–138. doi:10.1002/erv.2344.

Kakinami, L., Barnett, T. A., Seguin, L., & Paradis, G. (2015). Parenting style and obesity risk in children. *Prev Med, 75*, 18–22. doi:10.1016/j.ypmed.2015.03.005.

Kirk, S. F., Price, S. L., Penney, T. L., Rehman, L., Lyons, R. F., Piccinini-Vallis, H., … Aston, M. (2014). Blame, shame, and lack of support: A multilevel study on obesity management. *Qual Health Res, 24*(6), 790–800. doi:10.1177/1049732314529667.

Kurhe, Y., & Mahesh, R. (2015). Mechanisms linking depression co-morbid with obesity: An approach for serotonergic type 3 receptor antagonist as novel therapeutic intervention. *Asian J Psychiatr, 17*, 3–9. doi:10.1016/j.ajp.2015.07.007.

Leach, D., & Kranzler, H. R. (2013). An interpersonal model of addiction relapse. *Addict Disord Their Treat, 12*(4), 183–192. doi:10.1097/ADT.0b013e31826ac408.

Leahey, T. M., Doyle, C. Y., Xu, X., Bihuniak, J., & Wing, R. R. (2015). Social networks and social norms are associated with obesity treatment outcomes. *Obesity (Silver Spring), 23*(8), 1550–1554. doi:10.1002/oby.21074.

Lo Coco, G., Gullo, S., Scrima, F., & Bruno, V. (2012). Obesity and interpersonal problems: An analysis with the interpersonal circumplex. *Clin Psychol Psychother, 19*(5), 390–398. doi:10.1002/cpp.753.

Luppino, F. S., de Wit, L. M., Bouvy, P. F., Stijnen, T., Cuijpers, P., Penninx, B. W., & Zitman, F. G. (2010). Overweight, obesity, and depression: A systematic review and meta-analysis of longitudinal studies. *Arch Gen Psychiatry, 67*(3), 220–229. doi:10.1001/archgenpsychiatry.2010.2.

Marmorstein, N. R., Iacono, W. G., & Legrand, L. (2014). Obesity and depression in adolescence and beyond: Reciprocal risks. *Int J Obes (Lond), 38*(7), 906–911. doi:10.1038/ijo.2014.19.

Midei, A. J., & Matthews, K. A. (2011). Interpersonal violence in childhood as a risk factor for obesity: A systematic review of the literature and proposed pathways. *Obes Rev, 12*(5), e159–e172. doi:10.1111/j.1467-789X.2010.00823.x.

Midei, A. J., Matthews, K. A., & Bromberger, J. T. (2010). Childhood abuse is associated with adiposity in midlife women: Possible pathways through trait anger and reproductive hormones. *Psychosom Med, 72*(2), 215–223. doi:10.1097/PSY.0b013e3181cb5c24.

Mihalopoulos, N. L., & Spigarelli, M. G. (2015). Comanagement of pediatric depression and obesity: A clear need for evidence. *Clin Ther, 37*(9), 1933–1937. doi:10.1016/j.clinthera.2015.08.009.

Mills, J. K. (1995). A note on interpersonal sensitivity and psychotic symptomatology in obese adult outpatients with a history of childhood obesity. *J Psychol, 129*(3), 345–348. doi:10.1080/00223980.1995.9914970.

Neumark-Sztainer, D. (2005). Preventing the broad spectrum of weight-related problems: Working with parents to help teens achieve a healthy weight and a positive body image. *J Nutr Educ Behav, 37*(Suppl. 2), S133–S140.

Oliveira, A. J., Rostila, M., de Leon, A. P., & Lopes, C. S. (2013). The influence of social relationships on obesity: Sex differences in a longitudinal study. *Obesity (Silver Spring), 21*(8), 1540–1547. doi:10.1002/oby.20286.

Olvera, R. L., Williamson, D. E., Fisher-Hoch, S. P., Vatcheva, K. P., & McCormick, J. B. (2015). Depression, obesity, and metabolic syndrome: Prevalence and risks of comorbidity in a population-based representative sample of Mexican Americans. *J Clin Psychiatry, 76*(10), e1300–e1305. doi:10.4088/JCP.14m09118.

Palmeira, L., Pinto-Gouveia, J., Cunha, M., & Carvalho, S. (2017). Finding the link between internalized weight-stigma and binge eating behaviors in Portuguese adult women with overweight and obesity: The mediator role of self-criticism and self-reassurance. *Eat Behav, 26*, 50–54. doi:10.1016/j.eatbeh.2017.01.006.

Papazoglou, I. K., Jean, A., Gertler, A., Taouis, M., & Vacher, C. M. (2015). Hippocampal GSK3beta as a molecular link between obesity and depression. *Mol Neurobiol, 52*(1), 363–374. doi:10.1007/s12035-014-8863-x.

Parran, T., McCormick, R., & Delos Reyes, C. (2014). Assessment. In R. K. Reis, D. A. Fiellin, S. C. Miller, & R. Saitz (Eds.), *Principles of Addiction Medicine*, pp. 344–352, Philadelphia, PA: American Society of Addiction Medicine.

Pasco, J. A., Williams, L. J., Jacka, F. N., Brennan, S. L., & Berk, M. (2013). Obesity and the relationship with positive and negative affect. *Aust N Z J Psychiatry, 47*(5), 477–482. doi:10.1177/0004867413483371.

Petroni, M. L., Villanova, N., Avagnina, S., Fusco, M. A., Fatati, G., Compare, A., & Marchesini, G. (2007). Psychological distress in morbid obesity in relation to weight history. *Obes Surg, 17*(3), 391–399. doi:10.1007/s11695-007-9069-3.

Pila, E., Sabiston, C. M., Brunet, J., Castonguay, A. L., & O'Loughlin, J. (2015). Do body-related shame and guilt mediate the association between weight status and self-esteem? *J Health Psychol, 20*(5), 659–669. doi:10.1177/1359105315573449.

Pratt, L. A., & Brody, D. J. (2014). Depression and obesity in the U.S. adult household population, 2005–2010. *NCHS Data Brief* 167, 1–8.

Preiss, K., Brennan, L., & Clarke, D. (2013). A systematic review of variables associated with the relationship between obesity and depression. *Obes Rev, 14*(11), 906–918. doi:10.1111/obr.12052.

Rhee, K. E., Dickstein, S., Jelalian, E., Boutelle, K., Seifer, R., & Wing, R. (2015). Development of the General Parenting Observational Scale to assess parenting during family meals. *Int J Behav Nutr Phys Act, 12*, 49. doi:10.1186/s12966-015-0207-3.

Roberts, R. E., & Duong, H. T. (2015). Does major depression affect risk for adolescent obesity? *J Affect Disord, 186*, 162–167. doi:10.1016/j.jad.2015.06.030.

Saltzman, J. A., & Liechty, J. M. (2016). Family correlates of childhood binge eating: A systematic review. *Eat Behav, 22*, 62–71. doi:10.1016/j.eatbeh.2016.03.027.

Saltzman, J. A., Pineros-Leano, M., Liechty, J. M., Bost, K. K., Fiese, B. H., & Team, S. K. (2016). Eating, feeding, and feeling: Emotional responsiveness mediates longitudinal associations between maternal binge eating, feeding practices, and child weight. *Int J Behav Nutr Phys Act, 13*, 89. doi:10.1186/s12966-016-0415-5.

Salwen, J. K., Hymowitz, G. F., Vivian, D., & O'Leary, K. D. (2014). Childhood abuse, adult interpersonal abuse, and depression in individuals with extreme obesity. *Child Abuse Negl, 38*(3), 425–433. doi:10.1016/j.chiabu.2013.12.005.

Schneider, K. L., Appelhans, B. M., Whited, M. C., Oleski, J., & Pagoto, S. L. (2010). Trait anxiety, but not trait anger, predisposes obese individuals to emotional eating. *Appetite, 55*(3), 701–706. doi:10.1016/j.appet.2010.10.006.

Seacat, J. D., Dougal, S. C., & Roy, D. (2016). A daily diary assessment of female weight stigmatization. *J Health Psychol, 21*(2), 228–240. doi:10.1177/1359105314525067.

Sinha, R. (2007). The role of stress in addiction relapse. *Curr Psychiatry Rep, 9*(5), 388–395.

Sjoberg, R. L., Nilsson, K. W., & Leppert, J. (2005). Obesity, shame, and depression in school-aged children: A population-based study. *Pediatrics, 116*(3), e389–e392. doi:10.1542/peds.2005-0170.

Tuominen, L., Tuulari, J., Karlsson, H., Hirvonen, J., Helin, S., Salminen, P., … Nummenmaa, L. (2015). Aberrant mesolimbic dopamine-opiate interaction in obesity. *NeuroImage, 122*, 80–86. doi:10.1016/j.neuroimage.2015.08.001.

Van Niel, C., Pachter, L. M., Wade, R., Jr., Felitti, V. J., & Stein, M. T. (2014). Adverse events in children: Predictors of adult physical and mental conditions. *J Dev Behav Pediatr, 35*(8), 549–551. doi:10.1097/dbp.0000000000000102.

Wang, G. J., Tomasi, D., Convit, A., Logan, J., Wong, C. T., Shumay, E., … Volkow, N. D. (2014). BMI modulates calorie-dependent dopamine changes in accumbens from glucose intake. *PLoS One, 9*(7), e101585. doi:10.1371/journal.pone.0101585.

Weiss, F. (2004). Group psychotherapy with obese disordered-eating adults with body-image disturbances: An integrated model. *Am J Psychother, 58*(3), 281–303.

Westermann, S., Rief, W., Euteneuer, F., & Kohlmann, S. (2015). Social exclusion and shame in obesity. *Eat Behav, 17*, 74–76. doi:10.1016/j.eatbeh.2015.01.001.

Westermeyer, J. (2013). Historical understandings of addiction. In P. M. Miller (Ed.), *Principles of Addiction: Comprehensive Addictive Behaviors and Disorders*, pp. 3–12, New York: Elsevier.

Wurtman, R.J., & Wurtman, J. J. (1986). Carbohydrate craving, obesity and brain serotonin. *Appetite, 7*(Suppl.), 99–103.

17 DSM 5 SUD Criterion 7 *Activities Given Up*

Joan Ifland
Food Addiction Training, LLC
Cincinnati, OH

Rhona L. Epstein
Private Practice
Philadelphia, PA

CONTENTS

Important social, occupational, or recreational activities are given up or reduced because of processed food use. (American Psychiatric Association, 2013, p. 491)

17.1 INTRODUCTION

Criterion 7 illuminates a distressing consequence of processed food addiction (PFA), i.e., withdrawal from people and activities. The demands of the addiction can be a driving force in giving up activities, as could be the case in any addiction. However, in the case of PFA, the additional factor of weight gain can make the drive to isolate even more powerful through the mechanism of stigmatization. Fear of losing control over food in front of other people can also be a reason to isolate. Fatigue, brain fog, and mobility issues may also play a role in giving up activities. Activities given up may be a more important criterion for PFA relative to other addictions because food-addicted clients do not need to engage with suppliers to obtain addictive substances. It may be easier for food-addicted clients to isolate in their homes compared to other addictions.

Thus Criterion 7 presents an opportunity for the practitioner to gain in-depth information about the client. Information about activities that the client has given up can lead to discussions about physical limitations as well as emotional distress related to relationships and being lonely. Exploring activities given up can help the practitioner build a treatment plan for resuming a more satisfying and interesting life.

17.1.1 Importance

Learning about the activities that food-addicted clients have given up gives the practitioner a picture of the disintegration of lifestyle associated with PFA. Factors such as cognitive impairment, fatigue, and a body shape that attracts stigmatization conspire to isolate food-addicted clients. As the Food Addicts Anonymous manual states, "In an effort to hide the fat, we may hide from others" (Food Addicts Anonymous, 2010, p. 4). Food-addicted clients of any size may suffer from body dissatisfaction (Pearl & Puhl, 2014) so it is important for practitioners to pursue this line in inquiry regardless of clients' body shape.

The feeling of loneliness can be quite painful for food-addicted clients. The feeling may derive from low self-esteem and be experienced even when around people. This internal effect may make the prospect of being around other people unattractive, as food-addicted clients may not experience relief from loneliness by doing so. This quote describes the situation.

> It feels as if I've been alone all of my life, with just me for guidance, and that's being totally alone because I didn't know my own path. I used to wonder if I was the only one with such a sense of estrangement and unconnectedness. Everyone around me seemed so self-contained. Sometimes I felt like a nobody … a tiny puff of air. When everyone's around me, I'm just not there. Empty is how it feels to be lonely. When I feel loneliness, I feel totally abandoned and completely isolated in a group. (Food Addicts Anonymous, 2010, p. 135)

Of course not every food-addicted client's condition has progressed in the direction of isolation. Food-addicted clients may still be engaged in social events. They certainly may still go to a workplace. Practitioners may need to go back in time to find activities that may have been given up as weight, stigmatization, immobility, and negative affect increased. The process of giving up activities may be subtle and have taken place gradually, possibly without coming to awareness. Work problems may include concentration related to the inability to focus because of distracting food and body obsession (Field et al., 2016). This kind of preoccupation may affect the ability to work. There may also be fatigue from late-night binges (Harb et al., 2012) and effects of food on energy and mood (Jacka et al., 2010). Parenting activities including doing homework with children can suffer from food/mood issues. This can lead to pulling away from responsibilities with kids and caring for home (Roth, Munsch, Meyer, Isler, & Schneider, 2008). Marital, relationship, and sexual activities can be diminished (Carr & Jaffe, 2012). Food-addicted clients may withdraw from relationships due to negative body image and feeling ill (Guh et al., 2009; Palmeira, Pinto-Gouveia, & Cunha, 2016).

17.1.2 Evidence for the Syndrome

There is significant evidence for a number of factors driving the process of giving up activities. The roles of stigmatization, medical consequences, and mood disorders are demonstrated and can contribute to the syndrome of activities given up.

There is evidence for physical and emotional consequences of chronic processed food consumption that could lead to isolation and loss of activities. These include pain, fatigue, immobility, frequent illness, heart disease, amputations, muscle loss, and excess adipose tissue (Paulis, Silva, Koes, & Van Middelkoop, 2014; Wannamethee & Atkins, 2015). That emotional distress from teasing associated with childhood obesity can extend into adulthood is well documented (Rankin et al., 2016; Sanders, Han, Baker, & Cobley, 2015). The changes in neurostructure associated with depression in obesity have been found. They include prefrontal areas involved in emotional regulation and impulse control as well as downregulation of serotonin pathways (Kurhe & Mahesh, 2015;

Opel et al., 2015). Depression has also been found in eating disorders even when obesity is not present (Fitzsimmons-Craft et al., 2014). Further, it may be stressful for food-addicted clients to be around people due to sensitized stress functions in the brain (Ulrich-Lai & Ryan, 2014).

In addition to the physical and emotional characteristics of chronic processed food use, there is significant evidence for stigmatization of the obese. Stigmatization has been researched extensively, resulting in a number of recent review articles (Brewis, 2014; Phelan et al., 2015; Puhl & King, 2013; Rankin et al., 2016; Ratcliffe & Ellison, 2015). Self-stigmatization has been demonstrated in eating disorders, not just obesity (Griffiths, Mond, Murray, Thornton, & Touyz, 2015). Stigmatization could play a significant role in decisions to give up activities. A broad range of symptoms are associated with stigmatization, including depression, anxiety, low self-esteem, body dissatisfaction, suicidal ideation, poor academic performance, lower physical activity, maladaptive eating behaviors, and avoidance of health care (Puhl & King, 2013). These can create barriers to occupational, social, and recreational activities.

Ratcliffe and Ellison developed a model for the internalization of external stigmatization. The model describes the impact of negative societal and interpersonal experiences on how the obese view themselves. Obese people see themselves as stigmatized and this self-perception is the core of the model. The self-stigmatization is maintained by a number of factors, including negative self-judgments about what it means to be obese, obsessional attention to the importance of weight to the exclusion of other attributes, as well as low self-esteem and depression. Avoidance of activities including exercise is described as reinforcing self-stigmatization. The negative affect from instances of weight stigmatization can develop into fear, which can prompt safety behaviors consisting of avoiding frightening places. The isolation then prevents repair of the feelings. In a synergistic cycle, under the stress of internalized stigmatization, eating and weight management behaviors can become deregulated, which maintains both the obesity and the weight stigma (Ratcliffe & Ellison, 2015).

Brewis et al. found evidence for four mechanisms by which stigmatization could promote obesity. These four factors could also promote isolation.

- Feeling judged could encourage clients to avoid people in general.
- Social network changes based on stigmatizing actions and decisions by others could encourage clients to avoid particular groups of people.
- Psychosocial stress from feeling stigmatized could be associated with debilitating depression.
- Structural effects of discrimination could cause job loss or low-paying jobs that consume time and energy (Brewis, Brennhofer, Van Woerden, & Bruening, 2016).

Other evidence supports the link between obesity, stigma, and avoidance of activities. Westermann et al. found that when faced with social exclusion, individuals with obesity do not respond with more intensive negative emotions in general compared to controls but with a specific increase in shame (Westermann, Rief, Euteneuer, & Kohlmann, 2015). Wee et al. found in a cross-sectional telephone interview of an obese Caucasian female population that weight-related social stigma impacted quality of life more than any other factor (Wee, Davis, Chiodi, Huskey, & Hamel, 2015). Brewis et al. found that women and children suffered more from weight-related stigma more than men (Brewis, 2014). Stigma was found to be a barrier to participation in a community weight-management program for families (Kelleher et al., 2017). Rivera and Paredez found that self-stereotyping correlated with lower self-esteem and higher BMI in an Hispanic population (Rivera & Paredez, 2014).

Stigmatization by authority figures could contribute disproportionately to debilitating shame and isolation. Stigmatization of the obese by medical professionals has been demonstrated (Murphy & Gardner, 2016; Phelan et al., 2015). Discrimination against obesity is so pervasive in employment that legal measures are being considered to prevent it (Flint & Snook, 2015). Stigmatization of eating disorders in general has been found (Ebneter & Latner, 2013).

There is also a potential factor of financial distress that could lead to giving up activities. Patel et al. found that obese people are more likely to sleep during the day, work several jobs, and work at night, which could interfere with activities (Patel, Spaeth, & Basner, 2016).

The evidence shows a range of factors such as stigmatization, immobility, debilitating mood disorders, poor health, and financial demands, which can result in food-addicted clients giving up activities.

17.1.3 Use in Motivation

The ability to resume activities could be a good motivator for food addicts. As the quotes below illustrate, some obese people suffer from loneliness. They expect to be rejected, ridiculed, or even bullied by other people. They may have learned to expect abuse from experiences in childhood. Or, they may have learned to fit in by using drugs or engaging in sex. Thus the prospect of recovering the ability to be comfortable around other people could be appealing.

17.1.4 Use in Treatment

The realization that obese people have withdrawn from occupational, social, and recreational activities gives the practitioner the opportunity to write restoration of activities into a plan for recovery from PFA. The practitioner can work with the client to find venues where the client will be safe. For reasons of relationships sensitivity, it is important for the practitioner to recommend activities that involve people who accept overweight and obese clients without judgment. These venues may not be readily available in physical settings. Practitioners may start out by recommending social contact over the telephone in telephone conference calls offered by recovery groups. Online groups may also be attractive. In all cases, practitioners will need to make sure that the group is not advocating the use of processed foods, restricted dieting, or other practices that may be harmful to food-addicted clients. Resources for finding groups can be found at www.foodaddictionresources.com.

Gathering information about abandoned activities including the circumstances, reasons, and people involved will give the practitioner valuable insights, which can be incorporated into a treatment plan.

17.2 MANIFESTATIONS

Manifestations of abandoned activities are numerous. Possibly the most prevalent is the stigmatization related to obesity and overweight. However, the consuming properties of PFA can also play a role. These quotes are taken from the 12-step manuals for two recovery fellowships, Food Addicts Anonymous and Food Addicts in Recovery Anonymous (Food Addicts Anonymous, 2010; Food Addicts in Recovery Anonymous, 2013).

17.2.1 Behaviors

Isolation can begin at a young age. Children may choose isolation, but it may also be the result of being ignored by other children. Behaviors associated with PFA such as bingeing can propel food addicts to avoid being seen by other people. Attending events may also interfere with the ability to address the intense cravings and urges that characterize PFA. And the time required to obtain food can preclude involvement in other activities.

> For my first communion I wore a beautiful nylon and lace dress and felt ashamed that it had taken enough fabric for two dresses to make my one. My obesity gave rise to social isolation; the social isolation perpetuated the obesity. I was a very shy child. I didn't have the courage to join in with the other kids in the schoolyard, and it was rare that anyone approached me and asked me to join. I spent most of recess standing on the sidelines watching other kids playing and having fun—waiting for the bell to ring. (Food Addicts Anonymous, 2010, p. 95)
>
> No one ever witnessed my bingeing. The level of shame was too great to bear the scrutiny of another being. This is a disease of isolation. I did the dirty deed without corroboration. (Food Addicts Anonymous, 2010, p. 192)

> My disease progressed beyond my wildest imagination. Food became more important than my daughter, my husband, my integrity or anything else in my life. I would sneak food, hide food, leave the house at ungodly hours for it, stash it, and so on. I manipulated people, places and things so that I could be alone with my fix. (Food Addicts Anonymous, 2010, p. 235)
>
> … thinking only of how I needed to get to the pancake house. Little did I know that I was becoming so dependent on this treat that nothing could stop me. After six months I needed them twice a day. In the afternoon I would drive about 15 miles to the other side of town to a different pancake house than I had gone to in the morning. (Food Addicts Anonymous, 2010, p. 164)

17.2.2 Mental

Food-addicted clients can develop obsessional thought patterns that create barriers to participating in activities, even to making a phone call.

> In less than a year I was 92 pounds heavier. I had surrendered to the disease of food addiction. Now began a period of intense shame, depression and isolation. I imagined people were looking at me and condemning me for my lack of self-control. (pp 112-113; Food Addicts Anonymous, 2010)
>
> What is clear to me in the relapse is that this is not really about the food at all; it is in the thinking around the food, which is the horror of this disease. I developed a mental obsession and a hopelessness that was frightening in its intensity. I lost the ability to pray, to pick up the phone, to e-mail, to ask for help, to make abstinent decisions. (Food Addicts Anonymous, 2010, p. 41)
>
> Ultimately, I went into a state of clinical depression. I wasn't actually suicidal, but I did have a sense that even if I knew I was going to die that very day, I didn't care. The depression didn't stop me from eating, though. Amazing! I was too depressed to answer the phone, but I still managed to overeat. (Food Addicts Anonymous, 2010, p. 97)

17.2.3 Emotional

The distress of the behaviors, loss of health, and stigmatization can create a reluctance to attend activities. The emotional distress can begin in childhood and continue unabated into adulthood.

> Lonely, fat, and shy, my only friend was food. Food loved me. I loved food. Buying an ice cream bar after eating what was in my lunch box became a great event for me that I repeated over and over again. I got fatter and the loneliness only got worse. Classrooms were over-crowded. I was quiet and shy. It was easy for teachers to pay minimal attention to me. I was ridiculed because of my size. Kids made fun of me. Adults made fun of me. I remember the saleslady who laughed as she stretched a tape measure around my waist; the dentist who commented on my excessive weight and then laughed; the brother who tormented me daily, adding physical abuse to the laughter. My parents did very little to stop him. (Food Addicts Anonymous, 2010, p. 95)
>
> I suffered from anxiety attacks and periods of undiagnosed depression. In isolation, I fought for sanity and used poetry as my only therapeutic outlet. (Food Addicts Anonymous, 2010, p. 124)
>
> So there I was in a new town with no friends, newly sober, and terrified of people. I did what any good food addict would do. I began to camp out in the bakery of my neighborhood grocery store. As I struggled to stay sober and deal with my isolation and loneliness, I turned increasingly to food instead of the fellowship of AA. (Food Addicts Anonymous, 2010, p. 243)
>
> The holidays were always big affairs with an overabundance of food. I looked forward to them for the food, not for the pleasure of being with my relatives or celebrating the holiday itself. (Food Addicts Anonymous, 2010, p. 173)

17.2.4 Physical

Physical barriers to attending events can be a significant factor in manifestation of Criterion 7. These can pertain to consequences related to weight, dental problems, and skin eruptions.

I couldn't stand too long because my ankles would swell up. There was so much weight on my body that the blood couldn't circulate. I couldn't go places without getting out of breath. (Food Addicts Anonymous, 2010, p. 141)

As I threw back the sheets and lifted my obese legs off to one side of the bed, it was a struggle to move just a few inches. I knew I had responsibilities to face; pets to take care of and housework to do. I faced a 12-hour routine to keep my job in the federal government. But this day was different; I just couldn't do it anymore. (Food Addicts Anonymous, 2010, p. 225)

The sugars in my blood caused me to lose most of my teeth. My face was a mess with acne. My self-esteem was so low and there were long periods of time that I never bathed or took care of my home. I neglected my children. I always said I wanted a close-knit family, but in reality, I wanted everyone away from me so I could eat. I wanted to eat alone. I didn't want to share my food with anyone. When I was bingeing myself into oblivion, there was too much shame to let anyone see how much and how I ate. (Food Addicts Anonymous, 2010, p. 141)

17.3 APPLICATION

17.3.1 Care in Approach

Practitioners can carefully examine their own attitudes for prejudices toward both obese and addicted clients. The attitudes of medical professionals toward obese clients have been shown to be prejudicial in a number of studies (Buxton & Snethen, 2013; Mold & Forbes, 2013; Mulherin, Miller, Barlow, Diedrichs, & Thompson, 2013; Phelan et al., 2015). There are similarities to discriminatory attitudes toward clients with drug addiction.

Education about the extensive alterations in brain function underpinning PFA is a means for turning judgmental attitudes into compassionate, constructive attitudes. Practitioners can ask themselves if, in the past, they might have blamed clients for failure to progress when perhaps the program being offered was inconsistent with new developments in the science of PFA. Examples of advances include findings for the roles of stress, cues, and the addictive properties of high-fat/high-sugar foods. Examining past attitudes can help practitioners wipe the slate clean and begin using new techniques based on what is now known about PFA as a mental illness. This quote illustrates both the problem and the opportunity.

Case: A female patient at the Mass General Weight Management Center presented for a telephone consultation. She reported distress arising from a bariatric preoperative evaluation during which she was characterized as a drug addict because of her medication history that included naltrexone. The drug was prescribed in combination with bupropion to treat her obesity, not a drug or alcohol addiction. (Alfaris, Kyle, Nadai, & Stanford, 2016)

The attitudes of the obese can deteriorate under long-term misunderstanding from health professionals and families alike. The quote shown below illustrates the importance of educating the client's family. Using educational handouts from www.foodaddictionresources.com could help clients reintegrate into their families and begin to use their families for support. This reintegration could serve as a foundation for venturing back into social and recreational activities. This quote is excerpted from a study of an obese population referred for bariatric surgery:

Prior to being referred to specialist obesity services, participants identified that healthcare professionals had also been judgmental regarding their weight. Participants reported how their families did not understand their weight struggles, and viewed the surgery as an easy or soft option. This lack of understanding from the healthcare profession and of those closest to them meant that participants felt increasingly marginalized from networks they regarded as their support. (Homer, Tod, Thompson, Allmark, & Goyder, 2016)

Including families in education about PFA can provide relief to clients. Educational handouts may be found at www.foodaddictionresources.com.

Practitioners may also want to spend time positioning the label of PFA positively as a way of helping clients gain confidence about being around people. Addictions are viewed unfavorably in general (Ahern, Stuber, & Galea, 2007), although the label of PFA is not judged as severely as other addictions (DePierre, Puhl, & Luedicke, 2013). It is possible that PFA is common but undiagnosed in the general population. This could be the case because many people could be meeting common DSM 5 SRAD criteria such as unintended use, failure to cut back, cravings, and use in spite of knowledge of consequences.

The practitioner can explain that the diagnosis of PFA could be a breakthrough for the client insofar as the focus of recovery can shift away from exerting willpower to gradually eliminating the unprocessed foods, cues, and stressors associated with cravings and loss of control. Attaching hope to the diagnosis could help the client accept the diagnosis positively and regain the courage to be around people. Practitioners can discuss ways to explain PFA in social situations as a possibly common problem. Of course, clients will also benefit from learning how to avoid the topic with people who are unsafe in terms of teasing and bullying.

Practitioners will realize that food-addicted clients may suffer from relationship sensitivity. They may be acutely uncomfortable around other people because of real-life experience with stigmatization (Seacat, Dougal, & Roy, 2016). Being around other people may be stressful for neurochemical reasons, as processed foods and cues have been shown to sensitize the stress pathways in the brain (Cottone et al., 2009). For these reasons, it is helpful for practitioners to be unfailingly courteous and patient with clients. To give clients the courage to reengage with people in social, occupational, and recreational activities, practitioners can dwell on positive attributes. Practitioners can work to resolve clients' negative self-perceptions that may inhibit the desire to be among people. Practitioners can also prioritize developing resiliency in clients who are sensitive to other people's negativity.

The practitioner can also repeatedly tell clients how nice it is to have them in the practice, with simple phrases such as, "It's nice to have you here. I'm glad you're here. It's a pleasure to have you here." These small gestures can help the client heal from the numerous times when they might have been teased or rejected. The challenge is to change the internalized self-blame into self-appreciation for surviving an obesogenic environment.

17.3.2 Developing Goals

This is an area where restoration of self-esteem and disassociating self-value from weight status are valuable outcomes. Teaching the client that the weight gain and loss of control are engineered by neuroscientists in the food industry can move the client away from self-loathing to a place of self-esteem. Acceptance and commitment therapy has been shown to be effective to this end (Lillis, Hayes, Bunting, & Masuda, 2009). This is the shift that will allow the client to choose safe places in which to socialize.

There is also a need to develop goals around stigmatization. Detachment from others' derogatory comments can be practiced. Teaching clients about the neuroanomalies associated with exposure to processed food and cues can help clients let go of others' uneducated attitudes. This can lead to reductions in internalization of others' judgments that the client is lazy, sloppy, or lacks self-will (Alfaris et al., 2016). Gradually reducing exposure to stigmatizing media may also be a productive goal (Puhl, Luedicke, & Heuer, 2013).

17.3.3 Tracking Progress

Making progress in restoring activities is complicated. "Clearly there is a delicate balance to strike between intervention approaches that focus on decreasing avoidance whilst simultaneously increasing resilience due to the potential reality of the weight stigmatizing social environment" (Ratcliffe & Ellison, 2015).

The client can report on progress in establishing contact with safe people in welcoming environments. The phone and Internet are good places to start, as judgments about weight are not a risk in these methods of socializing that limit exposure of the body. As the client regains mobility, they can venture out to in-person support meetings and possibly to faith organizations where appropriate attitudes may be more prevalent. The challenges to progress in this area is illustrated by this quote.

> On Monday, I drove to the meeting place, sat in my car, and drove home without ever opening the car door. On Wednesday, I tried again. I told myself, "You've got to go, no matter what," and I followed through. (Food Addicts in Recovery Anonymous, 2013, p. 24)

The ability to speak up to people who stigmatize the obese is progress in being able to thrive in spite of a discriminatory environment.

17.4 CONCLUSION

Criterion 7 is an important criterion to explore with the client. Going back into the client's history can reveal jobs, social events, and recreational pleasures that have been given up as the addiction progressed into depression, fatigue, loss of control over food, and immobility. Integrating clients into activities can be a slow but rewarding process. As clients regain control of and reduce reactivity to cues, they can develop confidence that they can eat normally in front of other people. Similarly, as physical problems such as joint pain and excess adipose tissue resolve, clients can regain the ability to move around and rejoin events. In cases where low self-esteem has prevented clients from believing that they are desirable at events, the development of confidence can be a significant milestone in recovery.

REFERENCES

Ahern, J., Stuber, J., & Galea, S. (2007). Stigma, discrimination and the health of illicit drug users. *Drug Alcohol Depend, 88*(2–3), 188–196. doi:10.1016/j.drugalcdep.2006.10.014.

Alfaris, N., Kyle, T. K., Nadai, J., & Stanford, F. C. (2016). A new era of addiction treatment amplifies the stigma of disease and treatment for individuals with obesity. *Int J Obes (Lond), 40*(9), 1335–1336. doi:10.1038/ijo.2016.101.

American Psychiatric Association. (2013). *The Diagnostic and Statistical Manual of Mental Disorders, Fifth Edition* (Vol. 5).

Brewis, A., Brennhofer, S., van Woerden, I., & Bruening, M. (2016). Weight stigma and eating behaviors on a college campus: Are students immune to stigma's effects? *Prev Med Rep, 4*, 578–584. doi:10.1016/j.pmedr.2016.10.005.

Brewis, A. A. (2014). Stigma and the perpetuation of obesity. *Soc Sci Med, 118*, 152–158. doi:10.1016/j.socscimed.2014.08.003.

Buxton, B. K., & Snethen, J. (2013). Obese women's perceptions and experiences of healthcare and primary care providers: A phenomenological study. *Nurs Res, 62*(4), 252–259. doi:10.1097/NNR.0b013e318299a6ba.

Carr, D., & Jaffe, K. (2012). The psychological consequences of weight change trajectories: Evidence from quantitative and qualitative data. *Econ Hum Biol, 10*(4), 419–430. doi:10.1016/j.ehb.2012.04.007.

Cottone, P., Sabino, V., Roberto, M., Bajo, M., Pockros, L., Frihauf, J. B., … Zorrilla, E. P. (2009). CRF system recruitment mediates dark side of compulsive eating. *Proc Natl Acad Sci U S A, 106*(47), 20016–20020. doi:10.1073/pnas.0908789106.

DePierre, J. A., Puhl, R. M., & Luedicke, J. (2013). A new stigmatized identity? Comparisons of a "Food Addict" label with other stigmatized health conditions. *Basic and Applied Social Psychology, 35*(1), 10–21. doi:10.1080/01973533.2012.746148.

Ebneter, D. S., & Latner, J. D. (2013). Stigmatizing attitudes differ across mental health disorders: A comparison of stigma across eating disorders, obesity, and major depressive disorder. *J Nerv Ment Dis, 201*(4), 281–285. doi:10.1097/NMD.0b013e318288e23f.

Field, M., Werthmann, J., Franken, I., Hofmann, W., Hogarth, L., & Roefs, A. (2016). The role of attentional bias in obesity and addiction. *Health Psychol, 35*(8), 767–780. doi:10.1037/hea0000405.

Fitzsimmons-Craft, E. E., Ciao, A. C., Accurso, E. C., Pisetsky, E. M., Peterson, C. B., Byrne, C. E., & Le Grange, D. (2014). Subjective and objective binge eating in relation to eating disorder symptomatology, depressive symptoms, and self-esteem among treatment-seeking adolescents with bulimia nervosa. *Eur Eat Disord Rev, 22*(4), 230–236. doi:10.1002/erv.2297.

Flint, S. W., & Snook, J. (2015). Disability discrimination and obesity: The big questions? *Curr Obes Rep, 4*(4), 504–509. doi:10.1007/s13679-015-0182-7.

Food Addicts Anonymous. (2010). *Food Addicts Anonymous.* Port St. Lucie, FL: Food Addicts Anonymous.

Food Addicts in Recovery Anonymous. (2013). *Food Addicts in Recovery Anonymous.* Woburn, MA: Food Addicts in Recovery Anonymous.

Griffiths, S., Mond, J. M., Murray, S. B., Thornton, C., & Touyz, S. (2015). Stigma resistance in eating disorders. *Soc Psychiatry Psychiatr Epidemiol, 50*(2), 279–287. doi:10.1007/s00127-014-0923-z.

Guh, D. P., Zhang, W., Bansback, N., Amarsi, Z., Birmingham, C. L., & Anis, A. H. (2009). The incidence of co-morbidities related to obesity and overweight: A systematic review and meta-analysis. *BMC Public Health, 9*, 88. doi:10.1186/1471-2458-9-88.

Harb, A., Levandovski, R., Oliveira, C., Caumo, W., Allison, K. C., Stunkard, A., & Hidalgo, M. P. (2012). Night eating patterns and chronotypes: A correlation with binge eating behaviors. *Psychiatry Res, 200*(2–3), 489–493. doi:10.1016/j.psychres.2012.07.004.

Homer, C. V., Tod, A. M., Thompson, A. R., Allmark, P., & Goyder, E. (2016). Expectations and patients' experiences of obesity prior to bariatric surgery: A qualitative study. *BMJ Open, 6*(2), e009389. doi:10.1136/bmjopen-2015-009389.

Jacka, F. N., Pasco, J. A., Mykletun, A., Williams, L. J., Hodge, A. M., O'Reilly, S. L., … Berk, M. (2010). Association of Western and traditional diets with depression and anxiety in women. *Am J Psychiatry, 167*(3), 305–311. doi:10.1176/appi.ajp.2009.09060881.

Kelleher, E., Davoren, M. P., Harrington, J. M., Shiely, F., Perry, I. J., & McHugh, S. M. (2017). Barriers and facilitators to initial and continued attendance at community-based lifestyle programmes among families of overweight and obese children: A systematic review. *Obes Rev, 18*(2), 183–194. doi:10.1111/obr.12478.

Kurhe, Y., & Mahesh, R. (2015). Mechanisms linking depression co-morbid with obesity: An approach for serotonergic type 3 receptor antagonist as novel therapeutic intervention. *Asian J Psychiatr,* 17, 3–9. doi:10.1016/j.ajp.2015.07.007.

Lillis, J., Hayes, S. C., Bunting, K., & Masuda, A. (2009). Teaching acceptance and mindfulness to improve the lives of the obese: A preliminary test of a theoretical model. *Ann Behav Med, 37*(1), 58–69. doi:10.1007/s12160-009-9083-x.

Mold, F., & Forbes, A. (2013). Patients' and professionals experiences and perspectives of obesity in health-care settings: A synthesis of current research. *Health Expect, 16*(2), 119–142. doi:10.1111/j.1369-7625.2011.00699.x.

Mulherin, K., Miller, Y. D., Barlow, F. K., Diedrichs, P. C., & Thompson, R. (2013). Weight stigma in maternity care: Women's experiences and care providers' attitudes. *BMC Pregnancy Childbirth, 13*, 19. doi:10.1186/1471-2393-13-19.

Murphy, A. L., & Gardner, D. M. (2016). A scoping review of weight bias by community pharmacists towards people with obesity and mental illness. *Can Pharm J (Ott), 149*(4), 226–235. doi:10.1177/1715163516651242.

Opel, N., Redlich, R., Grotegerd, D., Dohm, K., Heindel, W., Kugel, H., … Dannlowski, U. (2015). Obesity and major depression: Body-mass index (BMI) is associated with a severe course of disease and specific neurostructural alterations. *Psychoneuroendocrinology, 51*, 219–226. doi:10.1016/j.psyneuen.2014.10.001.

Palmeira, L., Pinto-Gouveia, J., & Cunha, M. (2016). The role of weight self-stigma on the quality of life of women with overweight and obesity: A multi-group comparison between binge eaters and non-binge eaters. *Appetite, 105*, 782–789. doi:10.1016/j.appet.2016.07.015.

Patel, V. C., Spaeth, A. M., & Basner, M. (2016). Relationships between time use and obesity in a representative sample of Americans. *Obesity (Silver Spring), 24*(10), 2164–2175. doi:10.1002/oby.21596.

Paulis, W. D., Silva, S., Koes, B. W., & van Middelkoop, M. (2014). Overweight and obesity are associated with musculoskeletal complaints as early as childhood: A systematic review. *Obes Rev, 15*(1), 52–67. doi:10.1111/obr.12067.

Pearl, R. L., & Puhl, R. M. (2014). Measuring internalized weight attitudes across body weight categories: Validation of the modified weight bias internalization scale. *Body Image, 11*(1), 89–92. doi:10.1016/j.bodyim.2013.09.005.

Phelan, S. M., Burgess, D. J., Yeazel, M. W., Hellerstedt, W. L., Griffin, J. M., & van Ryn, M. (2015). Impact of weight bias and stigma on quality of care and outcomes for patients with obesity. *Obes Rev, 16*(4), 319–326. doi:10.1111/obr.12266.

Puhl, R. M., & King, K. M. (2013). Weight discrimination and bullying. *Best Pract Res Clin Endocrinol Metab, 27*(2), 117–127. doi:10.1016/j.beem.2012.12.002.

Puhl, R. M., Luedicke, J., & Heuer, C. A. (2013). The stigmatizing effect of visual media portrayals of obese persons on public attitudes: Does race or gender matter? *J Health Commun, 18*(7), 805–826. doi:10.1080/10810730.2012.757393.

Rankin, J., Matthews, L., Cobley, S., Han, A., Sanders, R., Wiltshire, H. D., & Baker, J. S. (2016). Psychological consequences of childhood obesity: Psychiatric comorbidity and prevention. *Adolesc Health Med Ther, 7*, 125–146. doi:10.2147/ahmt.s101631.

Ratcliffe, D., & Ellison, N. (2015). Obesity and internalized weight stigma: A formulation model for an emerging psychological problem. *Behav Cogn Psychother, 43*(2), 239–252. doi:10.1017/s1352465813000763.

Rivera, L. M., & Paredez, S. M. (2014). Stereotypes can "Get Under the Skin": Testing a self-stereotyping and psychological resource model of overweight and obesity. *J Soc Issues, 70*(2), 226–240. doi:10.1111/josi.12057.

Roth, B., Munsch, S., Meyer, A., Isler, E., & Schneider, S. (2008). The association between mothers' psychopathology, childrens' competences and psychological well-being in obese children. *Eat Weight Disord, 13*(3), 129–136.

Sanders, R. H., Han, A., Baker, J. S., & Cobley, S. (2015). Childhood obesity and its physical and psychological co-morbidities: A systematic review of Australian children and adolescents. *Eur J Pediatr, 174*(6), 715–746. doi:10.1007/s00431-015-2551-3.

Seacat, J. D., Dougal, S. C., & Roy, D. (2016). A daily diary assessment of female weight stigmatization. *J Health Psychol, 21*(2), 228–240. doi:10.1177/1359105314525067.

Ulrich-Lai, Y. M., & Ryan, K. K. (2014). Neuroendocrine circuits governing energy balance and stress regulation: Functional overlap and therapeutic implications. *Cell Metab, 19*(6), 910–925. doi:10.1016/j.cmet.2014.01.020.

Wannamethee, S. G., & Atkins, J. L. (2015). Muscle loss and obesity: The health implications of sarcopenia and sarcopenic obesity. *Proc Nutr Soc, 74*(4), 405–412. doi:10.1017/s002966511500169x.

Wee, C. C., Davis, R. B., Chiodi, S., Huskey, K. W., & Hamel, M. B. (2015). Sex, race, and the adverse effects of social stigma vs. other quality of life factors among primary care patients with moderate to severe obesity. *J Gen Intern Med, 30*(2), 229–235. doi:10.1007/s11606-014-3041-4.

Westermann, S., Rief, W., Euteneuer, F., & Kohlmann, S. (2015). Social exclusion and shame in obesity. *Eat Behav, 17*, 74–76. doi:10.1016/j.eatbeh.2015.01.001.

18 DSM 5 SUD Criterion 8 *Hazardous Use*

Joan Ifland
Food Addiction Training, LLC
Cincinnati, OH

Jennifer M. Cross
Authentic Living & Wellness - Life Coaching, Inc.
Downers Grove, IL

CONTENTS

Recurrent processed food use in situations in which it is physically hazardous. (American Psychiatric Association, 2013, p. 491)

18.1 INTRODUCTION

The physical hazards of processed food addiction (PFA) may not come to mind immediately. However, given the extensive similarities between drug and food abuse, it is not surprising that processed food abuse can be hazardous to the food addict. Indeed, comparisons can be made to classical scenarios of alcohol and alcohol-related hazards including operating machinery while impaired, fights, sexual consequences, suicide, and domestic violence (Vaca & D'Onofrio, 2014). The surprise at the similarities between drug and processed food abuse may come from stereotyping. Alcoholics may be stereotyped as violent (Schomerus et al., 2011), while the obese are stereotyped as sedentary (Hinman, Burmeister, Kiefner, Borushok, & Carels, 2015) but not vulnerable to physical dangers.

It is possible that stigmatization and judgment blind society to the dangers that food-addicted clients face (Seacat, Dougal, & Roy, 2016). Nonetheless, there is evidence that food-addicted clients are exposed to danger through physical limitations, compulsive behaviors, cognitive deficits, as well as low self-esteem that prolongs exposure to abusive relationships and promotes thoughts of suicide. A danger that is not necessarily shared with drug addicts is the consequences of being denied appropriate medical attention due to discrimination against the obese, lack of training in the special problems of the obese, and harmful medical treatment for weight loss (Bleich, Bandara, Bennett, Cooper, & Gudzune, 2014; Concors et al., 2016; Khandalavala, Rojanala, Geske, Koran-Scholl, & Guck, 2014).

As with other diagnostic criteria for substance use disorders (SUD), hazardous use may be easy to overlook or may be dismissed as not a serious indicator of severity of addiction. In this chapter, practitioners will gain insight into possible sources of danger in the lives of food-addicted clients. As with a number of the SUD diagnostic criteria, practitioners will want to carefully assess the safety of children in the food addict's house. With these insights, a solid scope of problem can be developed. It may be surprising to food-addicted clients themselves to see the extent of food-related hazards in their lives. As such, learning about the physical dangers of PFA may help clients find the motivation they need to undertake recovery and stay with it.

18.2 MANIFESTATIONS

The types of hazards that food-addicted clients endure are diverse and numerous. They include accidents, falls, interpersonal violence, suicide, defective food consumption, neglect, and barriers to effective medical treatment.

18.2.1 Accidents

Obese populations have been shown to have a higher rate of accidents than lean populations (Hoff et al., 2013; Kouvonen et al., 2013; Wang et al., 2015). Fast food outlets have drive-throughs, which are attractive to the obese, who may not be mobile or may feel too unsightly to appear in public. This encourages the distraction of eating in the car and may trigger lack of attention while driving (Kemps, Tiggemann, & Hollitt, 2014). Obese professional drivers have higher accident rates and obesity is an occupational hazard among professional drivers (Rosso, Perotto, Feola, Bruno, & Caramella, 2015; Sieber et al., 2014). The obese are disproportionately represented in mortality rates from motor vehicle accidents (Donnelly, Griffin, Sathiakumar, & McGwin, 2014). Poorly fitting seatbelts may be a factor (Reed, Ebert-Hamilton, & Rupp, 2012).

Impaired functioning may play a role in the accident rates of the obese. Sleepiness while driving may also be an issue. The obese have been shown to suffer from daytime sleepiness and related cognitive dysfunction (Igelstrom, Emtner, Lindberg, & Asenlof, 2013; Patel, Spaeth, & Basner, 2016). Sleepiness while driving may be related to consumption of sugary drinks (Horne & Baulk, 2004). Food-addicted clients also report suffering from "brain fog," described as slow thinking, difficulty focusing, confusion, lack of concentration, forgetfulness, or a haziness in thought processes (Ocon, 2013). Brain fog may be a contributor to accidents as well as other hazardous situations. A population with eating disorders versus a non–eating-disordered population displayed poor judgment about engaging in distracting behaviors while driving, such as changing clothes, reading, applying makeup, and combing/brushing their hair while driving (Glass et al., 2004).

Like drug addicts, processed food-addicted clients suffer from blackouts, although this phenomenon has not been studied. Food-addicted clients may leave home under dangerous circumstances in order to get a "fix." They may pursue processed foods in spite of storms and icy road conditions. They may also go out at dangerous times of the night. Although this syndrome is recognized in recovery communities, it does not appear to have been addressed in research.

A number of quotes from the food addiction 12-step manuals illustrate the nature of accidents that food-addicted clients may endure.

> More than once I drove in a blackout after stopping at a drive-through restaurant. I stayed too busy to go home because I knew I would eat too much and flop on the couch or into bed in a comatose state. (Food Addicts Anonymous, p. 181)

I fought my way into college, but I still lived with my parents. I prolonged going home while attending college and often stayed up late to binge in the coffee shops to the point of blacking out. I knew no other way of life. (Food Addicts Anonymous, p. 183)

I went back into the store and bought all the cakes I wanted and proceeded to make my way back home. I knew from experience that when I binged I got sleepy and would pass out. Usually when I did heavy bingeing I was home alone on the couch in front of the television. Now I was in my car, and I was scared. How was I going to eat all the food and get home without falling asleep behind the wheel? (Food Addicts Anonymous, p. 139)

The focal point of my food addiction during an entire year was pancakes. It began very quietly one day when I ordered a short stack (three pancakes) and then found myself having a short stack daily for six months. I remember a day in mid-winter when all of the roads were icy and many businesses were closed. I called the pancake house five miles away and they were open. Icy roads wouldn't stop me. I got in my car, and about half a mile down the main road, a station wagon collided with my car. I hurriedly exchanged information with the driver, thinking only of how I needed to get to the pancake house. Little did I know that I was becoming so dependent on this treat that nothing could stop me. (Food Addicts Anonymous, p. 164)

The mental anguish that food addiction created for me was so painful that:

I can't remember.
My thought process stops midstream.
My eyes are unable to focus.
My body can't operate at its potential.
I become numb and I create a fantasy world. (Food Addicts Anonymous, p. 166)

I used a lot of sugar to make me laugh and to fog out throughout my entire life. (Food Addicts Anonymous, p. 198)

The disease of PFA puts food-addicted clients at risk for accidents. Practitioners can ask for a history of accidents as well as periods of lost consciousness to develop the assessment of severity for this area.

18.2.2 Falls

The danger of falling is also higher for food-addicted clients due to complications of obesity. They may suffer fainting and dizziness (Lin & Bhattacharyya, 2014). They may also experience weak bone, muscles, and joints (Mignardot, Olivier, Promayon, & Nougier, 2013; Scott, Daly, Sanders, & Ebeling, 2015; Zhang, Peterson, Su, & Wang, 2015). In some cases, they fall from breaking a hip (Meyer, Willett, Flint, & Feskanich, 2016). Further, pain may put food-addicted clients off balance (Mitchell, Lord, Harvey, & Close, 2015). Neuropathy can also affect balance (Toosizadeh, Mohler, Armstrong, Talal, & Najafi, 2015). For a number of reasons, food-addicted clients may be at risk for falling.

18.2.3 Interpersonal Violence

Interpersonal violence is correlated with obesity. Using HARK (humiliate–afraid–rape–kick), an interpersonal violence (IVP) screening tool, Davies et al. found that the obese suffered from IVP at a rate of 30% versus 20% for nonobese. Among women who reported IVP, the odds were 1.67 times greater for obesity than non-IVP women (Davies, Lehman, Perry, & McCall-Hosenfeld, 2015). Possible explanations for the tolerance and attraction of IVP among the obese are low self-esteem and impaired general capabilities, which would otherwise have enabled the food addict to get help, resolve the situation, or leave. Low self-esteem leads to staying in abusive relationships (Bosch, Weaver, Arnold, & Clark, 2015).

These quotes illustrate the syndrome:

My father had beaten me and after our marriage, my husband began physically abusing me. I was in a bad situation. I had such low self-esteem, I thought I'd done something to deserve the violence, and, again, I felt I had nowhere to turn. I left my parents' home in September, and by December, I'd gained 30 pounds. (Food Addicts in Recovery Anonymous, p. 179)

The anticipation and the desire always seemed greatest when this little boy was made fun of, pinched, hit, or ignored by classmates and teachers. I could not wait to run home to my best friend, food. (Food Addicts Anonymous, p. 259)

In about a year, I went from 135 pounds to 198 pounds. I felt awful. I kept trying to diet and I would promise my husband that I would lose weight, yet I could not stick to a diet. My life was really falling apart. I was angry all the time. My husband and I had vicious fights that often resulted in physical abuse, initiated by either one of us. I was just as guilty as he was. (Food Addicts Anonymous, p. 242)

I should have died the night I kicked the man I was living with. I was retaliating for his beating, and he took a knife to me. (Food Addicts in Recovery Anonymous, p. 167)

Interpersonal violence may be difficult to surface during the assessment. Food-addicted clients may be too ashamed to talk about it. Or they may be prone to minimizing its importance. Practitioners may wait for several sessions before clients are able to talk about violence at home.

18.2.4 Suicide

Danger from suicide should not be a surprise to practitioners. Suicide has been shown to be more prevalent in obese populations (Brewer-Smyth, 2014). Dutton et al. found that the greater the BMI, the greater the likelihood of suicide ideation in a population of college students, and that a sense of being burdensome was a mediator (Dutton, Bodell, Smith, & Joiner, 2013). Chen et al. found that suicide ideation correlated with lack of college education, a history of suicide ideation and/or behavior, psychological distress, hopelessness, loneliness, history of physical and/or sexual abuse, and lifetime major depression (Chen et al., 2012). In a study of bariatric surgery patients, the suicide rate was found to be three times higher than the general population (Tindle et al., 2010). Shin et al. found that poor body image was a factor in suicide ideation among participants with a higher BMI (Shin et al., 2015). Christiansen et al. found an association between use of diet pills and suicide (Christensen, Kristensen, Bartels, Bliddal, & Astrup, 2007). Co-addictions such as workaholism, sex, drinking, and smoking (Olsen, 2011) can also encourage suicide.

These quotes show the profound distress that can precede a suicide attempt.

The years marched on and my disease progressed. Twice I attempted suicide because I could not live with the depression that always followed a binge. (Food Addicts Anonymous, p. 143)

My weight was now approximately 275 pounds. The doctor stopped the Pondamin prescription because I was gaining weight. I was bingeing on sugar, flour and wheat at least once a week and sometimes more often than that. At 68" inches tall, I was as wide as I was tall. I lost all hope and contemplated suicide as the only way out of my situation. (Food Addicts Anonymous, p. 245)

After nine months of shaky abstinence, I picked up sugar and binged and purged non-stop for four days. I was having spontaneous nosebleeds, alarming my therapist and thinking constantly about suicide. (Food Addicts Anonymous, p. 263)

I used to think that food addiction was just a physical illness, but it's a mental and spiritual illness, as well. It's deadly. I tried to kill myself with an overdose of pills one night. (Food Addicts in Recovery Anonymous, p. 162)

I never felt like I was enough. At one point, I tried to throw myself out of a moving car and was admitted to the hospital in a straitjacket. (Food Addicts in Recovery Anonymous, p. 297)

As might be obvious, assessing for current suicide plans and past attempts gives important information about the severity of the condition. The self-administered Patient Health Questionnaire (PHQ-9) includes a one-question assessment for suicidal ideation: "Have you thought that you would be better off dead or that you wanted to hurt yourself in some way?" (Kroenke, Spitzer, & Williams, 2001).

18.2.5 Defective Foods

Research shows that obese populations have a muted neuroresponse to disgust, including in response to contaminated foods (Watkins et al., 2015). Reduced disgust has been shown to be accompanied by reduced restraint (Houben & Havermans, 2012). It is possible that this lack of restraint, coupled with severe compulsion and loss of decision-making and memory, creates the circumstances under which a food addict might eat defective foods. The following quotes illustrate the problem.

> When we didn't have a bottle-opener, we were so determined to have some that we smashed the top and tried to drink through the jagged glass. (Food Addicts in Recovery Anonymous, p. 211)
>
> Normal people don't eat food that is stale or that has fallen on the floor. They don't eat until they burn their mouths with things that are too hot. (Food Addicts in Recovery Anonymous, p. 202)
>
> I ate burnt or frozen foods. Binge foods consumed my every thought and feeling. (Food Addicts Anonymous, p. 105)
>
> Instead of eating it, I gave the ice cream to the dog, and then got the rest out from the freezer and threw it in the trash. I went to bed, trying to resist the temptation. I even called a few people for support. But the disease was stronger and I went back to the kitchen, got the ice cream out of the trash and ate that bite I had wanted in the first place—a new low for me. (Food Addicts Anonymous, p. 23)
>
> I learned in the rehabilitation center that food addiction is a disease. I came to admit and accept that I stole, lied and cheated to get to my substance. I ate off the floor and out of garbage cans. (Food Addicts Anonymous, p. 192)

Finding out if the client is eating contaminated foods may be difficult for the practitioner initially, as shame may be a barrier to sharing about this behavior. However, the behavior is generally known in recovery communities and the practitioner may be able to explain the adaptation in the brain. This may prove to be a relief to the client.

18.2.6 Neglected Children

Child neglect in households with obese parents is well documented (Harper, 2014; Helton & Liechty, 2014; Neumark-Sztainer et al., 2014). Children are more likely to be unsupervised in households where processed foods are readily available (Helton & Liechty, 2014). Parents and siblings with raging and depressive symptoms contribute to home violence, which is associated with increased likelihood of developing obesity (Sumner et al., 2015). Children of obese parents are more likely to suffer adult obesity and other diseases (Sumner et al., 2015; Vickers, 2014).

It is possible that clients are too deeply compromised by their addiction to attend to children (Lydecker & Grilo, 2016). Parents may be too tired to provide healthy foods and may rely on convenient processed foods. Their self-esteem may be too low to withstand children's demands for addictive foods (Shloim, Edelson, Martin, & Hetherington, 2015). Obese children are more likely to have been present to violence than lean children (Midei & Matthews, 2011).

Parents may be well intentioned but impaired mobility may curtail their ability to care for children (Daviaux, Mignardot, Cornu, & Deschamps, 2014). Obesity during pregnancy can also present a threat to the well-being of the baby (Wojcicki, Young, Perham-Hester, de Schweinitz, & Gessner, 2015). Sexually abused women are more likely to be obese at their first pregnancy (Gisladottir et al., 2014).

These quotes show how the demands and consequences of PFA may put children in hazardous situations.

> I was now alone with my primary addiction, food. My husband, children, job and other relationships all took a back seat to my disease of food addiction. The pain of who I was, the shame of who I had

become, and the insanity caught up with me. I was forty-one years old and hated myself and almost everyone else. (Food Addicts Anonymous, p. 118)

My self-esteem was so low and there were long periods of time that I never bathed or took care of my home. I neglected my children. I always said I wanted a close-knit family, but in reality, I wanted everyone away from me so I could eat. I wanted to eat alone. I didn't want to share my food with anyone. When I was bingeing myself into oblivion, there was too much shame to let anyone see how much and how I ate. (Food Addicts Anonymous, pp. 141–142)

[*As a child*] I was appeased with food to keep me quiet, occupied and calm during the turmoil. (Food Addicts Anonymous, p. 145)

One day I was eating a meal when my son started howling. Without thinking, I hit him with my fist and knocked the wind out of him. He looked at me with his big eyes and cried. We were both stunned. I was never raised with violence, and yet I hit my child. I realized then that I had the alcoholic rage described in Alcoholics Anonymous. My fury came from nowhere. I never thought that I would be capable of abusing one of my children, but whatever made child abusers harm their children lived in me. (Food Addicts in Recovery Anonymous, p. 94)

I ate until I blacked out. I would wake up on top of and surrounded by boxes and bags. (Food Addicts Anonymous, p. 130)

The day started like any other, without breakfast, for my stomach was distended from the binge of candy, cookies, and carbohydrates from which I had passed out the night before. (Food Addicts Anonymous, p. 152)

Another major insight came to me while I was detoxifying. I actually had blackouts from sugar, wheat and flour. I started remembering how, at night, I would fix myself a stack of pancakes and sit down in front of the television with my plate. I would look into the plate and it would be empty. I must have eaten them but I couldn't remember even putting one forkful in my mouth. (Food Addicts Anonymous, pp.139–140)

Practitioners need to assess for the safety of children under the care of food-addicted clients. As food-addicted clients make more healthy foods for the household, children may become better nourished and easier to handle. The process of describing the scope of problem as far as children are concerned is tricky due to shame issues, yet the practitioner can find a way to present improvements in child care as a relief to the client, rather than an indication of failure.

18.2.7 Harmful Medical Practices

Research shows that obese populations experience barriers to medical care (Aleem, Lasky, Brooks, & Batsis, 2015). Health professionals have been shown to provide poor care to obese patients: "Many healthcare providers hold strong negative attitudes and stereotypes about people with obesity. There is considerable evidence that such attitudes influence person-perceptions, judgment, interpersonal behaviour and decision-making." Such attitudes may discourage the obese from seeking medical care (Phelan et al., 2015). Excess fat interferes with medical procedures in general and evaluation of assault (Byard, 2012; Kramer, 2013). A study of Australian students showed that health students were as prejudiced as non–health students (Robinson, Ball, & Leveritt, 2014). Bias may occur because health professionals are not trained in the environment as a cause of obesity nor in the difficulties of losing weight (Khandalavala et al., 2014; O'Brien, Puhl, Latner, Mir, & Hunter, 2010).

Another source of hazards for the obese come from the possibility that medical professionals may engage in harmful practices in treating food-addicted clients for "weight loss" instead of PFA. Research suggests that medical care is lacking when weight regain starts to occur after bariatric surgery (Jones, Cleator, & Yorke, 2016). Bariatric surgery patients exhibit slow weight regain (Magro et al., 2008; Sjostrom et al., 2004) and a tendency to develop alcoholism (Svensson et al., 2013). Pharmaceuticals add to the distress with side effects such as weight regain (Goldstein & Potvin, 1994), heart disease with fenfluramine and dexfenfluramine (Connolly & McGoon, 1999), suicide ideation with rimonabant (Christensen et al., 2007), memory loss and heightened anxiety from lorcaserin and phentermine–topiramate (Woloshin & Schwartz, 2014), hypertension from sibutramine (Rich, Rubin, Walker, Schneeweiss, & Abenhaim, 2000), and bowel leakage from orlistat (Hollywood & Ogden, 2011).

Food-addicted clients may also suffer financial depletion, leading to inability to seek medical care (Jorm et al., 2003).

These quotes illustrate the kinds of hazards that food-addicted clients can experience from medical practices.

> Two years later, when we decided to have another baby, I was seeing a doctor who was very strict. He put me on a starvation diet, and every time I went in, he yelled at me. He said I was gaining weight. I couldn't believe it, because I was following the diet. I could hardly walk and was having a hard time, but no one sympathized. … It turned out that I had twins. (Food Addicts in Recovery Anonymous, p. 53)
>
> Three pills worked, so four, and then five, seemed better. The pills made me want to drink more, which made me want to smoke more. In the end, they made me do everything faster. That included eating faster, and I took diet pills all the way up to where I weighed more than 350 pounds. (Food Addicts in Recovery Anonymous, p. 64)
>
> Fifty pounds later, I heard about the stomach stapling surgery. I was depressed; I was the largest I had ever been in my whole life—353 pounds. The doctor said I was morbidly obese and would qualify for the surgery. … I was driven with the fact that I was going to lose the weight this time and be thin. Well one year later I still wasn't thin. I was down to 213 pounds and couldn't lose any more. I eventually broke open the staples and was able to consume more food. (Food Addicts Anonymous, p. 169)

To conclude the Introduction, food-addicted clients face a surprising variety of dangers. Practitioners can adopt gentle yet perceptive approaches to assessing for hazardous use. By assessing for the role of fat tissue, the practitioner may look for hazards related to balance as well as hazards related to inadequate medical care. If the practitioner assesses positive for sleepiness, then hazards related to driving and caring for children can be discussed.

Dangers may be hidden. Shame and memory loss may interfere with disclosure of dangerous behavior (Kemps & Tiggemann, 2005). For the assessment, it is helpful for the professional to carefully examine their own attitudes toward obese clients. Health professionals may be judgmental and critical and miss dangers (Aleem et al., 2015).

Including hazards in the scope of problem may open the client to a new way of thinking about food abuse. The client may not recognize dangers as being related to processed PFA (Young, Mahfoud, Walker, Jenkins, & Stanton, 2008). The practitioner has the opportunity to significantly improve the safety of the client by assessing thoroughly for hazardous use.

18.2.8 Limitations of the Chapter

Physical hazards related to failure to cut back are covered in Criterion 2. Dangerous weight-loss behavior can include diet drugs (addiction, suicide, heart damage, eating and taking the pills, laxative), anorexia (death), inappropriate surgery (burst stomach, breaking open staples, premature skin removal surgery), bulimia (damage to internal organs), excessive exercise (damage to bones), and periodic starvation. Physically dangerous health consequences will be covered in Criterion 9, use in spite of knowledge of consequences. Cardiovascular disease, hypertension, diabetes (including harmful use of insulin to maintain addiction), cancer, Alzheimer's, excess fat tissue. Physical problems related to withdrawal will be covered in Criterion 11.

18.3 EVIDENCE FOR MECHANISMS OF HAZARDOUS USE

An overview of the impairments of obese populations helps fill in the picture for hazards of chronic processed food use. Several manifestations of vulnerability to hazardous use share common dysfunctions in basic neurological and physical impairments. In general, obese populations have been found to make poor decisions, have little memory of mistakes, and exhibit an inability to learn from mistakes (Yesavage et al., 2014). This can set up a tendency for accidents and neglect. Involvement in dangerous relationships may stem from intense cravings which impair attention to care and safety of self and children (Werthmann, Jansen, & Roefs, 2014).

Further, impaired disgust centers can promote the rapid ingestion of unsafe foods (Carnell, Gibson, Benson, Ochner, & Geliebter, 2012). There is also biochemistry, which is relevant to personality disorders. These include unstable glucose and downregulated neurotransmitter pathways (Fontes-Villalba et al., 2014; Stanfill et al., 2015). Physical disabilities limit capacity to prevent accidents and to care for self and children. Weak bone and musculature (Ormsbee et al., 2014), excessive fat tissue, dim vision, and blindness (D'Hondt et al., 2011) can also be factors in the inability to avoid hazards. Muscle strength rather than muscle mass is a key factor (Scott et al., 2014). Shortness of breath (Bernhardt & Babb, 2014) and joint mobility (Belczak, de Godoy, Belzack, Ramos, & Caffaro, 2014) can also contribute to physical vulnerabilities in a number of ways.

Fatigue and disturbed sleep (Jarosz et al., 2014; Kim, Kim, Lee, & Park, 2014) impairs the ability to pay attention and provide care. This can come from sleep apnea (Vijayan, 2012), night eating (Cleator et al., 2014; de Zwaan, Roerig, Crosby, Karaz, & Mitchell, 2006; Nolan & Geliebter, 2016), and sitting up to sleep to prevent choking on bile (Gilani, Quan, Pynnonen, & Shin, 2016). In general, too much or too little sleep is also associated with unintentional injuries (Kim et al., 2014).

There is also an issue of the relative severity of injuries. Obese populations may sustain more severe injury in terms of bone fractures (Meyer et al., 2016) and joint injuries, including dislocation (Ranavolo et al., 2013).

Food-addicted clients may also overestimate their capabilities. They may overestimate physical capabilities from poor judgment or lack of awareness of condition of body (Nikolas et al., 2016; Yesavage et al., 2014). This can occur in sports, recreation, exercise, and lifting.

There is evidence for general and varied impairment in capabilities in the obese. By impairing physical abilities, judgment, and mental alertness, these consequences of chronic processed food abuse can make food-addicted clients vulnerable to injuries under hazardous use.

18.4 APPLICATION

18.4.1 EDUCATION

As with all aspects of recovery from addiction, education is the key. Practitioners can connect processed foods with general risk of injury. Educating clients about the nature of the mental and emotional impairment related to processed foods can be the beginning of a process of awareness that eventually can help keep the addict safe from hazards (Jauch-Chara & Oltmanns, 2014; Yesavage et al., 2014). Clients may be surprised to learn about the difference between addictive processed and unprocessed foods and the impact on the brain, hormones, and peptides. Clients may already be aware that some foods are associated with drowsiness but may not have considered the hazards of driving while eating.

A valuable early-stage effort would be to reduce harm from hazardous driving while distracted or sleepy. A brief intervention has been shown to work in alcohol (Harris, Louis-Jacques, & Knight, 2014), so just raising the issue might be enough to reduce the risk of harm from driving while impaired or distracted.

The practitioner can also connect joint, gait, and balance issues to fall risk (Mignardot, Olivier, Promayon, & Nougier, 2010). Encouraging the client to pay attention while moving about can help here. Relief from joint pain has been reported as early as the first few weeks of eliminating processed foods. This prospect can be a good motivator, which can be reinforced by the opportunity to reduce the risk of a fall.

Similarly, the practitioner can encourage restoration of muscle and bone strength (Scott et al., 2015) through the use of YouTube exercise videos. These videos have a number of advantages.

They are free and they come in all lengths. They also cover many types of exercise, from yoga to walking to chair exercises to more strenuous aerobic exercises. The key is to start very slowly. Ten minutes of chair exercise may be all that a client can handle. If the client is very attached to television, these exercises can be learned and executed while watching another program.

In cases of thoughts of suicide and distorted body weight perception (Shin et al., 2015), the practitioner will want to educate the client about how processed foods can cause chemical reactions in the brain that are associated with despair and hopelessness. Although thoughts can certainly be associated with real life and childhood conditioning, the client can be encouraged to hang on until abstinence from mood-altering food and cues is achieved.

Harm to children can be reduced through education and monitoring. Cognitive behavioral therapy has been shown to help children regain functioning (Tsiros et al., 2008).

The practitioner can tie intense cravings to dangerous use of food. With cravings under control, the overwhelming urge to eat can be curtailed and eating contaminated foods, scaling foods, or frozen foods can be contained. Clients can be encouraged to prepare enough foods in advance that eating dangerously is avoided.

The practitioner can also serve clients by researching health professionals who are prepared to treat the obese appropriately, effectively, and with dignity. Food-addicted clients can be persuaded to avoid bariatric surgery and other harmful weight-loss recommendations in lieu of effective recovery from processed PFA.

18.4.2 Cultural Influences

The issue of hazardous use can be shameful to addicts. It is helpful to explain that the addict did not bring the disease upon themselves. PFA has been loosely correlated with BMI. There are now over 2 billion people with elevated BMI. Emphasizing that the disease is spread by the food industry just as addictive smoking was spread by the tobacco companies may give clients some room to talk about their hazardous use. Complications related to hazardous use may be unique to PFA because of the nature of the disease.

The most pronounced cultural factor in hazardous use in PFA is the presence of excess fat tissue. It contributes to low self-esteem, which can contribute to both hazards from violent interpersonal relationships and inability to demand appropriate medical care.

Another prominent feature of PFA is the intense availability of substances. This means that cue-induced cognitive impairment can be virtually constant. And the dense availability of drive-throughs is an ever-present temptation to drive dangerously.

The pain of condemnation from the culture is not unique to PFA. However, it contributes to self-blame and self-neglect, which increases the chance of physical harm.

18.5 CONCLUSION

Physical hazards are associated with addiction to processed foods. It is worthwhile to probe for them. Clinical practice shows a reversal of factors associated with risk of injury when processed foods are eliminated from the diet and range of cognitive and physical capabilities are restored. Risk of injury is a surprising element of addiction to processed food but it can be managed.

REFERENCES

Aleem, S., Lasky, R., Brooks, W. B., & Batsis, J. A. (2015). Obesity perceptions and documentation among primary care clinicians at a rural academic health center. *Obes Res Clin Pract*, *9*(4), 408–415. doi:10.1016/j.orcp.2015.08.014.

American Psychiatric Association. (2013). *The Diagnostic and Statistical Manual of Mental Disorders, Fifth Edition* (Vol. 5).

Belczak, C. E., de Godoy, J. M., Belzack, S. Q., Ramos, R. N., & Caffaro, R. A. (2014). Obesity and worsening of chronic venous disease and joint mobility. *Phlebology*, *29*(8), 500–504. doi:10.1177/0268355513492510.

Bernhardt, V., & Babb, T. G. (2014). Weight loss reduces dyspnea on exertion in obese women. *Respir Physiol Neurobiol*, *204*, 86–92. doi:10.1016/j.resp.2014.09.004.

Bleich, S. N., Bandara, S., Bennett, W. L., Cooper, L. A., & Gudzune, K. A. (2014). Impact of non-physician health professionals' BMI on obesity care and beliefs. *Obesity (Silver Spring)*, *22*(12), 2476–2480. doi:10.1002/oby.20881.

Bosch, J., Weaver, T. L., Arnold, L. D., & Clark, E. M. (2015). The impact of intimate partner violence on women's physical health: Findings from the Missouri behavioral risk factor surveillance system. *J Interpers Violence*. doi:10.1177/0886260515599162.

Brewer-Smyth, K. (2014). Obesity, traumatic brain injury, childhood abuse, and suicide attempts in females at risk. *Rehabil Nurs*, *39*(4), 183–191. doi:10.1002/rnj.150.

Byard, R. W. (2012). The complex spectrum of forensic issues arising from obesity. *Forensic Sci Med Pathol*, *8*(4), 402–413. doi:10.1007/s12024-012-9322-5.

Carnell, S., Gibson, C., Benson, L., Ochner, C. N., & Geliebter, A. (2012). Neuroimaging and obesity: Current knowledge and future directions. *Obes Rev*, *13*(1), 43–56. doi:10.1111/j.1467-789X.2011.00927.x.

Chen, E. Y., Fettich, K. C., Tierney, M., Cummings, H., Berona, J., Weissman, J., … Coccaro, E. (2012). Factors associated with suicide ideation in severely obese bariatric surgery-seeking individuals. *Suicide Life Threat Behav*, *42*(5), 541–549. doi:10.1111/j.1943-278X.2012.00110.x.

Christensen, R., Kristensen, P. K., Bartels, E. M., Bliddal, H., & Astrup, A. (2007). Efficacy and safety of the weight-loss drug rimonabant: A meta-analysis of randomised trials. *Lancet*, *370*(9600), 1706–1713. doi:10.1016/s0140-6736(07)61721-8.

Cleator, J., Judd, P., James, M., Abbott, J., Sutton, C. J., & Wilding, J. P. (2014). Characteristics and perspectives of night-eating behaviour in a severely obese population. *Clin Obes*, *4*(1), 30–38. doi:10.1111/cob.12037.

Concors, S. J., Ecker, B. L., Maduka, R., Furukawa, A., Raper, S. E., Dempsey, D. D., … Dumon, K. R. (2016). Complications and surveillance after bariatric surgery. *Curr Treat Options Neurol*, *18*(1), 5. doi:10.1007/s11940-015-0383-0.

Connolly, H. M., & McGoon, M. D. (1999). Obesity drugs and the heart. *Curr Probl Cardiol*, *24*(12), 745–792.

Daviaux, Y., Mignardot, J. B., Cornu, C., & Deschamps, T. (2014). Effects of total sleep deprivation on the perception of action capabilities. *Exp Brain Res*, *232*(7), 2243–2253. doi:10.1007/s00221-014-3915-z.

Davies, R., Lehman, E., Perry, A., & McCall-Hosenfeld, J. S. (2015). Association of intimate partner violence and health-care provider-identified obesity. *Women Health*, *56*(5), 561–575. doi:10.1080/03630242.2015.1101741.

de Zwaan, M., Roerig, D. B., Crosby, R. D., Karaz, S., & Mitchell, J. E. (2006). Nighttime eating: A descriptive study. *Int J Eat Disord*, *39*(3), 224–232. doi:10.1002/eat.20246.

D'Hondt, E., Segers, V., Deforche, B., Shultz, S. P., Tanghe, A., Gentier, I., … Lenoir, M. (2011). The role of vision in obese and normal-weight children's gait control. *Gait Posture*, *33*(2), 179–184. doi:10.1016/j.gaitpost.2010.10.090.

Donnelly, J. P., Griffin, R. L., Sathiakumar, N., & McGwin, G., Jr. (2014). Obesity and vehicle type as risk factors for injury caused by motor vehicle collision. *J Trauma Acute Care Surg*, *76*(4), 1116–1121. doi:10.1097/ta.0000000000000168.

Dutton, G. R., Bodell, L. P., Smith, A. R., & Joiner, T. E. (2013). Examination of the relationship between obesity and suicidal ideation. *Int J Obes (Lond)*, *37*(9), 1282–1286. doi:10.1038/ijo.2012.224.

Fontes-Villalba, M., Jonsson, T., Granfeldt, Y., Frassetto, L. A., Sundquist, J., Sundquist, K., … Lindeberg, S. (2014). A healthy diet with and without cereal grains and dairy products in patients with type 2 diabetes: Study protocol for a random-order cross-over pilot study—Alimentation and Diabetes in Lanzarote—ADILAN. *Trials*, *15*, 2. doi:10.1186/1745-6215-15-2.

Gilani, S., Quan, S. F., Pynnonen, M. A., & Shin, J. J. (2016). Obstructive sleep apnea and gastroesophageal reflux: A multivariate population-level analysis. *Otolaryngol Head Neck Surg*, *154*(2), 390–395. doi:10.1177/0194599815621557.

Gisladottir, A,, Harlow, B. L., Gudmundsdottir, B., Bjarnadottir, R. I., Jonsdottir, E., Aspelund, T., … Valdimarsdottir, U. A. (2014). Risk factors and health during pregnancy among women previously exposed to sexual violence. *Acta Obstet Gynecol Scand*, *93*(4), 351–358. doi:10.1111/aogs.12331.

Glass, J., Mitchell, J. E., de Zwaan, M., Wonderlich, S., Crosby, R. D., Roerig, J., … Voxland, J. (2004). Eating behavior and other distracting behaviors while driving among patients with eating disorders. *Compr Psychiatry*, *45*(3), 235–237. doi:10.1016/j.comppsych.2003.12.006.

Goldstein, D. J., & Potvin, J. H. (1994). Long-term weight loss: The effect of pharmacologic agents. *Am J Clin Nutr*, *60*(5), 647–657; discussion 658–649.

Harper, N. S. (2014). Neglect: Failure to thrive and obesity. *Pediatr Clin North Am, 61*(5), 937–957. doi:10.1016/j.pcl.2014.06.006.

Harris, S. K., Louis-Jacques, J., & Knight, J. R. (2014). Screening and brief intervention for alcohol and other abuse. *Adolesc Med State Art Rev, 25*(1), 126–156.

Helton, J. J., & Liechty, J. M. (2014). Obesity prevalence among youth investigated for maltreatment in the United States. *Child Abuse Negl, 38*(4), 768–775. doi:10.1016/j.chiabu.2013.08.011.

Hinman, N. G., Burmeister, J. M., Kiefner, A. E., Borushok, J., & Carels, R. A. (2015). Stereotypical portrayals of obesity and the expression of implicit weight bias. *Body Image, 12*, 32–35. doi:10.1016/j.bodyim.2014.09.002.

Hoff, J., Grell, J., Lohrman, N., Stehly, C., Stoltzfus, J., Wainwright, G., & Hoff, W. S. (2013). Distracted driving and implications for injury prevention in adults. *J Trauma Nurs, 20*(1), 31–34; quiz 35–36. doi:10.1097/JTN.0b013e318286616c.

Hollywood, A., & Ogden, J. (2011). Taking Orlistat: Predicting weight loss over 6 months. *J Obes, 2011*, 806896. doi:10.1155/2011/806896.

Horne, J. A., & Baulk, S. D. (2004). Awareness of sleepiness when driving. *Psychophysiology, 41*(1), 161–165. doi:10.1046/j.1469-8986.2003.00130.x.

Houben, K., & Havermans, R. C. (2012). A delicious fly in the soup. The relationship between disgust, obesity, and restraint. *Appetite, 58*(3), 827–830. doi:10.1016/j.appet.2012.01.018.

Igelstrom, H., Emtner, M., Lindberg, E., & Asenlof, P. (2013). Level of agreement between methods for measuring moderate to vigorous physical activity and sedentary time in people with obstructive sleep apnea and obesity. *Phys Ther, 93*(1), 50–59. doi:10.2522/ptj.20120123.

Jarosz, P. A., Davis, J. E., Yarandi, H. N., Farkas, R., Feingold, E., Shippings, S. H., … Williams, D. (2014). Obesity in urban women: Associations with sleep and sleepiness, fatigue and activity. *Womens Health Issues, 24*(4), e447–e454. doi:10.1016/j.whi.2014.04.005.

Jauch-Chara, K., & Oltmanns, K. M. (2014). Obesity—A neuropsychological disease? Systematic review and neuropsychological model. *Prog Neurobiol, 114*, 84–101. doi:10.1016/j.pneurobio.2013.12.001.

Jones, L., Cleator, J., & Yorke, J. (2016). Maintaining weight loss after bariatric surgery: When the spectator role is no longer enough. *Clin Obes, 6*(4), 249–258. doi:10.1111/cob.12152.

Jorm, A. F., Korten, A. E., Christensen, H., Jacomb, P. A., Rodgers, B., & Parslow, R. A. (2003). Association of obesity with anxiety, depression and emotional well-being: A community survey. *Aust N Z J Public Health, 27*(4), 434–440.

Kemps, E., & Tiggemann, M. (2005). Working memory performance and preoccupying thoughts in female dieters: Evidence for a selective central executive impairment. *Br J Clin Psychol, 44*(Pt 3), 357–366. doi:10.1348/014466505X35272.

Kemps, E., Tiggemann, M., & Hollitt, S. (2014). Biased attentional processing of food cues and modification in obese individuals. *Health Psychol, 33*(11), 1391–1401. doi:10.1037/hea0000069.

Khandalavala, B. N., Rojanala, A., Geske, J. A., Koran-Scholl, J. B., & Guck, T. P. (2014). Obesity bias in primary care providers. *Fam Med, 46*(7), 532–535.

Kim, Y. Y., Kim, U. N., Lee, J. S., & Park, J. H. (2014). The effect of sleep duration on the risk of unintentional injury in Korean adults. *J Prev Med Public Health, 47*(3), 150–157. doi:10.3961/jpmph.2014.47.3.150.

Kouvonen, A., Kivimaki, M., Oksanen, T., Pentti, J., De Vogli, R., Virtanen, M., & Vahtera, J. (2013). Obesity and occupational injury: A prospective cohort study of 69,515 public sector employees. *PLoS One, 8*(10), e77178. doi:10.1371/journal.pone.0077178.

Kramer, K. (2013). Overweight and the sexual assault forensic medical examination: A pressing problem. *J Forensic Leg Med, 20*(4), 207–210. doi:10.1016/j.jflm.2012.07.013.

Kroenke, K., Spitzer, R. L., & Williams, J. B. (2001). The PHQ-9: Validity of a brief depression severity measure. *J Gen Intern Med, 16*(9), 606–613.

Lin, H. W., & Bhattacharyya, N. (2014). Impact of dizziness and obesity on the prevalence of falls and fall-related injuries. *Laryngoscope, 124*(12), 2797–2801. doi:10.1002/lary.24806.

Lydecker, J. A., & Grilo, C. M. (2016). Children of parents with BED have more eating behavior disturbance than children of parents with obesity or healthy weight. *Int J Eat Disord, 50*(6), 648–656. doi:10.1002/eat.22648.

Magro, D. O., Geloneze, B., Delfini, R., Pareja, B. C., Callejas, F., & Pareja, J. C. (2008). Long-term weight regain after gastric bypass: A 5-year prospective study. *Obes Surg, 18*(6), 648–651. doi:10.1007/s11695-007-9265-1.

Meyer, H. E., Willett, W. C., Flint, A. J., & Feskanich, D. (2016). Abdominal obesity and hip fracture: Results from the Nurses' Health Study and the Health Professionals Follow-up Study. *Osteoporos Int, 27*(6), 2127–2136. doi:10.1007/s00198-016-3508-8.

Midei, A. J., & Matthews, K. A. (2011). Interpersonal violence in childhood as a risk factor for obesity: A systematic review of the literature and proposed pathways. *Obes Rev, 12*(5), e159–e172. doi:10.1111/j.1467-789X.2010.00823.x.

Mignardot, J. B., Olivier, I., Promayon, E., & Nougier, V. (2010). Obesity impact on the attentional cost for controlling posture. *PLoS One*, *5*(12), e14387. doi:10.1371/journal.pone.0014387.

Mignardot, J. B., Olivier, I., Promayon, E., & Nougier, V. (2013). Origins of balance disorders during a daily living movement in obese: Can biomechanical factors explain everything? *PLoS One*, *8*(4), e60491. doi:10.1371/journal.pone.0060491.

Mitchell, R. J., Lord, S. R., Harvey, L. A., & Close, J. C. (2015). Obesity and falls in older people: Mediating effects of disease, sedentary behavior, mood, pain and medication use. *Arch Gerontol Geriatr*, *60*(1), 52–58. doi:10.1016/j.archger.2014.09.006.

Neumark-Sztainer, D., MacLehose, R., Loth, K., Fulkerson, J. A., Eisenberg, M. E., & Berge, J. (2014). What's for dinner? Types of food served at family dinner differ across parent and family characteristics. *Public Health Nutr*, *17*(1), 145–155. doi:10.1017/s1368980012004594.

Nikolas, M. A., Elmore, A. L., Franzen, L., O'Neal, E., Kearney, J. K., & Plumert, J. M. (2016). Risky bicycling behavior among youth with and without attention-deficit hyperactivity disorder. *J Child Psychol Psychiatry*, *57*(2), 141–148. doi:10.1111/jcpp.12491.

Nolan, L. J., & Geliebter, A. (2016). "Food addiction" is associated with night eating severity. *Appetite*, *98*, 89–94. doi:10.1016/j.appet.2015.12.025.

O'Brien, K. S., Puhl, R. M., Latner, J. D., Mir, A. S., & Hunter, J. A. (2010). Reducing anti-fat prejudice in preservice health students: A randomized trial. *Obesity (Silver Spring)*, *18*(11), 2138–2144. doi:10.1038/oby.2010.79.

Ocon, A. J. (2013). Caught in the thickness of brain fog: Exploring the cognitive symptoms of Chronic Fatigue Syndrome. *Front Physiol*, *4*, 63. doi:10.3389/fphys.2013.00063.

Olsen, C. M. (2011). Natural rewards, neuroplasticity, and non-drug addictions. *Neuropharmacology*, *61*(7), 1109–1122. doi:10.1016/j.neuropharm.2011.03.010.

Ormsbee, M. J., Prado, C. M., Ilich, J. Z., Purcell, S., Siervo, M., Folsom, A., & Panton, L. (2014). Osteosarcopenic obesity: The role of bone, muscle, and fat on health. *J Cachexia Sarcopenia Muscle*, *5*(3), 183–192. doi:10.1007/s13539-014-0146-x.

Patel, V. C., Spaeth, A. M., & Basner, M. (2016). Relationships between time use and obesity in a representative sample of Americans. *Obesity (Silver Spring)*, *24*(10), 2164–2175. doi:10.1002/oby.21596.

Phelan, S. M., Burgess, D. J., Yeazel, M. W., Hellerstedt, W. L., Griffin, J. M., & van Ryn, M. (2015). Impact of weight bias and stigma on quality of care and outcomes for patients with obesity. *Obes Rev*, *16*(4), 319–326. doi:10.1111/obr.12266.

Ranavolo, A., Donini, L. M., Mari, S., Serrao, M., Silvetti, A., Iavicoli, S., … Draicchio, F. (2013). Lower-limb joint coordination pattern in obese subjects. *Biomed Res Int*, *2013*, 142323. doi:10.1155/2013/142323.

Reed, M. P., Ebert-Hamilton, S. M., & Rupp, J. D. (2012). Effects of obesity on seat belt fit. *Traffic Inj Prev*, *13*(4), 364–372. doi:10.1080/15389588.2012.659363.

Rich, S., Rubin, L., Walker, A. M., Schneeweiss, S., & Abenhaim, L. (2000). Anorexigens and pulmonary hypertension in the United States: Results from the surveillance of North American pulmonary hypertension. *Chest*, *117*(3), 870–874.

Robinson, E. L., Ball, L. E., & Leveritt, M. D. (2014). Obesity bias among health and non-health students attending an Australian university and their perceived obesity education. *J Nutr Educ Behav*, *46*(5), 390–395. doi:10.1016/j.jneb.2013.12.003.

Rosso, G. L., Perotto, M., Feola, M., Bruno, G., & Caramella, M. (2015). Investigating obesity among professional drivers: The high risk professional driver study. *Am J Ind Med*, *58*(2), 212–219. doi:10.1002/ajim.22400.

Schomerus, G., Lucht, M., Holzinger, A., Matschinger, H., Carta, M. G., & Angermeyer, M. C. (2011). The stigma of alcohol dependence compared with other mental disorders: A review of population studies. *Alcohol Alcohol*, *46*(2), 105–112. doi:10.1093/alcalc/agq089.

Scott, D., Daly, R. M., Sanders, K. M., & Ebeling, P. R. (2015). Fall and fracture risk in sarcopenia and dynapenia with and without obesity: The role of lifestyle interventions. *Curr Osteoporos Rep*, *13*(4), 235–244. doi:10.1007/s11914-015-0274-z.

Scott, D., Sanders, K. M., Aitken, D., Hayes, A., Ebeling, P. R., & Jones, G. (2014). Sarcopenic obesity and dynapenic obesity: 5-year associations with falls risk in middle-aged and older adults. *Obesity (Silver Spring)*, *22*(6), 1568–1574. doi:10.1002/oby.20734.

Seacat, J. D., Dougal, S. C., & Roy, D. (2016). A daily diary assessment of female weight stigmatization. *J Health Psychol*, *21*(2), 228–240. doi:10.1177/1359105314525067.

Shin, J., Choi, Y., Han, K. T., Cheon, S. Y., Kim, J. H., Lee, S. G., & Park, E. C. (2015). The combined effect of subjective body image and body mass index (distorted body weight perception) on suicidal ideation. *J Prev Med Public Health*, *48*(2), 94–104. doi:10.3961/jpmph.14.055.

Shloim, N., Edelson, L. R., Martin, N., & Hetherington, M. M. (2015). Parenting styles, feeding styles, feeding practices, and weight status in 4–12 year-old children: A systematic review of the literature. *Front Psychol*, *6*, 1849. doi:10.3389/fpsyg.2015.01849.

Sieber, W. K., Robinson, C. F., Birdsey, J., Chen, G. X., Hitchcock, E. M., Lincoln, J. E., … Sweeney, M. H. (2014). Obesity and other risk factors: The National Survey of U.S. long-haul truck driver health and injury. *Am J Ind Med*, *57*(6), 615–626. doi:10.1002/ajim.22293.

Sjostrom, L., Lindroos, A. K., Peltonen, M., Torgerson, J., Bouchard, C., Carlsson, B., … Wedel, H. (2004). Lifestyle, diabetes, and cardiovascular risk factors 10 years after bariatric surgery. *N Engl J Med*, *351*(26), 2683–2693. doi:10.1056/NEJMoa035622.

Stanfill, A. G., Conley, Y., Cashion, A., Thompson, C., Homayouni, R., Cowan, P., & Hathaway, D. (2015). Neurogenetic and neuroimaging evidence for a conceptual model of dopaminergic contributions to obesity. *Biol Res Nurs*, *17*(4), 413–421. doi:10.1177/1099800414565170.

Sumner, S. A., Mercy, J. A., Dahlberg, L. L., Hillis, S. D., Klevens, J., & Houry, D. (2015). Violence in the United States: Status, challenges, and opportunities. *JAMA*, *314*(5), 478–488. doi:10.1001/jama.2015.8371.

Svensson, P. A., Anveden, A., Romeo, S., Peltonen, M., Ahlin, S., Burza, M. A., … Carlsson, L. M. (2013). Alcohol consumption and alcohol problems after bariatric surgery in the Swedish obese subjects study. *Obesity (Silver Spring)*, *21*(12), 2444–2451. doi:10.1002/oby.20397.

Tindle, H. A., Omalu, B., Courcoulas, A., Marcus, M., Hammers, J., & Kuller, L. H. (2010). Risk of suicide after long-term follow-up from bariatric surgery. *Am J Med*, *123*(11), 1036–1042. doi:10.1016/j.amjmed.2010.06.016.

Toosizadeh, N., Mohler, J., Armstrong, D. G., Talal, T. K., & Najafi, B. (2015). The influence of diabetic peripheral neuropathy on local postural muscle and central sensory feedback balance control. *PLoS One*, *10*(8), e0135255. doi:10.1371/journal.pone.0135255.

Tsiros, M. D., Sinn, N., Brennan, L., Coates, A. M., Walkley, J. W., Petkov, J., … Buckley, J. D. (2008). Cognitive behavioral therapy improves diet and body composition in overweight and obese adolescents. *Am J Clin Nutr*, *87*(5), 1134–1140.

Vaca, F. E., & D'Onofrio, G. (2014). Traumatic injuries related to alcohol and other drug use: Epidemiology, screening and prevention. In R. K. Reis & D. A. Fiellin (Eds.), *The ASAM principles of addiction medicine* (5th ed., pp. 1795), pp. 1231–1238. Wolters Kluwer Health.

Vickers, M. H. (2014). Early life nutrition, epigenetics and programming of later life disease. *Nutrients*, *6*(6), 2165–2178. doi:10.3390/nu6062165.

Vijayan, V. K. (2012). Morbidities associated with obstructive sleep apnea. *Expert Rev Respir Med*, *6*(5), 557–566. doi:10.1586/ers.12.44.

Wang, W., Obi, J. C., Engida, S., Carter, E. R., Yan, F., & Zhang, J. (2015). The relationship between excess body weight and the risk of death from unnatural causes. *Accid Anal Prev*, *80*, 229–235. doi:10.1016/j.aap.2015.04.020.

Watkins, T. J., Di Iorio, C. R., Olatunji, B. O., Benningfield, M. M., Blackford, J. U., Dietrich, M. S., … Cowan, R. L. (2015). Disgust proneness and associated neural substrates in obesity. *Soc Cogn Affect Neurosci*, *11*(3), 458–465. doi:10.1093/scan/nsv129.

Werthmann, J., Jansen, A., & Roefs, A. (2014). Worry or craving? A selective review of evidence for food-related attention biases in obese individuals, eating-disorder patients, restrained eaters and healthy samples. *Proc Nutr Soc*, 1–16. doi:10.1017/s0029665114001451.

Wojcicki, J. M., Young, M. B., Perham-Hester, K. A., de Schweinitz, P., & Gessner, B. D. (2015). Risk factors for obesity at age 3 in Alaskan children, including the role of beverage consumption: Results from Alaska PRAMS 2005–2006 and its three-year follow-up survey, CUBS, 2008–2009. *PLoS One*, *10*(3), e0118711. doi:10.1371/journal.pone.0118711.

Woloshin, S., & Schwartz, L. M. (2014). The new weight-loss drugs, lorcaserin and phentermine-topiramate: slim pickings? *JAMA Intern Med*, *174*(4), 615–619. doi:10.1001/jamainternmed.2013.14629.

Yesavage, J. A., Kinoshita, L. M., Noda, A., Lazzeroni, L. C., Fairchild, J. K., Taylor, J., … O'Hara, R. (2014). Effects of body mass index-related disorders on cognition: Preliminary results. *Diabetes Metab Syndr Obes*, *7*, 145–151. doi:10.2147/dmso.s60294.

Young, M. S., Mahfoud, J. M., Walker, G. H., Jenkins, D. P., & Stanton, N. A. (2008). Crash dieting: The effects of eating and drinking on driving performance. *Accid Anal Prev*, *40*(1), 142–148. doi:10.1016/j.aap.2007.04.012.

Zhang, P., Peterson, M., Su, G. L., & Wang, S. C. (2015). Visceral adiposity is negatively associated with bone density and muscle attenuation. *Am J Clin Nutr*, *101*(2), 337–343. doi:10.3945/ajcn.113.081778.

19 DSM 5 SUD Criterion 9 *Use in Spite of Consequences*

Joan Ifland
Food Addiction Training, LLC
Cincinnati, OH

R. Sue Roselle
Roselle Center for Healing
Oakton, VA

CONTENTS

19.1 INTRODUCTION

Processed food use is continued despite knowledge of having a persistent or recurrent physical or psychological problem that is likely to have been caused or exacerbated by processed foods.

19.1.1 Importance

Identifying the consequences of addictions is important across the board. Using in spite of knowledge of consequences shows that the processed food addiction (PFA) has caused the client to engage in a kind of pathological self-harming. Early stage consequences such as a slight weight gain, prediabetes, or an upward trending cholesterol reading may encourage both practitioner and client alike to begin a preventive intervention. The assessment may reveal consequences that need medical attention. Failure to address consequences such as immobility, cognitive impairment, and mood disorders may prevent the addict from making progress in recovery.

The link between some consequences and processed foods may be novel information for the addict. This could apply to consequences such as fatigue, brain fog, confusion, and memory loss. As such, learning about the link between these less obvious consequences and processed foods might motivate the client to realize that the benefits of undertaking recovery are more worthwhile than previously thought. And, early stage recovery from consequences could be a motivator to stick with the recovery plan.

While clients may be overly focused about the consequence of weight gain, over time they may come to value recovery from other consequences even more than weight loss. Describing the full range of consequences can help the client overcome minimizing consequences to rationalize a lapse. There is much to be gained from thoroughly assessing for the full range of consequences.

19.1.2 Evidence for the Syndrome

Some consequences of PFA are well known, while others can be surprising to both practitioner and client. The well-known elements of the metabolic syndrome are excess adipose tissue, diabetes, high cholesterol/cardiovascular disease, and elevated glucose levels/diabetes. Less-recognized consequences may include thought disorders such as cravings, brain fog, and racing thoughts, as well as learning difficulties, inability to make decisions, and memory loss. Mood disorders such as depression, irritability, and anxiety are also not always understood to be linked to processed food consumption. Behavioral problems such as lethargy, hyperactivity in children, and violence are also not generally understood to be a possible consequence of processed food use.

Physical, mental, and behavioral diseases have been shown to be associated with processed foods. The list below describes a range of problems (Bray and Bellanger 2006; Guh et al. 2009; Ifland et al. 2012). Not every processed food user develops every disease, but repeated use of processed foods increases the risk of these consequences. It is important to note that weight status may correlate with these conditions, but this is not always the case. Practitioners should probe for consequences even in normally weighted clients.

19.1.2.1 Physical Diseases

Extensive physical disabilities have been demonstrated to be associated with obesity, including diabetes (Feinman et al. 2014), heart disease (Manzel et al. 2014), stroke (Danaei et al. 2009), excessive fat (Wells 2013), infection (Myles 2014), cancer (Caren et al. 2013), joint and bone disease (Tsanzi et al. 2008), and inflammation (Rai and Sandell 2011). The physical problems are extensive.

19.1.2.2 Mental Illnesses

A variety of mental illnesses have also been shown to be present in chronic overconsumption of processed foods. These include ADD (Johnson et al. 2011), Alzheimer's (McGregor et al. 2015), dementia (Nguyen et al. 2014), binge eating disorder (Castellini et al. 2014), and addiction (Caprioli et al. 2015).

19.1.2.3 Emotional Illnesses

Emotional issues may also manifest, including depression (Peters et al. 2014; Weltens et al. 2014), irritability (Amianto et al. 2012), and anxiety (Labarthe et al. 2014).

19.1.2.4 Behavioral Disorders

Behavioral problems are present as poor impulse control/disruptive behavior (Barry et al. 2009), fatigue (Maloney et al. 2010), poor quality of life (Keating et al. 2013), binge eating (Meule and Platte 2015), and sleep disorders (Young et al. 2005).

19.1.2.5 Failed Weight-Loss Attempts

Practitioners may consider that failed treatment for weight loss may be a consequence of PFA. Failed attempts to cut back have been described in DSM SUD Criterion 2. The failure of weight-loss schemes is measured at 95% and above (Foster et al. 2005; Ochner et al. 2013). Weight-loss surgery patients exhibit slow weight regain (Sjostrom et al. 2004; Magro et al. 2008) and a tendency to develop alcoholism (Svensson et al. 2013). Reactions to pharmaceuticals may also be a consequence (Goldstein and Potvin 1994), including heart disease with fenfluramine and dexfenfluramine (Connolly and McGoon 1999), suicide ideation with rimonabant (Christensen et al. 2007), memory loss and heightened anxiety from lorcaserin and phentermine–topiramate (Woloshin and Schwartz 2014), hypertension from sibutramine (Rich et al. 2000), and bowel leakage from orlistat (Hollywood and Ogden 2011).

Research shows extensive consequences from chronic use of processed foods. Although the pathology is distressing, educating clients about the link between compulsive chronic consumption of processed foods and relief from so many conditions can create a positive attitude toward recovery.

19.1.3 Use in Motivation

Clients may present for diagnosis and assessment with the intention of achieving weight loss after multiple failed attempts. Thus they may already be motivated to undertake a program. However, they may be embracing the framework of a short-term diet rather than long-term recovery involving extensive lifestyle changes. The practitioner can be challenged to persuade clients to build a recovery program that is comprehensive enough to protect against relapse into processed foods. Being able to describe benefits in addition to weight loss could encourage the client to undertake a more comprehensive program.

From the client's perspective, the possibility of putting a broad range of consequences into remission could steer the client away from another failed weight-loss attempt toward long-term success at a healthy lifestyle. It is good to remember that an unprocessed food plan is only one element of a recovery program. Clients will also need to develop extensive cue avoidance and negotiate with household members to contain food cues within the home. Clients may need to extensively restructure how they spend time in terms of disengaging from triggering television and replacing it with exercise, healthy sleep, phone calls, cognitive restoration, etc. It could take up to a year to build a program that is comprehensive enough to consistently prevent painful lapses. As with addictions in general, a lifetime of maintenance is also indicated.

The reward of weight loss alone might not be enough to keep the client motivated. Without awareness of the range of links between consequences and PFA, clients might be tempted to assume that when weight normalizes, they can go back to consuming processed foods. Having the whole picture of consequences of processed food use helps clients stay the course for the long term.

19.1.4 Use in Treatment

Knowledge of the full range of consequences allows the practitioner to incorporate recovery from the consequences into a treatment plan. Practitioners will be able to match financial and health insurance resources with the need for medical attention. To prepare for medical treatment issues, practitioners will want to identify health professionals who are qualified to treat the obese. Health professionals have been shown to discriminate against the obese. Humiliating encounters with health professionals may have traumatized clients and created barriers to seeking medical treatment (Phelan et al. 2015). Practitioners can find out if clients are comfortable with their current health professionals or if they need referrals.

Similarly, counseling and therapy for the resolution of abuse and trauma may be indicated. Cognitive behavioral therapy and dialectical behavior therapy have been shown to be effective in supporting behavior change (Schwartz et al. 2015; Montesi et al. 2016). Family therapy may be helpful to families where children have become addicted to processed foods (Altman and Wilfley 2015). In all cases, practitioners will need to research referrals to ascertain that the health professional is comfortable with the concepts of abstinence from processed foods that PFA recovery entails.

19.2 MANIFESTATIONS

The consequences of chronic processed food use are numerous across behavioral, mental, emotional, and physical domains. The illustrations included below describe the distress of suffering consequences without being able to stop the overconsumption of food.

19.2.1 Behaviors

The behaviors in Criterion 9 are generally that clients are aware that consuming processed foods is detrimental to their health and yet they continue to do so. With high rates of obesity, it is possible that use in spite of knowledge of weight gain is common. Overeaters may be engaged in rationalizing consumption frequently throughout their days. In severe cases, clients may be obsessing about their weight virtually continually but be unable to stop the overconsumption of processed foods.

Use can also continue in spite of financial and relationship consequences. Avoidance of medical services is another behavior that may need to be addressed. Compliance with diet recommendations has been shown to be low for diabetics (Rivellese et al. 2008).

This quote from the food addiction 12-step manuals illustrates behaviors related to use in spite of consequences, particularly around knowledge of weight gain.

> How high is this scale going to go? I wondered. I could easily imagine it reading 200 pounds, but I knew it wouldn't stop there. Would it stop at 250? What would happen to me when none of my clothes fit and I could no longer buy the professional outfits required for my job? And when my weight doubled my husband's? What was going to become of me? (Food Addicts in Recovery Anonymous, 2013, 23)

This quote illustrates use in spite of a behavioral cycle of bingeing, starvation, and loss of control.

> Most of the time, I binged on the weekends and tried to undo the damage by starving on Monday and Tuesday. I remember fasting all day one Monday until by four o'clock in the afternoon I couldn't bear it. I had a little piece of cheese and some lettuce, and that opened the floodgates. I went from fast-food restaurants to grocery stores, and I ate straight into the night. (Food Addicts in Recovery Anonymous, 2013, 110–112)

This quote illustrates the financial consequences of PFA.

> She gave me the apartment on the third floor, and I moved in. All of my resources went to support my addictions. I didn't pay rent or bills. The gas meter was taken out for nonpayment of my gas bills, and many times I was without heating oil. (Food Addicts in Recovery Anonymous, 2013, 64)

Relationship issues can also be a consequence of processed food consumption.

> Food addiction, panic and depression contributed to the breakup of our marriage … For three years after the divorce I enrolled myself in some traditional and not-so-traditional therapy. I learned many mood and negative-voice-fighting skills as well as relaxation techniques. Antidepressants made a world of difference in my overall mood. Still, the obsession with food and weight was out of control. (Food Addicts Anonymous, 2010, 126)

19.2.2 Mental Manifestations

The mental basis for use in spite of consequences may stem from use in spite of brain fog (Theoharides et al. 2015). Indeed, this illustration shows use while driving, in spite of knowledge of blackouts from eating processed foods.

> I knew from experience that when I binged I got sleepy and would pass out. Usually when I did heavy bingeing I was home alone on the couch in front of the television. Now I was in my car, and I was scared. How was I going to eat all the food and get home without falling asleep behind the wheel? (Food Addicts Anonymous, 2010, 139)

Practitioners may have trouble with conformance to Criterion 9 if clients do not know that a particular consequence is related to processed foods. Research shows impaired cognitive abilities in the frontal cortex of drug-addicted people (Volkow et al. 2016). In spite of research showing that decision-making pathways are hypoactive in the obese (Stice and Yokum 2016), clients may not be aware of the connection of learning difficulties, confused decisions, and memory loss with processed foods. Once educated, if the client continues to consume processed foods, then the practitioner may find that the behavior conforms to Criterion 9.

The practitioner may discover manifestations of this in terms of rationalizing. The client might think that the consequences of their consumption are not as serious as they are. As clients may also experience memory loss, they may not be able to remember how much processed food is being consumed. At the moment of consumption, they may not be able to recall consequences.

In a rat study, processed foods were shown to sensitize the stress pathways in the brain (Moore et al. 2017). These illustrations show how processed foods affect PFA clients mentally. This issue may be especially prominent when PFA clients are pursuing educations, as shown in these quotes.

> I gained 20 pounds my first semester, which terrified me. I had a mental breakdown that fall. I didn't do my assignments. I just partied, drank, started doing drugs, and ate and ate and ate—not happily. (Food Addicts in Recovery Anonymous 2013, 110)
>
> I was obsessed with my body. I might as well have weighed 300 pounds. I hated how I felt and barely passed my exams and clinical rotations. (Food Addicts in Recovery Anonymous 2013, 111)

19.2.3 Emotional Manifestations

The emotional manifestations of use in spite of consequences may be use in spite of self-loathing, as in this example.

> All the while, I kept telling myself I wasn't really fat. I wasn't 200 pounds, after all. I was only 190. I didn't like my appearance, but the real truth was that I loathed myself, not really because of how I looked or what I ate but because I wasn't who I thought I should be. I should have been someone who would be able to open the front door, walk out, and live in the world successfully. My deepest, darkest secret was that I couldn't open that door. I could not walk out into the world, much less live in it successfully. (Food Addicts in Recovery Anonymous 2013, 90)

19.2.4 Physical Manifestations

Of course the most prominent physical manifestation is use in spite of gaining weight. However, clients may be continuing use in spite of other physical problems, as well.

> Somehow, at 248 pounds, I had been willing to accept that there would be diabetes in my future. To my food-addicted mind, that was manageable, even though my friend's mother had just died of the disease after having both of her feet amputated. But I wasn't prepared to be on medication for blood pressure. Was this insane thinking, or what? (Food Addicts Anonymous, 2010, 157)

Practitioners may find common manifestations of use in spite of knowledge of consequences in the diagnosis of PFA. Criterion 9 can indicate the loss of important cognitive functions such as learning, decision-making, memory, and restraint. Cataloging consequences as well as the degree to which such consequences are of concern to the client can help shape the list of options to begin recovery. Practitioners can probe until they feel that they have a complete picture of the consequences that clients are enduring.

19.3 APPLICATION

19.3.1 Care in Approach

Practitioners will want to carefully inventory consequences. The DSM 5 SUD criteria will surface some pathology, which the practitioner can continue to develop during collection of data for the ASI. Clients may be experiencing shame about their loss of control. They may have experienced deep humiliation, which has developed into painful self-loathing.

During the collection of information about use in spite of consequences, clients may feel stupid and despairing about themselves. This is an opportunity for practitioners to reassure clients that such behavior is a normal element of addictions. Practitioners can reassure clients that an aggressive, sophisticated food industry may have had a role in provoking the development of the disease. In short, it is not the fault of the client. Focusing blame on the environment will help clients feel safe while they talk about consequences, and this will help develop trust.

19.3.2 Developing Goals

Practitioners may be tempted to allow clients to focus on weight loss as a central goal of recovery from food addiction. This is not necessarily helpful, as it may be a cue for the client to engage in unhealthy weight-loss behaviors such as undereating and weighing. These behaviors can in turn trigger self-judgment and stress, which can lead to relapse.

Goals that can be set under Criterion 9, use in spite of consequences, can instead focus on improvements in cognitive abilities, emotional stability, reductions in cravings, ability to withstand exposure to cues, adherence to an orderly eating schedule, compliance with medical recommendations, and improvements in general health.

19.3.3 Tracking Progress

Again, it is important to avoid tracking weight loss. Research shows that the obese can suffer from muscle and bone loss (Compston 2015; Lee et al. 2016), which may be reversed on a healthy food plan. The gain in mass from replenishing muscle and bone are reflected on the scale as weight gain and could trigger anxiety about failing, which could lead to relapse to either under- or overeating. Clients may wish to report being able to wear smaller sizes as a means of tracking progress rather than weight.

Important progress may be that the client may be able to avoid sleeping during the day. Progress could also be tracked in terms of recommendations to reduce medications from prescribing health professionals. The gradual elimination of processed foods from the home is another useful way to track progress. Sufficient energy to exercise is a positive development in recovery.

Keeping the client's focus on a comprehensive recovery program rather than weight loss will help the client recognize and enjoy the broad range of benefits of recovering from food addiction.

19.4 CONCLUSION

Probing for the extensive consequences of food addiction motivates clients to start recovery and stay with it. Extensive consequences also show practitioners more reasons to show compassion to food-addicted clients. Addictive overeaters have developed physical, mental, emotional, and behavioral conditions that add to the distress of food addiction. Gently guiding clients through the process of uncovering the extent of consequences may be distressing, but as the myriad of conditions moves into remission clients can be reinforced in their determination to stick to a program of recovery.

REFERENCES

Altman, M. and D. E. Wilfley (2015). Evidence update on the treatment of overweight and obesity in children and adolescents. *J Clin Child Adolesc Psychol* **44**(4): 521–537.

Amianto, F., S. Siccardi, G. Abbate-Daga, L. Marech, M. Barosio and S. Fassino (2012). Does anger mediate between personality and eating symptoms in bulimia nervosa? *Psychiatry Res* **200**(2–3): 502–512.

Barry, D., M. Clarke and N. M. Petry (2009). Obesity and its relationship to addictions: Is overeating a form of addictive behavior? *Am J Addict* **18**(6): 439–451.

Bray, G. A. and T. Bellanger (2006). Epidemiology, trends, and morbidities of obesity and the metabolic syndrome. *Endocrine* **29**(1): 109–117.

Caprioli, D., T. Zeric, E. B. Thorndike and M. Venniro (2015). Persistent palatable food preference in rats with a history of limited and extended access to methamphetamine self-administration. *Addict Biol* **20**(5): 913–928.

Caren, H., S. M. Pollard and S. Beck (2013). The good, the bad and the ugly: Epigenetic mechanisms in glioblastoma. *Mol Aspects Med* **34**(4): 849–862.

Castellini, G., L. Godini, S. G. Amedei, V. Galli, G. Alpigiano, E. Mugnaini, M. Veltri, et al. (2014). Psychopathological similarities and differences between obese patients seeking surgical and non-surgical overweight treatments. *Eat Weight Disord* **19**(1): 95–102.

Christensen, R., P. K. Kristensen, E. M. Bartels, H. Bliddal and A. Astrup (2007). Efficacy and safety of the weight-loss drug rimonabant: A meta-analysis of randomised trials. *Lancet* **370**(9600): 1706–1713.

Compston, J. (2015). Obesity and fractures in postmenopausal women. *Curr Opin Rheumatol* **27**(4): 414–419.

Connolly, H. M. and M. D. McGoon (1999). Obesity drugs and the heart. *Curr Probl Cardiol* **24**(12): 745–792.

Danaei, G., E. L. Ding, D. Mozaffarian, B. Taylor, J. Rehm, C. J. Murray and M. Ezzati (2009). The preventable causes of death in the United States: Comparative risk assessment of dietary, lifestyle, and metabolic risk factors. *PLoS Med* **6**(4): e1000058.

Feinman, R. D., W. K. Pogozelski, A. Astrup, R. K. Bernstein, E. J. Fine, E. C. Westman, A. Accurso, et al. (2014). Dietary carbohydrate restriction as the first approach in diabetes management: Critical review and evidence base. *Nutrition* **31**(1): 1–13.

Food Addicts Anonymous (2010). *Food Addicts Anonymous*. Port St. Lucie, FL, Food Addicts Anonymous, Inc.

Food Addicts in Recovery Anonymous (2013). *Food Addicts in Recovery Anonymous*. Woburn, MA, Food Addicts in Recovery Anonymous.

Foster, G. D., A. P. Makris and B. A. Bailer (2005). Behavioral treatment of obesity. *Am J Clin Nutr* **82**(1 Suppl): 230s–235s.

Goldstein, D. J. and J. H. Potvin (1994). Long-term weight loss: The effect of pharmacologic agents. *Am J Clin Nutr* **60**(5): 647–657; discussion 658–649.

Guh, D. P., W. Zhang, N. Bansback, Z. Amarsi, C. L. Birmingham and A. H. Anis (2009). The incidence of co-morbidities related to obesity and overweight: A systematic review and meta-analysis. *BMC Public Health* **9**: 88.

Hollywood, A. and J. Ogden (2011). Taking orlistat: Predicting weight loss over 6 months. *J Obes* 2011: 806896.

Ifland, J. R., K. Sheppard and H. T. Wright (2012). From the front lines: The impact of refined food addiction on well-being. *Food and Addiction: A Comprehensive Handbook*. In K. Brownell and M. Gold (eds.), Oxford, Oxford University Press.

Johnson, R. J., M. S. Gold, D. R. Johnson, T. Ishimoto, M. A. Lanaspa, N. R. Zahniser and N. M. Avena (2011). Attention-deficit/hyperactivity disorder: Is it time to reappraise the role of sugar consumption? *Postgrad Med* **123**(5): 39–49.

Keating, C. L., A. Peeters, B. A. Swinburn, D. J. Magliano and M. L. Moodie (2013). Utility-based quality of life associated with overweight and obesity: The Australian diabetes, obesity, and lifestyle study. *Obesity (Silver Spring)* **21**(3): 652–655.

Labarthe, A., O. Fiquet, R. Hassouna, P. Zizzari, L. Lanfumey, N. Ramoz, D. Grouselle, J. Epelbaum and V. Tolle (2014). Ghrelin-derived peptides: A link between appetite/reward, GH axis, and psychiatric disorders? *Front Endocrinol (Lausanne)* **5**: 163.

Lee, J., Y. P. Hong, H. J. Shin and W. Lee (2016). Associations of sarcopenia and sarcopenic obesity with metabolic syndrome considering both muscle mass and muscle strength. *J Prev Med Public Health* **49**(1): 35–44.

Magro, D. O., B. Geloneze, R. Delfini, B. C. Pareja, F. Callejas and J. C. Pareja (2008). Long-term weight regain after gastric bypass: A 5-year prospective study. *Obes Surg* **18**(6): 648–651.

Maloney, E. M., R. S. Boneva, J. M. Lin and W. C. Reeves (2010). Chronic fatigue syndrome is associated with metabolic syndrome: Results from a case-control study in Georgia. *Metabolism* **59**(9): 1351–1357.

Manzel, A., D. N. Muller, D. A. Hafler, S. E. Erdman, R. A. Linker and M. Kleinewietfeld (2014). Role of "Western diet" in inflammatory autoimmune diseases. *Curr Allergy Asthma Rep* **14**(1): 404.

McGregor, G., Y. Malekizadeh and J. Harvey (2015). Minireview: Food for thought: Regulation of synaptic function by metabolic hormones. *Mol Endocrinol* **29**(1): 3–13.

Meule, A. and P. Platte (2015). Facets of impulsivity interactively predict body fat and binge eating in young women. *Appetite* **87**: 352–357.

Montesi, L., M. El Ghoch, L. Brodosi, S. Calugi, G. Marchesini and R. Dalle Grave (2016). Long-term weight loss maintenance for obesity: A multidisciplinary approach. *Diabetes Metab Syndr Obes* **9**: 37–46.

Moore, C. F., V. Sabino, G. F. Koob and P. Cottone (2017). Pathological overeating: Emerging evidence for a compulsivity construct. *Neuropsychopharmacology* **42**(7): 1375–1389.

Myles, I. A. (2014). Fast food fever: Reviewing the impacts of the Western diet on immunity. *Nutr J* **13**: 61.

Nguyen, J. C., A. S. Killcross and T. A. Jenkins (2014). Obesity and cognitive decline: Role of inflammation and vascular changes. *Front Neurosci* **8**: 375.

Ochner, C. N., D. M. Barrios, C. D. Lee and F. X. Pi-Sunyer (2013). Biological mechanisms that promote weight regain following weight loss in obese humans. *Physiol Behav* **120**: 106–113.

Peters, S. L., J. R. Biesiekierski, G. W. Yelland, J. G. Muir and P. R. Gibson (2014). Randomised clinical trial: Gluten may cause depression in subjects with non-coeliac gluten sensitivity - An exploratory clinical study. *Aliment Pharmacol Ther* **39**(10): 1104–1112.

Phelan, S. M., D. J. Burgess, M. W. Yeazel, W. L. Hellerstedt, J. M. Griffin and M. van Ryn (2015). Impact of weight bias and stigma on quality of care and outcomes for patients with obesity. *Obes Rev* **16**(4): 319–326.

Rai, M. F. and L. J. Sandell (2011). Inflammatory mediators: Tracing links between obesity and osteoarthritis. *Crit Rev Eukaryot Gene Expr* **21**(2): 131–142.

Rich, S., L. Rubin, A. M. Walker, S. Schneeweiss and L. Abenhaim (2000). Anorexigens and pulmonary hypertension in the United States: Results from the surveillance of North American pulmonary hypertension. *Chest* **117**(3): 870–874.

Rivellese, A. A., M. Boemi, F. Cavalot, L. Costagliola, P. De Feo, R. Miccoli, L. Patti, M. Trovati, O. Vaccaro and I. Zavaroni (2008). Dietary habits in type II diabetes mellitus: How is adherence to dietary recommendations? *Eur J Clin Nutr* **62**(5): 660–664.

Schwartz, D. C., M. S. Nickow, R. Arseneau and M. T. Gisslow (2015). A substance called food: Long-term psychodynamic group treatment for compulsive overeating. *Int J Group Psychother* **65**(3): 386–409.

Sjostrom, L., A. K. Lindroos, M. Peltonen, J. Torgerson, C. Bouchard, B. Carlsson, S. Dahlgren, et al. (2004). Lifestyle, diabetes, and cardiovascular risk factors 10 years after bariatric surgery. *N Engl J Med* **351**(26): 2683–2693.

Stice, E. and S. Yokum (2016). Neural vulnerability factors that increase risk for future weight gain. *Psychol Bull* **142**(5): 447–471.

Svensson, P. A., A. Anveden, S. Romeo, M. Peltonen, S. Ahlin, M. A. Burza, B. Carlsson, et al. (2013). Alcohol consumption and alcohol problems after bariatric surgery in the Swedish obese subjects study. *Obesity (Silver Spring)* **21**(12): 2444–2451.

Theoharides, T. C., J. M. Stewart, E. Hatziagelaki and G. Kolaitis (2015). Brain "fog," inflammation and obesity: Key aspects of neuropsychiatric disorders improved by luteolin. *Front Neurosci* **9**: 225.

Tsanzi, E., H. R. Light and J. C. Tou (2008). The effect of feeding different sugar-sweetened beverages to growing female Sprague-Dawley rats on bone mass and strength. *Bone* **42**(5): 960–968.

Volkow, N. D., G. F. Koob and A. T. McLellan (2016). Neurobiologic advances from the brain disease model of addiction. *N Engl J Med* **374**(4): 363–371.

Wells, J. C. (2013). Obesity as malnutrition: The dimensions beyond energy balance. *Eur J Clin Nutr* **67**(5): 507–512.

Weltens, N., D. Zhao and L. Van Oudenhove (2014). Where is the comfort in comfort foods? Mechanisms linking fat signaling, reward, and emotion. *Neurogastroenterol Motil* **26**(3): 303–315.

Woloshin, S. and L. M. Schwartz (2014). The new weight-loss drugs, lorcaserin and phentermine-topiramate: Slim pickings? *JAMA Intern Med* **174**(4): 615–619.

Young, T., P. E. Peppard and S. Taheri (2005). Excess weight and sleep-disordered breathing. *J Appl Physiol (1985)* **99**(4): 1592–1599.

20 DSM 5 SUD Criterion 10 *Tolerance*

Joan Ifland
Food Addiction Training, LLC
Cincinnati, OH

Carrie L. Willey
Shades of Hope Treatment Center
Buffalo Gap, TX

CONTENTS

Tolerance, as defined by either of the following:

1. A need for markedly increased amounts of processed foods to achieve intoxication or desired effect.
2. A markedly diminished effect with continued use of the same amount of processed food. (American Psychiatric Association, 2013, 491)

20.1 INTRODUCTION

Tolerance, like withdrawal, is a broadly recognized characteristic of addiction. Although its presence is not required for diagnosing an addiction, it is a characteristic that many health professionals look for in assessing for the presence of an addiction. In the early stages of the disease, progression may not have yet manifested. So even if tolerance has not yet appeared, the practitioner may still diagnose positively, assess for needs, describe a scope of problem, and encourage the client to undertake a program of recovery.

Food-addicted clients may be able to recognize the behavior in themselves. They may know that they are buying larger containers of processed foods, or more containers of processed foods. They may recognize that they're eating processed foods more and more often throughout the day. They may know that they're hiding foods in more different places around their homes. They may be stopping at more processed food outlets while on the road or visiting grocery and convenience stores more often. This increase in volume can be frightening and shameful. Clients may be relieved to learn that progression is a normal characteristic of addiction. Knowing that progression cannot be controlled without treatment may reassure clients that it is unrealistic to think that they could have controlled it on their own.

Progression in processed food addiction (PFA) can be gradual. The addict may be unaware of the full extent of the pattern. It may be necessary to ask about credit card bills and spending to surface the scope of progression. Volumes used in bingeing may be an indication of progression, but bingeing is not necessary to exhibit progressive use. There may be progression in grazing where small amounts are being eaten more and more often through the day. The pattern may also be weekly. Compulsive use may be kept in check through the week but show progression on the weekends, with more time gradually spent eating, sleeping, isolating, and watching television. Further, progression may shift from one food to another. A client may give up sugar but gradually replace it with wheat flour, fat, excessive salt, or dairy.

The fields of addiction and pathological eating have developed neurological descriptions of tolerance through animal studies and brain-imaging research. The downregulation of pleasure pathways, combined with the sensitization of stress pathways, recruitment of habit-forming functions, as well as the suppression of cognitive pathways, combine to drive increasing use of processed foods. The negative effect of sensitized stress pathways becomes more pronounced while the compensating pleasure decreases and the ability to put on the brakes deteriorates (Volkow, Koob, & McLellan, 2016). These characteristics have also been described in pathological use of fat and sugar (Cottone, Sabino, Roberto, et al., 2009; Cottone, Sabino, Steardo, & Zorrilla, 2009; Moore, Sabino, Koob, & Cottone, 2017; Stice & Yokum, 2016).

The food addict may initially turn to food for pleasure. However, as stress pathways become increasingly active, processed food use can shift from the pursuit of pleasure to the relief of stress. The experience of eating processed foods may stop being enjoyable and become comforting instead. As the disease progresses, the ability of food to numb continues to decline while the sensation of stress increases. Nonetheless, the food addict remembers that at one time, the food served to improve mood and so the addict pursues the elusive effect by eating more and more (Moore et al., 2017).

At the same time that pleasure is declining and stress is increasing, cognitive pathways are increasingly impaired. Deteriorating cognitive functions include learning, decision-making, memory, and especially restraint (Yau, Kang, Javier, & Convit, 2014; Zhu et al., 2015). The decline of these parts of the brain, which might otherwise help the food addict think through the problem and take a different course, help explain the irrationality of chronic overeating (Moore et al., 2017).

As the neurology shows, in the course of progression, there may come a point where processed foods are not bringing comfort at all. In cases of advanced downregulation of pleasure pathways, the addict may be driven to use greater quantities in a desperate attempt to feel better. However, the lack of response from dopamine, opiate, serotonin, and endocannabinoid pathways and sensitized stress pathways conspire to deprive the addict of relief. As an example, an addict might experience a day with high psychosocial stressors and decide to eat a half-cup serving of ice cream, which had eased the stress in the past due to the dopamine response. However, this time, because of progression in the sensitization of stress pathways and downregulation of pleasure pathways, the half-cup serving is not enough. The negative self-talk continues after eating the half cup. This increases the stress level and an attempt to reduce stress may be made by eating the whole pint of ice cream. Understanding the distress, fright, and despair of this situation will help practitioners establish a relationship of trust with clients who otherwise could shut down with shame.

With understanding of the neurological processes of downregulation and sensitization, tolerance in food-addicted clients can be addressed with compassion. No longer do professionals need to judge the food addict's behavior as disgusting or repulsive when evaluating large amounts of processed foods consumed. The practitioner can attach such reports to the deterioration of pleasure and cognitive functions concomitant with the hyperactivation of stress. From this foundation, the practitioner can comfort the food addict, assure the client that the behavior is not their fault, and describe a course of recovery that restores control.

As this chapter will describe, tolerance can be quelled through techniques used in classic substance use recovery. These include abstaining from addictive foods, avoiding cues, and engaging in cognitive restoration. These techniques generally reduce cue reactivity and cravings, as well as strengthen restraint and decision-making. They are also designed to reduce the sensitivity of stress pathways.

20.1.1 Importance

Tolerance is important for several reasons. It is very helpful to be able to explain to clients why they're eating so much. The pattern of behavior can be distressing to food-addicted clients, and overeating can significantly damage self-esteem through self-disgust and self-blame. The stress of these self-judgments can perpetuate the addiction by further activating the stress pathways, which can lead to cravings (Gibson, 2006), loss of cognitive control, and overeating.

It's also important for practitioners to grasp the mechanisms of progression so that they can assess for severity. Perhaps out of all the diagnostic criteria for addictions, tolerance is the most revealing in terms of loss of control and dysfunction in the brain.

Another reason to study tolerance is to help clients understand what the progress of the disease might be if they decide not to proceed with recovery. The quantity and expense of foods will continue to increase. The consequences will also progress. This could include worsening loss of control, additional weight gain, worsening diabetes, risk of stroke, etc. Family and work relationships might also deteriorate.

It is also important to be able to explain the progression of PFA as distinct from weight gain. Because Westernized cultures emphasize weight loss, clients may equate PFA with their BMI. However, although severity of progression may be evaluated in terms of the progression of consequences, it is also important to look at patterns of consumption. Frequency and volume of use are the key factors in progression. Great volumes and great frequency are not required to assess positively for progression. What is important is an *increase* in use. Even a small increase in use may indicate that the client's brain has begun to develop the malfunctions of the addiction, including downregulated pleasure pathways, sensitized stress pathways, and impaired cognitive functions.

Distinguishing PFA from weight issues is especially important in children. Parents may think that their children do not have PFA because their weight is normal. However, if the practitioner is able to describe increases in instances of interest in food, such as asking for processed foods between meals or an increasing refusal to eat unprocessed foods in the "picky eater," then parents may awake to the possibility that their child exhibits characteristics of PFA and that the disease is progressing.

It is important for practitioners to determine how far the disease has progressed. In early stage, consequences may not have materialized and mental deterioration may not yet be significant. In the later stages, practitioners may find serious deterioration in the physical, mental, and emotional capabilities of the client. Understanding consumption patterns allows practitioners to assess capabilities, devise an accurate scope of problem, help the client prepare for withdrawal, and make appropriate referrals for more evaluation.

20.2 EVIDENCE FOR PROGRESSION IN ADDICTIVE EATING

With the advent of brain-imaging technology, an explanation for the phenomenon of progression in drug addiction has emerged. A number of pathways in the brain become downregulated, including pleasure pathways and cognitive functions. At the same time, stress pathways are sensitized. Furthermore, the sequence of reactions shifts from consumption to associated cues. These alterations in brain function occur gradually in response to cues and repeated use. The addict may be unaware of the progression of the disease until a practitioner develops an assessment and a statement of the scope of the problem.

20.2.1 Evidence for a Syndrome of Progressive Use in Addiction

Advances in brain-imaging research have demonstrated new elements in the progression of addictions. The shifts in brain function as the addiction progresses are extensive. Several review articles describe them in detail (Koob & Volkow, 2016; Volkow et al., 2016). For the purposes of this chapter, key dysfunctions are summarized from these review articles below.

20.2.1.1 Incentive Salience

In the progression of the addiction, one of the shifting states in the brain is the development of increasingly urgent responses to cues for addictive drugs. *Incentive salience* can be defined as motivation for rewards derived from both the client's physiological state and learned associations about a reward cue. This response is mediated by the mesocorticolimbic dopamine system. Increasing sensitivity and reactivity to cues, which are experienced as intense urges that override rational thought, are important elements in the progression of addictions.

20.2.1.2 Phases of Dopamine Release

The timing of dopamine releases shifts from responding to drugs themselves to responding to cues for the drugs. This shift allows previously neutral cues to activate the addiction. Cue reactivity strengthens with repeated exposure to newly associated cues and creates strong motivation to use the drug (Volkow et al., 2016).

20.2.1.3 Decreased Reward and Escalation of Use

In animal models of the transition to addiction, decreased rewards in the dopamine pathways occur that temporally precede and are highly correlated with escalation in drug intake (Koob et al., 2014).

20.2.1.4 Reduction in Endocannabinoid Function

With chronic exposure to addictive substances, downregulation in the endocannabinoid system, which modulates stress responses, might contribute to enhanced stress reactivity. Human brain imaging studies have reported reductions of cannabinoid receptors in cannabis abusers and alcoholics (Ceccarini et al., 2014; Hirvonen et al., 2012).

20.2.1.5 Reduced Dopamine Responses during Withdrawal

Repeated exposure can neutralize the effect of addictive substances by downregulating pleasure pathways. This is seen in brain imaging studies in humans in which amphetamine-induced or methylphenidate-induced striatal dopamine responses are 50% lower in detoxified abusers and 80% lower in active abusers. The condition of reduced dopamine responses is accompanied by lower self-reports of the drug's rewarding effects relative to non–drug-abusing controls (Martinez et al., 2007; Volkow et al., 2007).

20.2.1.6 Increased Stress Response

As tolerance and withdrawal develop, brain stress systems, such as corticotropin-releasing factor (CRF), norepinephrine, and dynorphin, are recruited in the extended amygdala and contribute to the development of negative emotional states in withdrawal and protracted abstinence (Koob et al., 2014).

20.2.1.7 Antireward

The increasing activity in CRF in response to increases in dopamine responses is labeled the *antireward effect*. Multiple circuits are likely to contribute to the hypothesized opponent-like processes. Antireward circuits are engaged as neuroadaptations during the development of addiction, producing aversive or stress-like states (Koob et al., 2014).

20.2.1.8 Relationship of Tolerance to Withdrawal

Tolerance can be seen to be driven by an increasingly stressful withdrawal syndrome. In this way, tolerance and withdrawal are linked as the disease progresses in severity. The worse the symptoms of withdrawal, the greater the urge to use addictive substances to avoid withdrawal. Withdrawal can consist of chronic irritability, emotional pain, malaise, dysphoria, alexithymia, states of stress, and loss of motivation for natural rewards. Across all major drugs of abuse, this stage is characterized in laboratory animals by decreased reward during withdrawal. During acute and protracted withdrawal from chronic administration of all drugs of abuse, increases in stress and anxiety-like responses occur that contribute greatly to the malaise of abstinence and protracted abstinence (Koob & Le Moal, 2005).

20.2.1.9 Habit Formation

Triggered increases in dopamine levels recruit habit-forming pathways of the brain, resulting in reinforcement of addictive routines (Belin, Jonkman, Dickinson, Robbins, & Everitt, 2009).

20.2.1.10 Enhanced Avoidance Habits

The enhancement of avoidance habits describes the progression of desire to avoid withdrawal. It provides another basis for the relationship of activation of the stress pathways to intense urges that occur in response to addictive cues (Gillan et al., 2014).

20.2.1.11 Persistence of Effects

The effects of withdrawal can become more persistent as the addiction progresses. Teaching addicts how to cope with stress helps build recovery and reduce the risk of relapse. Sensitivity in stress pathways can leave the client vulnerable to stress insofar as the sensitized addict could experience greater stress than a person who has never had an addiction (Koob & Bloom, 1988).

20.2.1.12 Reduced Response to Natural Rewards

Human brain imaging studies have demonstrated decreases in the sensitivity of brain reward circuits to stimulation by natural rewards during withdrawal. There is a loss of interest in normal, nondrug rewards, which can be thought of as a narrowing of the range of normal behavior and a growing expansion of focus on drugs and drug-related cues (Garavan et al., 2000).

20.2.1.13 Impaired Cognitive Function

Deficits in executive function worsen as the addiction progresses. Deficits are reflected in decreases in frontal cortex activity that indicate problems with decision making, self-regulation, inhibitory control, and working memory and might involve disrupted GABAergic activity (Volkow, Wang, Fowler, Tomasi, & Telang, 2011).

The science of addiction has taken significant strides toward describing the progression of the disease. The extent of neuroadaptations to chronic drug use is widespread, involving pleasure, reward, habit, stress, and cognition. With this research, it becomes possible to devise focused methods to prevent the development of addiction with earlier interventions and recognition of the role of cues. The science of overeating has also uncovered similar dysfunctions in chronic overeaters. These are shown in the next section.

20.2.2 Evidence for Progression in PFA

As is increasingly evident, chronic overeating shares characteristics with drug and alcohol addiction. In recent years, evidence has been developed that makes a case for progressive use or tolerance of processed foods. Using the categories shown above for new discoveries in progression in drug addiction, similar dysfunctions can be described for progressive use of processed foods. Two recent review articles describing progression in overeating are summarized below (Moore et al., 2017; Stice & Yokum, 2016).

20.2.2.1 Incentive Salience

Researchers have shown that repeated receipt of a milkshake increased dopamine responses in a population of women (Burger & Stice, 2014).

20.2.2.2 Phases of Dopamine Release

Research has shown that repeated receipt of a milkshake resulted in dopamine responses shifting from the taste of the milkshake to cues preceding receipt of the milkshake (Burger & Stice, 2014).

20.2.2.3 Decreased Reward and Escalation of Use

A study of rats fed a cafeteria diet over 15 weeks showed decreased dopamine releases and increases in obesity as compared to chow-fed rats, which showed normal dopamine levels and no weight gain (Geiger et al., 2009).

20.2.2.4 Reduction in Endocannabinoid Function

In a rat study, after 10 or 15 weeks of a processed food diet, the endocannabinoid system was found to be widely downregulated (Harrold, Elliott, King, Widdowson, & Williams, 2002; Timofeeva, Baraboi, Poulin, & Richard, 2009). A rat study demonstrated that brains in withdrawal from sugar/fat recruited the endocannabinoid system possibly to dampen withdrawal (Blasio et al., 2013). These findings suggest that downregulation of endocannabinoid receptors would increase the severity of withdrawal and possibly promote the habit of avoiding withdrawal from processed foods.

20.2.2.5 Reduced Dopamine Responses during Withdrawal

In animal models, high-fat and high-sugar diets induce downregulated dopamine throughout the brain. Over time, the once-rewarding properties of palatable food are diminished. Progressive overeating may therefore reflect the urge to reactivate progressively downregulated reward circuits (Geiger et al., 2009).

20.2.2.6 Antireward/Increased Stress

Extended access to drugs and palatable food engages the CRF system (Cottone, Sabino, Roberto, et al., 2009; Iemolo et al., 2013; Koob, 2010). During palatable food withdrawal, CRF expression is increased in the central amygdala and is accompanied by anxiety-like behavior (Cottone, Sabino, Roberto, et al., 2009; Iemolo et al., 2013; Teegarden & Bale, 2007; Teegarden, Nestler, & Bale, 2008). Individuals reporting chronic stress showed less engagement of cognitive pathways in response to images of high-calorie foods and showed greater caloric intake (Stice & Yokum, 2016).

20.2.2.7 Relationship of Tolerance to Withdrawal

Animal research showed that a CRF antagonist did not affect feeding after the first withdrawal from palatable food but did so after rats were exposed to a sugary diet for 7 weeks. This progression in the activity of stress pathways was reflected in increased eating of the sugar diet after withdrawal and upon return to access (Cottone, Sabino, Roberto, et al., 2009).

20.2.2.8 Habit Formation

In a human study using fMRI, researchers found decreased activation of goal-directed pathways and increased activity in habit-responding pathways in response to palatable food tastes in obese subjects as compared to healthy weight controls (Babbs et al., 2013). This suggests a greater reliance on habit than goals in the obese. A study found obese subjects engage in habit-based responding (Voon et al., 2015). Both drug-addicted and obese individuals show abnormal activation of prefrontal cortex regions following cue exposure. In compulsive eating, this increased activation is thought to reengage the basal ganglia circuitry involved in habitual overeating (Moore et al., 2017).

20.2.2.9 Enhanced Avoidance Habits

Animal studies have shown that rats cycled between palatable chow and regular chow show increasingly active stress pathways in the brain. As the sensation of stress increases, the drive to avoid withdrawal progresses and becomes a habit (Moore et al., 2017).

20.2.2.10 Persistence of Effects

Evidence shows that plasticity in the brain stress systems is triggered by acute excessive drug/palatable food intake. The stress pathways are sensitized by repeated withdrawal. The sensitization persists into protracted abstinence and contributes to the development and persistence of addiction (Koob, 2013). "Loss of control" is thought to result from deficits in restraint functions, which would otherwise suppress addictive eating. Impaired restraint likely increases risk of relapse. Impaired restraint emerges from persistent and prolonged drug use or palatable food overconsumption (Lubman, Yucel, & Pantelis, 2004; Volkow, Wang, Tomasi, & Baler, 2013). Habits can be considered compulsive when they persist despite devaluation (reduced pleasure) of the reward (Everitt & Robbins, 2016). Analogously to what is observed in drug addiction, in chronic overconsumption of processed foods, the inability to adapt reduce eating in the face of reduced pleasure may reflect the development of a compulsive habit (Everitt & Robbins, 2016; Moore et al., 2017; Voon, 2015).

20.2.2.11 Reduced Response to Natural Rewards

Intermittent, extended access to palatable food progressively leads to undereating of less preferred diets when palatable food is not available (Blasio, Rice, Sabino, & Cottone, 2014). This may be the underlying dysfunction that manifests as a "picky eater."

20.2.2.12 Impaired Cognitive Function

Balodis et al. found that binge eating individuals had lower striatal and prefrontal activation to anticipation of a monetary reward, and this decrease was associated with increased incidence of binge eating (Balodis et al., 2014; Moore et al., 2017). Further, lower prefrontal cortex response to high-calorie food images predicted greater ad lib food intake over the next 3 days (Cornier, Salzberg, Endly, Bessesen, & Tregellas, 2010). Stice et al. replicated this finding (Stice & Yokum, 2016).

The parallels in descriptions of progression in drug addicts and in chronic overeaters support the concept that progression is a valid diagnostic criterion in PFA. The descriptions also serve to portray the extensive nature of the neuroanomalies. Where a practitioner finds that clients describe progression in their consumption of processed foods, it would seem appropriate to be concerned about the scope of the brain dysfunction, whether the description is early stage without severe consequences, or late stage when the disease is manifesting as widespread reduction in quality of life.

20.3 MANIFESTATIONS

The illustrations of progressive use below are taken from the manuals of two 12-step groups: Food Addicts Anonymous and Food Addicts in Recovery Anonymous. As the research demonstrates, food-addicted clients can progress in terms of cravings, behaviors, loss of interest in nonaddictive foods, and consequences. The progressive loss of interest in natural rewards can be seen as food-addicted clients lose interest in natural nonaddictive foods. This progression might manifest in children as a picky eater who will not eat nonaddictive foods. There is also progression in terms of perceptions of futility and responses to stress.

> I also bought baguettes at the supermarket—the long, thin French breads. They came in three-loaf packages. I figured I'd buy extra for the kids, who'd be bringing their friends home. Of course, my children never got the baguettes, because I ate them all. After a while, I started buying two packages of baguettes—six loaves of bread. (Food Addicts in Recovery Anonymous, 2013, 5)

In the next two examples, it may be postulated that the feelings of inadequacy and anger may be exacerbated by progressively more sensitive stress pathways.

> When I ate, I felt better. This caused a bad cycle. My feelings of inadequacy made me eat, but the eating made me fat. Fatness made me feel more inadequate, which increased my drive to eat. (Food Addicts in Recovery Anonymous, 2013, 20–21)
>
> As an adult working woman, I was getting bigger and bigger, and angrier and angrier. My rage scared me. I knew if I ate, it would numb my anger a little, so I went ahead and ate. Because I ate, I got bigger, which infuriated me, and that made me eat more. I felt like a gerbil in a cage. (Food Addicts in Recovery Anonymous, 2013, 150)
>
> I felt like I was being chased by a demon and the only way to keep it at bay was to do more and more—more food, more drugs. (Food Addicts Anonymous, 2010, 119)
>
> I ate and was very smug and satisfied with myself. As my core issues surfaced more and more, my behavior escalated until I was buying a pound of chocolates to take home and pints of sugar-free yogurt and ice cream. Then I decided that after all the time I had in recovery and all the weight I had lost, I would introduce bread back into my food plan. When I finally admitted I was eating out of control again, I dove into the food like never before. I now ate a bucket of fried chicken at a time. (Food Addicts Anonymous, 2010, 120–121)

I had no idea that by now my addiction to sugar, flour and wheat had progressed even further and that I was physically addicted to these substances, forever craving more and more. (Food Addicts Anonymous, 2010, 126)

As I became more preoccupied with food, my body was becoming increasingly addicted to those abusive substances. I began to use exercise to purge myself of the calories I ingested. At a skinny ninety-eight pounds, my self-worth was based on how diligently I adhered to my caloric allotment, which generally encompassed candy all day with one normal meal. At age sixteen, I began to abuse alcohol, which I now believe is correlated to my sugar addiction. I frequently lost control of what I ate during those inebriated periods. My collegiate years illustrate the serious progression of my disease into exercise bulimia. Gaining fifteen pounds at the beginning of each new school year, I continued the cycle of drinking, bingeing and exercising compulsively. I ran in rain, sleet, or snow, and averaged six miles daily. During one winter vacation, I trained to become an aerobics instructor and overdid it so severely that I caused a stress fracture in my leg. My exercise addiction and preoccupation with having the "perfect" body became so severe at this time that, despite doctor's suggestions, I continued exercising on my hurt leg.

I nearly forced a complete fracture, but I simply could not stop. My fear of gaining weight overpowered my fear of breaking my leg. Food had turned on me several years before and now exercise had let me down as well. Because most of my waking hours were spent figuring how I would "get rid of" the calories I had ingested, managing my food and exercise became my primary purpose in college and gaining an education was secondary. In addition, my ability to concentrate was minimal as a result of the substances I put into my body.

Reflecting on those collegiate years and the two-and-a-half years following, I compare myself to a gerbil on a treadmill, not knowing how to get off. This vicious cycle of drinking, bingeing, and purging through exercise continued as my physical well-being became severely affected. My heart was telling me it was over-working, yet my compulsion forced me to shut out that information. I know now I was very close to a heart attack.

By the grace of God, I got sober in AA, yet my food addiction escalated. My body craved the sugar it had gotten from alcohol and I was forced to replace it, particularly with simple carbohydrates. I could no longer exercise enough to maintain my "normal," thin figure. (Food Addicts Anonymous, 2010, 133–134)

I longed to be able to eat delicately, but once I began I was an eating machine. One of my binges landed me in the hospital with acute pancreatitis. Another cost me my appendix. The years marched on and my disease progressed. Twice I attempted suicide because I could not live with the depression that always followed a binge. (Food Addicts Anonymous, 2010, 143)

I first found a support group that suggested a food plan that was free of white flour and sugar. I had some relief but I am addicted to wheat, too. Use of wheat products triggered my physical craving, and my mental obsession became more intense. I have a disease that is progressive. (Food Addicts Anonymous, 2010, 166)

I felt very lucky. He did not seem to mind my size, so of course, I ate all the more. (Food Addicts Anonymous, 2010, 168)

At the age of thirteen, I worked "off the books" for $1 an hour as a dishwasher at a local diner. I ate everything I could get my hands on. I saw myself "beating the system," which was always an important game I played, by eating free food and participating in my favorite activity. Eating for free gave me a truly euphoric feeling. The better it made me feel, the more I ate. (Food Addicts Anonymous, 2010, 190)

Food and eating were better than sex, more loyal than a friend, and truer than a wife. Food was heaven. Bingeing was seventh heaven. It was a sick and pathetic cycle. As I grew deeper and deeper into food, my functioning in life, work, and relationships became increasingly difficult. I was out of control and desperate. (Food Addicts Anonymous, 2010, 192)

As I reached puberty, the tables turned for me. I began to eat more and more food. I had the responsibility of cleaning up the kitchen after dinner. I cleaned up all right—I was the garbage can. Then of course, it was time for dessert. I started stealing food from the store across the street from our house. (Food Addicts Anonymous, 2010, 194)

I tried dieting, exercising, praying, reading books, reading my Bible and going to bed early only to wake up during the night for my donut binge. The compulsion inside me for food just escalated. (Food Addicts Anonymous, 2010, 213)

Breakfast consisted of donuts, cookies, or eggs and bacon, depending upon whether or not there was time to cook. Lunch was a sandwich with various sweets and carbohydrates. More sweets and carbohydrates followed protein and vegetables at dinner. Things had gotten so bad that I couldn't make it more than an hour or two at work without leaving the office to get something to eat. Some days, when things were really stressful, I would turn to the desk drawer full of sweets to help me cope.

Sometimes it seemed like I ate non-stop. I looked forward to work for the chance to eat at my desk without anyone knowing about it and I looked forward to getting home to eat before, during, and after dinner. I looked forward to time spent at my in-laws' house on the weekend where there was always food and alcohol galore. I looked forward to shopping by myself because I could get all kinds of sweets at the mall, but I dreaded shopping for clothes. I was becoming more mean and irritable. The sweets seemed to sedate me. (Food Addicts Anonymous, 2010, 225–226)

I guess I loved to help out in the kitchen because it meant extra food after meals. As I got older and needed more "fixes," I would sneak to the refrigerator and eat slices of raw butter or drink maple syrup out of the bottle. If there was ice cream in the freezer, I'd be there with a spoon. I began sneaking snacks and jars of peanut butter into my bedroom. I was actually hiding wrappers under my bed. (Food Addicts Anonymous, 2010, 229)

My disease progressed beyond my wildest imagination. Food became more important than my daughter, my husband, my integrity or anything else in my life. I would sneak food, hide food, leave the house at ungodly hours for it, stash it, and so on. I manipulated people, places and things so that I could be alone with my fix. One time, while my husband was paying our dinner check, I snuck back and ate the leftover food on his plate. My life consisted of bingeing, purging and exercising. It was nothing for me to do intense aerobic exercise for four hours a day. (Food Addicts Anonymous, 2010, 235–236)

However, one day my frustrations and anger got the better of me and I walked off the job. Suddenly I was alone 12–16 hours a day while my husband worked. I started drinking more, and I began to eat almost constantly. (Food Addicts Anonymous, 2010, 242)

As these quotes show, progression in PFA can take different forms of more frequent episodes of greater quantities of processed foods. As the disease escalates, the behavior and the consequences become more distressing to the addict. The research suggests this increasing stress activates and exacerbates the drive to consume.

20.4 APPLICATION

The evidence for and manifestations of progression in PFA describe widespread alterations in neurofunction upon repeated exposure to processed foods and cues. The combination of decreasing pleasure, increasing stress, stronger habits, decreasing interest in natural foods, as well as decreasing restraint, learning, memory, and decision-making offer an explanation for increasing use. The evidence suggests that food-addicted clients are attempting to deal with stress in an irrational way. The compensating pleasure pathways are decreasing in effectiveness, but the addict no longer has the ability to think through the problem and realize that increasing use is a harmful method for addressing stress. With conflicting information from media, diet, and health industries explaining the problem as one of "weight loss" rather than a progressive mental illness, the progression model offers a possible rationale for why people continue to experience higher and higher BMI.

20.4.1 Using Progression to Motivate Clients

The phenomenon of progression allows the practitioner to describe the course of the disease. The practitioner can help the client see that the disease has worsened over time. With this information, the practitioner can extend the trajectory of deterioration into the future. Clients in the early stages of PFA can be motivated by education about how the disease can progress.

Elements of progression can also help the practitioner describe severity in the statement of the scope of the problem. Food-addicted clients can be challenged in believing that they have a severe mental illness. Putting the problem in the context of progression could help clarify the seriousness of the condition to clients. Progression in terms of volume and frequency is a descriptor. Loss of cognitive abilities is also indicative. Clients may recognize difficulties in focusing, decision-making, and memory, but they may not have realized that these are related to the progression of PFA.

In the realm of PFA, loss of interest in natural rewards could be important. Clients may have developed an aversion to healthy unprocessed foods in the progression of the addiction. They may profess to being picky eaters. This could be especially true for children. Framing this loss of interest in nonaddictive foods as an element of the progression of the disease could be important information for the client.

20.4.2 Use in Treatment

The practitioner can use information about the client's progressive use and the diagnostic and assessment processes. Information about the severity of progress can help the client build a program that prevents relapse and promotes sobriety. By understanding the circumstances that supported progression, practitioners can work with clients to build specific protections against cues and stress into their programs. For example, if isolation permitted the progression, then community activities might be important. If a job loss led to progression, finding volunteer work might be helpful.

Practitioners will also want to know about progression because it will impact in three ways: (1) the distress of withdrawal; (2) impaired capabilities that could impact meal preparation; and (3) consequences that could require medical attention. Nutritional consultations might be recommended if progression has precluded the consumption of nutritious foods for a period of time.

Reductions in dopamine and endocannabinoid function can be addressed by adding activities that are associated with the production of endorphins. These include exercise, meditation, music, healthy sleep, etc.

Given the central role of the hyperactive stress pathways, stress management could be a priority. Teaching the client how to self-soothe as a replacement for the urge to use processed foods could improve outcomes. This is covered in Chapter 7, "Mindfulness Therapies for Food Addiction," in Part I, "Foundations."

The progression model describes the recruitment of habit-formation functions in the development of chronic overeating. This suggests the value of using habit-formation approaches in recovery from PFA. Efficacy has been demonstrated in a study of parenting and another of obesity (Lally, Chipperfield, & Wardle, 2008; McGowan et al., 2013).

Cognitive impairment is described in the progression model. Given the need to learn complex tasks such as meal preparation, cue avoidance, and relationship management, cognitive restoration could be a high priority in recovery from PFA. Online brain training has been shown to be effective in this regard (Hardy et al., 2015). The lack of interest in natural rewards could be addressed by having clients look at pictures of unprocessed foods.

Education about the nature of withdrawal could help clients reduce their aversion to withdrawal. Clients may be avoiding withdrawal without being conscious of doing so. They may be using processed foods to relieve stress as a habit without the awareness that the stress could be caused by the processed foods and, further, that paradoxically stress could be relieved by giving up addictive processed foods altogether. Understanding the nature of the progression of PFA can be helpful in the development of a treatment plan.

20.5 CONCLUSION

Progression is now a well-researched phenomenon in drug and alcohol addiction. As understanding has been developed for classic drug addiction, progression has now been documented in use of processed foods as well. The neuroadaptations are extensive, including downregulation of pleasure, cognitive, and natural reward pathways in conjunction with sensitization of stress and habit pathways. The scientific evidence is corroborated by cases from the stories found in the 12-step manuals of the food addiction fellowships.

A grounding in understanding of progression in PFA helps the practitioner diagnose PFA, even in early-stage cases where increases may be small. It also gives the practitioner the ability to counsel, comfort, and encourage clients. Learning about progression helps practitioners feel grounded in the PFA model and incorporate helpful recovery protocols into their practice.

REFERENCES

American Psychiatric Association. (2013). *The Diagnostic and Statistical Manual of Mental Disorders,* Fifth Edition (Vol. 5).

Babbs, R. K., Sun, X., Felsted, J., Chouinard-Decorte, F., Veldhuizen, M. G., & Small, D. M. (2013). Decreased caudate response to milkshake is associated with higher body mass index and greater impulsivity. *Physiol Behav, 121,* 103–111. doi:10.1016/j.physbeh.2013.03.025.

Balodis, I. M., Grilo, C. M., Kober, H., Worhunsky, P. D., White, M. A., Stevens, M. C., … Potenza, M. N. (2014). A pilot study linking reduced fronto-striatal recruitment during reward processing to persistent bingeing following treatment for binge-eating disorder. *Int J Eat Disord, 47*(4), 376–384. doi:10.1002/eat.22204.

Belin, D., Jonkman, S., Dickinson, A., Robbins, T. W., & Everitt, B. J. (2009). Parallel and interactive learning processes within the basal ganglia: Relevance for the understanding of addiction. *Behav Brain Res, 199*(1), 89–102. doi:10.1016/j.bbr.2008.09.027.

Blasio, A., Iemolo, A., Sabino, V., Petrosino, S., Steardo, L., Rice, K. C., … Cottone, P. (2013). Rimonabant precipitates anxiety in rats withdrawn from palatable food: Role of the central amygdala. *Neuropsychopharmacology, 38*(12), 2498–2507. doi:10.1038/npp.2013.153.

Blasio, A., Rice, K. C., Sabino, V., & Cottone, P. (2014). Characterization of a shortened model of diet alternation in female rats: Effects of the CB1 receptor antagonist rimonabant on food intake and anxiety-like behavior. *Behav Pharmacol, 25*(7), 609–617. doi:10.1097/fbp.0000000000000059.

Burger, K. S., & Stice, E. (2014). Greater striatopallidal adaptive coding during cue-reward learning and food reward habituation predict future weight gain. *NeuroImage, 99,* 122–128. doi:10.1016/j.neuroimage.2014.05.066.

Ceccarini, J., Hompes, T., Verhaeghen, A., Casteels, C., Peuskens, H., Bormans, G., … Van Laere, K. (2014). Changes in cerebral CB1 receptor availability after acute and chronic alcohol abuse and monitored abstinence. *J Neurosci, 34*(8), 2822–2831. doi:10.1523/jneurosci.0849-13.2014.

Cornier, M. A., Salzberg, A. K., Endly, D. C., Bessesen, D. H., & Tregellas, J. R. (2010). Sex-based differences in the behavioral and neuronal responses to food. *Physiol Behav, 99*(4), 538–543. doi:10.1016/j.physbeh.2010.01.008.

Cottone, P., Sabino, V., Roberto, M., Bajo, M., Pockros, L., Frihauf, J. B., … Zorrilla, E. P. (2009). CRF system recruitment mediates dark side of compulsive eating. *Proc Natl Acad Sci U S A, 106*(47), 20016–20020. doi:10.1073/pnas.0908789106.

Cottone, P., Sabino, V., Steardo, L., & Zorrilla, E. P. (2009). Consummatory, anxiety-related and metabolic adaptations in female rats with alternating access to preferred food. *Psychoneuroendocrinology, 34*(1), 38–49. doi:10.1016/j.psyneuen.2008.08.010.

Everitt, B. J., & Robbins, T. W. (2016). Drug addiction: Updating actions to habits to compulsions ten years on. *Annu Rev Psychol, 67,* 23–50. doi:10.1146/annurev-psych-122414-033457.

Food Addicts Anonymous. (2010). *Food Addicts Anonymous.* Port St. Lucie, FL: Food Addicts Anonymous, Inc.

Food Addicts in Recovery Anonymous. (2013). *Food Addicts in Recovery Anonymous.* Woburn, MA: Food Addicts in Recovery Anonymous.

Garavan, H., Pankiewicz, J., Bloom, A., Cho, J. K., Sperry, L., Ross, T. J., … Stein, E. A. (2000). Cue-induced cocaine craving: Neuroanatomical specificity for drug users and drug stimuli. *Am J Psychiatry, 157*(11), 1789–1798. doi:10.1176/appi.ajp.157.11.1789.

Geiger, B. M., Haburcak, M., Avena, N. M., Moyer, M. C., Hoebel, B. G., & Pothos, E. N. (2009). Deficits of mesolimbic dopamine neurotransmission in rat dietary obesity. *Neuroscience, 159*(4), 1193–1199. doi:10.1016/j.neuroscience.2009.02.007.

Gibson, E. L. (2006). Emotional influences on food choice: Sensory, physiological and psychological pathways. *Physiol Behav, 89*(1), 53–61.

Gillan, C. M., Morein-Zamir, S., Urcelay, G. P., Sule, A., Voon, V., Apergis-Schoute, A. M., … Robbins, T. W. (2014). Enhanced avoidance habits in obsessive-compulsive disorder. *Biol Psychiatry, 75*(8), 631–638. doi:10.1016/j.biopsych.2013.02.002.

Hardy, J. L., Nelson, R. A., Thomason, M. E., Sternberg, D. A., Katovich, K., Farzin, F., & Scanlon, M. (2015). Enhancing cognitive abilities with comprehensive training: A large, online, randomized, active-controlled trial. *PLoS One, 10*(9), e0134467. doi:10.1371/journal.pone.0134467.

Harrold, J. A., Elliott, J. C., King, P. J., Widdowson, P. S., & Williams, G. (2002). Down-regulation of cannabinoid-1 (CB-1) receptors in specific extrahypothalamic regions of rats with dietary obesity: A role for endogenous cannabinoids in driving appetite for palatable food? *Brain Res, 952*(2), 232–238.

Hirvonen, J., Goodwin, R. S., Li, C. T., Terry, G. E., Zoghbi, S. S., Morse, C., … Innis, R. B. (2012). Reversible and regionally selective downregulation of brain cannabinoid CB1 receptors in chronic daily cannabis smokers. *Mol Psychiatry, 17*(6), 642–649. doi:10.1038/mp.2011.82.

Iemolo, A., Blasio, A., St Cyr, S. A., Jiang, F., Rice, K. C., Sabino, V., & Cottone, P. (2013). CRF-CRF1 receptor system in the central and basolateral nuclei of the amygdala differentially mediates excessive eating of palatable food. *Neuropsychopharmacology, 38*(12), 2456–2466. doi:10.1038/npp.2013.147.

Koob, G. F. (2010). The role of CRF and CRF-related peptides in the dark side of addiction. *Brain Res, 1314*, 3–14. doi:10.1016/j.brainres.2009.11.008.

Koob, G. F. (2013). Negative reinforcement in drug addiction: The darkness within. *Curr Opin Neurobiol, 23*(4), 559–563. doi:10.1016/j.conb.2013.03.011.

Koob, G. F., & Bloom, F. E. (1988). Cellular and molecular mechanisms of drug dependence. *Science, 242*(4879), 715–723.

Koob, G. F., Buck, C. L., Cohen, A., Edwards, S., Park, P. E., Schlosburg, J. E., … George, O. (2014). Addiction as a stress surfeit disorder. *Neuropharmacology, 76 Pt B*, 370–382. doi:10.1016/j.neuropharm.2013.05.024.

Koob, G. F., & Le Moal, M. (2005). Plasticity of reward neurocircuitry and the 'dark side' of drug addiction. *Nat Neurosci, 8*(11), 1442–1444. doi:10.1038/nn1105-1442

Koob, G. F., & Volkow, N. D. (2016). Neurobiology of addiction: A neurocircuitry analysis. *Lancet Psychiatry, 3*(8), 760–773. doi:10.1016/s2215-0366(16)00104-8.

Lally, P., Chipperfield, A., & Wardle, J. (2008). Healthy habits: Efficacy of simple advice on weight control based on a habit-formation model. *Int J Obes (Lond), 32*(4), 700–707. doi:10.1038/sj.ijo.0803771.

Lubman, D. I., Yucel, M., & Pantelis, C. (2004). Addiction, a condition of compulsive behaviour? Neuroimaging and neuropsychological evidence of inhibitory dysregulation. *Addiction, 99*(12), 1491–1502. doi:10.1111/j.1360-0443.2004.00808.x.

Martinez, D., Narendran, R., Foltin, R. W., Slifstein, M., Hwang, D. R., Broft, A., … Laruelle, M. (2007). Amphetamine-induced dopamine release: Markedly blunted in cocaine dependence and predictive of the choice to self-administer cocaine. *Am J Psychiatry, 164*(4), 622–629. doi:10.1176/ajp.2007.164.4.622.

McGowan, L., Cooke, L. J., Gardner, B., Beeken, R. J., Croker, H., & Wardle, J. (2013). Healthy feeding habits: Efficacy results from a cluster-randomized, controlled exploratory trial of a novel, habit-based intervention with parents. *Am J Clin Nutr, 98*(3), 769–777. doi:10.3945/ajcn.112.052159.

Moore, C. F., Sabino, V., Koob, G. F., & Cottone, P. (2017). Pathological overeating: Emerging evidence for a compulsivity construct. *Neuropsychopharmacology*, *42*(7), 1375–1389. doi:10.1038/npp.2016.269.

Stice, E., & Yokum, S. (2016). Neural vulnerability factors that increase risk for future weight gain. *Psychol Bull, 142*(5), 447–471. doi:10.1037/bul0000044.

Teegarden, S. L., & Bale, T. L. (2007). Decreases in dietary preference produce increased emotionality and risk for dietary relapse. *Biol Psychiatry, 61*(9), 1021–1029. doi:10.1016/j.biopsych.2006.09.032.

Teegarden, S. L., Nestler, E. J., & Bale, T. L. (2008). Delta FosB-mediated alterations in dopamine signaling are normalized by a palatable high-fat diet. *Biol Psychiatry, 64*(11), 941–950. doi:10.1016/j.biopsych.2008.06.007.

Timofeeva, E., Baraboi, E. D., Poulin, A. M., & Richard, D. (2009). Palatable high-energy diet decreases the expression of cannabinoid type 1 receptor messenger RNA in specific brain regions in the rat. *J Neuroendocrinol, 21*(12), 982–992. doi:10.1111/j.1365-2826.2009.01921.x.

Volkow, N. D., Koob, G. F., & McLellan, A. T. (2016). Neurobiologic advances from the brain disease model of addiction. *N Engl J Med, 374*(4), 363–371. doi:10.1056/NEJMra1511480.

Volkow, N. D., Wang, G. J., Fowler, J. S., Tomasi, D., & Telang, F. (2011). Addiction: Beyond dopamine reward circuitry. *Proc Natl Acad Sci U S A, 108*(37), 15037–15042. doi:10.1073/pnas.1010654108.

Volkow, N. D., Wang, G. J., Telang, F., Fowler, J. S., Logan, J., Jayne, M., … Wong, C. (2007). Profound decreases in dopamine release in striatum in detoxified alcoholics: Possible orbitofrontal involvement. *J Neurosci, 27*(46), 12700–12706. doi:10.1523/jneurosci.3371-07.2007.

Volkow, N. D., Wang, G. J., Tomasi, D., & Baler, R. D. (2013). The addictive dimensionality of obesity. *Biol Psychiatry, 73*(9), 811–818. doi:10.1016/j.biopsych.2012.12.020.

Voon, V. (2015). Cognitive biases in binge eating disorder: The hijacking of decision making. *CNS Spectr, 20*(6), 566–573. doi:10.1017/s1092852915000681.

Voon, V., Derbyshire, K., Ruck, C., Irvine, M. A., Worbe, Y., Enander, J., … Bullmore, E. T. (2015). Disorders of compulsivity: A common bias towards learning habits. *Mol Psychiatry, 20*(3), 345–352. doi:10.1038/mp.2014.44.

Yau, P. L., Kang, E. H., Javier, D. C., & Convit, A. (2014). Preliminary evidence of cognitive and brain abnormalities in uncomplicated adolescent obesity. *Obesity (Silver Spring), 22*(8), 1865–1871. doi:10.1002/oby.20801.

Zhu, N., Jacobs, D. R., Meyer, K. A., He, K., Launer, L., Reis, J. P., … Steffen, L. M. (2015). Cognitive function in a middle aged cohort is related to higher quality dietary pattern 5 and 25 years earlier: The CARDIA study. *J Nutr Health Aging, 19*(1), 33–38. doi:10.1007/s12603-014-0491-7.

21 DSM 5 SUD Criterion 11 *Withdrawal*

Joan Ifland
Food Addiction Training, LLC
Cincinnati, OH

H. Theresa Wright
Renaissance Nutrition
East Norriton, PA

CONTENTS

Withdrawal, as manifested by either of the following:

1. The characteristic withdrawal syndrome for processed foods.
2. Processed foods are eaten to relieve or avoid withdrawal symptoms. (American Psychiatric Association, 2013, 491)

21.1 INTRODUCTION

Substance withdrawal has been defined by the American Psychiatric Association as "the development of a substance-specific maladaptive behavioral change, usually with uncomfortable physiological and cognitive consequences, that is the result of a cessation of, or reduction in, heavy and prolonged substance use. More severe withdrawal is associated with greater functional impairment and poor prognosis" (American Society of Addiction Medicine, 2014, 625). This was written for substance use disorders, but it is true for PFA clients in withdrawal from processed foods as well.

Withdrawal is one of the most important diagnostic criteria for addictions. Some professionals believe that without a withdrawal syndrome, a substance cannot be considered to be addictive. This is based on the belief that withdrawal perpetuates the addiction by creating a drive to avoid the distress of withdrawal. Indeed, some people believe that processed food addiction (PFA) does not exist because there is no withdrawal syndrome. This chapter describes evidence to the contrary.

Some experts include a withdrawal syndrome in the definition of PFA. "Food addicts usually present both a tolerance (i.e., a need to increase participation in their harmful relationships with food over space and time) as well as a form of withdrawal (i.e., an inability to escape their addiction with food without suffering undue anxiety, craving, or other adverse neurochemical reactivity [which may include depression or anger]) when deprived of access to addictive foods (Gold & Shriner, 2013, 785).

The DSM 5 does not require withdrawal to assess positively for the presence of an addiction. Only 50% of middle-class, high-functional individuals with alcohol use disorder will have ever experienced a full alcohol withdrawal syndrome (American Psychiatric Association, 2013, 501). Adolescents exhibit fewer alcohol withdrawal symptoms than adults (Martin & Winters, 1998). Children PFA clients may not exhibit withdrawal other than pleading for processed foods. So withdrawal is not a prerequisite for diagnosing PFA.

Nonetheless, as this chapter shows, there is evidence for a processed food withdrawal syndrome. Research is emerging on this topic. A number of laboratories have reported a syndrome of withdrawal from high-fat, high-sugar foods in animals (Cottone, Sabino, Roberto, et al., 2009; Cottone, Sabino, Steardo, & Zorrilla, 2008a, 2008b, 2009; Iemolo et al., 2012; Martire et al., 2014; Martire, Westbrook, & Morris, 2015; Moore, Sabino, Koob, & Cottone, 2017; Morris, Beilharz, Maniam, Reichelt, & Westbrook, 2014; Parylak, Koob, & Zorrilla, 2011; Smith & Robbins, 2013; South, Westbrook, & Morris, 2012; Teegarden & Bale, 2007). A hospital clinic treating PFA is reporting on a withdrawal syndrome related to processed foods (Shriner, 2013). And the 12-step manuals contain qualitative descriptions of the syndrome. In this chapter, practitioners will learn how to manage withdrawal and prepare clients for the process.

Withdrawal from processed foods is more difficult to organize into a syndrome because of the variety of addictive substances involved. "Substances in a given pharmacologic class produce similar withdrawal syndromes; however, the onset, duration, and intensity are variable, depending on the particular agent used, the duration of use, and the degree of neuroadaptation" (American Society of Addiction Medicine, 2014, 624). Because processed foods may contain combinations of sugar, artificial sweeteners, high fructose corn syrup, caffeine, processed fats, dairy, and excessive salt, withdrawal symptoms may vary with the type of foods and drinks most heavily used by the food addict.

For example, a food addict who is abusing caffeine and artificial sweetener in the form of diet sodas could experience different symptoms from a food addict who is abusing ice cream, which is high in sugar and fat. Baked sweet goods, which are high in sugar and gluteomorphin, can produce yet another set of symptoms. Bread, processed fats, and dairy may also have different withdrawal symptomology. The quantity of processed food being consumed could also affect severity and duration of withdrawal. A past history of drug abuse and the presence of mental illness may also make withdrawal from processed foods more severe.

21.1.1 Importance

It is very important to learn about withdrawal from processed foods. For some practitioners and clients, it is persuasive evidence that processed foods are addictive. For clients who doubt whether they have PFA, withdrawal can provide convincing evidence and help motivate the client to commit to building a recovery program.

For the practitioner, learning about withdrawal is vital to preparing clients to go through the process. For heavy users, withdrawal may mean 4–8 days of headache, nausea, fatigue, depression, disorientation, and intense cravings. Unless clients understand that they're going through withdrawal and that the distress is short term, they may give up and reintroduce the addictive food or drink to relieve symptoms. It's possible that increased cravings stemming from withdrawal could be a factor in the failure to cut back, as described in Criterion 2. If clients know that sometime after the fourth day of withdrawal, the symptoms will stop, they are more likely to fight through and complete withdrawal. They can then learn how to abstain from addictive foods and avoid lapsing with the distress of a return to bingeing.

Throughout the process of withdrawal or detoxification, the practitioner can offer encouragement and education about the long-term process of recovery to help motivate the client to complete withdrawal.

21.2 EVIDENCE

In recent years, researchers seem to have developed interest in the processed food withdrawal syndrome. They have devised both animal and human studies that demonstrate a withdrawal syndrome that is consistent with the characteristics of withdrawal from drugs.

21.2.1 Evidence for a Syndrome of Withdrawal from Processed Foods

There is growing evidence in research for a withdrawal syndrome related to processed foods. Both animal and human studies are emerging.

Of all processed foods, caffeine withdrawal is perhaps the most well documented. The DSM 5 contains diagnostic criteria for caffeine withdrawal, including:

1. Headache
2. Fatigue or drowsiness
3. Dysphoric mood, depressed mood, or irritability
4. Difficulty concentrating
5. Flu-like symptoms (nausea, vomiting, or muscle pain/stiffness) (American Psychiatric Association, 2013, 506)

Practitioners may be tempted to dismiss the seriousness of caffeine use because it is so common. "The ubiquitous use of caffeine and its integration in daily customs and routines (e.g., coffee break) may result in a lack of appreciation for the role that caffeine plays in one's daily subjective experiences, thus making the recognition and treatment of caffeine-associated problems particularly challenging" (Juliano, Ferre, & Griffiths, 2014, 182). Practitioners may wish to delay caffeine withdrawal until withdrawal from other addictive foods is complete. Caffeine withdrawal, especially headache, may take up to 21 days (American Psychiatric Association, 2013, 507). Because the acute phase of withdrawal from processed foods is only 4–8 days, it is better to allow the food addict to start feeling better and be reinforced in the experience of sobriety. Caffeine withdrawal can be accomplished in the third or fourth month of recovery.

21.2.1.1 Evidence from Animal Studies

There is evidence for a withdrawal syndrome for sugar in rats (Avena, Bocarsly, & Hoebel, 2012). Rats that had been bingeing on sugar showed withdrawal symptoms similar to those of morphine withdrawal, including paw tremoring, teeth chattering, and anxiety-related squeaks.

A withdrawal syndrome for high-fructose corn syrup has also been described based on addictive properties for fructose (Lustig, 2013). A study using fruit punch versus a protein drink demonstrated that the carbohydrate drink elevated mood (Corsica & Spring, 2008). This is evidence that sweet drinks can reverse the distress of withdrawal.

A number of animal studies have demonstrated symptoms of withdrawal from a combination of sugar and fat. Symptomology of depression, anxiety, cravings, and altered motor activity have been found.

Depression during withdrawal from a sugar/fat combination has been shown in a rat study. It was found that rats withdrawn from a highly palatable diet showed increased immobility time in the forced swim test, which is considered to be a demonstration of depression (Iemolo et al., 2012).

It was found that cravings and anxiety increased in rats when taken off of a palatable food plan and given regular chow. In withdrawal after 4 weeks of high-fat, high-sugar (HFHS) diet, obesity prone animals increased their motivation (i.e., craving) during the second withdrawal week and reduced time spent in the center of an open field (increased anxiety) compared to obesity-resistant animals.

Obesity-prone individuals may have withdrawal symptoms that are similar to those induced by addictive drugs (Pickering, Alsio, Hulting, & Schioth, 2009).

Another rat study focused on motor activity in withdrawal from HSHF food. After 10 weeks, rats that were cycled between palatable food and regular chow showed less diurnal motor activity than rats maintained on regular chow, regardless of what diet they were currently receiving. Cycled rats were significantly more active on the first day of withdrawal from the palatable foods, suggesting food-seeking behavior. In withdrawal from the palatable diet, rats also exhibited reduced open arm time, indicating increased anxiety, and increased closed arm entries, indicating hyperactivity. In withdrawal, rats also withdrew more into the sheltered chamber of the defensive withdrawal test than did rats consuming only regular chow. This is demonstration of increased anxiety in withdrawal (Cottone, Sabino, Steardo, et al., 2009). This research shows increased anxiety and activity in withdrawal from sugar and fat.

Evidence for a withdrawal syndrome for fat has also been developed. In a rat study, withdrawal from a high-fat, but not a low-fat, diet potentiated anxiety and basal corticosterone levels and enhanced motivation for sucrose and high-fat food rewards (Sharma, Fernandes, & Fulton, 2013).

21.2.1.2 Evidence in Humans

In terms of evidence in humans, there are reports of obese people who experienced not only irritability and nervousness but also intense anxiety upon starting a diet (Keys et al., 1950; Silverstone and Lascelles, 1966; Stunkard, 1957; Moore et al., 2017). This phenomenon may also be related to reducing calories.

While drug users may quit drugs, in PFA, abstinence from certain foods is achieved by "dieting." Dieting may include a reduction in calories ingested and/or a shift from energy-dense, highly palatable "forbidden" foods to energy-diffuse, less palatable "safe" foods. There is evidence that switching from a high- to low-fat diet can have adverse effects on mood (Wells, Read, Laugharne, & Ahluwalia, 1998). Dietary restraint is known to correlate with stress and depressive symptoms (Eldredge et al., 1990; Kagan and Squires, 1983; Rosen et al., 1990; Rosen et al., 1987), and these correlate with overeating in response to stress (Greeno and Wing, 1994; Heatherton et al., 1991), perhaps reflecting an attempt to self-soothe or self-medicate with "comfort" foods (Macht, 2008; Tomiyama et al., 2011) as this eating can effectively dampen down the body's stress response (Pecoraro et al., 2004). In (Iemolo et al., 2012), While withdrawal from palatable food is responsible for the emergence of negative affect and, in turn, hypothesized to drive compulsive eating through a negative reinforcement mechanism, abstaining from calorie-dense food also often implicates caloric restriction, which has well-known effects on rebound binge-eating and weight gain (Stice et al., 2008; Mann et al., 2007). Another demonstration of withdrawal involves showing that substances can reverse the distress of withdrawal. Renewing access to palatable food … is able to relieve withdrawal-induced depressive and anxiety-like behaviors. (Iemolo et al., 2012)

Evidence exists that adaptations in the brain stress systems are triggered by acute excessive palatable food intake. Stress systems are sensitized during repeated withdrawal, the sensitization persists into protracted abstinence and contributes to the development and persistence of addiction (Koob, 2013).

21.2.2 Evidence for the Neurological Basis of Withdrawal

Animal and brain-imaging research has demonstrated the neurological underpinning of withdrawal. In a review article, Koob and Volkow described addiction as a three-stage, recurring cycle of intoxication, withdrawal/negative affect, and preoccupation/anticipation (craving). They note that the cycle worsens over time. Addictions occur because of dysfunctional neuroplastic changes in reward, stress, and executive functions in response to repeated use and cues.

The review article goes on to describe withdrawal across all substances as characterized by chronic irritability, emotional pain, malaise, dysphoria, alexithymia, states of stress, and loss of motivation for natural rewards. In laboratory animals, withdrawal is characterized by decreased rewards. In animal models of the transition to addiction, decreased rewards precede and are highly correlated with escalation in drug intake. During acute and protracted withdrawal from chronic administration of all drugs of abuse, increases in stress and anxiety-like responses also occur that contribute greatly to the malaise of abstinence and protracted abstinence (Koobs).

Research showing changes in circuits during withdrawal is summarized as follows:

Increased Activity	**Decreased Activity**
Corticotropin-releasing factor	Dopamine
Dynorphin	Serotonin
Norepinephrine	Opioid Peptide Receptors
Hypocretin (orexin)	Neuropeptide Y
Substance P	Nociceptin
	Endocannabinoids
	Oxytocin

The substances showing increased activity are associated with stress, while the substances showing decreased activity are associated with pleasure. When the substance is withdrawn, pleasurable neuroactivity decreases while stressful activity increases. This is the neurological basis for the discomfort of withdrawal. Research suggests that while the addictive substances are provoking pleasurable responses, the brain is developing opposing stress responses to keep the brain in balance.

Persistence of the opposing effects after the drug is withdrawn produces the withdrawal response. Decreases in reward system function might persist in the form of long-term biochemical changes that contribute to the clinical syndrome of acute withdrawal and protracted abstinence and could also explain the loss of interest in normal, nondrug rewards (Koob & Volkow, 2010). In the case of PFA, the loss of interest in normal, nondrug rewards manifests as loss of interest in nonaddictive, unprocessed foods.

Koob and Volkow point out that both the hypothalamic–pituitary–adrenal (HPA) axis and brain stress system mediated by CRF are dysregulated by the chronic administration of all major drugs with dependence or abuse potential. There is a common response of elevated adrenocorticotropic hormone, corticosterone, and amygdala CRF during acute withdrawal (Koob et al., 2014; Piazza & Le Moal, 1996). As tolerance and withdrawal develop, brain stress systems, such as CRF, norepinephrine, and dynorphin, are recruited. The dysfunction in stress systems can manifest as negative emotional states in withdrawal and protracted abstinence (Delfs, Zhu, Druhan, & Aston-Jones, 2000; Koob et al., 2014).

The findings of increased activity in stress pathways is labeled as the "antireward" concept (Koob & Le Moal, 2008). It is based on the proposal that opponent processes act to limit reward stimulated by the drugs of abuse (Koob & Le Moal, 1997). Multiple circuits are likely to contribute to the hypothesized opponent-like processes. Decreases in the release of dopamine in the nucleus accumbens can also be driven by increases in the activity of the dynorphin-κ opioid receptor system in the ventral striatum and possibly increases in the activity of CRF in the ventral tegmental area. These dysfunctions contribute to the negative emotional state associated with withdrawal and protracted abstinence (Koob et al., 2014).

Koob and Volkow also pointed out the role of a decrease in the reinforcing value of rewards. Introduction of Cyclic adenosine monophosphate (cAMP) response element binding protein in the nucleus accumbens decreases the reinforcing value of natural and drug rewards, and this change plausibly contributes to withdrawal/negative affect stage-related decreases in reward pathway function. Reductions in the value of reward leave a drug-abstinent individual in an unmotivated, dysphoric, or depressed-like state (Carlezon et al., 1998; Nestler, 2004). These substance-related changes in susceptibility to negative emotional states might begin early: alcohol use during adolescence might lead to epigenetic modifications that alter amygdalar gene expression and dendritic density, increasing susceptibility to anxiety-like behaviors and alcohol ingestion in adulthood (Pandey, Sakharkar, Tang, & Zhang, 2015). In (Koob & Volkow, 2016). Of course, in the case of PFA, use and abuse of processed foods can begin in toddlerhood.

In addition to resetting the brain's reward system, repeated exposure to the dopamine-enhancing effects of most drugs leads to adaptations in the circuitry of the extended amygdala in the basal forebrain. These adaptations result in increases in a person's reactivity to stress and lead to the emergence of negative emotions (Davis, Walker, Miles, & Grillon, 2010; Jennings et al., 2013). This antireward system is fueled by the neurotransmitters involved in the stress response, such as corticotropin-releasing factor (CRF) and dynorphin, which ordinarily help to maintain homeostasis. However, in the addicted brain, the antireward system becomes overactive, giving rise to the highly dysphoric phase of drug addiction that ensues when the direct effects of the drug wear off or the drug is withdrawn and to the decreased reactivity of dopamine cells in the brain's reward circuitry (Volkow, Koob, & McLellan, 2016).

This research into the neurology of withdrawal in drug addiction finds parallels in research into withdrawal from processed foods. In a rat study, a possible explanation for the increased anxiety in withdrawal from processed foods was found in a role for CRF. Rats that had withdrawn from 7 weeks of cycling of chow and palatable foods exhibited less open arm time than chow-fed controls, reflecting an anxiety-inducing effect. CRF peptide immunoreactivity in the central nucleus of the amygdala of animals withdrawn from the palatable diet was 70% higher than in chow-fed animals. This condition was reversed with access to the palatable diet. The results also suggest that palatable food might acquire negative reinforcing properties by relieving negative affective consequences of abstinence (Wells et al., 1998; Cottone, Sabino, Roberto, et al., 2009).

In another study design, rimonabant administration showed a compensatory role for the cannabinoid system. Administration of rimonabant precipitated anxiety-like behavior and anorexia of the regular chow diet in rats withdrawn from palatable diet cycling, independent from the degree of adrenocortical activation. These behavioral observations were accompanied by increased cannabinoid receptor mRNA and protein levels selectively in the central nucleus of the amygdala. Finally, rimonabant, microinfused directly into the central nucleus of the amygdala, precipitated anxiety-like behavior and anorexia (Blasio et al., 2013). This study demonstrates that the brain will try to protect against stress.

In another rat study, 15 weeks of cafeteria diet exposure tended to increase corticotropin-releasing hormone (CRH) expression in the dorsal hypothalamus (DH), which was accompanied by increased glucocorticoid receptor (GR) expression in the amygdala. Six-week cafeteria-fed rats exhibited reduced brain-derived neurotrophic factor expression, an effect that has been associated with stress. Finally, switching to chow following 15 weeks of cafeteria diet resulted in elevated CRH mRNA expression in the DH, while switching to the cafeteria diet produced a reduction in amygdala GR expression. These findings have implications for dieting in humans, as they suggest that withdrawal from a palatable diet is associated with heightened HPA axis activity, whereas acute exposure to a palatable diet may dampen stress levels. Obese humans who binge eat often report being chronically stressed, and preference for "comfort foods" (e.g., rich in fat/sugar) is likely a consequence of their ability to alter glucocorticoid and CRH activity (Dallman et al., 2003). Thus, activation of stress systems upon palatable food withdrawal, and potential dampening of stress when access to the diet is renewed, would likely encourage continuous intake (Martire et al., 2014).

These findings are summarized in a review article. Rats that were taken off a palatable diet showed increased activity in the HPA access and an increase in CRH in the hypothalamic paraventricular nucleus in a cascade that releases pituitary adrenocorticotropic hormone, corticosterone from the adrenal glands, and activates GR in the hypothalamus, hippocampus, and amygdala. An increase in amygdala CRH mRNA expression also occurred in rats switched from the palatable diet to chow compared to rats continuously fed chow. Increased CRH in this area has been associated with the dysphoria-like state seen following drug and palatable food withdrawal (Bruijnzeel, Small, Pasek, & Yamada, 2010; Teegarden & Bale, 2007). Reinstatement of palatable food following a period of withdrawal has been shown to normalize previously high CRH levels in the central amygdala (Cottone,

Sabino, Roberto, et al., 2009; Cottone, Sabino, Steardo, et al., 2009). The attendant normalization is associated with binge-like behavior when rats are given access to palatable food following a period of withdrawal (Cottone, Sabino, Steardo, et al., 2009). It is possible that increases in CRH may be a driver for this binge-like behavior following withdrawal, and CRH1 receptor antagonism has been shown to reduce stress-induced palatable food seeking and the hypophagia seen following palatable food withdrawal (Cottone, Sabino, Roberto, et al., 2009; Ghitza, Gray, Epstein, Rice, & Shaham, 2006). This implies that increases in CRH expression in the amygdala may be a driver to reinstate reward-seeking behavior following withdrawal of a rewarding substance such as drugs of abuse or palatable food. These reactions are consistent with an increase in the experience of stress. It was also found that rats eat less when removed from a palatable diet and put onto regular chow. This is consistent with the loss of interest in natural rewards observed in drug addicts in South et al. (2012).

The evidence for a syndrome of distress upon withdrawal from sugars and fats has developed into a coherent body of findings. Increased activation of stress pathways in combination with decreased activation of reward/pleasure pathways becomes more pronounced in the absence of processed foods. This is a plausible explanation for the emotional symptomology exhibited by PFA clients in withdrawal as described below.

21.3 MANIFESTATIONS

Manifestations of PFA withdrawal are varied in terms of symptoms, duration, and severity. Clients may insist that they've had a flu and not withdrawal.

A popular description of the withdrawal syndrome was published in 1993, in *Food Addiction: The Body Knows*: "The symptoms of withdrawal may include dizziness, chills, nausea or vomiting, food craving, severe headache, lethargy and poor concentration. These may appear to be flu-like symptoms. After long periods of eating high carbohydrate foods, it will take a period of three to ten days or more to complete the acute withdrawal stage. The intensity of withdrawal differs from individual to individual. Some people are bedridden during the course of withdrawal, while others experience less severe symptoms which barely interfere with daily routine" (Sheppard, 1993).

Quotes from the food addiction manuals illustrate the symptoms of withdrawal. These quotes also illustrate some of the range of severity from no symptoms to weeks of distress.

> The initial withdrawal from sugar, flour and wheat was hell. I was so tired and depressed. (Food Addicts Anonymous, 2010, p. 99)
>
> My initial reaction was an overwhelming hunger, which made no sense because I had just eaten. Then came crabbiness, followed by nausea and a headache so terrible that I had to take a nap. (Food Addicts Anonymous, 2010, p. 150)
>
> Because I was suffering through a tremendous amount of detoxification and withdrawal, I could hardly read or write. (Food Addicts Anonymous, 2010, p. 184)
>
> The first two years of my abstinence were very hard. I was going through heavy withdrawal. I didn't know that post-acute withdrawal syndrome can last for two years. During my first year I became disabled and lost my income. Although I was highly suicidal, I kept on going. (Food Addicts Anonymous, 2010, p. 185)
>
> Day three is when it all broke loose. I had been warned about this: WITHDRAWAL! I somehow made it through the next four days on the strength of the warning and also because the physical manifestations were quite severe for me. I had the shakes, night sweats, and could not concentrate. I was irritable and constantly "hungry" or angry. My counselor, who was a recovering food addict, had explained the physical effects of the disease and had tried to prepare me for the denial, rationalization and addictive thinking that would try to undermine my commitment to abstinence. The body was craving its substance of choice—sugar. I had undergone this agony when I became sober; I knew it was real. (Food Addicts Anonymous, 2010, pp. 222–223)
>
> The physical symptoms of withdrawal were my proof that food addiction was not just talk. This was indeed a biological disease. The fear of these symptoms carried me through the next six months.

> I remember saying to myself, "I will stay abstinent because I don't want to go through withdrawal again." (Food Addicts Anonymous, 2010, p. 223)
>
> About day four, I sat in a few hours of traffic getting home from work and my husband and I decided to run errands before dinner. … I sat there staring at my salad with oil and vinegar on it. I tried to eat, but I suddenly burst out crying. I must have cried for half an hour. (Food Addicts Anonymous, 2010, p. 227)
>
> I had no withdrawal symptoms, and a few months into abstinence, my energy level dramatically increased. I no longer sleep 10 hours a day. (Food Addicts Anonymous, 2010, p. 251)

As can be seen from this qualitative evidence, withdrawal can manifest differently in individual clients. Educating clients about the range of possibilities prepares them for the experience and increases the likelihood that they will complete withdrawal without lapsing.

21.4 APPLICATION

Managing withdrawal helps the client move through the process with dignity and with a minimum of discomfort. Heavy users can be encouraged to take a few days off of work. Severe symptoms may include a flu-like condition. Clients should not be expected to care for children in this condition. Clients who have already tapered may go through withdrawal without symptoms. Clients may also choose to eliminate addictive foods one by one to reduce withdrawal symptoms. For example, the client might eliminate sugars for 4 days, then artificial sweeteners, then gluten, then dairy, then excessive salt, then processed fats.

Caffeine withdrawal may wait for several months after withdrawal from processed foods. Caffeine withdrawal may be more severe and prolonged than withdrawal from processed foods. Separating out caffeine withdrawal from food withdrawal means that the client can appreciate a meaningful improvement in well-being at the end of 4–8 days of food withdrawal. Enjoying the improvement in mental clarity and energy while reducing cravings and bloating are powerful motivators for the food addict. However, caffeine withdrawal can overshadow these enjoyable improvements and block perception of the value of sobriety. Thus, scheduling caffeine withdrawal to coincide with food withdrawal could mean that an important motivator could be lost.

Practitioners are advised to assess the client for medicated conditions that may improve significantly in the course of withdrawal, even possibly starting on the first day. These include diabetes, hypertension, and rapid heartbeat. In the case of diabetes, it is thought that the meal combinations suggested in the recovery food plan can start to stabilize glucose even with the first meal. The theory is that the unprocessed carbohydrate combined with protein, a small quantity of fat, and lots of fiber serves to modulate the release of carbohydrate into the gut. In other words, glucose no longer peaks and falls because the food combinations are stabilizing glucose. Thus the need to reduce diabetic medication may come early, even on the first day of withdrawal. Practitioners should confirm with diabetic clients that they are monitoring their glucose levels and that they know how to adjust their medications. If clients fail to adjust medications at the direction of their prescribing professional, their glucose could drop too low.

As glucose levels are tied to blood pressure, clients taking medications to lower blood pressure should also be questioned about their ability to monitor blood pressure and their knowledge of how to adjust medication. It may be difficult to persuade clients that changes could occur in the first few days of recovery. However, if clients do not monitor and adjust blood pressure medication and their blood pressure becomes too low, they are at risk of becoming light-headed and falling.

In the case of rapid heartbeat, if a client is being medicated for this condition and the condition improves in recovery, the client's heartbeat could be too slow. Again, this needs to be monitored starting early in withdrawal.

Other conditions such as cholesterol levels, endocrine-related conditions, and mood disorders seem to improve more slowly. Clients should be aware of the possibility of improvement and encouraged to work with their prescribing health professionals to adjust medications as indicated.

21.4.1 Using Withdrawal in Motivating the Client

It is likely that clients have experienced withdrawal without knowing that they are doing so. Use of processed foods in a snacking or grazing routine may be driven by withdrawal avoidance. Clients may or may not be able to describe why they seek processed foods. They may need help connecting withdrawal avoidance with the urge to stop a craving, get energy, clear brain fog, relieve a headache, assuage a stomachache, and reduce anxiety, depression, or anger. Educating clients about the possibility that the overwhelming urge to eat processed foods could be an attempt to avoid withdrawal might be an eye-opener for clients. Of importance, framing overeating as withdrawal avoidance might help relieve self-blame.

The possibility of relieving the syndrome of eating to avoid withdrawal could be a motivator for undertaking recovery. In general, the prospect of relief from the compulsion and self-blame is a strong motivator for clients who have suffered internalized stigmatization (Ratcliffe & Ellison, 2015).

21.4.2 Use in Treatment

Withdrawal may be used in several ways in treatment.

Withdrawal may be used as a deterrent to relapse. The practitioner may make extensive notes about the distress of withdrawal and reiterate these with the client. Bearing in mind that at the moment of exposure to food cues, triggered cravings can co-occur with loss of memory, the practitioner may even write down the withdrawal experience and encourage the PFA client to keep it handy should they need to remind themselves of why they don't eat processed foods. The limitation to using withdrawal as a relapse deterrent is, of course, that the client will not remember the experience under the influence of cravings.

There are two schools of thought about managing withdrawal symptoms. One school suggests letting the client feel the full impact of withdrawal as a deterrent to relapse. This approach has the limitation that the client could forget about withdrawal distress during a craving. Research shows that memory loss occurs during a craving. The second approach is to ease the symptoms of withdrawal with analgesics, hot and cold compresses, rest, a hot bath, and medication for nausea. The argument in favor of mitigation of symptoms is based on the high likelihood that the client will lapse. The proliferation of food cues and availability of processed foods argue for a higher risk of an incidence of craving triggers than other addictions. If the client lapses, then memory of a painful withdrawal could be a deterrent to eliminating the addictive foods and becoming sober again.

The withdrawal syndrome may also be used to break through denial about whether the client really has PFA. Because it is rarely diagnosed, and it is possible that the general population has PFA to some degree, PFA clients may not understand why they have to work for recovery when few others must. It may appear to the PFA client that all other people are able to eat processed foods without problems. For these reasons, it may be difficult for PFA clients to accept that they have the disease and that abstinence and cue avoidance are necessary for recovery. Reviewing the withdrawal experience can help cut through the confusion on this point.

Education about withdrawal can also help clients let go of self-blame. If clients understand that withdrawal symptoms may have been propelling use of processed foods, they may be able to shift from thinking that they were weak-willed. Clients are likely to be unaware that using processed foods to alter a mental state, boost energy, and stop a physical pain could be considered as avoiding withdrawal, rather than lacking morals.

Making these points to PFA clients during withdrawal can help them tie their behavior to the disease of addiction. It can improve motivation to undertake recovery and then to stick with a program.

21.5 CONCLUSION

Withdrawal from processed foods and drinks is a painful but valuable experience. It teaches the client that processed foods are addictive. Managed properly, it can also deter the client from lapsing.

Further, the early appearance of results can encourage and motivate the client to stick to an abstinent food plan. Withdrawal should be carefully monitored for the need to reduce medications for diet-related diseases. The need for adjustment can come quite early in the withdrawal process, even starting on the first day.

REFERENCES

American Psychiatric Association. (2013). *The Diagnostic and Statistical Manual of Mental Disorders, Fifth Edition* (Vol. 5).

American Society of Addiction Medicine. (2014). *The ASAM Principles of Addiction Medicine* (Fifth ed.). Alphen aan den Rijn, Netherlands: Wolters Kluwer.

Avena, N. M., Bocarsly, M. E., & Hoebel, B. G. (2012). Animal models of sugar and fat bingeing: Relationship to food addiction and increased body weight. *Methods Mol Biol, 829*, 351–365. doi:10.1007/978-1-61779-458-2_23.

Blasio, A., Iemolo, A., Sabino, V., Petrosino, S., Steardo, L., Rice, K. C., . . . Cottone, P. (2013). Rimonabant precipitates anxiety in rats withdrawn from palatable food: Role of the central amygdala. *Neuropsychopharmacology, 38*(12), 2498–2507. doi:10.1038/npp.2013.153.

Bruijnzeel, A. W., Small, E., Pasek, T. M., & Yamada, H. (2010). Corticotropin-releasing factor mediates the dysphoria-like state associated with alcohol withdrawal in rats. *Behav Brain Res, 210*(2), 288–291. doi:10.1016/j.bbr.2010.02.043.

Carlezon, W. A., Jr., Thome, J., Olson, V. G., Lane-Ladd, S. B., Brodkin, E. S., Hiroi, N., . . . Nestler, E. J. (1998). Regulation of cocaine reward by CREB. *Science, 282*(5397), 2272–2275.

Corsica, J. A., & Spring, B. J. (2008). Carbohydrate craving: A double-blind, placebo-controlled test of the self-medication hypothesis. *Eat Behav, 9*(4), 447–454. doi:10.1016/j.eatbeh.2008.07.004.

Cottone, P., Sabino, V., Roberto, M., Bajo, M., Pockros, L., Frihauf, J. B., . . . Zorrilla, E. P. (2009). CRF system recruitment mediates dark side of compulsive eating. *Proc Natl Acad Sci U S A, 106*(47), 20016–20020. doi:10.1073/pnas.0908789106.

Cottone, P., Sabino, V., Steardo, L., & Zorrilla, E. P. (2008a). Intermittent access to preferred food reduces the reinforcing efficacy of chow in rats. *Am J Physiol Regul Integr Comp Physiol, 295*(4), R1066–1076. doi:10.1152/ajpregu.90309.2008.

Cottone, P., Sabino, V., Steardo, L., & Zorrilla, E. P. (2008b). Opioid-dependent anticipatory negative contrast and binge-like eating in rats with limited access to highly preferred food. *Neuropsychopharmacology, 33*(3), 524–535. doi:10.1038/sj.npp.1301430.

Cottone, P., Sabino, V., Steardo, L., & Zorrilla, E. P. (2009). Consummatory, anxiety-related and metabolic adaptations in female rats with alternating access to preferred food. *Psychoneuroendocrinology, 34*(1), 38–49. doi:10.1016/j.psyneuen.2008.08.010.

Dallman, M. F., Pecoraro, N., Akana, S. F., La Fleur, S. E., Gomez, F., Houshyar, H., . . . Manalo, S. (2003). Chronic stress and obesity: A new view of "comfort food". *Proc Natl Acad Sci U S A, 100*(20), 11696–11701. doi:10.1073/pnas.1934666100.

Davis, M., Walker, D. L., Miles, L., & Grillon, C. (2010). Phasic vs sustained fear in rats and humans: Role of the extended amygdala in fear vs anxiety. *Neuropsychopharmacology, 35*(1), 105–135. doi:10.1038/npp.2009.109.

Delfs, J. M., Zhu, Y., Druhan, J. P., & Aston-Jones, G. (2000). Noradrenaline in the ventral forebrain is critical for opiate withdrawal-induced aversion. *Nature, 403*(6768), 430–434. doi:10.1038/35000212.

Food Addicts Anonymous. (2010). Port St. Lucie, FL: Food Addicts Anonymous, Inc.

Ghitza, U. E., Gray, S. M., Epstein, D. H., Rice, K. C., & Shaham, Y. (2006). The anxiogenic drug yohimbine reinstates palatable food seeking in a rat relapse model: A role of CRF1 receptors. *Neuropsychopharmacology, 31*(10), 2188–2196. doi:10.1038/sj.npp.1300964.

Gold, M. S., & Shriner, R. L. (2013). Food addictions. In P. M. Miller (Ed.), *Principles of Addiction: Comprehensive Addictive Behaviors and Disorders* (Vol. 1), pp. 787–796. Waltham, MA: Elsevier.

Iemolo, A., Valenza, M., Tozier, L., Knapp, C. M., Kornetsky, C., Steardo, L., . . . Cottone, P. (2012). Withdrawal from chronic, intermittent access to a highly palatable food induces depressive-like behavior in compulsive eating rats. *Behav Pharmacol, 23*(5–6), 593–602. doi:10.1097/FBP.0b013e328357697f.

Jennings, J. H., Sparta, D. R., Stamatakis, A. M., Ung, R. L., Pleil, K. E., Kash, T. L., & Stuber, G. D. (2013). Distinct extended amygdala circuits for divergent motivational states. *Nature, 496*(7444), 224–228. doi:10.1038/nature12041.

Juliano, L. M., Ferre, S., & Griffiths, R. R. (2014). The pharmacology of caffeine. In R. M. Ries, Shannon; Fiellin, David.; Saitz, Richard (Ed.), *ASAM Principles of Addiction Medicine* (5th ed.). Washington, DC: American Society of Addiction Medicine.

Koob, G. F. (2013). Negative reinforcement in drug addiction: The darkness within. *Curr Opin Neurobiol, 23*(4), 559–563. doi:10.1016/j.conb.2013.03.011.

Koob, G. F., Buck, C. L., Cohen, A., Edwards, S., Park, P. E., Schlosburg, J. E., . . . George, O. (2014). Addiction as a stress surfeit disorder. *Neuropharmacology, 76* Pt B, 370–382. doi:10.1016/j.neuropharm.2013.05.024.

Koob, G. F., & Le Moal, M. (1997). Drug abuse: Hedonic homeostatic dysregulation. *Science, 278*(5335), 52–58.

Koob, G. F., & Le Moal, M. (2008). Addiction and the brain antireward system. *Annu Rev Psychol, 59*, 29–53. doi:10.1146/annurev.psych.59.103006.093548.

Koob, G. F., & Volkow, N. D. (2010). Neurocircuitry of addiction. *Neuropsychopharmacology, 35*(1), 217–238. doi:10.1038/npp.2009.110.

Koob, G. F., & Volkow, N. D. (2016). Neurobiology of addiction: A neurocircuitry analysis. *Lancet Psychiatry, 3*(8), 760–773. doi:10.1016/s2215-0366(16)00104-8.

Lustig, R. H. (2013). Fructose: It's "alcohol without the buzz". *Adv Nutr, 4*(2), 226–235. doi:10.3945/an.112.002998.

Martin, C. S., & Winters, K. C. (1998). Diagnosis and assessment of alcohol use disorders among adolescents. *Alcohol Health Res World, 22*(2), 95–105.

Martire, S. I., Maniam, J., South, T., Holmes, N., Westbrook, R. F., & Morris, M. J. (2014). Extended exposure to a palatable cafeteria diet alters gene expression in brain regions implicated in reward, and withdrawal from this diet alters gene expression in brain regions associated with stress. *Behav Brain Res, 265*, 132–141. doi:10.1016/j.bbr.2014.02.027.

Martire, S. I., Westbrook, R. F., & Morris, M. J. (2015). Effects of long-term cycling between palatable cafeteria diet and regular chow on intake, eating patterns, and response to saccharin and sucrose. *Physiol Behav, 139*, 80–88. doi:10.1016/j.physbeh.2014.11.006.

Moore, C. F., Sabino, V., Koob, G. F., & Cottone, P. (2017). Pathological overeating: Emerging evidence for a compulsivity construct. *Neuropsychopharmacology, 42*(7), 1375–1389. doi:10.1038/npp.2016.269.

Morris, M. J., Beilharz, J., Maniam, J., Reichelt, A., & Westbrook, R. F. (2014). Why is obesity such a problem in the 21st century? The intersection of palatable food, cues and reward pathways, stress, and cognition. *J Neurosci, 58*, 36–45. doi:10.1523/jneurosci.2013-14.2014 10.1016/j.neubiorev.2014.12.002.

Nestler, E. J. (2004). Molecular mechanisms of drug addiction. *Neuropharmacology, 47 Suppl 1*, 24–32. doi:10.1016/j.neuropharm.2004.06.031.

Pandey, S. C., Sakharkar, A. J., Tang, L., & Zhang, H. (2015). Potential role of adolescent alcohol exposure-induced amygdaloid histone modifications in anxiety and alcohol intake during adulthood. *Neurobiol Dis, 82*, 607–619. doi:10.1016/j.nbd.2015.03.019.

Parylak, S. L., Koob, G. F., & Zorrilla, E. P. (2011). The dark side of food addiction. *Physiol Behav, 104*(1), 149–156. doi:10.1016/j.physbeh.2011.04.063.

Piazza, P. V., & Le Moal, M. L. (1996). Pathophysiological basis of vulnerability to drug abuse: Role of an interaction between stress, glucocorticoids, and dopaminergic neurons. *Annu Rev Pharmacol Toxicol, 36*, 359–378. doi:10.1146/annurev.pa.36.040196.002043.

Pickering, C., Alsio, J., Hulting, A. L., & Schioth, H. B. (2009). Withdrawal from free-choice high-fat high-sugar diet induces craving only in obesity-prone animals. *Psychopharmacology (Berl), 204*(3), 431–443. doi:10.1007/s00213-009-1474-y [doi].

Ratcliffe, D., & Ellison, N. (2015). Obesity and internalized weight stigma: A formulation model for an emerging psychological problem. *Behav Cogn Psychother, 43*(2), 239–252. doi:10.1017/s1352465813000763.

Sharma, S., Fernandes, M. F., & Fulton, S. (2013). Adaptations in brain reward circuitry underlie palatable food cravings and anxiety induced by high-fat diet withdrawal. *Int J Obes (Lond), 37*(9), 1183–1191. doi:10.1038/ijo.2012.197.

Sheppard, K. (1993). *Food Addiction: The Body Knows*. Deerfield Beach, FL: Health Communications.

Shriner, R. L. (2013). Food addiction: Detox and abstinence reinterpreted? *Exp Gerontol, 48*(10), 1068–1074. doi:10.1016/j.exger.2012.12.005.

Smith, D. G., & Robbins, T. W. (2013). The neurobiological underpinnings of obesity and binge eating: A rationale for adopting the food addiction model. *Biol Psychiatry, 73*(9), 804–810. doi:10.1016/j.biopsych.2012.08.026.

South, T., Westbrook, F., & Morris, M. J. (2012). Neurological and stress related effects of shifting obese rats from a palatable diet to chow and lean rats from chow to a palatable diet. *Physiol Behav, 105*(4), 1052–1057. doi:10.1016/j.physbeh.2011.11.019.

Teegarden, S. L., & Bale, T. L. (2007). Decreases in dietary preference produce increased emotionality and risk for dietary relapse. *Biol Psychiatry, 61*(9), 1021–1029. doi:10.1016/j.biopsych.2006.09.032.

Volkow, N. D., Koob, G. F., & McLellan, A. T. (2016). Neurobiologic advances from the brain disease model of addiction. *N Engl J Med, 374*(4), 363–371. doi:10.1056/NEJMra1511480.

Wells, A. S., Read, N. W., Laugharne, J. D., & Ahluwalia, N. S. (1998). Alterations in mood after changing to a low-fat diet. *Br J Nutr, 79*(1), 23–30.

22 The Addiction Severity Index in the Assessment of Processed Food Addiction

Joan Ifland
Food Addiction Training, LLC
Cincinnati, OH

Kathryn K. Sheppard
Private Practice
Palm Bay, FL

H. Theresa Wright
Renaissance Nutrition
East Norriton, PA

CONTENTS

22.1 INTRODUCTION

Addicts often suffer from addiction in all areas of their lives. The addict's mental, physical, and emotional health and ability to cope with life's stressors are significantly compromised as the addict's brain and body chemistry adapt to the addictive process. Compromised health progressively erodes relationships and creates financial and legal complications, which leave the addict overwhelmed with problems. The stress of multiple problems coupled with limited coping skills can lead to relapse for the recovering addict. A key element of an effective recovery plan provides resources for handling problems in line with the client's abilities and concerns. The Addiction

Severity Index (ASI) provides practitioners an effective instrument to collect information to support an individualized treatment plan that addresses the full scope of identified problems, reduces vulnerability to relapse, and improves outcomes. The complete ASI can be found at http://www.tresearch.org/wp-content/uploads/2012/09/ASI_5th_Ed.pdf.

The ASI has been in use since 1980 (McLellan, Cacciola, Alterman, Rikoon, & Carise, 2006). The ASI gives practitioners a method for collecting comprehensive data from clients about their well-being and surfacing problems that need to be addressed in treatment planning. Chronic overconsumption of processed foods can result in a myriad of conditions that affect clients in many areas. In severe cases, most areas of their lives may be adversely affected. Through the process of diagnosing using the DSM 5 SUD criteria, the practitioner may develop an idea about processed food addiction (PFA) clients' abilities to cope with problems and how severely clients are compromised by physical, mental, emotional, and behavioral limitations. The ASI provides information that aids in the development of the treatment plan, which includes the resources needed to restore PFA clients to healthy living. With data from the ASI, the practitioner can organize resources to help PFA clients manage problems and avoid triggering relapse.

PFA is comparable to other addictions in terms of the development of limited capabilities in combination with a variety of problems. The comorbidities of obesity, which loosely correlates with PFA (Gearhardt, Corbin, & Brownell, 2016), are extensive (Guh et al., 2009). Evidence for physical comorbidities includes type 2 diabetes, all cancers except esophageal (female), pancreatic and prostate cancer, all cardiovascular diseases (except congestive heart failure), asthma, gallbladder disease, osteoarthritis, and chronic back pain (Guh et al., 2009). Limitations on cognitive functions include learning, decision-making, memory, and restraint (Voon, 2015; Wang et al., 2014; Yau, Kang, Javier, & Convit, 2014; Zhu et al., 2015). Mood disorders are also present, including depression, irritability, anxiety, and shame (Koball et al., 2016). Because PFA has been framed as a weight-loss problem, comorbidities have been missed. Failure to consider the burden of physical, mental, and emotional disorders experienced by the obese may partially explain the almost universal failure of weight-loss approaches (Turk et al., 2009).

Evidence suggests that PFA impacts people as extensively as other addictions. Yet, because of the distracting characteristic of weight gain and obesity, the nature and scope of PFA have been overlooked. In decades past, the extent of adverse consequences associated with addiction in general was also largely unrecognized in PFA clients. This lack of awareness gave rise to the use of the ASI, which serves as an instrument for gathering data on the full scope of consequences of addiction. Considered the gold standard for assessing addiction severity, the ASI is broadly accepted and validated for a variety of addictions across cultures (Makela, 2004; McLellan et al., 2006). Thus, the ASI provides an appropriate vehicle for organizing a comprehensive description of PFA. The ASI helps illustrate that obesity is only one consequence of this disorder, and not necessarily the most important.

The ASI is designed to be used after the diagnosis has been made. Through the process of diagnosing, practitioners will have also made a determination of severity based on how many DSM 5 SUD criteria are met. If an in-depth interview was possible in the development of the diagnosis, the practitioner may already be able to start to organize information into the ASI format.

22.2 ASI CATEGORIES

Consequences of PFA are organized according to six ASI categories—medical; employment; alcohol, drug, and processed food use; legal; family/social; and psychiatric. A section on other considerations is provided for issues specific to PFA. The term *abstinence* is defined as the elimination from the diet of addictive foods that cause loss of control over eating for that individual. The consequences described in this section apply to PFA clients as a group; the particular constellation of consequences for any given client is highly variable and comprises only a subset of the potential consequences.

22.2.1 Medical

The medical consequences of PFA are diverse and can be extensive. The ASI asks a number of questions in the medical section.

- How many times hospitalized and how long ago?
- Chronic medical problems that interfere with life?
- Prescribed medications?
- Pension for disability?
- Number of days of medical problems out of the last 30 days?

Practitioners may find that clients have been hospitalized for diabetes, heart disease, depression (including suicide attempts), cancer, bariatric surgery, and complications from these conditions (Guh et al., 2009). In recent years, complications of bariatric surgery have been noted such as binging and vomiting, compromised nutrient absorption, and weight regain (Boules et al., 2016; Magro et al., 2008; Pataky, Locatelli, Jung, & Golay, 2016; Sevincer, Konuk, Bozkurt, & Coskun, 2016; Surve et al., 2016; Thibault & Pichard, 2016; Tran et al., 2016).

Psychiatric hospitalization may also be found for a variety of symptoms. Clients may report that over years of processed food consumption irritability has progressed to rage, sadness to depression, anxiety to panic, and guilt to debilitating shame (Rankin et al., 2016). Practitioners may find that as abstinence from processed foods progresses, client could report diminishment or even elimination of these symptoms.

Endocrine system issues include hyper- or hypothyroidism, diabetes, polycystic ovarian syndrome, and infertility (Kulshreshtha, Singh, & Arora, 2013; Zhang et al., 2014). In abstinence, clients may report being restored to regular menses and fertility. Rheumatologic conditions reported most commonly are fibromyalgia, arthralgia, and joint swelling (e.g., ankles, knees) (Iannone et al., 2016; Theoharides, Stewart, Hatziagelaki, & Kolaitis, 2015). Common immune system issues include recurring infections such as sinusitis, pharyngitis, and even pneumonia, as well as yeast infections in the digestive system, reproductive system, and skin folds (Manzel et al., 2014; Myles, 2014). Infections and inflammatory conditions also tend to remit in abstinence from processed foods and to recur in relapse.

Clients may present with chronic digestive system conditions, including irritable bowel syndrome, diverticulitis, and gluten intolerance, that often clear up in the first month of abstinence and recur in relapse. Circulatory system issues include rapid heartbeat and hypertension (Espeland et al., 2015; Park, Huynh, Schell, & Baker, 2015). These conditions may show significant improvement in the first 10 days of abstinence and clients should work with prescribing health professionals to adjust medications. The syndromes should be closely monitored in relapse. Cholesterol may normalize and should also be monitored (Varbo et al., 2015). We find that excessive weight is associated with a wide range of musculoskeletal disorders, such as sciatica; neck, shoulder, and back pain; as well as osteoarthritis (Lee, Hong, Shin, & Lee, 2016; Wertli, Held, Campello, & Schecter Weiner, 2016; Zhang, Peterson, Su, & Wang, 2015). Osteoporosis is also commonly observed (Batsis et al., 2015).

Practitioners may find that clients are taking a variety of medications. Medications may have been prescribed for depression, anxiety, dyspepsia, pain, thyroid disease, diabetes, hypercholesterolemia, and/or hypertension. Practitioners may want to ascertain that clients are working with prescribing health professionals to monitor medications insofar as requirements for medications may decrease rapidly in abstinence, often unrelated to the rate of weight loss. If clients fail to adjust diabetes or hypertension medications, they may experience glucose or blood pressure that is too low. Medications regulating heart beat may also need to be monitored.

Practitioners can help clients interface with medical services. Obese people have been shown to avoid seeking medical care because of experience with stigmatism (Phelan, Burgess, Yeazel, et al., 2015). Practitioners may want to research medical services within their geographic area of practice to identify health professionals who are trained to manage obese clients. With the use of "safe" referrals, practitioners may be able to persuade clients to seek medical care. Practitioners may also encourage clients to undertake recovery from processed foods as research shows that symptoms of the metabolic syndrome can be put into remission using an unprocessed food plan (Boers et al., 2014).

Awareness of diet-related conditions will also help practitioners help their clients manage lapses. Due to sensitivity of craving neuropathways (Boswell & Kober, 2016), availability of processed foods (Ifland et al., 2009), and a proliferation of food cues (Lifshitz & Lifshitz, 2014), clients are prone to lapsing. Lapses may require adjustments in medications. Clients would benefit from learning how to care for themselves during lapses.

22.2.2 Employment/Support Status

The ASI asks a number of questions about the employment status of clients as well as how they are supported financially (Treatment Research Institute, 2017). Practitioners may already be familiar with the answers to some of these questions from information gathered under Criterion 3, time spent; Criterion 5, failure to fulfill roles; and Criterion 7, activities given up.

- Education completed?
- Training or technical education completed?
- Valid driver's license?
- Automobile available for use?
- Length of longest full-time job?
- Usual or last occupation?
- Does someone support you?
- Is this the majority of your support?
- Usual employment pattern: full- or part-time, student, retired, disability, unemployed, in a controlled environment.
- Paid days out of last 30 days?
- Income from employment, unemployment compensation, public assistance, pension, benefits, friend/family, illegal?
- How many dependents?
- Days of problems in employment?

As described under several DSM 5 SUD criteria, PFA clients may have given up on education, employment, and career advancement. Clients may be disabled from some combination of the medical and psychiatric disorders described in the DSM SUD criteria. In particular, depression, arthritis, and obesity contribute directly to disability (Colmegna, Hitchon, Bardales, Puri, & Bartlett, 2016; Sirtori et al., 2016; Wertli et al., 2016). Moreover, learning disabilities, "brain fog," fatigue, and somnolence seriously interfere with the ability to function at work (Theoharides et al., 2015). Those clients who are able to hold jobs or go to school may be absent often (Howard & Potter, 2014; Pan, Sherry, Park, & Blanck, 2013). Clients describe a distress syndrome that could reduce productivity, including nonspecific gastrointestinal symptoms, headache, and generalized malaise. These kinds of symptoms could be early stage withdrawal (Addicott, 2014; Caprioli, Zeric, Thorndike, & Venniro, 2015; Martire et al., 2014; Mental Health Blog, 2017; Morris, Beilharz, Maniam, Reichelt, & Westbrook, 2014; Schulte, Grilo, & Gearhardt, 2016). Such symptoms may abate after 4–8 days of withdrawal from processed foods.

In studies of how obese people spend time, it was found that they are more likely to be in low-paying jobs, be working at night, or working several jobs (Griep et al., 2014; Patel, Spaeth, & Basner, 2016).

In recovery, clients may be able to return to school, return to work, or try for better jobs. These goals could be reflected in treatment plans based on the interests of the client. The client's educational and employment history that reflect marketable skills, aptitudes, and preferences may guide the practitioner in incorporating employment strategies into the treatment plan. Consideration should be given to the client's ability to stand and move, as well as limited cognitive functions. There is evidence that the presence of food cues should rule out a potential workplace (Sample, Jones, Hargrave, Jarrard, & Davidson, 2016; Sample, Martin, Jones, Hargrave, & Davidson, 2015; Zoon, He, de Wijk, de Graaf, & Boesveldt, 2014). This will rule out food-related jobs, which could make the job hunt more difficult.

Practitioners should exercise care in developing treatment plans in the area of school and employment. PFA clients are vulnerable to relapse due to stress. The experience of stress could be exacerbated in school or work environments (Phelan, Burgess, Puhl, et al., 2015; Phelan, Burgess, Yeazel, et al., 2015). Cognitive functions can improve in recovery (Pina-Camacho, Jensen, Gaysina, & Barker, 2015). Practitioners should ascertain that clients are ready to resist stigmatization and discrimination in addition to being cognitively, emotionally, and physically comfortable with a school or workplace.

22.2.3 Substance Use: Processed Food and Drugs/Alcohol

The ASI asks a number of questions about drug and alcohol use. The ASI is designed for drug and alcohol addicts, but here it is adapted to include PFA.

- What is drug use in the last 30 days and the last year for alcohol (use vs. intoxication), heroin, methadone, other opiates, analgesics, barbiturates, other sedatives, hypnotics, tranquilizers, cocaine, amphetamines, cannabis, hallucinogens, inhalants? PFA clients can be asked about their use of processed foods including baked goods, ice cream, frozen products, sweets, fast food, candy, snacks, crackers, cheese, and any foods used in grazing or bingeing.
- Are there days when more than one substance or type of substance is used?
- Which substance or food is the major problem? Is more than one a problem?
- How long was the last period of voluntary abstinence from the problem drug or food?
- How many months ago did the abstinence end?
- How many times have you had withdrawal from the food or substance?
- Have you ever overdosed, blacked out, or had to go to the emergency room because of volumes consumed?
- How many times in your life have you been treated for overeating, or alcohol abuse, or drug abuse?
- How many of these times were for detox only? Alcohol, drugs, processed foods?
- How much money have you spent in the last 30 days on alcohol, drugs, processed foods?
- How many days have you been treated in an outpatient setting for drug, alcohol, or processed foods in the last 30 days? (Include 12-step meetings, counseling, online groups, etc.)
- How many days in the last 30 have you experienced alcohol, drug, or processed food problems?
- Specifically for PFA clients, what is use of these substances in the last 30 days and the last year: laxatives, diuretics, appetite suppressants, artificial sweeteners, caffeine, nicotine, insulin, ADHD medications, levothyroxine, and steroids (Dennis & Pryor, 2014)?

In the case of PFA, practitioners are assessing the severity of use. PFA clients may be ashamed of episodes of bingeing so practitioners may want to preface this phase of the ASI with assurances that development of binge eating is not the fault of the client. There is evidence that binge eating is the result of genetics (Stice & Yokum, 2016), as well as the practices of the food industry (Kraak & Story, 2015) and inept approaches to weight loss (Moore, Sabino, Koob, & Cottone, 2017; Turk et al., 2009).

At first glance, questions about use of hard drugs may seem inappropriate for a PFA client; however, substance use disorders and eating disorder can co-occur (Dennis & Pryor, 2014). There are some instances where a drug/alcohol problem may have developed from attempts to control overconsumption of processed foods. The PFA client may have developed a problem with amphetamines (diet pills) prescribed for weight loss (Bray, 2014; Hendricks et al., 2014). It is also possible that PFA clients may have developed a problem with alcohol following bariatric surgery (Bak, Seibold-Simpson, & Darling, 2016; Steffen, Engel, Wonderlich, Pollert, & Sondag, 2015). Cocaine has been shown to be used in weight control (Cochrane, Malcolm, & Brewerton, 1998). Pain-related complications of obesity such as bone deterioration are also a possibility, which could have led to a problem with opiates (Narouze & Souzdalnitski, 2015).

Dennis and Pryor described use of substances by overeaters to control weight gain (Dennis & Pryor, 2014). PFA clients may abuse over-the-counter medications in an attempt to control weight. These could include laxatives, diuretics, and appetite suppressants. They may also be abusing artificial sweeteners, nicotine, and caffeine. In diabetics, doses of insulin may be skipped to achieve weight loss. ADHD medications have a side effect of reduced appetite and could be misused to control weight. Similarly, overuse of the thyroid medication levothyroxine can promote weight loss and so is vulnerable to misuse. Steroids may be abused by athletes to build muscle and reduce fat (Dennis & Pryor, 2014). PFA can be seen to open the door to drug addiction.

Conversely, PFA may stem from drug or alcohol addiction. A drug/alcohol addict in recovery may have been encouraged to switch from the substance of abuse to sugar or other processed foods and have developed PFA as a result (Bluml et al., 2012; Hodgkins, Cahill, Seraphine, Frost-Pineda, & Gold, 2004; Hodgkins, Frost-Pineda, & Gold, 2007; Kleiner et al., 2004; McIntyre et al., 2007; Orsini et al., 2014; Warren, Frost-Pineda, & Gold, 2005). Ex-smokers have been shown to gain weight, which could be interpreted as switching addictive substances from nicotine to processed foods (Berg, Park, Chang, & Rigotti, 2008; Farley, Hajek, Lycett, & Aveyard, 2012). Patients who have been prescribed antipsychotics may also develop obesity (Alvarez-Jimenez et al., 2006).

With regard to food abuse, PFA clients report two general eating patterns: eating frequently throughout the day or episodic binging, with many variations on each theme. Some may have a weekly pattern of restricting calories monday through thursday to compensate for overconsuming on the weekend. Regardless of the temporal pattern, clients characteristically eat refined carbohydrates, foods cooked in large amounts of cooking oil (e.g., french fries), refined foods high in salt content or heavily salted, and high-fat dairy (e.g., ice cream). In addition, they drink caffeinated, artificially or sugar-sweetened drinks. Just as drug addicts use substances in order to change how they feel, PFA clients also seek a change in mood. PFA clients may have turned to the use of other substances because they have been unable to establish adequate abstinence from addictive foods to prevent relapses. They have extensive experience with failed attempts at partial abstinence in the form of diets, fasts, or moderate consumption of refined foods. In our opinion, these diets fail due to the stimulation of cravings—followed by uncontrolled eating—that are caused by ingestion of processed foods, cues for processed foods, and stress.

PFA clients may have extensive residential and outpatient treatment histories. They may report a broad range of treatment failures including eating only a specific food (e.g., the grapefruit diet), restricted calories, diet pills, prepared meal plans, 12-step groups, eating disorder treatment, exercise, fasting, hypnosis, bariatric surgery, and purging (Turk et al., 2009). They have been blamed for these failures by uninformed health professionals (Phelan, Burgess, Yeazel, et al., 2015). The experience of failure exacerbates the cycle of shame and food abuse and can drive the decision to use substances to relieve negative affect or control appetite.

Clients underestimate how much they spend on food. They take advantage of cheap sources such as discount ice cream, baked goods, and cookies. Nonetheless, working clients may report vending machine expenditures of $70 or more per week. Fast food seems inexpensive until volume spending is considered. One client reported spending "the entire day driving from one restaurant to the next." Others have reported thousands of dollars of credit card debt for food.

22.2.4 Legal

The ASI is designed to gather information from users of illegal drugs and from alcoholics who may have disorderly conduct resulting from intoxication. Many of the questions will not apply to PFA clients.

- Was the referral from the legal system?
- Probation or parole?

- Shoplifting, parole violation, drug charges, forgery, weapons offense, burglary, larceny, robbery, assault, arson, rape, homicide, manslaughter, prostitution, contempt of court, other?
- Convictions, disorderly conduct, vagrancy, public intoxication, driving while intoxicated, driving violations, months of incarceration, length of last incarceration, reason for incarceration, awaiting trial, for what, days of incarceration in last 30 days, days of engagement in illegal activities out of last 30 days?

Legal problems among PFA clients may be less frequent as compared to drug addiction because virtually no aspect of PFA is illegal (except for stealing food). Further, even though PFA clients may be too impaired to drive, driving under the influence of processed foods is not illegal as is the case with alcohol. In general, obesity is not associated with aggressive behavior (Belsare et al., 2010). However, recidivist criminals have been found to have hypoglycemia (Virkkunen, De Jong, Bartko, Goodwin, & Linnoila, 1989), which may also be symptomatic of PFA (Xi, Cheng, Chen, Zhao, & Mi, 2016).

PFA clients may report legal problems related to divorce if their health profile differs from that of their spouse (Torvik, Gustavson, Roysamb, & Tambs, 2015). In the future, clients may begin to engage in legal recourse related to discrimination in the workplace and bullying (Puhl, Suh, & Li, 2016a, 2016b). As PFA clients increasingly turn to weight-loss surgery, there is a possibility that legal problems related to malpractice will increase (Weber et al., 2013). Concerns about neglect of obese children are also beginning to surface (Garrahan & Eichner, 2012).

22.2.5 Family/Social

Family and social problems are common in PFA clients as described in DSM 5 SUD Criterion 3, time spent, and Criterion 5, failure to fulfill roles. Questions from the ASI that can surface the extent of problems in family and social areas are as follows:

- Marital status and satisfaction with marital status.
- Usual living arrangement: with sexual partner and children, sexual partner alone, children alone, parents, family, friends, alone, controlled environment (hospital, jail), no stable arrangements.
- How long in these living arrangements and degree of satisfaction?
- Do you live with anyone who has an alcohol problem, nonprescription drugs?
- Who do you spend the most time with: family, friends, alone? How many close friends do you have?
- Would you say you have had close, long-lasting, personal relationships with any of the following people in your life: mother, father, brothers/sisters, sexual partner/spouse, children, friends?
- Have you had significant periods in which you have experienced serious problems getting along with mother, father, brothers/sisters, sexual partner/spouse, children, other significant family, close friends, neighbors, co-workers?
- Did any of these people abuse you emotionally, physically, sexually?
- How many days in the last 30 days have you had serious conflicts with family or other people?

For PFA, practitioners should also ascertain whether the client is pregnant.

PFA clients may have trouble managing family relationships. Blood relatives often have eating problems, alcoholism, or other addictions, as well as diet-related medical conditions such as heart disease or diabetes (Blum et al., 2011). Food abuse may be common in home and workplace environments. Finding out about unavoidable cueing will help practitioners include countering cues with cognitive restoration techniques. Some cueing may be reduced with negotiations with family members and colleagues, and this can also be included in treatment planning.

As discussed in Criterion 3, time spent, PFA clients spend time planning what to eat, obtaining food, eating it, and then recovering from the eating episode by sleeping or watching television. PFA clients may have acquaintances but few intimate friends (Palmeira, Pinto-Gouveia, & Cunha, 2016). They may have serious problems getting along with others, including family members (Davies, Lehman, Perry, & McCall-Hosenfeld, 2015). This may be in part because emotional, physical, and/or sexual abuse has found to correlate with obese adults' families of origin (Felitti, 1993).

Practitioners will want to ascertain that clients are safe in their current living situation. The treatment plan may gradually include activities with safe family members or friends or support groups specifically for obese people. As clients resolve shame issues regarding body shape, they may be ready to reengage friends. As with any aspect of recovery, the key is to go slow and ascertain that the client is resilient enough to withstand negativity from friends before reestablishing friendships.

A key issue is the safety of children who are under the care of a PFA client. Children in PFA-affected homes may be suffering from neglect, especially of distressing emotions and malnutrition (Harper, 2014; Saltzman et al., 2016). As the client gains food preparation skills, the practitioner can offer guidance about how to introduce unprocessed foods to children. The client may also need support in negotiations with adults in the household regarding reduced cueing related to the availability of processed foods in the home, as well as their visibility (Voon, 2015). Household members can keep processed foods out of sight in designated cabinets to reduce the impact of cues on the recovering PFA client.

Pregnancy is also an issue in PFA. Pregnant women may be accelerating their use of processed foods to assuage hunger related to the pregnancy. Poor diet during pregnancy has been shown to be correlated with psychological problems in the child (O'Neil et al., 2014; Pina-Camacho et al., 2015).

22.2.6 Psychiatric

Psychiatric problems are commonly associated with both addictions and chronic use of processed foods. Here are the questions from the ASI that elicit information about psychiatric problems.

- How many times treated for psychological or emotional problems in a hospital or outpatient?
- Receive a pension for psychiatric disability?
- A significant period of depression, anxiety or tension, hallucinations, trouble understanding, concentrating or remembering, trouble controlling violent behavior, serious thoughts of suicide, attempted suicide, medication for any psychological emotional problem?
- How many days out of last 30 days experienced psychological or emotional problems?

Although the determinants of mental health are complex, the emerging and compelling evidence for nutrition as a crucial factor in the high prevalence and incidence of mental disorders suggests that diet is as important to psychiatry as it is to cardiology, endocrinology, and gastroenterology (Sarris et al., 2015).

Not surprisingly, treatment for chronic psychological and emotional problems is common in obese populations (Mansur, Brietzke, & McIntyre, 2015; Soczynska et al., 2011), and the ASI will allow practitioners to assess for the medical services accessed as well as use of medications. Symptoms may slowly abate on an unprocessed food plan (Logan & Jacka, 2014).

Debilitating mood disorders found in obese populations are consistent with ASI criteria of a significant period of serious depression, sadness, hopelessness, loss of interest, difficulty with daily functioning, anxiety, worry, or inability to relax. Prevalence is high (Rankin et al., 2016). Poor impulse control over behaviors may be present (Sutin, Ferrucci, Zonderman, & Terracciano, 2011). Anger disorders can also be present (Tsenkova, Carr, Coe, & Ryff, 2014). Suicide ideation is prevalent (Wagner, Klinitzke, Brahler, & Kersting, 2013). Clients may be so troubled by their relationship with food and body image that they may have made plans for suicide, as has been described in other substance use disorders (Colon-Perez et al., 2016; Shin et al., 2015).

PFA clients may suffer from obsessive thinking about food, anxiety about others' opinions of them, and distorted ideas about the effects of eating (Sharma & Fulton, 2013). They may rationalize their self-destructive food choices, the resultant harmful consequences, and poor life choices (Koritzky, Dieterle, Rice, Jordan, & Bechara, 2014; Verbeken, Braet, Bosmans, & Goossens, 2014). They often have difficulty with comprehension, concentration, and memory (Noble & Kanoski, 2016). They may forget how to shop, prepare food, or navigate driving routes related to brain fog (Theoharides et al., 2015).

22.2.7 Other Considerations

22.2.7.1 Chronic Obesity

Usually, but not always, PFA clients are overweight or obese. In abstinence, weight loss occurs at 1–2 lbs. per week. Obesity limits mobility, affects hygiene, and is associated with internalized stigmatization (Ratcliffe & Ellison, 2015). In advanced stages of illness, PFA clients cannot fly in an airplane, drive a car, find and afford clothing, or even shoes that fit because their feet are so wide. The prominence of adipose tissue creates a distraction from the underlying addictive disease and limits the perception of required treatment.

22.2.7.2 Age of Onset

It is possible that PFA clients have been subjected to addictive food substances from infancy (Ng et al., 2014). PFA clients may report addictive behavior in early childhood such as manipulating adults, stealing, and hiding processed foods. PFA in early childhood may be a precursor to health problems later in life, in addition to persisting as PFA (Llewellyn, Simmonds, Owen, & Woolacott, 2016).

22.2.7.3 Remission and Reoccurrence

Symptoms associated with PFA may go into remission promptly after eliminating processed foods from the diet (Logan & Jacka, 2014). Recognizing this phenomenon can be helpful to practitioners in terms of how they might encourage the client to undertake new behaviors. For example, the practitioner may think that exercise could be severely limited for the long-term due to joint pain. However, it is possible that joint pain will readily abate as inflammation related to processed foods is reduced (Myles, 2014; Spreadbury, 2012). Practitioners can check for improvements during follow-up to gauge opportunities to introduce exercise. By the same token, practitioners can educate clients on the potential impact of relapse. Joint pain could flare up again promptly after a lapse. The symptoms of processed food use are varied and may reoccur rapidly in relapse.

22.3 DISCUSSION

In the society, tools are lacking to identify, assess, and treat PFA. Inappropriate, even harmful, treatment is a significant factor in PFA as opposed to other addictions because lose/gain cycles have been shown to contribute to weight gain in a rat study (Martire, Westbrook, & Morris, 2015) and to be associated with psychological distress (Petroni et al., 2007). Because neither the substances nor the consequences are illegal, the legal system does not intervene to stop the cycle of restriction followed by overconsumption.

If PFA is understood to be an addictive disorder, as presented here, then a more comprehensive, aggressive, and focused approach to the treatment of obesity can be undertaken. Although not all obesity is a result of PFA, and not all PFA clients are obese, we believe that the majority of obese individuals also suffer from PFA and need to be treated accordingly. Direction for effective public policy with regard to addictive refined food substances may be drawn from the experience of regulating tobacco. Such policies have included initiatives involving education, pricing, taxation, farm subsidies, availability, labeling, litigation, nonsmoking areas, and advertising.

22.4 CONCLUSION

In conclusion, the ASI was used to organize clinical observations regarding the phenomenology of PFA in humans. Further development of the ASI for PFA clients would be useful because it would facilitate the clinical documentation of this as-yet unrecognized disorder, leading to more effective assessment, treatment, and public policy. We have also argued that unless and until the obesity epidemic is understood to be primarily a consequence of PFA, afflicted individuals will continue to suffer from a litany of medical and psychiatric disorders that are refractory to current treatment approaches.

REFERENCES

Addicott, M. A. (2014). Caffeine use disorder: A review of the evidence and future implications. *Curr Addict Rep, 1*(3), 186–192. doi:10.1007/s40429-014-0024-9.

Alvarez-Jimenez, M., Gonzalez-Blanch, C., Vazquez-Barquero, J. L., Perez-Iglesias, R., Martinez-Garcia, O., Perez-Pardal, T., … Crespo-Facorro, B. (2006). Attenuation of antipsychotic-induced weight gain with early behavioral intervention in drug-naive first-episode psychosis patients: A randomized controlled trial. *J Clin Psychiatry, 67*(8), 1253–1260.

Bak, M., Seibold-Simpson, S. M., & Darling, R. (2016). The potential for cross-addiction in post-bariatric surgery patients: Considerations for primary care nurse practitioners. *J Am Assoc Nurse Pract, 28*(12), 675–682. doi:10.1002/2327-6924.12390.

Batsis, J. A., Zbehlik, A. J., Barre, L. K., Bynum, J. P., Pidgeon, D., & Bartels, S. J. (2015). Impact of obesity on disability, function, and physical activity: Data from the osteoarthritis initiative. *Scand J Rheumatol, 44*(6), 495–502. doi:10.3109/03009742.2015.1021376.

Belsare, P. V., Watve, M. G., Ghaskadbi, S. S., Bhat, D. S., Yajnik, C. S., & Jog, M. (2010). Metabolic syndrome: Aggression control mechanisms gone out of control. *Med Hypotheses, 74*(3), 578–589. doi:10.1016/j.mehy.2009.09.014.

Berg, C. J., Park, E. R., Chang, Y., & Rigotti, N. A. (2008). Is concern about post-cessation weight gain a barrier to smoking cessation among pregnant women? *Nicotine Tob Res, 10*(7), 1159–1163. doi:10.1080/14622200802163068.

Blum, K., Bailey, J., Gonzalez, A. M., Oscar-Berman, M., Liu, Y., Giordano, J., … Gold, M. (2011). Neuro-Genetics of Reward Deficiency Syndrome (RDS) as the root cause of "Addiction Transfer": A new phenomenon common after bariatric surgery. *J Genet Syndr Gene Ther, 2012*(1), 23. doi:10.4172/2157-7412.s2-001.

Bluml, V., Kapusta, N., Vyssoki, B., Kogoj, D., Walter, H., & Lesch, O. M. (2012). Relationship between substance use and body mass index in young males. *Am J Addict, 21*(1), 72–77. doi:10.1111/j.1521-0391.2011.00192.x.

Boers, I., Muskiet, F. A., Berkelaar, E., Schut, E., Penders, R., Hoenderdos, K., … Jong, M. C. (2014). Favourable effects of consuming a Palaeolithic-type diet on characteristics of the metabolic syndrome: A randomized controlled pilot-study. *Lipids Health Dis, 13*, 160. doi:10.1186/1476-511x-13-160

Boswell, R. G., & Kober, H. (2016). Food cue reactivity and craving predict eating and weight gain: A meta-analytic review. *Obes Rev, 17*(2), 159–177. doi:10.1111/obr.12354.

Boules, M., Chang, J., Haskins, I. N., Sharma, G., Froylich, D., El-Hayek, K., … Kroh, M. (2016). Endoscopic management of post-bariatric surgery complications. *World J Gastrointest Endosc, 8*(17), 591–599. doi:10.4253/wjge.v8.i17.591.

Bray, G. A. (2014). Medical treatment of obesity: The past, the present and the future. *Best Pract Res Clin Gastroenterol, 28*(4), 665–684. doi:10.1016/j.bpg.2014.07.015.

Caprioli, D., Zeric, T., Thorndike, E. B., & Venniro, M. (2015). Persistent palatable food preference in rats with a history of limited and extended access to methamphetamine self-administration. *Addict Biol, 20*(5), 913–926. doi:10.1111/adb.12220.

Cochrane, C., Malcolm, R., & Brewerton, T. (1998). The role of weight control as a motivation for cocaine abuse. *Addict Behav, 23*(2), 201–207.

Colmegna, I., Hitchon, C. A., Bardales, M. C., Puri, L., & Bartlett, S. J. (2016). High rates of obesity and greater associated disability among people with rheumatoid arthritis in Canada. *Clin Rheumatol, 35*(2), 457–460. doi:10.1007/s10067-015-3154-0.

Colon-Perez, L. M., Tran, K., Thompson, K., Pace, M. C., Blum, K., Goldberger, B. A., … Febo, M. (2016). The psychoactive designer drug and bath salt constituent MDPV causes widespread disruption of brain functional connectivity. *Neuropsychopharmacology, 41*(9), 2352–2365. doi:10.1038/npp.2016.40.

Davies, R., Lehman, E., Perry, A., & McCall-Hosenfeld, J. S. (2015). Association of intimate partner violence and health-care provider-identified obesity. *Women Health, 56*(5), 561–575. doi:10.1080/03630242.2015.1101741.

Dennis, A. B., & Pryor, T. (2014). Introduction to substance use disorders for the eating disorder specialist. In T. D. Brewerton & A. B. Dennis (Eds.), *Eating Disorders, Addictions, and Substance Use Disorders: Research, Clinical, and Treatment Perspectives*, pp. 226–266. New York: Springer.

Espeland, M. A., Probstfield, J., Hire, D., Redmon, J. B., Evans, G. W., Coday, M., … Cushman, W. C. (2015). Systolic blood pressure control among individuals with type 2 diabetes: A comparative effectiveness analysis of three interventions. *Am J Hypertens, 28*(8), 995–1009. doi:10.1093/ajh/hpu292.

Farley, A. C., Hajek, P., Lycett, D., & Aveyard, P. (2012). Interventions for preventing weight gain after smoking cessation. *Cochrane Database Syst Rev, 1*, Cd006219. doi:10.1002/14651858.CD006219.pub3.

Felitti, V. J. (1993). Childhood sexual abuse, depression, and family dysfunction in adult obese patients: A case control study. *South Med J, 86*(7), 732–736.

Garrahan, S. M., & Eichner, A. W, (2012). Tipping the scale: A place for childhood obesity in the evolving legal framework of child abuse and neglect. *Yale J Health Policy Law Ethics, 12*(2), 336–370.

Gearhardt, A. N., Corbin, W. R., & Brownell, K. D. (2016). Development of the Yale Food Addiction Scale Version 2.0. *Psychol Addict Behav, 30*(1), 113–121. doi:10.1037/adb0000136.

Griep, R. H., Bastos, L. S., Fonseca Mde, J., Silva-Costa, A., Portela, L. F., Toivanen, S., & Rotenberg, L. (2014). Years worked at night and body mass index among registered nurses from eighteen public hospitals in Rio de Janeiro, Brazil. *BMC Health Serv Res, 14*, 603. doi:10.1186/s12913-014-0603-4.

Guh, D. P., Zhang, W., Bansback, N., Amarsi, Z., Birmingham, C. L., & Anis, A. H. (2009). The incidence of co-morbidities related to obesity and overweight: A systematic review and meta-analysis. *BMC Public Health, 9*, 88. doi:10.1186/1471-2458-9-88.

Harper, N. S. (2014) Neglect: Failure to thrive and obesity. *Pediatr Clin North Am, 61*(5), 937–957. doi:10.1016/j.pcl.2014.06.006.

Hendricks, E. J., Srisurapanont, M., Schmidt, S. L., Haggard, M., Souter, S., Mitchell, C. L., … Greenway, F. L. (2014). Addiction potential of phentermine prescribed during long-term treatment of obesity. *Int J Obes (Lond), 38*(2), 292–298. doi:10.1038/ijo.2013.74.

Hodgkins, C. C., Cahill, K. S., Seraphine, A. E., Frost-Pineda, K., & Gold, M. S. (2004). Adolescent drug addiction treatment and weight gain. *J Addict Dis, 23*(3), 55–65.

Hodgkins, C., Frost-Pineda, K., & Gold, M. S. (2007). Weight gain during substance abuse treatment: The dual problem of addiction and overeating in an adolescent population. *J Addict Dis, 26* Suppl 1, 41–50. doi:10.1300/J069v26S01_05.

Howard, J. T., & Potter, L. B. (2014). An assessment of the relationships between overweight, obesity, related chronic health conditions and worker absenteeism. *Obes Res Clin Pract, 8*(1), e1–e15. doi:10.1016/j.orcp.2012.09.002.

Iannone, F., Lopalco, G., Rigante, D., Orlando, I., Cantarini, L., & Lapadula, G. (2016). Impact of obesity on the clinical outcome of rheumatologic patients in biotherapy. *Autoimmun Rev, 15*(5), 447–450. doi:10.1016/j.autrev.2016.01.010.

Ifland, J. R., Preuss, H. G., Marcus, M. T., Rourke, K. M., Taylor, W. C., Burau, K., … Manso, G. (2009). Refined food addiction: A classic substance use disorder. *Med Hypotheses, 72*(5), 518–526. doi:S0306-9877(08)00642-7 [pii]10.1016/j.mehy.2008.11.035 [doi].

Kleiner, K. D., Gold, M. S., Frost-Pineda, K., Lenz-Brunsman, B., Perri, M. G., & Jacobs, W. S. (2004). Body mass index and alcohol use. *J Addict Dis, 23*(3), 105–118. doi:10.1300/J069v23n03_08.

Koball, A. M., Clark, M. M., Collazo-Clavell, M., Kellogg, T., Ames, G., Ebbert, J., & Grothe, K. B. (2016). The relationship among food addiction, negative mood, and eating-disordered behaviors in patients seeking to have bariatric surgery. *Surg Obes Relat Dis, 12*(1), 165–170. doi:10.1016/j.soard.2015.04.009.

Koritzky, G., Dieterle, C., Rice, C., Jordan, K., & Bechara, A. (2014). Decision-making, sensitivity to reward and attrition in weight management. *Obesity (Silver Spring), 22*(8), 1904–1909. doi:10.1002/oby.20770.

Kraak, V. I., & Story, M. (2015). An accountability evaluation for the industry's responsible use of brand mascots and licensed media characters to market a healthy diet to American children. *Obes Rev, 16*(6), 433–453. doi:10.1111/obr.12279.

Kulshreshtha, B., Singh, S., & Arora, A. (2013). Family background of Diabetes Mellitus, obesity and hypertension affects the phenotype and first symptom of patients with PCOS. *Gynecol Endocrinol, 29*(12), 1040–1044. doi:10.3109/09513590.2013.829446.

Lee, J., Hong, Y. P., Shin, H. J., & Lee, W. (2016). Associations of sarcopenia and sarcopenic obesity with metabolic syndrome considering both muscle mass and muscle strength. *J Prev Med Public Health, 49*(1), 35–44. doi:10.3961/jpmph.15.055.

Lifshitz, F., & Lifshitz, J. Z. (2014). Globesity: The root causes of the obesity epidemic in the USA and now worldwide. *Pediatr Endocrinol Rev, 12*(1), 17–34.

Llewellyn, A., Simmonds, M., Owen, C. G., & Woolacott, N. (2016). Childhood obesity as a predictor of morbidity in adulthood: A systematic review and meta-analysis. *Obes Rev, 17*(1), 56–67. doi:10.1111/obr.12316.

Logan, A. C., & Jacka, F. N. (2014). Nutritional psychiatry research: An emerging discipline and its intersection with global urbanization, environmental challenges and the evolutionary mismatch. *J Physiol Anthropol, 33*, 22. doi:10.1186/1880-6805-33-22.

Magro, D. O., Geloneze, B., Delfini, R., Pareja, B. C., Callejas, F., & Pareja, J. C. (2008). Long-term weight regain after gastric bypass: A 5-year prospective study. *Obes Surg, 18*(6), 648–651. doi:10.1007/s11695-007-9265-1.

Makela, K. (2004). Studies of the reliability and validity of the Addiction Severity Index. *Addiction, 99*(4), 398–410; discussion 411–398. doi:10.1111/j.1360-0443.2003.00665.x.

Mansur, R. B., Brietzke, E., & McIntyre, R. S. (2015). Is there a "metabolic-mood syndrome"? A review of the relationship between obesity and mood disorders. *Neurosci Biobehav Rev, 52*, 89–104. doi:10.1016/j.neubiorev.2014.12.017.

Manzel, A., Muller, D. N., Hafler, D. A., Erdman, S. E., Linker, R. A., & Kleinewietfeld, M. (2014). Role of "Western diet" in inflammatory autoimmune diseases. *Curr Allergy Asthma Rep, 14*(1), 404. doi:10.1007/s11882-013-0404-6.

Martire, S. I., Maniam, J., South, T., Holmes, N., Westbrook, R. F., & Morris, M. J. (2014). Extended exposure to a palatable cafeteria diet alters gene expression in brain regions implicated in reward, and withdrawal from this diet alters gene expression in brain regions associated with stress. *Behav Brain Res, 265*, 132–141. doi:10.1016/j.bbr.2014.02.027.

Martire, S. I., Westbrook, R. F., & Morris, M. J. (2015). Effects of long-term cycling between palatable cafeteria diet and regular chow on intake, eating patterns, and response to saccharin and sucrose. *Physiol Behav, 139*, 80–88. doi:10.1016/j.physbeh.2014.11.006.

McIntyre, R. S., McElroy, S. L., Konarski, J. Z., Soczynska, J. K., Bottas, A., Castel, S., … Kennedy, S. H. (2007). Substance use disorders and overweight/obesity in bipolar I disorder: Preliminary evidence for competing addictions. *J Clin Psychiatry, 68*(9), 1352–1357.

McLellan, A. T., Cacciola, J. C., Alterman, A. I., Rikoon, S. H., & Carise, D. (2006). The Addiction Severity Index at 25: Origins, contributions and transitions. *Am J Addict, 15*(2), 113–124. doi:10.1080/10550490500528316.

Mental Health Blog. (2017). Gluten Withdrawal Symptoms + How Long do They Last? Retrieved from http://mentalhealthdaily.com/2015/03/27/gluten-withdrawal-symptoms-how-long-do-they-last/

Moore, C. F., Sabino, V., Koob, G. F., & Cottone, P. (2017). Pathological overeating: Emerging evidence for a compulsivity construct. *Neuropsychopharmacology, 42*(7), 1375–1389. doi:10.1038/npp.2016.269.

Morris, M. J., Beilharz, J., Maniam, J., Reichelt, A., & Westbrook, R. F. (2014). Why is obesity such a problem in the 21st century? The intersection of palatable food, cues and reward pathways, stress, and cognition. *J Neurosci, 58*, 36–45. doi:10.1523/jneurosci.2013-14.2014 10.1016/j.neubiorev.2014.12.002.

Myles, I. A. (2014). Fast food fever: Reviewing the impacts of the Western diet on immunity. *Nutr J, 13*, 61. doi:10.1186/1475-2891-13-61.

Narouze, S., & Souzdalnitski, D. (2015). Obesity and chronic pain: Systematic review of prevalence and implications for pain practice. *Reg Anesth Pain Med, 40*(2), 91–111. doi:10.1097/aap.0000000000000218.

Ng, M., Fleming, T., Robinson, M., Thomson, B., Graetz, N., Margono, C., … Gakidou, E. (2014). Global, regional, and national prevalence of overweight and obesity in children and adults during 1980–2013: A systematic analysis for the Global Burden of Disease Study 2013. *Lancet, 384*(9945), 766–781. doi:10.1016/s0140-6736(14)60460-8.

Noble, E. E., & Kanoski, S. E. (2016). Early life exposure to obesogenic diets and learning and memory dysfunction. *Curr Opin Behav Sci, 9*, 7–14. doi:10.1016/j.cobeha.2015.11.014.

O'Neil, A., Itsiopoulos, C., Skouteris, H., Opie, R. S., McPhie, S., Hill, B., & Jacka, F. N. (2014). Preventing mental health problems in offspring by targeting dietary intake of pregnant women. *BMC Med, 12*, 208. doi:10.1186/s12916-014-0208-0.

Orsini, C. A., Ginton, G., Shimp, K. G., Avena, N. M., Gold, M. S., & Setlow, B. (2014). Food consumption and weight gain after cessation of chronic amphetamine administration. *Appetite, 78*, 76–80. doi:10.1016/j.appet.2014.03.013.

Palmeira, L., Pinto-Gouveia, J., & Cunha, M. (2016). The role of weight self-stigma on the quality of life of women with overweight and obesity: A multi-group comparison between binge eaters and non-binge eaters. *Appetite, 105*, 782–789. doi:10.1016/j.appet.2016.07.015.

Pan, L., Sherry, B., Park, S., & Blanck, H. M. (2013). The association of obesity and school absenteeism attributed to illness or injury among adolescents in the United States, 2009. *J Adolesc Health, 52*(1), 64–69. doi:10.1016/j.jadohealth.2012.04.003.

Park, A. E., Huynh, P., Schell, A. M., & Baker, L. A. (2015). Relationship between obesity, negative affect and basal heart rate in predicting heart rate reactivity to psychological stress among adolescents. *Int J Psychophysiol, 97*(2), 139–144. doi:10.1016/j.ijpsycho.2015.05.016.

Pataky, Z., Locatelli, L., Jung, M., & Golay, A. (2016). Not all patients might benefit from gastric by-pass. *Rev Med Suisse, 12*(511), 597–598, 600–591.

Patel, V. C., Spaeth, A. M., & Basner, M. (2016). Relationships between time use and obesity in a representative sample of Americans. *Obesity (Silver Spring), 24*(10), 2164–2175. doi:10.1002/oby.21596.

Petroni, M. L., Villanova, N., Avagnina, S., Fusco, M. A., Fatati, G., Compare, A., & Marchesini, G. (2007). Psychological distress in morbid obesity in relation to weight history. *Obes Surg, 17*(3), 391–399. doi:10.1007/s11695-007-9069-3.

Phelan, S. M., Burgess, D. J., Puhl, R., Dyrbye, L. N., Dovidio, J. F., Yeazel, M., … van Ryn, M. (2015). The adverse effect of weight stigma on the well-being of medical students with overweight or obesity: Findings from a National Survey. *J Gen Intern Med, 30*(9), 1251–1258. doi:10.1007/s11606-015-3266-x.

Phelan, S. M., Burgess, D. J., Yeazel, M. W., Hellerstedt, W. L., Griffin, J. M., & van Ryn, M. (2015). Impact of weight bias and stigma on quality of care and outcomes for patients with obesity. *Obes Rev, 16*(4), 319–326. doi:10.1111/obr.12266.

Pina-Camacho, L., Jensen, S. K., Gaysina, D., & Barker, E. D. (2015). Maternal depression symptoms, unhealthy diet and child emotional-behavioural dysregulation. *Psychol Med, 45*(9), 1851–1860. doi:10.1017/s0033291714002955.

Puhl, R. M., Suh, Y., & Li, X. (2016a). Improving anti-bullying laws and policies to protect youth from weight-based victimization: Parental support for action. *Pediatr Obes, 12*(2), e14–e19. doi:10.1111/ijpo.12129.

Puhl, R. M., Suh, Y., & Li, X. (2016b). Legislating for weight-based equality: National trends in public support for laws to prohibit weight discrimination. *Int J Obes (Lond), 40*(8), 1320–1324. doi:10.1038/ijo.2016.49.

Rankin, J., Matthews, L., Cobley, S., Han, A., Sanders, R., Wiltshire, H. D., & Baker, J. S. (2016). Psychological consequences of childhood obesity: Psychiatric comorbidity and prevention. *Adolesc Health Med Ther, 7*, 125–146. doi:10.2147/ahmt.s101631.

Ratcliffe, D., & Ellison, N. (2015). Obesity and internalized weight stigma: A formulation model for an emerging psychological problem. *Behav Cogn Psychother, 43*(2), 239–252. doi:10.1017/s1352465813000763.

Saltzman, J. A., Pineros-Leano, M., Liechty, J. M., Bost, K. K., Fiese, B. H., & Team, S. K. (2016). Eating, feeding, and feeling: Emotional responsiveness mediates longitudinal associations between maternal binge eating, feeding practices, and child weight. *Int J Behav Nutr Phys Act, 13*, 89. doi:10.1186/s12966-016-0415-5.

Sample, C. H., Jones, S., Hargrave, S. L., Jarrard, L. E., & Davidson, T. L. (2016). Western diet and the weakening of the interoceptive stimulus control of appetitive behavior. *Behav Brain Res, 312*, 219–230. doi:10.1016/j.bbr.2016.06.020.

Sample, C. H., Martin, A. A., Jones, S., Hargrave, S. L., & Davidson, T. L. (2015). Western-style diet impairs stimulus control by food deprivation state cues: Implications for obesogenic environments. *Appetite, 93*, 13–23. doi:10.1016/j.appet.2015.05.018.

Sarris, J., Logan, A. C., Akbaraly, T. N., Amminger, G. P., Balanza-Martinez, V., Freeman, M. P., … Morris, M. C. (2015). Nutritional medicine as mainstream in psychiatry Mediterranean diet and depressive symptoms among older adults over time. *Lancet Psychiatry, 2*(3), 271–274. doi:10.3390/ijerph6031235.

Schulte, E. M., Grilo, C. M., & Gearhardt, A. N. (2016). Shared and unique mechanisms underlying binge eating disorder and addictive disorders. *Clin Psychol Rev, 44*, 125–139. doi:10.1016/j.cpr.2016.02.001.

Sevincer, G. M., Konuk, N., Bozkurt, S., & Coskun, H. (2016). Food addiction and the outcome of bariatric surgery at 1-year: Prospective observational study. *Psychiatry Res, 244*, 159–164. doi:10.1016/j.psychres.2016.07.022.

Sharma, S., & Fulton, S. (2013). Diet-induced obesity promotes depressive-like behaviour that is associated with neural adaptations in brain reward circuitry. *Int J Obes (Lond), 37*(3), 382–389. doi:10.1038/ijo.2012.48.

Shin, J., Choi, Y., Han, K. T., Cheon, S. Y., Kim, J. H., Lee, S. G., & Park, E. C. (2015). The combined effect of subjective body image and body mass index (*distorted body weight perception) on suicidal ideation. J Prev Med Public Health, 48*(2), 94–104. doi:10.3961/jpmph.14.055.

Sirtori, A., Brunani, A., Capodaglio, P., Berselli, M. E., Villa, V., Ceriani, F., … Raggi, A. (2016). Patients with obesity-related comorbidities have higher disability compared with those without obesity-related comorbidities: Results from a cross-sectional study. *Int J Rehabil Res, 39*(1), 63–69. doi:10.1097/mrr.0000000000000146.

Soczynska, J. K., Kennedy, S. H., Woldeyohannes, H. O., Liauw, S. S., Alsuwaidan, M., Yim, C. Y., & McIntyre, R. S. (2011). Mood disorders and obesity: Understanding inflammation as a pathophysiological nexus. *Neuromolecular Med, 13*(2), 93–116. doi:10.1007/s12017-010-8140-8.

Spreadbury, I. (2012). Comparison with ancestral diets suggests dense acellular carbohydrates promote an inflammatory microbiota, and may be the primary dietary cause of leptin resistance and obesity. *Diabetes Metab Syndr Obes, 5*, 175–189. doi:10.2147/dmso.s33473.

Steffen, K. J., Engel, S. G., Wonderlich, J. A., Pollert, G. A., & Sondag, C. (2015). Alcohol and other addictive disorders following bariatric surgery: Prevalence, risk factors and possible etiologies. *Eur Eat Disord Rev, 23*(6), 442–450. doi:10.1002/erv.2399.

Stice, E., & Yokum, S. (2016). Neural vulnerability factors that increase risk for future weight gain. *Psychol Bull, 142*(5), 447–471. doi:10.1037/bul0000044.

Surve, A., Zaveri, H., Cottam, D., Belnap, L., Medlin, W., & Cottam, A. (2016). Mid-term outcomes of gastric bypass weight loss failure to duodenal switch. *Surg Obes Relat Dis, 12*(9), 1663–1670. doi:10.1016/j.soard.2016.03.021

Sutin, A. R., Ferrucci, L., Zonderman, A. B., & Terracciano, A. (2011). Personality and obesity across the adult life span. *J Pers Soc Psychol, 101*(3), 579–592. doi:10.1037/a0024286.

Theoharides, T. C., Stewart, J. M., Hatziagelaki, E., & Kolaitis, G. (2015). Brain "fog," inflammation and obesity: Key aspects of neuropsychiatric disorders improved by luteolin. *Front Neurosci, 9*, 225. doi:10.3389/fnins.2015.00225.

Thibault, R., & Pichard, C. (2016). Overview on nutritional issues in bariatric surgery. *Curr Opin Clin Nutr Metab Care, 19*(6), 484–490. doi:10.1097/mco.0000000000000325.

Torvik, F. A., Gustavson, K., Roysamb, E., & Tambs, K. (2015). Health, health behaviors, and health dissimilarities predict divorce: Results from the HUNT study. *BMC Psychol, 3*(1), 13. doi:10.1186/s40359-015-0072-5.

Tran, D. D., Nwokeabia, I. D., Purnell, S., Zafar, S. N., Ortega, G., Hughes, K., & Fullum, T. M. (2016). Revision of Roux-En-Y gastric bypass for weight regain: A systematic review of techniques and outcomes. *Obes Surg, 26*(7), 1627–1634. doi:10.1007/s11695-016-2201-5.

Treatment Research Institute. (2017). Addiction Severity Index 5th. Accessed from http://www.tresearch.org/wp-content/uploads/2012/09/ASI_5th_Ed.pdf

Tsenkova, V. K., Carr, D., Coe, C. L., & Ryff, C. D. (2014). Anger, adiposity, and glucose control in nondiabetic adults: Findings from MIDUS II. *J Behav Med, 37*(1), 37–46. doi:10.1007/s10865-012-9460-y.

Turk, M. W., Yang, K., Hravnak, M., Sereika, S. M., Ewing, L. J., & Burke, L. E. (2009). Randomized clinical trials of weight loss maintenance: A review. *J Cardiovasc Nurs, 24*(1), 58–80. doi:10.1097/01.jcn.0000317471.58048.32.

Varbo, A., Benn, M., Smith, G. D., Timpson, N. J., Tybjaerg-Hansen, A., & Nordestgaard, B. G. (2015). Remnant cholesterol, low-density lipoprotein cholesterol, and blood pressure as mediators from obesity to ischemic heart disease. *Circ Res, 116*(4), 665–673. doi:10.1161/circresaha.116.304846.

Verbeken, S., Braet, C., Bosmans, G., & Goossens, L. (2014). Comparing decision making in average and overweight children and adolescents. *Int J Obes (Lond), 38*(4), 547–551. doi:10.1038/ijo.2013.235.

Virkkunen, M., De Jong, J., Bartko, J., Goodwin, F. K., & Linnoila, M. (1989). Relationship of psychobiological variables to recidivism in violent offenders and impulsive fire setters. A follow-up study. *Arch Gen Psychiatry, 46*(7), 600–603.

Voon, V. (2015). Cognitive biases in binge eating disorder: The hijacking of decision making. *CNS Spectr, 20*(6), 566–573. doi:10.1017/s1092852915000681.

Wagner, B., Klinitzke, G., Brahler, E., & Kersting, A. (2013). Extreme obesity is associated with suicidal behavior and suicide attempts in adults: Results of a population-based representative sample. *Depress Anxiety, 30*(10), 975–981. doi:10.1002/da.22105.

Wang, J., Freire, D., Knable, L., Zhao, W., Gong, B., Mazzola, P., … Pasinetti, G. M. (2014). Childhood/adolescent obesity and long term cognitive consequences during aging. *J Comp Neurol, 523*(5), 757–768. doi:10.1002/cne.23708

Warren, M., Frost-Pineda, K., & Gold, M. (2005). Body mass index and marijuana use. *J Addict Dis, 24*(3), 95–100. doi:10.1002/cne.23708.

Weber, C. E., Talbot, L. J., Geller, J. M., Kuo, M. C., Wai, P. Y., & Kuo, P. C. (2013). Obesity and trends in malpractice claims for physicians and surgeons. *Surgery, 154*(2), 299–304. doi:10.1016/j.surg.2013.04.026.

Wertli, M. M., Held, U., Campello, M., & Schecter Weiner, S. (2016). Obesity is associated with more disability at presentation and after treatment in low back pain but not in neck pain: Findings from the OIOC registry. *BMC Musculoskelet Disord, 17*, 140. doi:10.1186/s12891-016-0992-0.

Xi, B., Cheng, H., Chen, F., Zhao, X., & Mi, J. (2016). Joint effect of birth weight and obesity measures on abnormal glucose metabolism at adulthood. *Zhonghua Yu Fang Yi Xue Za Zhi, 50*(1), 17–22. doi:10.3760/cma.j.issn.0253-9624.2016.01.004.

Yau, P. L., Kang, E. H., Javier, D. C., & Convit, A. (2014). Preliminary evidence of cognitive and brain abnormalities in uncomplicated adolescent obesity. *Obesity (Silver Spring), 22*(8), 1865–1871. doi:10.1002/oby.20801.

Zhang, Y., Liu, J., Yao, J., Ji, G., Qian, L., Wang, J., … Liu, Y. (2014). Obesity: Pathophysiology and intervention. *Nutrients, 6*(11), 5153–5183. doi:10.3390/nu6115153.

Zhang, P., Peterson, M., Su, G. L., & Wang, S. C. (2015). Visceral adiposity is negatively associated with bone density and muscle attenuation. *Am J Clin Nutr, 101*(2), 337–343. doi:10.3945/ajcn.113.081778.

Zhu, N., Jacobs, D. R., Meyer, K. A., He, K., Launer, L., Reis, J. P., … Steffen, L. M. (2015). Cognitive function in a middle aged cohort is related to higher quality dietary pattern 5 and 25 years earlier: The CARDIA study. *J Nutr Health Aging, 19*(1), 33–38. doi:10.1007/s12603-014-0491-7.

Zoon, H. F., He, W., de Wijk, R. A., de Graaf, C., & Boesveldt, S. (2014). Food preference and intake in response to ambient odours in overweight and normal-weight females. *Physiol Behav, 133*, 190–196. doi:10.1016/j.physbeh.2014.05.026.

Section III

Recovery from Processed Food Addiction

23 Introduction to Recovery from Processed Food Addiction

Joan Ifland
Food Addiction Training, LLC
Cincinnati, OH

Douglas M. Ziedonis
University of California San Diego
San Diego, CA

CONTENTS

"We don't have protocols." This was the answer recently given by a researcher/clinician in a weight-loss surgery practice in response to a question about whether incoming patients were screened for processed food addiction (PFA) and whether treatment for PFA was offered. The researcher knew the growing literature on PFA and was clear that the brains of obese people show similar brain adaptations to those of drug- and alcohol-addicted people (Brownell & Gold, 2012; Carter et al., 2016; Criscitelli & Avena, 2016; Moore, Sabino, Koob, & Cottone, 2017; Schulte, Yokum, Potenza, & Gearhardt, 2016; Volkow & Baler, 2015). However, he was looking for practical advice on how to assess and treat PFA. He wanted to translate research and expert consensus into help for the potentially food-addicted people presenting at the weight-loss surgery clinic.

In addition, the researcher/clinician was getting little support from the clinic for introducing screening, assessment, and treatment for PFA. Some of the reasons were lack of knowledge of the research on this topic and what to do, limited staff training on this topic, and the uncertainty of how PFA-specific treatments might be reimbursed, including group treatments dedicated to this topic. He was concerned that his staff didn't understand the important consequences to treating a food addict only with surgery. This can be especially important if there is no other support to address the compulsive behaviors that might lead the food addict client to find that addictive liquids (ice cream, sodas, and alcohol) pass through the surgery easily. Turning to addictive liquids can result in a return of weight gain and a risk of developing an alcohol use disorder, which has additional consequences. By reverting to liquids, the addict can sustain the PFA, develop another addiction (Bak, Seibold-Simpson, & Darling, 2016; Steffen, Engel, Wonderlich, Pollert, & Sondag, 2015; Svensson et al., 2013), and thwart the purpose of the surgery.

While bariatric surgery can provide a quick fix, there is a high risk with the lack of screening and inappropriate treatment that the core driver for the obesity is ignored and the chronic overeating of processed foods will return. It can be argued that some part of the poor long-term outcomes (more than 2 years) of "weight loss" protocols are the result of a missed diagnosis of PFA

(Turk et al., 2009). Weight loss for a food addict can be an ineffective, potentially harmful treatment because it does not address the core addiction problem.

The nature of the missed diagnosis can be understood by imagining that obesity resulting from compulsive and excessive use of beer or other forms of alcohol (more than 1 drink per day or 7 per week for a woman or 2 drinks a day or 14 per week for a man) were treated only as a general weight-loss issue rather than high-risk alcohol use or potentially an alcohol use disorder. The frustration and abject sense of failure on the part of both client and practitioner would be expected if the practitioner failed to advise a period of time for abstinence or substantial reduction of the alcohol use as part of the further assessment of alcohol use disorder and the helpful advice to reduce liquid calories. All addicted people will benefit from a new healthy lifestyle of appropriate levels of abstinence, exercise, sleep, healthy foods, appropriate meal sizes, and other activities.

As was seen in Parts I and II of this textbook, the evidence supporting the perspective that chronic overeating of processed foods can be an addiction is extensive (Moore et al., 2017; Stice & Yokum, 2016; Wiss, Criscitelli, Gold, & Avena, 2017). In the DSM 5 diagnostic manual, addictions are both substance use disorders (SUDs; alcohol, tobacco, heroin, etc.) and addictive disorders (only gambling disorder in the DSM 5) that have a range of severity and manifest comprehensively as they progress. PFA shares the clinical characteristic of these other addictions, including changes in personal behaviors; physical, mental, and emotional consequences; and broader impacts on relationships, careers, and society (Barry, Clarke, & Petry, 2009; Ifland et al., 2012; Koball et al., 2016; Moore et al., 2017; Patel, Spaeth, & Basner, 2016; Saltzman et al., 2016). Addiction to processed foods in some ways is both a "substance" use disorder (similar to alcohol or other substances) and an addictive disorder (similar to gambling disorder and other compulsive behaviors). This extensive syndrome was described in Part II of this textbook which describes the 11 diagnostic criteria in the DSM 5 SUD category as they manifest in chronic overeating. As will be seen in Part III, in order for treatment of PFA to be effective, the treatment also needs to monitor a wide range of behaviors and other manifestations as would be the case with any addiction. As was seen in Chapter 22, "The Addiction Severity Index in the Assessment of Processed Food Addiction," a comprehensive approach that considers severity of the problem, medical and psychiatric comorbidities, and psychological and social determinants of health is the key to restoring the client to optimal functioning.

Only on rare occasion does the PFA research finds its way into mainstream media. Nonetheless, "food addiction" has become a commonly used term. In popular and even clinical use, PFA can be confused with behavioral addictions such as gambling, shopping, and sex addiction. It can also be mistaken for a binge eating disorder manifesting as a specific type of loss of control over just specific foods, although more research is needed on the potential relationship of these two conditions and emotional overeating. However, the model that fits the research closely and "explains" disordered eating logically is that of a classic SUD involving a broad range of processed foods. This points to use of classic SUD abstinence/reduced harm protocols including abstinence or reduced use, cue avoidance, and support in the treatment of PFA. When this model is considered, it is possible to see why treating PFA as a behavioral disorder alone and failing to provide for abstinence or reduced use from the addictive food-like substances would be problematic. Similarly, a binge eating disorder model that provides for abstinence only from foods involved in the binge eating behavior, or just the bingeing itself, could maintain the brain in an addictive, reactive state. It may also become apparent that trying to persuade binge eaters not to be afraid of processed foods could worsen the addiction.

In the 1960s, Overeaters Anonymous began successfully using abstinence concepts to help individuals shift from bingeing and grazing to three measured meals per day. At that time, sugar and white flour were identified as foods that triggered members' cravings (Rozanne 2005). Over the years, popular practitioners such as Kay Sheppard (1993) and Ann Katherine (1991) as well as 12-step food addiction fellowships found that any kind of wheat product and a range of sweeteners triggered cravings (Food Addicts Anonymous, 2010; Food Addicts in Recovery Anonymous, 2013). This led to the expansion of definitions of abstinence. In some fellowships, such as Overeaters Anonymous, members are given the opportunity to define abstinence for themselves (Overeaters

Anonymous, 2017). This has resulted in recovery circles hotly debating the definitions of abstinence as members argue that they are unaffected by some processed foods and therefore should be allowed to "enjoy" them (Rozanne 2005).

Part III takes the approach that PFA is a disease of varying severity with potentially serious consequences, and the disease is easy to activate given the pervasiveness of easily available processed foods and dense food cueing in Westernized obesogenic cultures. Thus, the orientation of Part III is to recommend that clinicians educate their clients about a broad range of processed foods and cues while providing extensive support for recovery as needed for supporting cognition (neurofunctioning), addressing comorbidities, enhancing relationships, and encouraging work careers. Part III offers specific protocols for consideration and recommends excluding foods described in Chapter 6, "Abstinent Food Plans for Processed Food Addiction." For example, regarding food lists, based on research showing the presence of a naturally occurring morphine in gluten and dairy, those substances were eliminated from the protocols offered in Chapter 6. Given the target population is individuals with addiction to processed food, Part III offers simple but beautiful and delicious meal plans that exclude almost all processed foods.

Because of increasing public familiarity with the term *food addiction*, coupled with poor long-term outcomes of existing treatment models for obesity, it can be imagined that many health professionals would like to learn how to effectively administer PFA protocols based on a classic SUD model. Part III is for that purpose.

23.1 GOALS OF "RECOVERY FROM PROCESSED FOOD ADDICTION"

There are three broad goals of Part III. The first is to translate generally accepted alcohol, tobacco, and other drug addiction treatment into recommendations for recovery from PFA. The second is to make the translation into highly practical and simple methods that are effective with PFA clients who may have learning difficulties, challenges in decision-making, limited memory, or impaired restraint (Noble & Kanoski, 2016; Restivo, McKinnon, Frey, Hall, & Taylor, 2016). The third is to guide practitioners in methods to help PFA clients rebuild their lives to be productive and happy.

The primary goal of Part III is to translate classic SUD addiction treatment into recommendations for recovery from addictive processed foods. This goal derives directly from the many types of evidence that overeating exhibits the same brain dysfunction as alcohol, tobacco, and other drug addictions, coupled with findings for addictive properties in processed foods (Beitscher-Campbell et al., 2016; Carter et al., 2016; Gold, Badgaiyan, & Blum, 2015; Hutsell, Negus, & Banks, 2015; Schulte, Joyner, Potenza, Grilo, & Gearhardt, 2015; Tomasi et al., 2015). Thus Part III describes how clinicians can educate consumers about the disease concept. It also educates about methods to quit or reduce use of addictive processed foods and manage the stress of withdrawal (Blasio et al., 2013; Blasio, Rice, Sabino, & Cottone, 2014; Cottone, Sabino, Steardo, & Zorrilla, 2009; Iemolo et al., 2012; Martire et al., 2014; Mental Health Blog, 2017; Moore et al., 2017; Morris, Beilharz, Maniam, Reichelt, & Westbrook, 2015; Sharma, Fernandes, & Fulton, 2013). As threads in the education process, Part III describes how to enhance client motivation to reduce and ultimately abstain from addictive processed foods and to stick with their program of recovery.

Part III advocates simple, delightful meals. The preparation techniques and the teaching methods take into consideration that PFA clients may suffer compromised cognitive function including attention deficit, impaired decision-making, memory loss, and poor impulse control (Zhu et al., 2015). Similar to other SUDs there can be compromised cognitive function in normal attention, memory, sleep, irritability, management of anger, and other symptoms of protracted withdrawal (Moore et al., 2017; Sharma et al., 2013). There is a risk for other cognitive difficulties during the active use phase that may be substance specific, such as drowsiness, limited attention span, and poor memory (Chastin, Palarea-Albaladejo, Dontje, & Skelton, 2015; Cox, Fadardi, Intriligator, & Klinger, 2014; Kemps, Tiggemann, & Hollitt, 2014; Patel et al., 2016; Yesavage et al., 2014). Of course Part III covers the topic of relapse prevention. Part III also discusses methods for accessing and using support for the individual with PFA.

The second goal of Part III is to offer solutions to issues of practicality that are specific to PFA recovery. Obtaining and consuming food is naturally at the center of life. Depending on how they are managed and filtered, food cues and associative cues can drive either healthy or disordered feeding behavior. Recovery from PFA is the only addiction that requires engagement in cued activities associated with the addiction such as grocery shopping, cooking, eating, and cleaning up. Even in recovery, food-related activities remain at the center of the addict's life, requiring time and attention to plan and execute.

Of particular concern is that food-preparation activities must proceed in spite of hyperreactive craving neuropathways (Boswell & Kober, 2016) co-occurring with compromised cognitive function (Zhu et al., 2015), various physical and emotional ailments (Guh et al., 2009), and an environment of uncooperative domestic, social, or professional relationships (Carr, Friedman, & Jaffe, 2007; Seacat, Dougal, & Roy, 2016). Often, the food addict must also succeed in spite of limited energy and finances (Lee, Andrew, Gebremariam, Lumeng, & Lee, 2014; Phelan et al., 2015). So one important goal of the book is to describe very simple, easy, practical solutions to the day-to-day mental, time, money, and energy challenges faced by the recovering food addict.

The third goal of Part III addresses the disruption in education, careers, and family life that may be associated with PFA (Knutson, Taber, Murray, Valles, & Koeppl, 2010; Patel et al., 2016). As was seen in Part II on manifestations of the DSM 5 SUD diagnostic criteria, PFA can erupt and accelerate in the stressful environments of school, career, and families. PFA clients may be quite intelligent and motivated to resume progress in these areas as the disease goes into remission. Providing encouragement and direction in these areas can help PFA clients achieve an enjoyable and productive life.

23.2 IMPORTANCE OF "RECOVERY FROM PROCESSED FOOD ADDICTION"

Part III is important for a number of reasons. The most obvious is that it provides an alternative addiction lens perspective to rethink solutions to the unresolved global epidemic of chronic overeating and associated serious consequences. Over a billion people around the world are now overweight or obese (Ng et al., 2014). The consequences of chronic overeating are grave. Diabetes, stroke, heart disease, dementia, Alzheimer's, cancer, and joint disease are major life-disrupting maladies that are associated with overuse of processed food (Guh et al., 2009). At the same time, treatment for chronic overeating has almost universally failed, possibly because the diagnosis of PFA is not identified or included in the problem list in addition to a diagnosis of obesity. Thus "weight loss" options focus on the obesity, but these strategies are not working for PFA and could make PFA worse. Without methods to identify and effectively treat PFA, it can be argued that there is no foreseeable stop to the spread of the epidemic of obesity. There also is a need to provide more education to health care workers in general about nutritional assessment and treatment in general.

The importance of Part III versus the overall textbook is that although there are literally thousands of studies demonstrating many aspects of PFA, there is a need for more academically oriented books that present evidence-based treatments and provide consensus information from experts in the field. Although lay practices can be found in overeating and food addiction 12-step groups, these practices are generally unaware of findings in the research and could be enhanced by increased collaboration amongst researchers and clinicians. More studies of treatment in the field of PFA is needed so that evidence-based treatment becomes routine in the treatment of obesity with precision, thoroughness, compassion, and patience.

Another reason that Part III is important is that the recommendations are grounded in the current research available and experienced wisdom of practitioners in the field. Part III recognizes that PFA is a serious disease fostered by obesogenic environments (Cordain et al., 2005; Morris et al., 2015). Thus, it takes a conservative stance on issues such as eliminating a broad range of processed foods and potentially addictive food additives. It identifies the crucial role of craving cues found in home, commercial, workplace, and entertainment environments. Craving is now one of the 11 DSM 5 SUD diagnostic criteria (American Psychiatric Association, 2013, p. 491). PFA also addresses the whole family system, including addicted children (Mogul, Irby, & Skelton, 2014), while educating about the relationship of relapse to relationship sensitivity (Carr et al., 2007).

Of note, clinicians must be aware of the broad range of consequences of chronic processed food use even in people who are not overweight nor obese. As described in Chapter 22, "The Addiction Severity Index in the Assessment of Processed Food Addiction," consequences of use can include extensive immune, inflammation, and digestive problems before appearing as a weight issue. Part III also emphasizes methods to restore compromised cognitive functions that have been shown to be associated with overweight and obesity although a weight issue is not always present (Voon, 2015; Wang et al., 2015; Yau, Kang, Javier, & Convit, 2014; Zhu et al., 2015). In summary, "Recovery from Processed Food Addiction" is the first document that constructs a comprehensive program to recover from a serious mental illness and protect against an extended array of relapse triggers related to chronic overeating.

23.3 STRENGTHS OF "RECOVERY FROM PROCESSED FOOD ADDICTION"

There are a number of strengths to Part III related primarily to the strength of the evidence for its underlying treatment constructs as adapted from treatment for drug addiction (Beitscher-Campbell et al., 2016; Carter et al., 2016; Hutsell et al., 2015; Schulte et al., 2015; Tomasi et al., 2015), as well as emerging evidence specifically for high-sugar/high-fat foods in the development of addictive adaptations in the brain (Moore et al., 2017; Stice & Yokum, 2016).

The foundation of evidence for overeating as an SUD is strong, extensive, consistent, and logical across research techniques including brain imaging (Stice & Yokum, 2016), animal studies (Moore et al., 2017; Wiss et al., 2017), crossover drug-to-food studies (Farley, Hajek, Lycett, & Aveyard, 2012; Michaelides et al., 2012), crossover food-to-drug in bariatric studies (Steffen et al., 2015), research with antagonists (Blasio et al., 2013; Caravaggio et al., 2015; Gòmez & Ryabinin, 2014; Scherma et al., 2013), and similarities of genetic anomalies between drug-addicted people and the obese (Blum et al., 2015). As shown in Part II of this textbook, researchers have found a strong association between obesity and the 11 DSM 5 SUD diagnostic criteria (Hone-Blanchet & Fecteau, 2014; Ifland et al., 2009; Meule & Gearhardt, 2014). There is consistent evidence that overeating is an addictive behavioral syndrome.

There is also evidence for the efficacy of applying classic drug addiction approaches to PFA. These include abstinence/reduced harm, support, cognitive restoration, relationship repair, mindfulness, cognitive therapy, dialectical therapy, family therapy, and exercise (Brewerton & Dennis, 2014). The findings have been supported across questionnaire studies, MRI research, animal research, and intervention projects. This supports Part III's goal of helping people to stop cravings and restore cognitive functions through classic addiction recovery approaches.

There is also substantial evidence for the efficacy of unprocessed food plans in the remission of symptoms of chronic overeating, as described in Chapter 6, "Abstinent Food Plans for Processed Food Addiction." Abstinence from processed foods has been used successfully in 12-step programs since the 1960s (Rozanne 2005). The use of abstinence/reduced use is supported by numerous studies showing benefits from eliminating processed foods. These include studies of the Mediterranean diet and the Paleo diet, both of which eliminate most processed foods. These food plans are similar to the recovery food plan recommended in Part III.

There is a body of research showing a relationship between the Mediterranean diet and mental/emotional health. Rienks found that the Mediterranean diet appears to protect middle-aged women from depression (Rienks, Dobson, & Mishra, 2013). Of particular interest to the resolution of mental disorders, Psaltopoulou found in a meta-analysis that the Mediterranean diet was associated with reduced stroke, depression, and compromised cognitive functions (Psaltopoulou et al., 2013). In a switch-over study of women, Lee et al. found that just 10 days of the Mediterranean diet improved mood and memory (Lee et al., 2015). In a prospective study of university graduates, Sanchez-Villegas found that adherence to the Mediterranean diet inversely correlated with depression after

4.4 years (Sanchez-Villegas et al., 2009). Similarly, Skarupski found in a prospective study of older adults over 7.7 years that closer adherence to a Mediterranean diet correlated with reduced risk of depression (Skarupski, Tangney, Li, Evans, & Morris, 2013).

In addition to protection against mental and emotional disorders, physical problems also seem to be inversely correlated with a Mediterranean diet. Koloverou et al. found that the Mediterranean diet correlated with decreased rates of diabetes (Koloverou, Esposito, Giugliano, & Panagiotakos, 2014). Richter et al. found in a review article that the Mediterranean diet reduces cardiovascular disease and associated risk factors (Richter, Skulas-Ray, & Kris-Etherton, 2014). It is important for PFA clients to regain physical as well as mental and emotional health.

Another body of evidence exists for the efficacy of the Paleo diet in restoring health. Like the Mediterranean diet, the Paleo diet also eliminates most processed foods and also shows a range of physical, mental, and emotional benefits. In a finding that directly impacts recovery from addiction, Jonsson et al. found greater satiety in a population of diabetics consuming the Paleo diet versus a diabetes diet that contained more processed foods (Jonsson, Granfeldt, Lindeberg, & Hallberg, 2013). The finding was replicated in a trial comparing the Paleo diet, which eliminates grains and dairy, versus the Mediterranean diet, which does not (Jonsson, Granfeldt, Erlanson-Albertsson, Ahren, & Lindeberg, 2010). In a population of Dutch 50-year-olds, the Paleo diet improved blood pressure, triglyceride levels, abdominal circumference, and cholesterol levels, more so than a "healthy" diet recommended by the Dutch government (Boers et al., 2014).

Lindeberg found in a review article that eliminating dairy products, margarine, oils, refined sugar, and cereal grains, which provide 70% or more of the dietary intake in northern European populations, was beneficial in recovery from the metabolic syndrome (Lindeberg, 2012). In a review article, Kowalski et al. found evidence that a diet of meat, fish, shellfish, fresh fruits and vegetables, roots, tubers, eggs, and nuts was effective in weight, waist circumference, C-reactive protein, glycated hemoglobin (HbAlc), blood pressure, glucose tolerance, insulin secretion, insulin sensitivity and lipid profiles, type 2 diabetes, cancer, acne vulgaris, and myopia (Kowalski & Bujko, 2012). In a review article, Konner et al. noted that in 25 years of research of the Paleo diet, recommendations have been sharpened and results have been widely confirmed (Konner & Eaton, 2010).

This evidence for the efficacy of food plans that eliminate processed foods is a strength of Part III. Chapter 6, "Abstinent Food Plans for Processed Food Addiction," describes the evidence for abstaining from various processed foods as an effective treatment protocol for a number of diet-related diseases.

"Recovery from Processed Food Addiction" is part of a textbook that describes the syndrome of PFA so practitioners and clients can learn more as desired. The disease of PFA has many facets. Clients present with many different kinds of challenges. With the textbook at hand, practitioners can turn to the science, the diagnostic criteria, and the assessment tool to learn more and inform treatment options as desired.

SUD treatment has excellent psychosocial and pharmacological evidence-based treatments. Concepts of abstinence have been used successfully since the founding of Alcoholics Anonymous in the 1930s; however, there can be differences in how to define abstinence in the context of food, which humans must consume to survive. Avoidance of triggers and cues, along with support, has been found to be effective in the treatment of alcohol, tobacco, and other drug addictions. So conceptual constructs and the efficacy of the treatment modalities offered in "Recovery from Processed Food Addiction" are aligned with the evidence-based treatments commonly used in alcohol, tobacco, and drug addiction treatment such as abstinence, support, and a long-term approach.

23.4 LIMITATIONS OF "RECOVERY FROM PROCESSED FOOD ADDICTION"

The limitations of Part III derive primarily from the need for more research focused on evaluating abstinent food plans, the teaching of abstinent meal preparation, and particularly means for helping food-addicted children. In addition, there is an extensive array of consequences of PFA that are not the focus of Part III. PFA is a disease that can severely affect clients physically, emotionally, mentally, and spiritually. Part III does not cover all disease consequences of chronic use of processed foods.

Depending on the background of the practitioner, clients may benefit from more in-depth treatment for specific comorbid conditions and the need to be referred for evaluation and treatment of conditions related to diabetes, heart disease, joint deterioration, excess skin, etc. Fatigue, hormonal imbalances, and mineral deficiencies may also benefit from outside consultation. Referrals for in-depth work may also be helpful in areas such as behavioral or cognitive therapy, spiritual counseling, codependency work, yoga, meditation, mindfulness, etc.

Clinicians may be able to integrate and address comorbid psychiatric disorders or may need to refer, including PTSD symptoms, trauma, depression, anxiety, and anger. Fertility issues may also need referral. Other issues such as body distortion and social phobia may well be treated within the structure described in this toolkit.

It should also be noted that evaluation of the specific portfolio of modalities offered in Part III has not been studied in a controlled intervention.

23.5 ORGANIZATION OF "RECOVERY FROM PROCESSED FOOD ADDICTION"

Part III is organized into eight chapters: "Introduction to Recovery from Processed Food Addiction," "Premises of Recovery for Adults," "Avenues to Success for the Practitioner," "Adaptation of APA Practice Guidelines for SUD to Processed Food Addiction," "Preparing Adults for Recovery," "Insights from the Field," "Adaptation of SUD and ED Practice Parameters to Adolescents and Children with PFA," and "Strategies for Helping Food-Addicted Children."

Chapter 24, "Premises of Recovery for Adults," lays out the foundation for much of the orientation of Part III. Four key premises lend structure to Part III, including the applicability of classic SUD treatment to PFA, the need for greater cue avoidance relative to other SUDs, the importance of evaluating severity, response to treatment, and the need for extended care. Part III also offers suggestions for the delivery of services in person as well as in online settings.

The first key premise is that classic SUD treatment approaches can be transferred to PFA. Treatment approaches are discussed, including abstinence, harm reduction, trigger avoidance, relapse prevention, recovery of health, relationship skills, support, career, and purpose in life. These approaches have been used in both SUD treatment and in recovery from disordered eating. As much of Part III concerns teaching strategies for abstaining from processed foods and managing exposure to processed food cues, it is important to describe the evidence for this orientation.

The second premise is that more training in cue avoidance, protection from exposure to cueing, and recovery from exposure to cues is indicated relative to other SUDs. This is due to the higher prevalence in Westernized cultures of processed food cues relative to smoking, alcohol, or illegal drug cues. The premise also derives from advances in biological and marketing techniques to provoke reactive craving neuropathways developed by commercial food companies. More comprehensive training in cue avoidance is also suggested by the sensitivity to stress that obese people endure in relationships, which can increase cue reactivity.

The third premise of treatment is that, because PFA is a chronic condition with many external cues for relapse, extended care will often be needed. In making the case for extended care, this section describes the seriousness of the disease, the extensive variety of dysfunction, and the complex culture in which recovery takes place. This subsection covers the ways in which most clients might meet criteria for severity including young age of onset, polysubstance use, endorsement of numerous DSM 5 SUD criteria, relationship sensitivity, comorbidities, and the challenges of caring for addicted children and adult household members. There may also be a history of repeated relapse, unavoidable exposure to intense cueing, likelihood of accidental ingestion, and easy availability of addictive processed foods. In addition, there may be a history of trauma and childhood abuse.

The extended-care model also covers the need to reeducate clients due to extensive misinformation about treatment stemming from the common misconception of the disease as a weight loss issue. As a corollary, treatment may need to follow clients through a year of significant changes in body shape. And it argues that skill acquisition in the management of preparing unprocessed, balanced meals (see Chapter 6) benefits from a long period of supervision. The case for extended care has many elements.

The fourth premise of treatment that shapes Part III is that home outreach and a support network are important to success. This section describes ways to enhance this support, including through family support, support networks, and use of web-based and mobile personal electronic devices. The reasons to consider mobile and web-based supports are issues of client mobility, ability to pay, limited cognitive function (easy-to-access information to accommodate impairment to learning, decision-making, memory, and restraint), need for frequent contact, ability to limit exposure to relationship sensitivities, and practitioner efficiencies.

The immobility of clients is a barrier to in-person treatment but is easily overcome with a home outreach component. Clients may have limited ability to pay and Internet options can reduce overhead expense as well as increase the number of clients who can be treated by a single practitioner. There is a need for research on these approaches. However, there is excellent evidence for tobacco use disorders in utilizing quit-times and some evidence for web-based and mobile applications (Buller et al., 2014; Graham et al., 2015). A home outreach program using personal electronic devices overcomes the problem of geographic disbursement of willing clients and increases the practitioner's access to the world population of PFA sufferers. The use of personal electronic devices also allows for the delivery of education in brief, easy-to-follow messages, which is crucial given the large amount of information that needs to be learned in a population suffering from limited cognitive function (Forman, Hoffman, Juarascio, Butryn, & Herbert, 2013; Voon, 2015; Yau et al., 2014; Zhu et al., 2015). There is a need for these messages to be developed and there are different methods to do this including texting, Twitter, Facebook, email, and other technologies.

There is also the problem of the moment-to-moment nature of the disease, i.e., the unpredictability of flare-ups of cravings and momentary loss of rational decision-making that accompanies a craving flare-up. There is constant potential for a rapid change in ability to fight the disease due to exposure to stress and fatigue and ease of access to processed foods. Having access to a support group via personal electronic devices means that help is available virtually constantly. Online communities run by a knowledgeable person have been shown to be effective (Stice, Durant, Rohde, & Shaw, 2014; Veling, van Koningsbruggen, Aarts, & Stroebe, 2014; Wagner et al., 2016).

Chapter 25 of Part III is "Avenues to Success for the Practitioner." Practitioner attitudes and what they choose to emphasize are key to effective encouragement of clients. The more practitioners understand the potential severity, natural history, and possibility for long-term recovery from PFA, the better their patience and ability to place a kind word with an insight to keep a wobbly client going. The issue of patience is also discussed in regard to accommodating compromised cognitive function. Grasping the nature and range of severity of the compromised cognitive function will remind the practitioner of the value of providing information in a manner that supports these difficulties. This might include repeating instructions, making suggestions very brief, using photographs or other visual aids, and pacing the amount of information given in the development of meal preparation, cue management, relationship repair, and workplace management skills. The successful practitioner will learn how to steer attention away from weight loss toward recovery of physical, mental, and emotional health and how to manage weight-loss discussions that might be the focus of the client.

The successful practitioner will also consider how incorporating recommendations to the client in their own lives will help their authenticity and remind them of the difficulties of the change process. Obesity is so common that some practitioners may be obese and need to consider how to help themselves address their own obesity. This is of course a personal decision, but clients are observant and will recognize this issue in others. Similarly, if a practitioner were a tobacco smoker they would lose credibility in leading a smoking cessation program; however, they could still be helpful in learning how to make referrals.

Chapter 26 describes practice parameters for adults. It is an adaptation of the American Psychiatric Association's parameters for treatment of SUDs to treatment of PFA. As such it reviews the process of evaluation and treatment planning as well as the kinds of healthy challenges PFA clients are likely to face.

Chapter 27 of Part III is titled, "Preparing Adults for Recovery." Initially, clients may benefit from motivational interviewing including careful listening, open-ended questions, and reflections. This process requires patience and providing personalized feedback that might arise from an initial assessment or a pros–cons discussion (cost–benefit) of seeking versus not seeking treatment as well as overcoming concerns about implementing a food plan that only includes unprocessed food. Phases of motivation defining the reasons for change, problem recognition, optimism about the change, commitment to the change, and choosing from a menu of options. Empathy and patience at this stage will pay off as the client knows the reasons for making decisions. Asking permission to "give advice" is an art in motivational interviewing and also requires follow-up discussion.

Chapter 28 of Part III is titled, "Insights from the Field." This section lays out what PFA clients may need to know in order to be successful in the complex obesogenic environments where most PFA clients will carry out their recovery. PFA clients may be interested in how their disease fits the criteria of the DSM 5 SUD diagnostic criteria. This can help them understand the complexity of their problem and the hope for a solution. Educating clients about the neurochemistry of addictions may relieve them of the shame and guilt about not being able to conquer the disease through weight-loss approaches that did not address PFA. PFA clients could need extensive training in meal planning and preparation. PFA clients will need strategies for limiting exposure to processed food cues. PFA clients will also need more help with cognitive restoration because of unavoidable exposure to cues and food decisions but also to difficult relationship adjustments and meal preparation. Relapse prevention skills will be needed, as well as knowledge about how and when to access support. Parents will need plans for managing addicted children and their caregivers. Like all addicted people, PFA clients may have abandoned educations and careers. They will need to develop steps to regaining their paths in these areas.

Although the material is divided into the sections "Orientation Materials for Adults" and "Building a Healthy Lifestyle," topics may be sequenced earlier or later according to the specific needs and progress of a group. The materials progress through topics such as the mechanics of an unprocessed food plan, relapse avoidance, PFA versus weight loss, relationships, physical healing, mental healing, emotional healing, spiritual healing, reclaiming careers, evaluating sources of support, and helping children. Practitioners can add and delete material according to their particular backgrounds and goals.

Chapter 29, which deals with practice parameters for children, is similar to the parameters described for adults. It is adapted from the APA's parameters for SUD in children, as well as other practice parameters for the treatment of pediatric obesity.

Chapter 30 is titled, "Strategies for Helping Food-Addicted Children." This is an extensive section that includes an introduction and sections on strengths, limitations, and premises of treatment. It then offers three stages of education for helping addicted children. The first is motivating parents and starts off with an assessment and the recommendation to change. Parents then explore the question of whether it's worth it to make indicated changes and any concerns about doing so. Parents can refine self-concepts and pick from a menu of options for starting. In the second stage, parents are trained in recognizing addictive reactions in their children, including cravings. They learn how to support remission of the addiction. The third stage regards how to teach children about PFA. The discussion is theoretical and is offered as research questions.

This introduction has oriented the practitioner to Part III. Although a great deal of material is included in Part III, it is hoped that the practitioner will gradually gain command of treatment processes. In order to achieve a healthy, productive life, PFA clients need nuanced pacing, information, strategies, and encouragement across many different tasks.

REFERENCES

American Psychiatric Association. (2013). *The diagnostic and statistical manual of mental disorders* (5th ed., Vol. 5).

Bak, M., Seibold-Simpson, S. M., & Darling, R. (2016). The potential for cross-addiction in post-bariatric surgery patients: Considerations for primary care nurse practitioners. *J Am Assoc Nurse Pract, 28*(12), 675–682. doi:10.1002/2327-6924.12390.

Barry, D., Clarke, M., & Petry, N. M. (2009). Obesity and its relationship to addictions: Is overeating a form of addictive behavior? *Am J Addict, 18*(6), 439–451. doi:10.3109/10550490903205579.

Beitscher-Campbell, H., Blum, K., Febo, M., Madigan, M. A., Giordano, J., Badgaiyan, R. D., … Gold, M. S. (2016). Pilot clinical observations between food and drug seeking derived from fifty cases attending an eating disorder clinic. *J Behav Addict, 5*(3), 533–541. doi:10.1556/2006.5.2016.055.

Blasio, A., Iemolo, A., Sabino, V., Petrosino, S., Steardo, L., Rice, K. C., … Cottone, P. (2013). Rimonabant precipitates anxiety in rats withdrawn from palatable food: Role of the central amygdala. *Neuropsychopharmacology, 38*(12), 2498–2507. doi:10.1038/npp.2013.153.

Blasio, A., Rice, K. C., Sabino, V., & Cottone, P. (2014). Characterization of a shortened model of diet alternation in female rats: Effects of the CB1 receptor antagonist rimonabant on food intake and anxiety-like behavior. *Behav Pharmacol, 25*(7), 609–617. doi:10.1097/fbp.0000000000000059.

Blum, K., Thanos, P. K., Oscar-Berman, M., Febo, M., Baron, D., Badgaiyan, R. D., … Gold, M. S. (2015). Dopamine in the brain: Hypothesizing surfeit or deficit links to reward and addiction. *J Reward Defic Syndr, 1*(3), 95–104. doi:10.17756/jrds.2015-016.

Boers, I., Muskiet, F. A., Berkelaar, E., Schut, E., Penders, R., Hoenderdos, K., … Jong, M. C. (2014). Favourable effects of consuming a palaeolithic-type diet on characteristics of the metabolic syndrome: A randomized controlled pilot-study. *Lipids Health Dis, 13*, 160. doi:10.1186/1476-511x-13-160.

Boswell, R. G., & Kober, H. (2016). Food cue reactivity and craving predict eating and weight gain: A meta-analytic review. *Obes Rev, 17*(2), 159–177. doi:10.1111/obr.12354.

Brewerton, T., & Dennis, A. B. (Eds.). (2014). *Eating disorders, addictions and substance use disorders*. Berlin: Springer-Verlag.

Brownell, K., & Gold, M. (Eds.). (2012). *Handbook of food and addiction*. Oxford: Oxford University Press.

Buller, D. B., Halperin, A., Severson, H. H., Borland, R., Slater, M. D., Bettinghaus, E. P., … Woodall, W. G. (2014). Effect of nicotine replacement therapy on quitting by young adults in a trial comparing cessation services. *J Public Health Manag Pract, 20*(2), E7–E15. doi:10.1097/PHH.0b013e3182a0b8c7.

Caravaggio, F., Raitsin, S., Gerretsen, P., Nakajima, S., Wilson, A., & Graff-Guerrero, A. (2015). Ventral striatum binding of a dopamine d2/3 receptor agonist but not antagonist predicts normal body mass index. *Biol Psychiatry, 77*(2), 196–202. doi:10.1016/j.biopsych.2013.02.017.

Carr, D., Friedman, M. A., & Jaffe, K. (2007). Understanding the relationship between obesity and positive and negative affect: The role of psychosocial mechanisms. *Body Image, 4*(2), 165–177. doi:10.1016/j.bodyim.2007.02.004.

Carter, A., Hendrikse, J., Lee, N., Yucel, M., Verdejo-Garcia, A., Andrews, Z., & Hall, W. (2016). The neurobiology of "food addiction" and its implications for obesity treatment and policy. *Annu Rev Nutr, 36*, 105–128. doi:10.1146/annurev-nutr-071715-050909.

Chastin, S. F., Palarea-Albaladejo, J., Dontje, M. L., & Skelton, D. A. (2015). Combined effects of time spent in physical activity, sedentary behaviors and sleep on obesity and cardio-metabolic health markers: A novel compositional data analysis approach. *PLoS One, 10*(10), e0139984. doi:10.1371/journal.pone.0139984.

Cordain, L., Eaton, S. B., Sebastian, A., Mann, N., Lindeberg, S., Watkins, B. A., … Brand-Miller, J. (2005). Origins and evolution of the Western diet: Health implications for the 21st century. *Am J Clin Nutr, 81*(2), 341–354.

Cottone, P., Sabino, V., Steardo, L., & Zorrilla, E. P. (2009). Consummatory, anxiety-related and metabolic adaptations in female rats with alternating access to preferred food. *Psychoneuroendocrinology, 34*(1), 38–49. doi:10.1016/j.psyneuen.2008.08.010.

Cox, W. M., Fadardi, J. S., Intriligator, J. M., & Klinger, E. (2014). Attentional bias modification for addictive behaviors: Clinical implications. *CNS Spectr, 19*(3), 215–224. doi:10.1017/s1092852914000091.

Criscitelli, K., & Avena, N. M. (2016). The neurobiological and behavioral overlaps of nicotine and food addiction. *Prev Med, 92*, 82–89. doi:10.1016/j.ypmed.2016.08.009.

Farley, A. C., Hajek, P., Lycett, D., & Aveyard, P. (2012). Interventions for preventing weight gain after smoking cessation. *Cochrane Database Syst Rev, 1*, Cd006219. doi:10.1002/14651858.CD006219.pub3.

Food Addicts Anonymous. (2010). *Food addicts anonymous*. Port St. Lucie, FL: Food Addicts Anonymous, Inc.

Food Addicts in Recovery Anonymous. (2013). *Food addicts in recovery anonymous*. Woburn, MA: Food Addicts in Recovery Anonymous.

Forman, E. M., Hoffman, K. L., Juarascio, A. S., Butryn, M. L., & Herbert, J. D. (2013). Comparison of acceptance-based and standard cognitive-based coping strategies for craving sweets in overweight and obese women. *Eat Behav, 14*(1), 64–68. doi:10.1016/j.eatbeh.2012.10.016.

Gold, M. S., Badgaiyan, R. D., & Blum, K. (2015). A shared molecular and genetic basis for food and drug addiction: Overcoming hypodopaminergic trait/state by incorporating dopamine agonistic therapy in psychiatry. *Psychiatr Clin North Am, 38*(3), 419–462. doi:10.1016/j.psc.2015.05.011.

Gomez, J. L., & Ryabinin, A. E. (2014). The effects of ghrelin antagonists [D-Lys(3)]-GHRP-6 or JMV2959 on ethanol, water, and food intake in C57BL/6J mice. *Alcohol Clin Exp Res, 38*(9), 2436–2444. doi:10.1111/acer.12499.

Graham, A. L., Papandonatos, G. D., Cobb, C. O., Cobb, N. K., Niaura, R. S., Abrams, D. B., & Tinkelman, D. G. (2015). Internet and telephone treatment for smoking cessation: Mediators and moderators of short-term abstinence. *Nicotine Tob Res, 17*(3), 299–308. doi:10.1093/ntr/ntu144.

Guh, D. P., Zhang, W., Bansback, N., Amarsi, Z., Birmingham, C. L., & Anis, A. H. (2009). The incidence of co-morbidities related to obesity and overweight: A systematic review and meta-analysis. *BMC Public Health, 9*, 88. doi:10.1186/1471-2458-9-88.

Hone-Blanchet, A., & Fecteau, S. (2014). Overlap of food addiction and substance use disorders definitions: Analysis of animal and human studies. *Neuropharmacology, 85*, 81–90. doi:10.1016/j.neuropharm.2014.05.019.

Hutsell, B. A., Negus, S. S., & Banks, M. L. (2015). A generalized matching law analysis of cocaine vs. food choice in rhesus monkeys: Effects of candidate "agonist-based" medications on sensitivity to reinforcement. *Drug Alcohol Depend, 146*, 52–60. doi:10.1016/j.drugalcdep.2014.11.003.

Iemolo, A., Valenza, M., Tozier, L., Knapp, C. M., Kornetsky, C., Steardo, L., … Cottone, P. (2012). Withdrawal from chronic, intermittent access to a highly palatable food induces depressive-like behavior in compulsive eating rats. *Behav Pharmacol, 23*(5–6), 593–602. doi:10.1097/FBP.0b013e328357697f.

Ifland, J. R., Preuss, H. G., Marcus, M. T., Rourke, K. M., Taylor, W. C., Burau, K., … Manso, G. (2009). Refined food addiction: A classic substance use disorder. *Med Hypotheses, 72*(5), 518–526. doi:10.1016/j.mehy.2008.11.035.

Ifland, J. R., Preuss, H. G., Marcus, M. T., Rourke, K. M., Taylor, W. C., & Lerner, M. (2012). The evidence for refined food addiction. In *Obesity: Epidemiology, pathophysiology and prevention* (2nd ed., pp. 53–72). Boca Ratan, FL: Taylor and Francis.

Jonsson, T., Granfeldt, Y., Erlanson-Albertsson, C., Ahren, B., & Lindeberg, S. (2010). A paleolithic diet is more satiating per calorie than a mediterranean-like diet in individuals with ischemic heart disease. *Nutr Metab (Lond), 7*, 85. doi:10.1186/1743-7075-7-85.

Jonsson, T., Granfeldt, Y., Lindeberg, S., & Hallberg, A. C. (2013). Subjective satiety and other experiences of a paleolithic diet compared to a diabetes diet in patients with type 2 diabetes. *Nutr J, 12*, 105. doi:10.1186/1475-2891-12-105.

Katherine, A. (1991). *Anatomy of a food addiction: The brain chemistry of overeating*. Carlsbad, CA: Gurze Books.

Kemps, E., Tiggemann, M., & Hollitt, S. (2014). Biased attentional processing of food cues and modification in obese individuals. *Health Psychol, 33*(11):1391–1401. doi:10.1037/hea0000069.

Knutson, J. F., Taber, S. M., Murray, A. J., Valles, N. L., & Koeppl, G. (2010). The role of care neglect and supervisory neglect in childhood obesity in a disadvantaged sample. *J Pediatr Psychol, 35*(5), 523–532. doi:10.1093/jpepsy/jsp115.

Koball, A. M., Clark, M. M., Collazo-Clavell, M., Kellogg, T., Ames, G., Ebbert, J., & Grothe, K. B. (2016). The relationship among food addiction, negative mood, and eating-disordered behaviors in patients seeking to have bariatric surgery. *Surg Obes Relat Dis, 12*(1), 165–170. doi:10.1016/j.soard.2015.04.009.

Koloverou, E., Esposito, K., Giugliano, D., & Panagiotakos, D. (2014). The effect of Mediterranean diet on the development of type 2 diabetes mellitus: A meta-analysis of 10 prospective studies and 136,846 participants. *Metabolism, 63*(7), 903–911. doi:10.1016/j.metabol.2014.04.010.

Konner, M., & Eaton, S. B. (2010). Paleolithic nutrition: Twenty-five years later. *Nutr Clin Pract, 25*(6), 594–602. doi:10.1177/0884533610385702.

Kowalski, L. M., & Bujko, J. (2012). Evaluation of biological and clinical potential of paleolithic diet. *Rocz Panstw Zakl Hig, 63*(1), 9–15.

Lee, H., Andrew, M., Gebremariam, A., Lumeng, J. C., & Lee, J. M. (2014). Longitudinal associations between poverty and obesity from birth through adolescence. *Am J Public Health, 104*(5), e70–76. doi:10.2105/AJPH.2013.301806.

Lee, J., Pase, M., Pipingas, A., Raubenheimer, J., Thurgood, M., Villalon, L., … Scholey, A. (2015). Switching to a 10-day Mediterranean-style diet improves mood and cardiovascular function in a controlled cross-over study. *Nutrition, 31*(5), 647–652. doi:10.1016/j.nut.2014.10.008.

Lindeberg, S. (2012). Paleolithic diets as a model for prevention and treatment of Western disease. *Am J Hum Biol, 24*(2), 110–115. doi:10.1002/ajhb.22218.

Martire, S. I., Maniam, J., South, T., Holmes, N., Westbrook, R. F., & Morris, M. J. (2014). Extended exposure to a palatable cafeteria diet alters gene expression in brain regions implicated in reward, and withdrawal from this diet alters gene expression in brain regions associated with stress. *Behav Brain Res, 265*, 132–141. doi:10.1016/j.bbr.2014.02.027.

Mental Health Blog. (2017). *Gluten withdrawal symptoms + how long do they last?* Retrieved from http://mentalhealthdaily.com/2015/03/27/gluten-withdrawal-symptoms-how-long-do-they-last/ (accessed on January 10, 2017).

Meule, A., & Gearhardt, A. N. (2014). Food addiction in the light of DSM-5. *Nutrients, 6*(9), 3653–3671. doi:10.3390/nu6093653.

Michaelides, M., Thanos, P. K., Kim, R., Cho, J., Ananth, M., Wang, G. J., & Volkow, N. D. (2012). PET imaging predicts future body weight and cocaine preference. *NeuroImage, 59*(2), 1508–1513. doi:10.1016/j.neuroimage.2011.08.028.

Mogul, A., Irby, M. B., & Skelton, J. A. (2014). A systematic review of pediatric obesity and family communication through the lens of addiction literature. *Child Obes, 10*(3), 197–206. doi:10.1089/chi.2013.0157.

Moore, C. F., Sabino, V., Koob, G. F., & Cottone, P. (2017). Pathological overeating: Emerging evidence for a compulsivity construct. *Neuropsychopharmacology, 42*(7), 1375–1389. doi:10.1038/npp.2016.269.

Morris, M. J., Beilharz, J., Maniam, J., Reichelt, A., & Westbrook, R. F. (2015). Why is obesity such a problem in the 21st century? The intersection of palatable food, cues and reward pathways, stress, and cognition. *Neurosci Biobehav Rev, 58*, 36–45. doi:10.1016/j.neubiorev.2014.12.002.

Ng, M., Fleming, T., Robinson, M., Thomson, B., Graetz, N., Margono, C., … Gakidou, E. (2014). Global, regional, and national prevalence of overweight and obesity in children and adults during 1980–2013: A systematic analysis for the Global Burden of Disease Study 2013. *Lancet, 384*(9945), 766–781. doi:10.1016/s0140-6736(14)60460-8.

Noble, E. E., & Kanoski, S. E. (2016). Early life exposure to obesogenic diets and learning and memory dysfunction. *Curr Opin Behav Sci, 9*, 7–14. doi:10.1016/j.cobeha.2015.11.014.

Overeaters Anonymous. (2017). *Difference between abstinence and a plan of eating workshop-handout.* Retrieved from https://oa.org/files/pdf/abstinence_and_plan_of_eating_handouts.pdf (accessed on February 10, 2107).

Patel, V. C., Spaeth, A. M., & Basner, M. (2016). Relationships between time use and obesity in a representative sample of Americans. *Obesity (Silver Spring), 24*(10), 2164–2175. doi:10.1002/oby.21596.

Phelan, S. M., Burgess, D. J., Puhl, R., Dyrbye, L. N., Dovidio, J. F., Yeazel, M., … van Ryn, M. (2015). The adverse effect of weight stigma on the well-being of medical students with overweight or obesity: Findings from a National Survey. *J Gen Intern Med, 30*(9), 1251–1258. doi:10.1007/s11606-015-3266-x.

Psaltopoulou, T., Sergentanis, T. N., Panagiotakos, D. B., Sergentanis, I. N., Kosti, R., & Scarmeas, N. (2013). Mediterranean diet, stroke, cognitive impairment, and depression: A meta-analysis. *Ann Neurol, 74*(4), 580–591. doi:10.1002/ana.23944.

Restivo, M. R., McKinnon, M. C., Frey, B. N., Hall, G. B., & Taylor, V. H. (2016). Effect of obesity on cognition in adults with and without a mood disorder: Study design and methods. *BMJ Open, 6*(2), e009347. doi:10.1136/bmjopen-2015-009347.

Richter, C. K., Skulas-Ray, A. C., & Kris-Etherton, P. M. (2014). Recent findings of studies on the Mediterranean diet: What are the implications for current dietary recommendations? *Endocrinol Metab Clin North Am, 43*(4), 963–980. doi:10.1016/j.ecl.2014.08.003.

Rienks, J., Dobson, A. J., & Mishra, G. D. (2013). Mediterranean dietary pattern and prevalence and incidence of depressive symptoms in mid-aged women: Results from a large community-based prospective study. *Eur J Clin Nutr, 67*(1), 75–82. doi:10.1038/ejcn.2012.193.

Rozanne, S. (2005). *Beyond our wildest dreams*. Rio Rancho, NM: Overeaters Anonymous.

Saltzman, J. A., Pineros-Leano, M., Liechty, J. M., Bost, K. K., Fiese, B. H., & Team, S. K. (2016). Eating, feeding, and feeling: Emotional responsiveness mediates longitudinal associations between maternal binge eating, feeding practices, and child weight. *Int J Behav Nutr Phys Act, 13*, 89. doi:10.1186/s12966-016-0415-5.

Sanchez-Villegas, A., Delgado-Rodriguez, M., Alonso, A., Schlatter, J., Lahortiga, F., Serra Majem, L., & Martinez-Gonzalez, M. A. (2009). Association of the Mediterranean dietary pattern with the incidence of depression: The Seguimiento Universidad de Navarra/University of Navarra follow-up (SUN) cohort. *Arch Gen Psychiatry, 66*(10), 1090–1098. doi:10.1001/archgenpsychiatry.2009.129.

Scherma, M., Fattore, L., Satta, V., Businco, F., Pigliacampo, B., Goldberg, S. R., … Fadda, P. (2013). Pharmacological modulation of the endocannabinoid signalling alters binge-type eating behaviour in female rats. *Br J Pharmacol, 169*(4), 820–833. doi:10.1111/bph.12014.

Schulte, E. M., Joyner, M. A., Potenza, M. N., Grilo, C. M., & Gearhardt, A. N. (2015). Current considerations regarding food addiction. *Curr Psychiatry Rep, 17*(4), 563. doi:10.1007/s11920-015-0563-3.

Schulte, E. M., Yokum, S., Potenza, M. N., & Gearhardt, A. N. (2016). Neural systems implicated in obesity as an addictive disorder: From biological to behavioral mechanisms. *Prog Brain Res, 223*, 329–346. doi:10.1016/bs.pbr.2015.07.011.

Seacat, J. D., Dougal, S. C., & Roy, D. (2016). A daily diary assessment of female weight stigmatization. *J Health Psychol, 21*(2), 228–240. doi:10.1177/1359105314525067.

Sharma, S., Fernandes, M. F., & Fulton, S. (2013). Adaptations in brain reward circuitry underlie palatable food cravings and anxiety induced by high-fat diet withdrawal. *Int J Obes (Lond), 37*(9), 1183–1191. doi:10.1038/ijo.2012.197.

Sheppard, K. (1993). *Food addiction: The body knows*. Deerfield Beach, FL: Health Communications.

Skarupski, K. A., Tangney, C. C., Li, H., Evans, D. A., & Morris, M. C. (2013). Mediterranean diet and depressive symptoms among older adults over time. *J Nutr Health Aging, 17*(5), 441–445. doi:10.1007/s12603-012-0437-x.

Steffen, K. J., Engel, S. G., Wonderlich, J. A., Pollert, G. A., & Sondag, C. (2015). Alcohol and other addictive disorders following bariatric surgery: Prevalence, risk factors and possible etiologies. *Eur Eat Disord Rev, 23*(6), 442–450. doi:10.1002/erv.2399.

Stice, E., Durant, S., Rohde, P., & Shaw, H. (2014). Effects of a prototype Internet dissonance-based eating disorder prevention program at 1- and 2-year follow-up. *Health Psychol*. doi:10.1037/hea0000090.

Stice, E., & Yokum, S. (2016). Neural vulnerability factors that increase risk for future weight gain. *Psychol Bull, 142*(5), 447–471. doi:10.1037/bul0000044.

Svensson, P. A., Anveden, A., Romeo, S., Peltonen, M., Ahlin, S., Burza, M. A., … Carlsson, L. M. (2013). Alcohol consumption and alcohol problems after bariatric surgery in the Swedish obese subjects study. *Obesity (Silver Spring), 21*(12), 2444–2451. doi:10.1002/oby.20397.

Tomasi, D., Wang, G. J., Wang, R., Caparelli, E. C., Logan, J., & Volkow, N. D. (2015). Overlapping patterns of brain activation to food and cocaine cues in cocaine abusers: Association to striatal D2/D3 receptors. *Hum Brain Mapp, 36*(1), 120–136. doi:10.1002/hbm.22617.

Turk, M. W., Yang, K., Hravnak, M., Sereika, S. M., Ewing, L. J., & Burke, L. E. (2009). Randomized clinical trials of weight loss maintenance: A review. *J Cardiovasc Nurs, 24*(1), 58–80. doi:10.1097/01.jcn.0000317471.58048.32.

Veling, H., van Koningsbruggen, G. M., Aarts, H., & Stroebe, W. (2014). Targeting impulsive processes of eating behavior via the internet. Effects on body weight. *Appetite, 78*, 102–109. doi:10.1016/j.appet.2014.03.014.

Volkow, N. D., & Baler, R. D. (2015). NOW vs LATER brain circuits: Implications for obesity and addiction. *Trends Neurosci, 38*(6), 345–352. doi:10.1016/j.tins.2015.04.002.

Voon, V. (2015). Cognitive biases in binge eating disorder: The hijacking of decision making. *CNS Spectr, 20*(6), 566–573. doi:10.1017/s1092852915000681.

Wagner, B., Nagl, M., Dolemeyer, R., Klinitzke, G., Steinig, J., Hilbert, A., & Kersting, A. (2016). Randomized controlled trial of an Internet-based cognitive-behavioral treatment program for binge-eating disorder. *Behav Ther, 47*(4), 500–514. doi:10.1016/j.beth.2016.01.006.

Wang, J., Freire, D., Knable, L., Zhao, W., Gong, B., Mazzola, P., … Pasinetti, G. M. (2015). Childhood/adolescent obesity and long term cognitive consequences during aging. *J Comp Neurol, 523*(5), 757–768. doi:10.1002/cne.23708.

Wiss, D. A., Criscitelli, K., Gold, M., & Avena, N. (2017). Preclinical evidence for the addiction potential of highly palatable foods: Current developments related to maternal influence. *Appetite, 115*, 19–27. doi:10.1016/j.appet.2016.12.019.

Yau, P. L., Kang, E. H., Javier, D. C., & Convit, A. (2014). Preliminary evidence of cognitive and brain abnormalities in uncomplicated adolescent obesity. *Obesity (Silver Spring), 22*(8), 1865–1871. doi:10.1002/oby.20801.

Yesavage, J. A., Kinoshita, L. M., Noda, A., Lazzeroni, L. C., Fairchild, J. K., Taylor, J., … O'Hara, R. (2014). Effects of body mass index-related disorders on cognition: Preliminary results. *Diabetes Metab Syndr Obes, 7,* 145–151. doi:10.2147/dmso.s60294.

Zhu, N., Jacobs, D. R., Meyer, K. A., He, K., Launer, L., Reis, J. P., … Steffen, L. M. (2015). Cognitive function in a middle aged cohort is related to higher quality dietary pattern 5 and 25 years earlier: The CARDIA study. *J Nutr Health Aging, 19*(1), 33–38. doi:10.1007/s12603-014-0491-7.

24 Premises of Recovery for Adults

Douglas M. Ziedonis
University of California San Diego
San Diego, CA

Joan Ifland
Food Addiction Training, LLC
Cincinnati, OH

CONTENTS

Processed food addiction (PFA) is a far-reaching and complex condition touching virtually every aspect of clients and the people around them. By understanding the premises of treatment, practitioners can accelerate their understanding of how to guide clients to successful recovery from PFA. Practitioners will more easily orient themselves to PFA practice techniques by recognizing similarities to their existing practices.

Whether general, diet-related, eating disorder, mental health, or addiction, all types of practices can incorporate information about PFA. By importing expertise in diets or substance use disorders (SUDs), practitioners can readily make themselves comfortable with identifying and helping PFA clients. For some readers, this textbook might be their first brush with PFA so grounding in treatment rationales can help practitioners grow confident about implementing principles. That is the purpose of this chapter.

24.1 THE THREE PREMISES

Three premises are covered in this discussion.

1. The first is the transferability of classic SUD treatment approaches to PFA. These approaches are lifelong abstinence or reduced use of addictive substances, comprehensive management of cues for the addictive substances, and restitution of mental, emotional, and behavioral health.
2. The second premise is that long-term care could often be appropriate in light of extensive needs for skill acquisition, restoration of a wide variety of neurofunctions, and support from a community of like-minded people for improvement in self-esteem and socializing.
3. The third premise is that the Internet and mobile devices could be helpful due to mobility issues, a high risk of relapse due to easy availability of processed foods, and pervasive cuing for processed foods in Westernized cultures. Frequent contact and reinforcement via electronic devices for clients can be instrumental in protecting them against temptation in obesogenic environments.

By grounding in these three premises, practitioners can become familiar with the "lay of the land" as they undertake to heal PFA. The premises give practitioners practical understanding of the reasons to structure effective treatment on a drug addiction recovery model.

Part I of the textbook lays out the science behind these premises. These three premises of transferability of SUD approaches, long-term care, and use of Internet and mobile devices are derived from research showing the addictive properties of processed foods (Ifland, Preuss, Marcus, Taylor, & Rourke, 2015b), which supports the concept of SUD-style abstinence. Cue reactivity in the brains of overeaters (Boswell & Kober, 2016) leads to the premise that cue avoidance will help with control of cravings. The broad extent of trauma in obese populations (Brewer-Smyth, Cornelius, & Pohlig, 2016; Mason et al., 2014) supports the premise that long-term membership in a recovery community could help restore self-esteem and social skills. Compromised cognitive functions in the obese (Abiles et al., 2013; Giuliani, Calcott, & Berkman, 2013; Voon, 2015; Wang et al., 2015; Yau, Kang, Javier, & Convit, 2014; Zhu et al., 2015) support recommendations to teach slowly in a long-term setting. The match between the disease of PFA and the structure of using the Internet and mobile devices for treatment is due primarily to mobility (Belczak, de Godoy, Belczack, Ramos, & Caffaro, 2014; McGregor, Cameron-Smith, & Poppitt, 2014) and stigmatization (Ratcliffe & Ellison, 2015), issues that can hamper the ability of clients to travel away from home. Research forms the basis for the premises of treatment and reassures practitioners that their approaches are effective.

24.2 PREMISE 1: APPROACHES USED IN SUD ARE TRANSFERRABLE TO PFA

The premise that classic SUD treatment modalities can be applied to PFA drives a fair share of the training material of this textbook insofar as abstinence/reduced use, cue management, and relapse prevention strategies require the acquisition of fairly extensive skills for the recovering PFA client.

The support for the application of classic SUD treatment protocols comes from Parts I and II of this textbook. Part I of the textbook lays out the similarities between processed food use and drug addiction in terms of neurofunctioning, behaviors, consequences, and addictive substances. The genesis of addictions are neuroadaptations in the brain as key neuropathways become hyperreactive to cues in environments. In PFA clients, this is seen in dopamine, opiate, serotonin, and endocannabinoid pathways (Fortuna, 2012). Reward pathways are downregulated (Johnson & Kenny, 2010). At the same time, cognitive centers in the brain are hypoactive including learning, decision-making, memory, restraint, and satiation (Yau et al., 2014). Overwhelming urges combined with the loss of impulse control have been shown to drive the self-destructive use of addictive substances, including processed foods (McLaren et al., 2014). These neuroadaptations shape recommendations for abstinence/reduced use, cue management, relapse prevention, cognitive restoration, and improvements in self-esteem in the treatment of PFA.

24.2.1 Abstinence/Reduced Use in Recovery from PFA

Findings of addictive neuroanomalies in the obese are not sufficient to convincingly argue for PFA as a *substance use disorder* as opposed to a *process addiction* such as gambling, sex, or shopping because there are similar neuroanomalies in all addictions regardless of the presence of addictive substances. However, in the case of PFA, addictive substances are present. As discussed in Chapter 6 of Part I, these include sugars, sweeteners, flour, gluten, excessive salt, processed fats, and caffeine (Ifland et al., 2015b). The addictive use of these substances moves PFA from a process addiction to an SUD. This concept is developed in Part II, which describes the conformance of processed food use to the DSM 5 SUD diagnostic criteria. Thus this textbook uses the SUD model in treatment of PFA by including guidelines for teaching lifetime abstinence/reduced use of addictive foods just as a drug/alcohol-addicted client would be taught to abstain from, or reduce use of, mood-altering drugs for a lifetime.

Most addictions are not confusing on the question of whether or not a substance is being used addictively. Addictive substances are described clearly in the DSM 5 including alcohol, cocaine, cannabis, heroin, club drugs, amphetamines, etc. As a class, practitioners generally do not counsel clients to abstain from just one kind of addictive substance due to the consequences of shifting to or maintaining use of others. The class of mood-altering substances are targeted for elimination or reduced use in the treatment of SUD (Witkiewitz et al., 2017). This extends even to pharmaceuticals such as pain medication. Where drugs are concerned, generally accepted treatment approaches consider all mood-altering substances (McLellan, Cacciola, Alterman, Rikoon, & Carise, 2006) in order to reduce cue reactivity, restore cognitive functioning, and allow for the establishment of healthy behaviors.

However, clarity has been absent on the question of whether addictive substances are being used in PFA (Ifland, Preuss, Marcus, Taylor, & Rourke, 2015a; Schulte, Potenza, & Gearhardt, 2016). The nature and classification of PFA has confused practitioners and clients alike. Is it a process addiction or an SUD? Part of the confusion may come from the broad range of commonly found processed foods used in PFA including sugars, gluten, flour, excessive salt, processed fats, caffeine, and possibly food additives. Part may come from the lack of public awareness. How could these "foods" be addictive without the public knowing? Contributing to the confusion is the widespread use of processed foods coupled with the virtual absence of government regulations that would reasonably be expected to be attached to addictive substances. The situation is similar to the lack of awareness about the harmful effects of tobacco in the mid-1900s (Brandt, 2007).

Like drug addiction, recovery from PFA calls for abstaining from or reducing use of a broad class of addictive processed substances including sugar, sweeteners, gluten, flour, excessive salt, processed fats, dairy, and caffeine. Although not processed, nuts and olives are also generally considered to be addictive foods (Ifland et al., 2015b). Some foods can be classified as less harmful or "marginal," such as white potatoes, high sugar fruits, and avocados, even though white potatoes are high in available glucose, high sugar fruits are high in fructose, and avocados are high in fat. The most conservative guidelines would provide for eliminating these foods. However, for ease of navigating situations outside the home, some PFA clients seem to be able to eat these marginal foods occasionally. Refer to Chapter 6 on food plans in Part I of the textbook for more detailed information about food plans. Handouts with food lists are available at http://www.foodaddictionresources.com/handouts.html.

The distinction between PFA as an SUD or as a process addiction is helped by considering the addictive properties of processed foods. This should help clarify the nature of PFA.

The failure to addresses the issue of abstinence/reduced use of addictive foods in "weight loss" regimens may explain their almost universal failure (Turk et al., 2009). Thus the premise of this textbook is that PFA should not be treated as a behavioral addiction alone. Abstinence from or reduced use of a broad range of addictive processed foods supports success. While there is good evidence that broad abstinence may be the key to success, eliminating thousands of processed foods and food additives for a lifetime might seem like an insurmountable challenge especially for a population with possibly limited cognitive abilities. Reduced use is an acceptable treatment outcome, as is the case with substance use (Witkiewitz et al., 2017).

An example of the efficacy of abstinence is the case of Heidi. She had undergone several therapies for her chronic overeating including cognitive behavioral therapy, mindfulness and hypnosis. However, her cravings often got the better of her and led to distressing episodes of bingeing. She joined a program that advocated abstinence and got her meals organized. Within a week, her cravings had subsided and she was satisfied with three unprocessed meals per day.

Abstinence or reduced use is made easier by treating processed foods as a single class of substances to be eliminated gradually. It is further helped by situating the PFA client in a group of people who are eating similarly even if it is a virtual group on an Internet, email, or telephone conference call platform. The process is facilitated by teaching very simple meal preparation through the use of pictures. These concepts will be developed in Chapter 28, "Insights from the Field."

24.2.2 Management of Triggering and Cueing

In classic SUD treatment protocols, abstinence is combined with cue avoidance to allow the brain to heal from both the bombardment of neurotransmitter receptors in pleasure and reward pathways, as well as from the suppression of activity in the cognitive pathways and sensitization of stress pathways (Cottone et al., 2009; Moore, Sabino, Koob, & Cottone, 2017; Sharma, Fernandes, & Fulton, 2013). Cue avoidance is commonly practiced in recovery from drug and alcohol addiction as addicts are trained to avoid people, places, and things that trigger cravings. Twelve-step fellowships use the acronym HALT to help members to remember not to become *hungry*, *angry*, *lonely*, or *tired*, as these conditions can also be triggers to relapse (Alcoholics Anonymous, 2017). Cue-avoidance protocols are supported by research showing that the cascade of addictive neurotransmitter adaptation often starts with exposure to a cue associated with use (Boswell & Kober, 2016).

Perhaps the greatest factor that distinguishes PFA from most other addictions is that recovery takes place in a heavily cued food environment (Lindberg, Dementieva, & Cavender, 2011). The situation is analogous to the influence of the tobacco industry in the 1900s, which persuaded about two-thirds of American adults to smoke (Brandt, 2007). Popular media showing the pleasure of smoking reinforced the development of nicotine addiction. A parallel can be seen today for processed foods for adults and especially for children. The diet industry exacerbates cravings through reduced calorie approaches that can cause hunger (Stice, Burger, & Yokum, 2013a). Teaching clients how to protect sensitive craving neuropathways from persistent and pervasive food cues can require extensive strategies.

The need to adopt new lifestyles to avoid exposure to cueing and effectuate recovery from PFA is much more extensive than most addictions. PFA clients are in a position similar to that of drug-addicted clients trying to recover in a drug-infested neighborhood. Food cues are everywhere.

The cued-craving issue is compounded by several important factors. Research shows that cue reactivity can be reinforced with repetition, compounding, and prolonged exposure (van den Akker, Havermans, Bouton, & Jansen, 2014). This would appear to be the case in patterns of exposure to processed food cues. Because processed food cues can be presented in volume to children over television, significant cue reactivity can develop at a young age (Kearns & Weiss, 2005). Over 500 processed food television commercials may be shown in a single Saturday morning on children's programming (Nestle, 2013). No other addictive substances are promoted to this degree at such a young age.

The use of *compounded* cues is an issue in PFA more so than other addictions. To grasp how this works from a red-hot, cue-reactive food addict's perspective, the following analogy is offered. Imagine that grocery stores were actually "drug" stores selling tens of thousands of variations of heroin, cocaine, methamphetamines, club drugs, cannabis, cigarettes, alcohol, etc. Children would be enticed to visit with free cookies. The smells of meth production and beer brewing along with cigarette crack, hash, and opium smoke would hit the visitor upon entering. Sample snorts, puffs, tokes, and sips would be pushed by friendly staff. Dance music would play. People would lounge around the café getting high. These huge stores would be numerous in all kinds of neighborhoods including family neighborhoods. Groceries would be for sale only around the perimeters of these stores.

To continue the image, visualize the drug-addicted client going home from buying groceries in this store environment and turning on the television to commercials for more drugs. When the drug-addicted client goes to a 12-step meeting, trays of drugs are out for the taking. The drug counselor recommends mindfulness to control the use of the drugs. The drug-addicted client's employer stocks drugs in the breakroom and vending machines and they are feely offered in staff meetings. Every gas station offers drugs and even faith organizations promote them after services. Family members become enraged and insulted when the drug-addicted client turns down their homemade drug concoctions. Online outlets deliver drugs within minutes of placing an order. Children sell recreational drugs door to door to raise money for their organizations. A family night takes place at fun-themed drug emporiums. Even the government designs healthy food pyramids that recommend the use of addictive drugs, albeit in small quantities.

Many practitioners would agree that recovery from drug addiction would be difficult in this environment. To a food-addicted client in the grips of heightened cue reactivity, Westernized life can appear this way.

The handouts at http://www.foodaddictionresources.com/handouts.html include information about the use of cueing guidelines to "counter condition" the brain to self-calm in the face of exposure to processed food cues. The evidence suggests that a focused counter-cueing program is useful because recovery from processed PFA is occurring in an intense food environment. In such a counter-cueing program, members can counteract the effects of cues to crave by building new conditioning to replace cued-craving responses with cued-calming when faced with relapse triggers.

An example of the role of food cues can be found in Zola. Zola came into a food addiction program with a love of shopping. She got to work on her food plan and was excited about the different foods she could try. She made many visits to grocery stores. And she went to restaurants with her family. For the first 6 months, she relapsed frequently, sometimes for as long as 3 weeks. Gradually, she stopped the restaurant visits and organized her grocery shopping to be done once per week. She is now free from lapsing.

In addition to associating calming cues with food cues, calming cues can also be associated with other relapse triggers such as stress, fatigue, and strong emotions. It may be helpful to go through a process of associating calming cues with commonly frequented places such as home, workplace, and especially the car. Calming cues may be portable objects, such as personal electronic devices, books, jewelry, photographs, and recovery literature. Smells such as a nonfood essential oil are also good cues to associate with calming activities (Weiss, 1972). Even a gesture such as tugging on the ear could be a conditioned cue to calm.

The nature of food cueing in Westernized cultures is intense. One theory is that a counter-cueing program might need to match unavoidable exposure to food cueing in variation, compounding, duration of exposure, and frequency of exposure in order to be effective at quelling cravings in intense environments (Bouton, 2011). Compounded visual, auditory, tactile, gustatory, and olfactory calming cues can be assembled in a quiet place where the client can be exposed for extended periods of time.

24.2.3 Other Goals of Classic Addiction Recovery in PFA

Under the SUD model, PFA recovery can embrace approaches that are generally found in SUD recovery programs but might be downplayed in eating disorders recovery and weight-loss programs. Comprehensive treatment for PFA can include recovering from health problems, including physical, mental, emotional, and behavioral conditions. Clients who started overusing in toddlerhood can acquire relationships skills that can be fruitfully practiced in a recovery community (Carr, Friedman, & Jaffe, 2007; Kakinami, Barnett, Seguin, & Paradis, 2015). Artistic pleasures can be reclaimed. Like all addicts, PFA clients can be encouraged to resume educations and careers and thereby recover financial vitality. Clients can find a purpose in life. When viewed as an SUD, treatment can flower into a comprehensive program that brings the client to a vigorous new life and a satisfying sense of purpose.

24.3 PREMISE 2: THE NEED FOR LONG-TERM CARE IN PFA

The second major premise of treatment for PFA is that long-term care may often be needed. There are a number of factors that indicate that long-term care may be productive. Borrowing from the drug addiction treatment literature, similar measures of severity and risk of relapse can be used to determine if long-term care is justified (Donovan, 2013). A high risk of future relapse may be indicated by a history of recurring relapses. In addition to risks in drug use, risk of relapse in PFA may be exacerbated by factors in the environment. This includes unavoidable exposure to prolonged compounded food cueing, pressure to use in social and professional situations, and easy availability of addictive processed foods.

In the context of these risk factors, clients may need to acquire and reinforce extensive skills related to the planning and preparation of abstinent meals and cue avoidance within dysfunctional families. Further, as weight loss occurs, there may be a need to acclimate the client to a new body shape over the course of a year or even several years. A new body shape can evoke possibly unsettling reactions from friends, family, and colleagues, as well as the public.

A good understanding of the factors involved in recommending long-term care can help practitioners motivate prospective clients to enter an extended program. Appreciation for the extensive needs of a PFA client can also help the practitioner envision and implement a sufficiently comprehensive program. Matching extent of need with length of treatment can improve outcomes.

24.3.1 Severity in Long-Term Care

In classic drug addiction treatment, an assessment of severity can include a number of factors. These guidelines can also be useful in assessing severity of PFA. Long-term care may also be justified by other severity factors such as:

- Age of onset
- Conformance to multiple DSM 5 SUD diagnostic criteria
- Polysubstance use (Donovan, 2013)
- Heightened emotions from relationship sensitivity (Verdejo-Garcia et al., 2015)
- Internalized stigmatization (Ratcliffe & Ellison, 2015)
- Painful physical comorbidities (Narouze & Souzdalnitski, 2015)
- Sleep-eating (Opolski, Chur-Hansen, & Wittert, 2015)
- The possibility of a stressful food-addicted family system including addicted children (Sigman-Grant, Hayes, VanBrackle, & Fiese, 2015)
- A history of trauma (Zeller et al., 2015)

Regarding young age of onset, research shows that children as young as toddlers exhibit the neuroanomalies associated with addiction including cued cravings, a willingness to work for food, and cognitive impairment (Rollins, Loken, Savage, & Birch, 2014). Children may meet multiple DSM 5 SUD diagnostic criteria including use in spite of trouble in relationships and school (Rankin et al., 2016), as well as unintended use (Matheson et al., 2015), time spent (Katzmarzyk et al., 2015), missed activities (Campbell, 2016), failure to cut back (Altman & Wilfley, 2015), and use in spite of knowledge of consequences (Sanders, Han, Baker, & Cobley, 2015). The young age of onset criteria in PFA may be compounded by severity at a young age as shown by meeting many of the DSM 5 SUD diagnostic criteria. An outline of children's behavior that can be construed to meet the DSM 5 SUD diagnostic criteria are found in Chapter 29, which focuses on food-addicted children.

Severity is also gauged by the number of DSM 5 SUD criteria met. As adults, PFA clients could meet all of the 11 DSM 5 diagnostic criteria, which would be an indication of severity. A PFA client whose daily routine is to avoid eating during the day but then visit a series of food outlets to binge, go out for more processed foods during the evening, sleep, get up in the night to eat more, and sleep again meets many SUD diagnostic criteria. Unintended use, failed efforts to cut back, time spent, cravings, failure to fulfill roles, relationship problems, missed activities, hazardous use, knowledge of consequences, progression, and withdrawal avoidance could all be manifesting simultaneously, albeit to different degrees, in a single client. Thus clients may be assessed as severely addicted through application of the DSM 5 SUD diagnostic criteria.

A third element of severity that factors into the decision to undergo extended treatment is the presence of polysubstance use. Research shows that polysubstance use is harder to treat than single substance use (Connor, Gullo, White, & Kelly, 2014). The greater the variety of substances, the more resistant is the disease to treatment. PFA clients are generally engaged in *de facto* polysubstance use by the formulation of processed food products (Martinez Steele et al., 2016). A fast food meal of cheeseburger, taco, or pizza generally contains sweeteners, gluten, flour, excessive salt, dairy (cheese), processed fat, and caffeine. Pastries might contain sweeteners, flour, processed fat, salt, and possibly dairy and caffeine. Caffeinated drinks contain sweetener and caffeine and, in the case of coffee, dairy may be added. Ice cream is another processed food that can contain sugar, high-fat dairy, and caffeine (chocolate). Further, food additives may have addictive properties (Warner, 2014). As discussed in Chapter 6, "Abstinent Food Plans for Processed Food Addiction," these processed foods activate a broad range of craving pathways. The polysubstance nature of use supports the argument for long-term care to treat more severe or stubborn addictions.

In addition to the traditional elements of severity assessment, there are characteristics of PFA clients that could exacerbate severity. PFA clients are likely to have some level of debilitating physical and cognitive limitations (Guh et al., 2009; Zhu et al., 2015). These may slow the progress of recovery because of restrictions on exercise and ability to stand to prepare meals. It may be also difficult to carry out instructions for meal preparation because of limited learning, decision-making, memory, and restraint. Impaired restraint centers may be unable to overcome cravings activated by cues in grocery stores. Issues with relationship sensitivity and shame may prevent some clients from recruiting a friend to go to the grocery store for them. It takes time for the client's brain to recover sufficiently to consistently prepare and consume meals on a regular schedule. Other nonphysical and noncognitive recovery activities such as crafts, music, and conference calls can contribute to restoration while the client works up to reliable abstinent meals, but important recovery benefits may not fully materialize until the client has withdrawn from processed foods.

Because of stigmatism related to excess adipose tissue, food-addicted clients may also benefit from long-term participation in a "safe" community where they can experience being normal and accepted (van der Kolk, 1994). Clients may have developed low self-esteem and internalized stigmatization since childhood (Ratcliffe & Ellison, 2015).

Fifi is an example of a client who used fast food outlets compulsively, which suggests a polysubstance dependency. She had been molested as a child and was using alcohol regularly when she came into recovery. She had a history of anorexia but was 50 pounds overweight. Fifi wanted recovery primarily for weight loss and felt that she just needed to work the food plan. However, with frequent lapses, her weight did not change. Over the course of 3 years, Fifi gradually built a diverse recovery program and reduced her lapses substantially.

A year may be seen as barely enough time when the extent of need is considered.

24.3.2 Elevated Risk of Relapse in Long-Term Care

Risk of relapse may be elevated for PFA clients for a number of reasons, including a history of relapse, unavoidable cue exposure, accidental ingestion of hidden addictive ingredients, relationship sensitivity, and internalized stigmatization. Addicted parents may have the additional risk factor of exposure to stressors related to their addicted children.

For chronic overeaters, there is likely to be an extensive history of relapse. This is described in Chapter 12, Criterion 2 of the DSM 5 SUD diagnostic criteria, failure to cut back. Research shows that all forms of treatment for chronic overeating have a history of failure (Foster, Makris, & Bailer, 2005;

Turk et al., 2009). Reasons for this history of relapse bear a closer look. Two different reasons for relapse may be present, each of which supports the need for long-term care in a different way. The first possibility is that relapses have occurred in spite of appropriate PFA treatment. As in classic drug addiction treatment, this history could indicate the presence of a relatively severe case needing extended treatment.

The second possibility is that the "relapses" were caused by misguided treatment aimed at weight loss rather than recovery from PFA. In this case, consideration should be given to the possibility that this type of failed attempt could have made the PFA worse. See the handout at http://www.foodaddictionresources.com/handouts.html, "'Weight-Loss' Schemes Can Make Food Addiction Worse." Weight-loss regimens may worsen PFA by intensifying cravings and cue reactivity stemming from malnourishment (Casas Patino, Rodriguez Torres, & Jarillo Soto, 2016), use of addictive foods (Stice, Burger, & Yokum, 2013b), and inadequate caloric intake (Stice et al., 2013a). So the supposition that repeated relapse indicates a need for long-term treatment would be valid in either case of repeated relapse whether the pattern of relapse occurred under appropriate treatment or weight-loss programs.

Elevated risk related to food cue exposure is covered above under "Premise 1: Approaches Used in SUD Are Transferrable to PFA."

Accidental ingestion of addictive foods or additives also increases risk of relapse. As discussed in Chapter 6, "Abstinent Food Plans for Processed Food Addiction," there is evidence that the processed food industry is using 15,000 food additives and that the industry is deliberately formulating products to stimulate cravings and bypass satiation functions in the brain (Moss, 2013). Like tobacco smoke was mixed into the air breathed by the public, addictive ingredients are mixed into the public food supply. Clients can be taught to cook from safe ingredients and to avoid packaged foods at home. However, visits to restaurants and to social events are inevitable. The risk of ingesting an addictive ingredient in these venues is high. Hosts are not likely to understand concepts of abstinence and restaurants are unlikely to be able to reliably produce meals with no addictive additives. Training in intuitive eating and other mindfulness techniques can help (Marcus et al., 2009).

The significance of this is that addicts are at greater risk of relapse from obesogenic environments. In this situation, the chances of reestablishing abstinence or regaining a routine of reduced harm are much greater if the PFA client is participating in a long-term recovery community either online or via in-person meetings. The longer the program, the greater stabilization, and thereby the greater the probability of being able to safely get back on plan after exposure to triggers in the environment.

Relationship sensitivity and internalized stigmatization can also factor into determining appropriate length of treatment. Obesity attracts condescension, judgment, ridicule, teasing, stigmatization, and bullying (Seacat, Dougal, & Roy, 2016). This emotional abuse not only comes from family but also friends, colleagues, strangers, and even medical professionals. Painful internal shame, sense of failure, and self-blame can develop and be easily triggered in interpersonal relationships (Ratcliffe & Ellison, 2015). Not surprisingly, relationship stressors have been shown to be a leading cause of relapse into self-destructive eating behavior as addicts seek to numb the pain (Grilo, Shiffman, & Wing, 1989). Sensitivities can be extensive and need a long-term program to repair.

Clients who are parents are likely to be grappling with issues related to food-addicted children (Matheson et al., 2015). These children may suffer from learning disabilities and erratic behavior (Mackenbach et al., 2012). These are stressors. Through a long-term program, parents can first achieve sobriety for themselves and then learn techniques for helping their food-addicted children through withdrawal and into the safety of recovery. These kinds of projects justify a long-term approach.

Another factor that increases the need for long-term care in PFA treatment is a history of trauma. PFA clients have often grown up in households with food and drug misuse. They may have endured abusive relationships because of low self-esteem and inability to support themselves outside of the abusive relationships (Stensland, Thoresen, Wentzel-Larsen, & Dyb, 2015). See Chapter 18, "DSM 5 Criterion 8: Hazardous Use," for a discussion of the physical dangers of PFA for evidence of trauma in relationships. Children in food-addicted households may suffer from neglect, witnessing abuse among adult members of the household, and may have endured physical and emotional abuse. Obesity in children has been found to be a barrier to parental acceptance of children (Radoszewska, 2014).

An example of a single parent who was at high risk of relapse is Bea. Bea came into recovery with a highly addicted child in the home. Bea was in a new relationship and working a demanding job, which interfered with her sleep. Although she was unable to organize a once-per-week shopping, Bea participated in an online community regularly. Gradually, she worked with her daughter to begin to eat a short list of unprocessed foods. As the weeks went by, Bea and her daughter ate more and more unprocessed foods. Food became orderly in the home. Both Bea and her daughter stopped overeating and became calm about their lives.

24.3.3 Need for Extensive Skill Acquisition in Long-Term Care

A final reason for long-term care is the need to acquire extensive recovery skills. The goals of recovery from PFA are quite a bit more complex and involved than a weight-loss program. Goals include:

- Cessation of cue-reactive cravings
- Establishment of food planning and preparation routines for wide variety of unprocessed foods
- Cessation of chaotic eating patterns
- Restoration of cognitive functions
- Ease of appearing in public
- Ability to set boundaries with food pushers
- Ability to identify and meet personal needs
- Ability to restore calm after emotional triggering
- Fluidity in social relationships
- Orderly family relationships
- Establishment of spiritual practices

In short, the extensive dysfunction described under the DSM 5 SUD diagnostic criteria in Part II of this textbook needs to be addressed and healed. Reaching these goals could easily take a year or more. Participation in a recovery community for a lifetime may be desirable, as has been found in recovery communities such as 12-step programs.

Planning, shopping, cooking, boundary-setting, creating a nonaddictive home environment, learning how to counter craving cues, and avoiding food triggers to the extent possible are all time-consuming tasks. When consideration is given to the limited cognitive functioning that food addicts may endure, it can be imagined that skill acquisition will be a cart-and-horse proposition until the clients' learning, decision-making, memory, and restraint functions are restored enough to consistently consume nonaddictive, unprocessed meals that in turn support better cognitive functioning. Skill acquisition enhances cognitive restoration but skill acquisition is rocky until cognitive restoration is accomplished. Bit by bit, the PFA client accumulates experiences that eventually will consolidate into effective defenses, but this can take months of trial and error as addicts learn from ill-fated attempts to manage use and to withstand exposure to food cues.

Similarly, relationship management skills are needed to set boundaries with household members, educate household members, graciously decline offers of processed foods, reduce exposure to triggering people, and navigate social events.

In addition to relationship and cooking skills, in a long-term program, clients have a safe environment in which to begin reclaiming marketable professional skills that may have fallen into disuse in the disease. Within the program, members may learn how to help others, assist in administrative tasks, take leadership roles, etc. With this intermediate stepping stone, members may gain the confidence needed to go back to work.

An example of a client who absorbed new information slowly but steadily was Lana. She came into the program with a history of overeating from a young age but no childhood trauma. She was unable to sleep for more than a few hours, engaged in no exercise, and did not have any routines around cognitive restoration. She participated in an online community but did not make any changes in her life for 6 months. Gradually she began to work on her sleep issues by setting a goal of staying in bed for 6–8 hours straight. Next, she started walking around her back yard. She also researched exercise videos at www.youtube.com. After about a year, she attempted a full day of abstinence. It took another 6 months of building a food routine to achieve somewhat consistence abstinence. Nonetheless, in that time she gained significant benefits in terms of energy and mental clarity.

The severity of PFA combined with the need to acquire extensive skills form the basic arguments for long-term care for clients. Severity manifests as a history of relapse, circumstances that increase the risk of relapse, exacerbated sources of stress, a history of trauma, and the need for extensive skill acquisition. Above all, PFA clients need to build their programs in a stress-free environment. As clients make mistakes, they need to be reassured that they have plenty of time in which to figure out a program that fits their needs and lifestyles as well as those of their household members. They need time to be able to make mistakes and to recover in a low-key environment of unremitting warmth, patience, and understanding. Any suggestion that goals need to be met within a time frame is counterproductive, as it could trigger fear of failure and stress.

24.4 PREMISE 3: USE OF INTERNET AND MOBILE DEVICES IN PFA

For PFA clients, hopeless cases may become manageable by increasing accessibility to support delivered through personal electronic devices such as smartphones and tablets, telephone, and computer. Research increasingly shows that weight-loss and addiction recovery services may be effectively delivered over the Internet (Gilmore, Duhe, Frost, & Redman, 2014; Murray, 2012). Smoking cessation services have been found to be more effective with telephone support (Skov-Ettrup, Dalum, Bech, & Tolstrup, 2016), and web-based alcohol treatment has been shown to be effective (Murray et al., 2012). For clients who are unable to appear for treatment in person, outreach can improve the chance of success (Wieland et al., 2012). Internet access also addresses barriers related to stigmatization of body shape (Hague & White, 2005; Kelleher et al., 2017). As will be seen in Chapter 28, "Insights from the Field," much of the material can be delivered over electronic devices (Murray, 2012). For clients who are able to access in-person services such as individual and group counseling, Internet, telephone, and email access to support groups can strengthen in-person programs by extending the scope of treatment from weekly to daily, even hourly support.

There are many reasons that Internet and mobile devices are a good match for PFA.

- Clients have limited mobility for a number of reasons, which can make reaching in-person services difficult (Belczak et al., 2014; McGregor et al., 2014).
- Because cue-induced cravings are a primary relapse trigger in PFA, accessing diversion from a handheld device is helpful.
- Handheld devices can provide education and support in easily understood messages virtually instantly regardless of time of day (Boswell & Kober, 2016; Brockmeyer, Hahn, Reetz, Schmidt, & Friederich, 2015).
- The delivery over electronic devices as opposed to in-person also reduces treatment resistance stemming from relationship sensitivities because the client has control over the amount of personal interface within the group (Broberg, Hjalmers, & Nevonen, 2001; Carr et al., 2007).

- On a practical level, delivery of support over mobile devices and telephone allows practitioners to reach a broad, disbursed population, literally worldwide at a low cost (ITU World Communication/ICT Indicators Database, 2015). Reducing cost of treatment per client is important for financially disadvantaged clients (Patel, Spaeth, & Basner, 2016).

Understanding the rationale for delivering services over personal electronic devices will help practitioners improve outcomes.

24.4.1 Limited Mobility as a Rationale for Internet and Mobile Devices

Limited physical mobility and financial resources as well as commitments to job and family create barriers to in-person treatment. Cognitive impairment (Wang et al., 2015) may make finding a meeting location challenging, while relationship phobia and body shame (Ratcliffe & Ellison, 2015) may stop a PFA client from appearing in public.

As seen in Chapter 19, under DSM 5 SUD Criterion 9, use in spite of consequences, PFA clients may be physically immobile. The range of physical barriers to mobility include excess adipose tissue, joint pain, fatigue, amputations, blindness, and shortness of breath (Gerlach, Williams, & Coates, 2013; Vincent, Adams, Vincent, & Hurley, 2013). The client may be able to walk only a short distance, which can make meeting rooms far from the parking lot inaccessible even if the client is able to drive. Furthermore, leaving the home to travel in a car is risky for PFA clients if the route takes them past triggering food outlets (Morris, Beilharz, Maniam, Reichelt, & Westbrook, 2014).

As discussed in Chapter 17, DSM 5 Criterion 7, activities given up, PFA clients may have limited financial resources to access in-person services (Flint & Snook, 2015; Patel et al., 2016). PFA may have cut short their educations and careers due to disabilities and cognitive impairment. PFA is found to be disproportionately prevalent in economically disadvantaged populations (Ali & Lindstrom, 2006). A weekly session with a professional counselor may be well beyond the means of a PFA client. Clients may have withdrawn from low-cost resources such as 12-step groups because of perceived judgment about body size and a history of failure (Ratcliffe & Ellison, 2015). Limited financial means may be a source of embarrassment to the PFA client, which further inhibits them from seeking help. Limited finances combined with a changing body size may mean that the client might not have appropriate clothing to wear to in-person services.

By contrast, delivery of services over electronic devices can be accomplished at a low cost overall and yet can serve a large number of clients. So the cost per client can be quite low. Clients who cannot pay initially can recover earning abilities and gradually improve ability to pay. A low cost, plus improvements in ability to pay, may make treatment possible for low-income PFA clients.

Clients may also be restrained by inflexible time commitments to care for family members. They may hold down several jobs or a night-shift job (Patel et al., 2016). Women are more likely to be caring for children or elders, which may create a barrier to in-person treatment due to the need to find babysitters or elder caregivers. In food-addicted households, children and elders may have challenging and demanding health and behavioral problems (Bauer et al., 2014; Braet, Claus, Verbeken, & Van Vlierberghe, 2007; Nguyen, Killcross, & Jenkins, 2014). Fortunately, it is easy for home-bound women to pick up a smartphone or tablet and engage in services even if just for a few minutes. Otherwise for in-person services, it could be difficult and stressful for them to arrange for a caregiver for children or elders in order to leave home and attend a program. Unpredictable schedules related to caregiving needs can be solved by personal electronic devices when support and conversation is available at all times, even late at night when the PFA client may finally be free from household demands. With electronic devices, PFA clients could be expected to access support services more consistently, more reliably, and for a longer period of time. Even clients who are at workplaces can improve access to support through online services.

Relationships can also create barriers to treatment. It is possible that the client may be forbidden to travel by a controlling parent or spouse. Clients may not have the relationship skills to negotiate treatment with a resistant family member. They may not want family members to know that treatment is being sought for fear of ridicule (Brewis, Trainer, Han, & Wutich, 2016). Further, social phobia may be a barrier to mobility. Home may feel like a safer place from which to access services. Mobility may be limited by emotional issues such as a fear of stigma. Employees may not want their boss or colleagues to know that they are absent for reasons of treatment.

In more severe cases of limited cognitive function, clients may be challenged to follow directions to a meeting place. Depression and fatigue could also result in the client abandoning the effort to go to a new place. Access to the Internet is available for free in libraries and community centers and inexpensive on cell phones. Even very financially disadvantaged people can participate as some welfare agencies provide cell phones to clients. There is no need for a car, gas, parking, etc.

24.4.2 Delivery of Information in PFA

Electronic outreach allows for the structuring of information in ways that could overcome specific aspects of cognitive challenges. Research shows that PFA is a neurodisorder characterized by hyperactive craving and stress pathways and hypoactive cognitive pathways (Moore et al., 2017; Stice & Yokum, 2016; Wang et al., 2015). For the purpose of delivering training and skills, hypoactivity of cognitive pathways is problematic. Evidence shows that clients are likely to have significant cognitive impairment in:

- Focus
- Learning
- Decision-making
- Memory
- Restraint

These capabilities are all important to acquiring essential skills (Martin & Davidson, 2014). Populations may also be relatively undereducated (Ali & Lindstrom, 2006). All of this suggests that short, repetitive educational messages delivered over mobile devices might be effective. Electronic access to support might reinforce and extend the benefits of counseling sessions.

An example of electronic support is learning meal assembly using the Facebook platform. Learning meal assembly through repetitive pictures of simple meals posted by members of the group requires less cognitive ability than the alternative of reading instructions, imagining what meals might look like, figuring out how to cook everything, and measuring out quantities. Instead, knowledge of meals can be absorbed from a personal device as pictures are uploaded by members. Members who are having trouble focusing on words can grasp the simplicity of unprocessed meals through pictures.

For the PFA client, written instructions can be difficult to execute:

- Learning quantities and combinations from a written page may be too confusing.
- Food lists may overwhelm the client.
- Cravings may be triggered just from reading the list of addictive foods to eliminate.
- Feelings of grief and loss can also be triggered by considering all of the processed foods that need to be eliminated in an unprocessed food plan.
- Memories of past failures and a feeling of being overwhelmed can wash over the food addict.

On the other hand, a picture of a simple, easy meal of, e.g., chicken, green beans, and sweet potato is lovely, attractive, calming, and memorable. Clients easily see how to make enjoyable meals.

Pictures reassure clients that they not only can make the meals but that they will be satisfied and pleased with the experience of eating them. Instead of faltering over loss of processed foods, meal pictures can help clients look forward to the pleasure of unprocessed meals.

In general, the use of pictures facilitates immediate feedback and encouragement related to meal preparation (Buckland, Finlayson, Edge, & Hetherington, 2014). It is easy for clients to upload pictures of their meals. And it is easy for the practitioner to comment as needed. Using this method facilitates repeating messages without being boring. Posting pictures just takes a few seconds so it may be easier for the cognitively impaired than writing down foods. Since members can see that everyone is doing it and being praised for it, they are more likely to join in.

Pictures of meals and activities may harness subconscious, primitive urges to eat like the rest of the "tribe" (Cohen, 2008). This may "normalize" the abstinent food plan for the PFA client, which could reduce stress related to eating differently from friends and family in obesogenic environments (Campbell, 2016; O'Dare Wilson, 2016). Identifying with the group through pictures gives the client the foundation to see processed foods for what they are. The client builds resistance to foods being eaten by members of the household (Buckland et al., 2014). The client has the chance to feel normal and to see that people who eat unprocessed foods are healthy. This replaces triggering feelings of being left out or feeling abnormal when eating healthy.

Mobile devices also give the practitioner the ability to manage the pace of learning. Information can be delivered in short segments that can be absorbed by a member whose learning capacity is limited (Ells et al., 2006). This reinforces material and accommodates members who may be better at either visual or auditory learning. Unlike a fixed workbook, uploading files to a website or Facebook or distributing files by email gives the practitioner the ability to rearrange the order of lessons according to the readiness of participants. For example, the practitioner might find out that there may be more enthusiasm for meditation than for exercise. So the practitioner might encourage meditation and let the lessons on exercise fall back in the schedule. Flexibility helps the practitioner match material with clients' readiness to absorb it.

Because of dense cueing in the environment and relationship sensitivity, cravings can be triggered anytime. This makes access to 24-hour group support delivered over electronic devices valuable. Diverting thoughts at the moment of a craving has been shown to help clients resist acting on the craving (Kemps, Tiggemann, & Hollitt, 2014). A Facebook group can incorporate many counter cues such as pictures of safe food, words, messages from friends, videos, and meditations. YouTube videos, PubMed research papers, brain training, and other sites to facilitate education and recovery can be easily found by impaired addicts. Because of fatigue and immobility issues, clients may already spend time on the Internet. They may be adept at basic Internet navigation including following links.

A periodic conference call can be recorded so members can listen at any time. A facility such as www.instantteleseminar.com can be accessed from local numbers or over the Internet worldwide. Slides can also be recorded with the phone call and replayed. Repeatedly listening and watching new material is helpful to members who suffer from learning disabilities and memory loss. The recordings can be accessed by smartphone, tablet, or computer so clients can work the replay into other activities such as meal preparation, driving, or exercise. In this way, practitioners can reach literally thousands of clients in a 1-hour call.

Deenee is a mother of two young children whose husband travels for business. Financial resources are limited. She is busy with children during the day but in the evening, she puts them to bed and then sits in their room until they fall asleep. At that time, she can access her online community quietly so she doesn't wake them up. In spite of having only a few minutes per day to work on recovery from PFA, she's able to use her mobile device to stay connected and make progress.

24.4.3 Pacing Relationship Development through Mobile Devices

PFA clients may suffer from relationship sensitivity (Carr et al., 2007; Ratcliffe & Ellison, 2015). This was covered in Chapter 16, under DSM 5 SUD Diagnostic Criteria 6, interpersonal relationships.

Relationship sensitivities can also be overcome through mobile devices. Outreach minimizes the impact of relationship sensitivities in two helpful ways. The anonymity of the Internet removes body size as an issue (Wang, Houshyar, & Prinstein, 2006). Electronic devices offer a range of communication formats to be in touch with other members. This allows members to fully control the pace of relationship development with other members.

Mobile devices allow clients to be present without being encumbered by shame about their bodies. They can flourish in their personalities without fearing reprisals or jokes about their bodies. They can leave behind the deep mortification of stigmatization (Seacat et al., 2016) and let their personalities be accepted, their behavior be praised, their meals be admired, and their emotions be honored, all free from fear of stigmatization.

By the same token, each client is protected from erecting their own personal judgmental barriers. As clients judge themselves, they also judge other people. In the absence of images of members' bodies, clients can move ahead and form relationships without judgments.

Communication via Internet and mobile devices lets participants manage relationship risk. They can form relationships at their own pace and deepen relationships as they gain confidence and trust. Different depths of communication channels include webinars, posts, private messaging, conference calls, small chat groups, texting, and email. If a member feels uncomfortable for any reason in any of those mediums, they can withdraw and fall back on other channels. If the client is socially phobic, they can just read messages and listen to conference call recordings, without appearing at all. They can still make progress. PFA clients may feel safer using Internet and mobile devices than in-person services.

Nina is a long-time PFA client who came into recovery then tried other approaches for 5 years before returning to an online PFA community. She is a good cook and was immediately able to organize her food. She participated with frequent posts in the online community. However, she had experienced extreme swings in weight between 200 and 600 pounds. She rarely left her house due to fear of stigmatization in public. Six months passed before she was able to join the phone calls. She is recovering at her own pace, using the resources of the online community to fit her remarkable capabilities.

24.4.4 Practitioner Efficiencies as a Rationale for Mobile Devices

Efficiencies for the practitioner might not seem like an important argument for using electronic outreach. However, in the case of addiction to processed foods, efficiencies are important for a number of reasons. Considering the evidence for a correlation between obesity and severity of PFA, it is possible to reframe the obesity epidemic as an epidemic of PFA (Gearhardt, Corbin, & Brownell, 2016). There are approximately 2 billion overweight and obese people worldwide (Ng et al., 2014). The consequences and suffering associated with PFA are severe, as can be seen in Part II of the textbook, covering the manifestations according to the DSM 5 SUD diagnostic criteria and the Addiction Severity Index (ASI). So helping every practitioner to be as efficient as possible is an important issue. Seeing clients in person would limit a practitioner to perhaps 40 clients at a time. Organizing groups might increase the practitioner's capacity to a maximum of a few hundred clients.

On the other hand, delivery of services over Internet and mobile devices can allow a single practitioner to help thousands of clients. Because of the ability to treat a large number of clients, fees can be set low enough to be affordable for private pay. Automated recurring fees can be collected through PayPal.

Regardless of the number of members, an online practice can let everyone see the practitioner's daily messages of encouragement, education, and assignments. Clients can post questions and all clients can benefit from reading the answers to the questions. Advanced clients can become volunteer monitors and help new clients. The practitioner or group monitors can scroll through meal pictures giving a few words of positive feedback. Similarly, conference calls can accommodate up to 1000 callers with unlimited access to recordings of the calls. Webcasts can accommodate tens of thousands of attendees and unlimited views of replays. Clients with varying needs would be able to access a range of levels of engagement.

In addition to improving access for the client, use of the Internet/phone also allows the practitioner to mesh work and home schedules. Practitioners can provide the bulk of services over a mobile device. The short responses required to monitor and support clients means that the practitioner can parcel out information throughout the day and evening. This is important for practitioners who are attending to family needs. This would allow more practitioners to work part-time while meeting family responsibilities. Practitioners have minimal overhead (no office needed) yet have the ability to monitor a large number of clients.

A writer in the field of children's fiction had trained as a counselor. She had a special-needs son at home and so had given up her counseling practice. She had been in successful recovery from PFA for 15 years. She set up a group on Facebook, established an account at PayPal, and signed up for a conference call service at www.instantteleseminar.com. She attracted PFA sufferers to her free Facebook group and eventually started offering a paid daily phone call subscription. Within 2 years, she had 300 clients while continuing to meet her responsibilities to her son and to her publisher.

The Internet/phone platform solves another important problem for practitioners: reaching PFA clients globally. At any given moment, PFA clients who are willing to start treatment may be widely disbursed (De Vogli, Kouvonen, & Gimeno, 2014), which makes finding enough participants to create viable in-person groups very difficult. Internet-based groups can be assembled from participants regardless of geographic location. Service providers who have a list of clients who quit in-person programs may be able to revive interest in treatment by making access easier and less expensive through electronic devices.

24.4.5 Integration of Internet/Phone Platforms with In-Person Treatment

Although electronic devices appear to be compatible with the needs of PFA clients, there are some aspects of PFA that require in-depth treatment. Further, there are successful in-person groups where mobility barriers have been overcome that could nonetheless benefit from the addition of an electronic component. It's helpful to know how to integrate outreach programs into existing in-person services.

Laila had been coming to in-person support for several years without meaningful success. Her clinic started offering online chats, texts, and twice-daily emails of support. With 24-hour access to her support group, Laila gradually turned to her group when she had a craving. With their continual support, she was able to work with her husband to clear the processed foods out of the house. She is now making balanced meals with infrequent lapses.

In conclusion, this section described rationales for an electronically based outreach component for recovery from PFA. The primary arguments are that outreach can overcome problems of immobility. And electronic platforms are a match for the nature of PFA insofar as the platforms permit the flexible delivery of information in manageable amounts, 24 hours per day. Electronic devices allow for the safe and controlled development of relationships. They also provide efficiencies for practitioners. And finally, outreach components can be integrated into in-person programs. Given the vast proportions of the epidemic of obesity, the ability to deliver services inexpensively, globally, effectively, and efficiently is crucial to improving the chances of halting the spread of the epidemic of chronic overeating.

24.5 CONCLUSION

This chapter, "Premises of Recovery for Adults," has laid out three fundamental concepts that shape the approaches to recovery from PFA. The core concept is that classic SUD treatment methods can be adapted to the treatment of PFA. Abstinence protocols, cue avoidance, relapse prevention, recovery of cognitive function, career, etc., are all well-developed SUD recovery techniques that can effectively be transferred to the treatment of PFA.

The second key premise is that long-term care of at least a year may often be indicated. The combination of a finding of severity, gravity of consequences, and the amount of training required to live safely in an obesogenic environment justifies an extended program.

The third premise is that electronic devices can be instrumental in achieving success. The ability to improve access to support and education is a rationale for using personal electronic devices for both client and practitioner. In addition, electronic platforms reduce barriers stemming from body shame and relationship sensitivity. And they permit the pacing of information to accommodate cognitive impairment.

Taken together, these three key premises explain the structure of much of the textbook. Regardless of whether the practitioner is administering an in-person, telephone, or online practice, the textbook offers a plethora of ideas and materials that can be incorporated into an existing program.

REFERENCES

Abiles, V., Abiles, J., Rodriguez-Ruiz, S., Luna, V., Martin, F., Gandara, N., & Fernandez-Santaella, M. C. (2013). Effectiveness of cognitive behavioral therapy on weight loss after two years of bariatric surgery in morbidly obese patients. *Nutr Hosp*, *28*(4), 1109–1114. doi:10.3305/nh.2013.28.4.6536.

Alcoholics Anonymous. (2017). Hungry, Angery, Lonely, Tired! (HALT). Retrieved from http://www.aa.activeboard.com/t50489159/halt/ (accessed on February 16, 2017).

Ali, S. M., & Lindstrom, M. (2006). Socioeconomic, psychosocial, behavioural, and psychological determinants of BMI among young women: Differing patterns for underweight and overweight/obesity. *Eur J Public Health*, *16*(3), 325–331. doi:10.1093/eurpub/cki187.

Altman, M., & Wilfley, D. E. (2015). Evidence update on the treatment of overweight and obesity in children and adolescents. *J Clin Child Adolesc Psychol*, *44*(4), 521–537. doi:10.1080/15374416.2014.963854.

Bauer, C. C., Moreno, B., Gonzalez-Santos, L., Concha, L., Barquera, S., & Barrios, F. A. (2015). Child overweight and obesity are associated with reduced executive cognitive performance and brain alterations: A magnetic resonance imaging study in Mexican children. *Pediatr Obes*, *10*(3), 196–204. doi:10.1111/ijpo.241.

Belczak, C. E., de Godoy, J. M., Belzack, S. Q., Ramos, R. N., & Caffaro, R. A. (2014). Obesity and worsening of chronic venous disease and joint mobility. *Phlebology*, *29*(8), 500–504. doi:10.1177/0268355513492510.

Born, J. M., Lemmens, S. G., Rutters, F., Nieuwenhuizen, A. G., Formisano, E., Goebel, R., & Westerterp-Plantenga, M. S. (2010). Acute stress and food-related reward activation in the brain during food choice during eating in the absence of hunger. *Int J Obes (Lond)*, *34*(1), 172–181. doi:10.1038/ijo.2009.221.

Boswell, R. G., & Kober, H. (2016). Food cue reactivity and craving predict eating and weight gain: A meta-analytic review. *Obes Rev*, *17*(2), 159–177. doi:10.1111/obr.12354.

Bouton, M. E. (2011). Learning and the persistence of appetite: Extinction and the motivation to eat and overeat. *Physiol Behav*, *103*(1), 51–58. doi:10.1016/j.physbeh.2010.11.025.

Braet, C., Claus, L., Verbeken, S., & Van Vlierberghe, L. (2007). Impulsivity in overweight children. *Eur Child Adolesc Psychiatry*, *16*(8), 473–483. doi:10.1007/s00787-007-0623-2.

Brandt, A. (2007). *The cigarette century: The rise, fall, and deadly persistence for the product that defined America.* New York: Basic Books.

Brewer-Smyth, K., Cornelius, M., & Pohlig, R. T. (2016). Childhood adversity and mental health correlates of obesity in a population at risk. *J Correct Health Care*, *22*(4), 367–382. doi:10.1177/1078345816670161.

Brewis, A., Trainer, S., Han, S., & Wutich, A. (2016). Publically misfitting: Extreme weight and the everyday production and reinforcement of felt stigma. *Med Anthropol Q.* doi:10.1111/maq.12309.

Broberg, A. G., Hjalmers, I., & Nevonen, L. (2001). Eating disorders, attachment and interpersonal difficulties: A comparison between 18- to 24-year-old patients and normal controls. *Eur Eat Disord Rev*, *9*(6), 381–396. doi:10.1002/ERV.421.

Brockmeyer, T., Hahn, C., Reetz, C., Schmidt, U., & Friederich, H. C. (2015). Approach bias and cue reactivity towards food in people with high versus low levels of food craving. *Appetite*, *95*, 197–202.

Buckland, N. J., Finlayson, G., Edge, R., & Hetherington, M. M. (2014). Resistance reminders: Dieters reduce energy intake after exposure to diet-congruent food images compared to control non-food images. *Appetite*, *73*, 189–196. doi:10.1016/j.appet.2013.10.022.

Campbell, M. K. (2016). Biological, environmental, and social influences on childhood obesity. *Pediatr Res*, *79*(1–2), 205–211. doi:10.1038/pr.2015.208.

Carr, D., Friedman, M. A., & Jaffe, K. (2007). Understanding the relationship between obesity and positive and negative affect: The role of psychosocial mechanisms. *Body Image*, *4*(2), 165–177. doi:10.1016/j.bodyim.2007.02.004.

Casas Patino, D., Rodriguez Torres, A., & Jarillo Soto, E. C. (2016). The feeding-nutrition connection, three aspects for its understanding. *Medwave*, *16*(3), e6424. doi:10.5867/medwave.2016.03.6424.

Cohen, D. A. (2008). Neurophysiological pathways to obesity: Below awareness and beyond individual control. *Diabetes*, *57*(7), 1768–1773. doi:10.2337/db08-0163.

Connor, J. P., Gullo, M. J., White, A., & Kelly, A. B. (2014). Polysubstance use: Diagnostic challenges, patterns of use and health. *Curr Opin Psychiatry*, *27*(4), 269–275. doi:10.1097/yco.0000000000000069.

Cottone, P., Sabino, V., Roberto, M., Bajo, M., Pockros, L., Frihauf, J. B., ... Zorrilla, E. P. (2009). CRF system recruitment mediates dark side of compulsive eating. *Proc Natl Acad Sci U S A*, *106*(47), 20016–20020. doi:10.1073/pnas.0908789106.

De Vogli, R., Kouvonen, A., & Gimeno, D. (2014). The influence of market deregulation on fast food consumption and body mass index: A cross-national time series analysis. *Bull World Health Organ*, *92*(2), 99–107, 107A. doi:10.2471/BLT.13.120287.

Donovan, D. M. (2013). Evidence-based assessment: Strategies and measures in addictive behaviors. In B. S. McCrady & E. E. Epstein (Eds.), *Addictions: A comprehensive guidebook*, pp. 311–351. Oxford: Oxford University Press.

Ells, L. J., Lang, R., Shield, J. P., Wilkinson, J. R., Lidstone, J. S., Coulton, S., & Summerbell, C. D. (2006). Obesity and disability—A short review. *Obes Rev*, *7*(4), 341–345. doi:10.1111/j.1467-789X.2006.00233.x.

Flint, S. W., & Snook, J. (2015). Disability discrimination and obesity: The big questions? *Curr Obes Rep*, *4*(4), 504–509. doi:10.1007/s13679-015-0182-7

Fortuna, J. L. (2012). The obesity epidemic and food addiction: Clinical similarities to drug dependence. *J Psychoactive Drugs*, *44*(1), 56–63. doi:10.1080/02791072.2012.662092.

Foster, G. D., Makris, A. P., & Bailer, B. A. (2005). Behavioral treatment of obesity. *Am J Clin Nutr*, *82*(1 Suppl), 230s–235s.

Gearhardt, A. N., Corbin, W. R., & Brownell, K. D. (2016). Development of the Yale Food Addiction Scale Version 2.0. *Psychol Addict Behav*, *30*(1), 113–121. doi:10.1037/adb0000136.

Gerlach, Y., Williams, M. T., & Coates, A. M. (2013). Weighing up the evidence—A systematic review of measures used for the sensation of breathlessness in obesity. *Int J Obes (Lond)*, *37*(3), 341–349. doi:10.1038/ijo.2012.49.

Gilmore, L. A., Duhe, A. F., Frost, E. A., & Redman, L. M. (2014). The technology boom: A new era in obesity management. *J Diabetes Sci Technol*, *8*(3), 596–608. doi:10.1177/1932296814525189.

Giuliani, N. R., Calcott, R. D., & Berkman, E. T. (2013). Piece of cake. *Cognitive reappraisal of food craving. Appetite*, *64*, 56–61. doi:10.1016/j.appet.2012.12.020.

Grilo, C. M., Shiffman, S., & Wing, R. R. (1989). Relapse crises and coping among dieters. *J Consult Clin Psychol*, *57*(4), 488–495.

Guh, D. P., Zhang, W., Bansback, N., Amarsi, Z., Birmingham, C. L., & Anis, A. H. (2009). The incidence of co-morbidities related to obesity and overweight: A systematic review and meta-analysis. *BMC Public Health*, *9*, 88. doi:10.1186/1471-2458-9-88.

Hague, A. L., & White, A. A. (2005). Web-based intervention for changing attitudes of obesity among current and future teachers. *J Nutr Educ Behav*, *37*(2), 58–66.

Ifland, J. R., Preuss, H. G., Marcus, M. T., Taylor, W. C., & Rourke, K. M. (2015a). Commentary: Clearing the confusion around food addiction. *J Am Coll Nutr*, *34*(3), 240–243.

Ifland, J. R., Preuss, H. G., Marcus, M. T., Taylor, W. C., & Rourke, K. M. (2015b). Food plans in the treatment of food addiction. In D. Bagchi, A. Swaroop, & P. H. G. (Eds.), *Nutraceuticals and functional foods in human health and disease prevention.* Boca Ratan, FL: CRC Press.

ITU World Communication/ICT Indicators Database. (2015). Core household Indicators: Access to and use of ICT by household and individuals. Retrieved from http://www.itu.int/en/ITU-D/Statistics/Documents/statistics/2016/CoreHouseholdIndicator.xls (accessed on November 18, 2017).

Johnson, P. M., & Kenny, P. J. (2010). Dopamine D2 receptors in addiction-like reward dysfunction and compulsive eating in obese rats. *Nat Neurosci*, *13*(5), 635–641. doi:10.1038/nn.2519.

Kakinami, L., Barnett, T. A., Seguin, L., & Paradis, G. (2015). Parenting style and obesity risk in children. *Prev Med*, *75*, 18–22. doi:10.1016/j.ypmed.2015.03.005.

Katzmarzyk, P. T., Barreira, T. V., Broyles, S. T., Champagne, C. M., Chaput, J. P., Fogelholm, M., ... Church, T. S. (2015). Physical activity, sedentary time, and obesity in an international sample of children. *Med Sci Sports Exerc*, *47*(10), 2062–2069. doi:10.1249/mss.0000000000000649.

Kearns, D. N., & Weiss, S. J. (2005). Reinstatement of a food-maintained operant produced by compounding discriminative stimuli. *Behav Processes*, *70*(2), 194–202. doi:10.1016/j.beproc.2005.04.007.

Kelleher, E., Davoren, M. P., Harrington, J. M., Shiely, F., Perry, I. J., & McHugh, S. M. (2017). Barriers and facilitators to initial and continued attendance at community-based lifestyle programmes among families of overweight and obese children: A systematic review. *Obes Rev*, *18*(2), 183–194. doi:10.1111/obr.12478.

Kemps, E., Tiggemann, M., & Hollitt, S. (2014). Biased attentional processing of food cues and modification in obese individuals. *Health Psychol*, *33*(11), 1391–1401. doi:10.1037/hea0000069.

Lindberg, M. A., Dementieva, Y., & Cavender, J. (2011). Why has the BMI gone up so drastically in the last 35 years? *J Addict Med*, *5*(4), 272–278. doi:10.1097/ADM.0b013e3182118d41.

Mackenbach, J. D., Tiemeier, H., Ende, J., Nijs, I. M., Jaddoe, V. W., Hofman, A., … Jansen, P. W. (2012). Relation of emotional and behavioral problems with body mass index in preschool children: The generation R study. *J Dev Behav Pediatr*, *33*(8), 641–648. doi:10.1097/DBP.0b013e31826419b8.

Marcus, M. T., Schmitz, J., Moeller, G., Liehr, P., Cron, S. G., Swank, P., … Granmayeh, L. K. (2009). Mindfulness-based stress reduction in therapeutic community treatment: A stage 1 trial. *Am J Drug Alcohol Abuse*, *35*(2), 103–108. doi:10.1080/00952990902823079.

Martin, A. A., & Davidson, T. L. (2014). Human cognitive function and the obesogenic environment. *Physiol Behav*, *136*, 185–193. doi:10.1016/j.physbeh.2014.02.062.

Martinez Steele, E., Baraldi, L. G., Louzada, M. L., Moubarac, J. C., Mozaffarian, D., & Monteiro, C. A. (2016). Ultra-processed foods and added sugars in the US diet: Evidence from a nationally representative cross-sectional study. *BMJ Open*, *6*(3), e009892. doi:10.1136/bmjopen-2015-009892.

Mason, S. M., Flint, A. J., Roberts, A. L., Agnew-Blais, J., Koenen, K. C., & Rich-Edwards, J. W. (2014). Posttraumatic stress disorder symptoms and food addiction in women by timing and type of trauma exposure. *JAMA Psychiatry*, *71*(11), 1271–1278. doi:10.1001/jamapsychiatry.2014.1208.

Matheson, B. E., Camacho, C., Peterson, C. B., Rhee, K. E., Rydell, S. A., Zucker, N. L., & Boutelle, K. N. (2015). The relationship between parent feeding styles and general parenting with loss of control eating in treatment-seeking overweight and obese children. *Int J Eat Disord*, *48*(7), 1047–1055. doi:10.1002/eat.22440.

McGregor, R. A., Cameron-Smith, D., & Poppitt, S. D. (2014). It is not just muscle mass: A review of muscle quality, composition and metabolism during ageing as determinants of muscle function and mobility in later life. *Longev Healthspan*, *3*(1), 9. doi:10.1186/2046-2395-3-9.

McLaren, I. P., Dunn, B. D., Lawrence, N. S., Milton, F. N., Verbruggen, F., Stevens, T., … Leknes, S. (2014). Why decision making may not require awareness. *Behav Brain Sci*, *37*(1), 35–36. doi:10.1017/s0140525x13000794.

McLellan, A. T., Cacciola, J. C., Alterman, A. I., Rikoon, S. H., & Carise, D. (2006). The addiction severity index at 25: Origins, contributions and transitions. *Am J Addict*, *15*(2), 113–124. doi:10.1080/10550490500528316.

Moore, C. F., Sabino, V., Koob, G. F., & Cottone, P. (2017). Pathological overeating: Emerging evidence for a compulsivity construct. *Neuropsychopharmacology*, *42*(7), 1375–1389. doi:10.1038/npp.2016.269.

Morris, M. J., Beilharz, J., Maniam, J., Reichelt, A., & Westbrook, R. F. (2014). Why is obesity such a problem in the 21st century? The intersection of palatable food, cues and reward pathways, stress, and cognition. *Neurosci Biobehav Rev*, *58*, 36–45. doi:10.1016/j.neubiorev.2014.12.002.

Moss, M. (2013). *Salt, sugar, fat: How the food giants hooked us*, New York: Random House.

Murray, E. (2012). Web-based interventions for behavior change and self-management: Potential, pitfalls, and progress. *Med 2 0*, *1*(2), e3. doi:10.2196/med20.1741.

Murray, E., Linke, S., Harwood, E., Conroy, S., Stevenson, F., & Godfrey, C. (2012). Widening access to treatment for alcohol misuse: Description and formative evaluation of an innovative web-based service in one primary care trust. *Alcohol Alcohol*, *47*(6), 697–701. doi:10.1093/alcalc/ags096.

Narouze, S., & Souzdalnitski, D. (2015). Obesity and chronic pain: Systematic review of prevalence and implications for pain practice. *Reg Anesth Pain Med*, *40*(2), 91–111. doi:10.1097/aap.0000000000000218.

Nestle, M. (2013). *Food politics*. Berkeley: University of California Press.

Ng, M., Fleming, T., Robinson, M., Thomson, B., Graetz, N., Margono, C., … Gakidou, E. (2014). Global, regional, and national prevalence of overweight and obesity in children and adults during 1980–2013: A systematic analysis for the Global Burden of Disease Study 2013. *Lancet*, *384*(9945), 766–781. doi:10.1016/s0140-6736(14)60460-8.

Nguyen, J. C., Killcross, A. S., & Jenkins, T. A. (2014). Obesity and cognitive decline: Role of inflammation and vascular changes. *Front Neurosci*, *8*, 375. doi:10.3389/fnins.2014.00375.

O'Dare Wilson, K. (2016). Place matters: Mitigating obesity with the person-in-environment approach. *Soc Work Health Care*, *55*(3), 214–230. doi:10.1080/00981389.2015.1107017.

Opolski, M., Chur-Hansen, A., & Wittert, G. (2015). The eating-related behaviours, disorders and expectations of candidates for bariatric surgery. *Clin Obes*, *5*(4), 165–197. doi:10.1111/cob.12104.

Patel, V. C., Spaeth, A. M., & Basner, M. (2016). Relationships between time use and obesity in a representative sample of Americans. *Obesity (Silver Spring)*, *24*(10), 2164–2175. doi:10.1002/oby.21596.

Radoszewska, J. (2014). Perception of the child's obesity in parents of girls and boys treated for obesity (preliminary study). *Dev Period Med*, *18*(2), 148–154.

Rankin, J., Matthews, L., Cobley, S., Han, A., Sanders, R., Wiltshire, H. D., & Baker, J. S. (2016). Psychological consequences of childhood obesity: Psychiatric comorbidity and prevention. *Adolesc Health Med Ther*, *7*, 125–146. doi:10.2147/ahmt.s101631.

Ratcliffe, D., & Ellison, N. (2015). Obesity and internalized weight stigma: A formulation model for an emerging psychological problem. *Behav Cogn Psychother*, *43*(2), 239–252. doi:10.1017/s13524658 13000763.

Rollins, B. Y., Loken, E., Savage, J. S., & Birch, L. L. (2014). Measurement of food reinforcement in preschool children. Associations with food intake, BMI, and reward sensitivity. *Appetite*, *72*, 21–27. doi:10.1016/j.appet.2013.09.018.

Sanders, R. H., Han, A., Baker, J. S., & Cobley, S. (2015). Childhood obesity and its physical and psychological co-morbidities: A systematic review of Australian children and adolescents. *Eur J Pediatr*, *174*(6), 715–746. doi:10.1007/s00431-015-2551-3.

Schulte, E. M., Potenza, M. N., & Gearhardt, A. N. (2016). A commentary on the "eating addiction" versus "food addiction" perspectives on addictive-like food consumption. *Appetite*, *115*, 9–15. doi:10.1016/j.appet.2016.10.033.

Seacat, J. D., Dougal, S. C., & Roy, D. (2016). A daily diary assessment of female weight stigmatization. *J Health Psychol*, *21*(2), 228–240. doi:10.1177/1359105314525067.

Sharma, S., Fernandes, M. F., & Fulton, S. (2013). Adaptations in brain reward circuitry underlie palatable food cravings and anxiety induced by high-fat diet withdrawal. *Int J Obes (Lond)*, *37*(9), 1183–1191. doi:10.1038/ijo.2012.197.

Sigman-Grant, M., Hayes, J., VanBrackle, A., & Fiese, B. (2015). Family resiliency: A neglected perspective in addressing obesity in young children. *Child Obes*, *11*(6), 664–673. doi:10.1089/chi.2014.0107.

Skov-Ettrup, L. S., Dalum, P., Bech, M., & Tolstrup, J. S. (2016). The effectiveness of telephone counselling and internet- and text-message-based support for smoking cessation: Results from a randomised controlled trial. *Addiction*, *111*(7), 1257–1266. doi:10.1111/add.13302.

Stensland, S. O., Thoresen, S., Wentzel-Larsen, T., & Dyb, G. (2015). Interpersonal violence and overweight in adolescents: The HUNT Study. *Scand J Public Health*, *43*(1), 18–26. doi:10.1177/1403 494814556176.

Stice, E., Burger, K., & Yokum, S. (2013a). Caloric deprivation increases responsivity of attention and reward brain regions to intake, anticipated intake, and images of palatable foods. *NeuroImage*, *67*, 322–330. doi:10.1016/j.neuroimage.2012.11.028.

Stice, E., Burger, K. S., & Yokum, S. (2013b). Relative ability of fat and sugar tastes to activate reward, gustatory, and somatosensory regions. *Am J Clin Nutr*, *98*(6), 1377–1384. doi:10.3945/ajcn.113.069443.

Stice, E., & Yokum, S. (2016). Neural vulnerability factors that increase risk for future weight gain. *Psychol Bull*, *142*(5), 447–471. doi:10.1037/bul0000044.

Turk, M. W., Yang, K., Hravnak, M., Sereika, S. M., Ewing, L. J., & Burke, L. E. (2009). Randomized clinical trials of weight loss maintenance: A review. *J Cardiovasc Nurs*, *24*(1), 58–80. doi:10.1097/01.jcn.0000317471.58048.32.

van den Akker, K., Havermans, R. C., Bouton, M. E., & Jansen, A. (2014). How partial reinforcement of food cues affects the extinction and reacquisition of appetitive responses. *A new model for dieting success? Appetite*, *81C*, 242–252. doi:10.1016/j.appet.2014.06.024.

van der Kolk, B. A. (1994). The body keeps the score: Memory and the evolving psychobiology of posttraumatic stress. *Harv Rev Psychiatry*, *1*(5), 253–265.

Verdejo-Garcia, A., Verdejo-Roman, J., Rio-Valle, J. S., Lacomba, J. A., Lagos, F. M., & Soriano-Mas, C. (2015). Dysfunctional involvement of emotion and reward brain regions on social decision making in excess weight adolescents. *Hum Brain Mapp*, *36*(1), 226–237. doi:10.1002/hbm.22625.

Vincent, H. K., Adams, M. C., Vincent, K. R., & Hurley, R. W. (2013). Musculoskeletal pain, fear avoidance behaviors, and functional decline in obesity: Potential interventions to manage pain and maintain function. *Reg Anesth Pain Med*, *38*(6), 481–491. doi:10.1097/aap.0000000000000013.

Voon, V. (2015). Cognitive biases in binge eating disorder: The hijacking of decision making. *CNS Spectr, 20*(6), 566–573. doi:10.1017/s1092852915000681.

Wang, J., Freire, D., Knable, L., Zhao, W., Gong, B., Mazzola, P., … Pasinetti, G. M. (2015). Childhood/adolescent obesity and long term cognitive consequences during aging. *J Comp Neurol, 523*(10), 1587. doi:10.1002/cne.23708.

Wang, S. S., Houshyar, S., & Prinstein, M. J. (2006). Adolescent girls' and boys' weight-related health behaviors and cognitions: Associations with reputation- and preference-based peer status. *Health Psychol, 25*(5), 658–663. doi:10.1037/0278-6133.25.5.658.

Warner, M. (2014). *Pandora's lunchbox.* New York: Scribner.

Weiss, S. J. (1972). Stimulus compounding in free-operant and classical conditioning. A review and analysis. *Psychol Bull, 78*(3), 189–208.

Wieland, L. S., Falzon, L., Sciamanna, C. N., Trudeau, K. J., Brodney, S., Schwartz, J. E., & Davidson, K. W. (2012). Interactive computer-based interventions for weight loss or weight maintenance in overweight or obese people. *Cochrane Database Syst Rev*, (8), CD007675. doi:10.1002/14651858.CD007675.pub2.

Witkiewitz, K., Hallgren, K. A., Kranzler, H. R., Mann, K. F., Hasin, D. S., Falk, D. E., … Anton, R. F. (2017). Clinical validation of reduced alcohol consumption after treatment for alcohol dependence using the World Health Organization risk drinking levels. *Alcohol Clin Exp Res, 41*(1), 179–186. doi:10.1111/acer.13272.

Yau, P. L., Kang, E. H., Javier, D. C., & Convit, A. (2014). Preliminary evidence of cognitive and brain abnormalities in uncomplicated adolescent obesity. *Obesity (Silver Spring), 22*(8), 1865–1871. doi:10.1002/oby.20801.

Zeller, M. H., Noll, J. G., Sarwer, D. B., Reiter-Purtill, J., Rofey, D. L., Baughcum, A. E., … Becnel, J. N. (2015). Child maltreatment and the adolescent patient with severe obesity: Implications for clinical care. *J Pediatr Psychol, 40*(7), 640–648. doi:10.1093/jpepsy/jsv011.

Zhu, N., Jacobs, D. R., Meyer, K. A., He, K., Launer, L., Reis, J. P., … Steffen, L. M. (2015). Cognitive function in a middle aged cohort is related to higher quality dietary pattern 5 and 25 years earlier: The CARDIA study. *J Nutr Health Aging, 19*(1), 33–38. doi:10.1007/s12603-014-0491-7.

25 Avenues to Success for the Practitioner

Douglas M. Ziedonis
University of California San Diego
San Diego, CA

Joan Ifland
Food Addiction Training, LLC
Cincinnati, OH

CONTENTS

Practitioners in the field of processed food addiction (PFA) need a variety of skills and knowledge, as well as a hopeful attitude that recovery is possible and sustainable. The recovery journey from PFA has additional challenges of acquiring recovery skills as well as sustaining abstinence in the context of an intensely cueing environment, where the marketing of processed food and the culture supporting a "fast food" mentality are designed to promote cravings for and regular intake of processed foods. Unfortunately, individuals with PFA have often been given only weight-loss advice without focusing on the deeper issue of addiction and the related biological, psychological, social, and even spiritual concerns. There can be value in understanding the range of guidance people have had in the past, including from lay, commercial, and professional practitioners, web-based products, and social media. Often people have become more frustrated and uncertain about the possibility of recovery from the ineffectiveness of the many different suggestions. Compassion and positive regard for an individual's willingness and persistence to try again can help to build trust and engagement.

There are six key areas that will help practitioners be successful in restoring PFA clients to full health:

1. A consistently compassionate, and positive attitude. Shame and guilt are often present, and even gentle feedback can be perceived as harsh criticism. Checking in after providing feedback helps clarify intent and enhance confidence [1,2].
2. Attention to learning styles. As with other addictions, individuals with PFA may have more cognitive challenges during the initial withdrawal or protracted abstinence phase. Some of these perceived cognitive challenges are symptomatic of what occurs with other

chronic addictions, including poor decision-making, overprioritizing of food consumption, memory loss, and impaired impulse control [3–6]. Slow, measured teaching is appropriate for this population.
3. Weight loss is not the primary goal. This means leaving weight loss out of the discussion in favor of focusing on the addiction and the benefits of recovery on brain repair [7]. This strategy will also help avoid triggering body obsession [8–10].
4. Exploring of the world of PFA. PFA is a singular addiction in that it requires a food plan. Exploring a personal food plan, support meetings, and food addiction social media will give practitioners hands-on experience with the world of food addiction [11,12]. Exploring the world of PFA will also help practitioners look for unexpected benefits in clients.
5. Optimizing abstinence. Practitioners can help client balance the consequences of taking a bite of processed food versus the ability to ease a social situation by joining in the consumption of a processed food.
6. Weaving education about PFA into existing practices. Practitioners can include information about PFA into practice approaches by using handouts found at www.foodaddictionresources.com.

Practitioners will find success by monitoring behaviors such as minimizing, denial, and rationalizing of problems as simply weight loss issues. An avenue to success is to watch whether clients make exceptions to their food plan or permit overexposure to high risk cues, as these can increase the risk of relapse [13]. PFA can be successfully treated with attention to how thoughts and feelings linger for the individual and how that affects their behaviors.

25.1 ADOPT A CONSISTENTLY COMPASSIONATE AND CONSTRUCTIVE ATTITUDE

Individuals with PFA often feel frustrated, demoralized, and not confident as they reenter treatment. Many have suffered from repeat "failures" to lose weight [7], jeers and insults related to body size [14], perception of condescension from some health professionals [15], abuse and neglect in childhood [16], and isolation [17]. And they are perceiving and interpreting these experiences through downregulated pleasure and sensitized stress neuropathways, which intensifies the distress [18,19]. Taken all together, one can understand their mistrust and fears in new relationships [20]. For the practitioner, this emotional profile translates into an approach to treatment of assessing how one is perceived as being judgmental or critical. Even gentle feedback can be perceived as painful criticism. Help individuals frame "setbacks" in a positive way as routine, normal opportunities to discover more about the disease and to increase their own self-awareness of triggers and ways to cope.

The avenue to success is most important when helping the client learn to protect against lapsing. Framing lapses as positive contributions to the process sets a warm tone that supports the PFA client in rebuilding self-esteem and staying open to continuing to build a recovery program. There will be lots of bumps along the way for these clients. Cognitive challenges, protracted abstinence [6], and the diminished ability to protect themselves from food-cueing environments of this particular addiction [21] could make skill acquisition slow and uneven. How clients interpret and internalize likely lapses is crucial to success. If they fall into the mindset that a mistake indicates failure and is personalized as shameful, their progress may be slowed or it may be too painful for them to stay with the program at all [22].

On the other hand, if clients can be persuaded that mistakes are somewhat expected and a behavior that can be readjusted, even a valuable lesson learned, then they may be able to learn from the lapse and see this as new "data" about their program. With this approach, they can gradually reframe these "mistakes" in behavior as part of the normal learning experience. Maintaining self-compassion in the context of these events is a goal. Examples of reassuring ways to respond to mistakes are:

- PFA can be a challenging disease. Learning together can be helpful. This is normal.
- We all have sensitive brains, and PFA can hijack the brain. Learning how to protect your brain in the context of an aggressive processed food (PF) environment is needed.
- This is not your "fault"—and the journey of recovery can help find the path. We can't know what we'll need until we try.
- You just got overexposed to a cue. That's all. It's not your fault. You're just in the process of exploring how much cue exposure your individual brain can handle.
- Yes, I'm sorry that happened. Lapses can be scary. It's just the nature of the disease and we're all learning together for each of us what our individual program is going to look like.
- I heard you say that you know better. But after exposure to a cue we get cravings, and our knowledge is suppressed by cravings. It's not your fault that this happened. It's just the nature of the disease.
- You're in the right place having the right experiences and the right thoughts. Everything's OK.
- These are hard behaviors to change. You aren't defined by your thoughts. It's very hard to believe that this could be the case because it's the first time that you've experienced this.

There isn't just one way to provide feedback about mistakes and lapses. Having an increased sensitivity and inquiry on how your feedback is heard is important. Even a straightforward question of, "What did you learn?" can feel reprimanding to some. "Why did you do that?" may sound accusatory; however, the tone and context can influence what is said. At some point the individual will have more confidence and accept personal responsibility; however, a gentle reminder of the many factors that influence relapses in early recovery can be reviewed to assure clients that relapses are not entirely their fault. These include:

- Food industry marketing [23]
- Cue reactivity in early recovery [13]
- The difficulty of living in a provocative environment
- The social nature of food
- The fast pace of life that has increased processed food choices [24]

In truth, from a profound understanding of the disease and the environment, lapses are anticipated. With consistent support, encouragement, understanding, and education, each client will learn through their own trials how to structure their days to avoid activating the disease. Clients can learn how to enhance their own brain's abilities and internal resilience.

A compassionate attitude also helps success during withdrawal after a lapse. It is compassionate to teach PFA clients to manage the discomfort of withdrawal. Clients may have the idea that increasing the suffering of withdrawal could create a deterrent to relapsing. However, suffering through withdrawal can create a barrier to going through withdrawal after a lapse. Clients could be sick with headache, cravings, fatigue, nausea, depression, grogginess, etc. [25–27]. The value of lapses is that they have built-in negative reinforcement. Practitioners can use this to the client's advantage by acknowledging the symptoms and expressing compassion and empathy. This models kindness to themselves and supports improvements in self-compassion and self-esteem. By associating emotional discomfort with processed foods with new learning in a positive, constructive environment, clients can develop a natural aversion to processed foods.

Compassion also helps clients accept the pace of recovery in terms of how quickly lapses are brought under control. This can vary widely from client to client. Clients can present with a diverse range of capabilities across a wide range of severity [28]. There may be times when the client feels inadequate. Based on past experiences, they may fear that the practitioner thinks they're not trying hard enough. Clients can be reassured that they're working to the best of their abilities and their task is challenging but doable.

Positive concepts of recovery can be reinforced. This moves the discussion beyond mere symptom reduction to discussions of mobilizing their personal resources to help them better find meaning and purpose in their lives. Practitioners can help clients see that they're courageous and determined. Clients will learn to take the needed small steps and trust their instincts and feelings to manage feelings and thoughts as they arise, including enhancing their ability to manage difficult emotions of anger, shame, guilt, and confusion. Deep listening, compassion, and encouragement gives clients the opportunity to internalize confidence. Understanding the nature of PFA facilitates the process of acquiring skills to protect against food cues and emotional triggers that lead to relapse.

By understanding and adapting to the severity of PFA, the practitioner naturally develops compassion for the suffering of normal lapses and "setbacks" while slowly establishing protective routines. How many lapses and of what nature for each client is hard to predict. It could be months before a client recognizes the danger of going into a grocery store when tired or attending a heavily cued family event when stressed. Clients are able to enhance their resilience to the culture of ubiquitous processed foods through encouragement and acceptance of the difficulty of a disease that is easily activated by provocative food environments and relationships.

At any given moment, clients are sorting out complex decisions about what's needed to protect their brains from stimulation. It is rational that they will take the path of least resistance and greatest outcome in their own view. Figuring out the best course of action is challenging in the early stages of recovery as cognitive functions are restoring. Patience, expressing confidence, and planting seeds will yield satisfying results. Clients may respond well to an attitude that learning at an individual pace is the norm. This is as opposed to setting goals, deadlines, agendas, etc., which could be experienced as stressful and counterproductive for many (but not all) PFA clients. The pace of recovery will be different for each client. Whatever the pace, it is gratifying to watch the PFA client gently soak up new experiences and perceptions about a difficult disease and slowly build a foundation of new knowledge and capabilities.

Clients will also respond to having dignity and space in which to absorb guidance as shared information as opposed to correcting a problem. Lapses can be handled by consistent encouragement and reinforcement to restore self-confidence in clients. Some PFA clients could readily blame themselves for lapses, which could increase stress and can activate cravings [29]. Even a seemingly small step in the right direction is worthy of notice and praise. Periods of low motivation can be normal. Clients can be taught that patience and taking breaks is fine. There's no specific time when anything needs to be done. This approach encourages the client to relax, which reduces stress and allows the client to move forward.

Examples of lapses that occur because of lack of experience with managing cues and stressors follow:

- Frank allows guests to bring desserts into his home. He does not ask the guests to take the desserts home at the end of the evening. He's tired and argues with his wife about cleaning up. Frank eats the leftover processed foods until they're finished. The next day at work, he's sick with a headache and brain fog. The compassionate practitioner reminds Frank to use hot and cold compresses on the headache and to try 1-minute meditations for the brain fog.
- Mavis has an upsetting day at work because a colleague has been arrested for drug possession and a client is mad about an order. Candy is kept at a table in the office and she eats some. The next day she has cravings and is terrified of losing control again. The empathetic practitioner sends her the handout "Recover from a Cravings Flare-Up" from www.foodaddictionresources.com and encourages her to believe that she can reduce the cravings.

- Anna continues to watch television for hours at a time and lapses frequently. The patient practitioner shares about the benefits of other activities, touching on the research that correlates watching television with weight gain. Exercise videos are reviewed. Meditation apps can be downloaded in the office. Online stores with puzzles are identified. The practitioner reassures Anna that it takes time to wind down triggering activities. She has all the time in the world to pick out other activities. She can really think about what else she might enjoy. There is no hurry.

Here are some general approaches that emphasize skill development as a means for reducing lapsing. This is as opposed to criticizing the client for failing or leading the client to believe that the cause might be an emotional issue.

Problem	Compassionate Approach
Something isn't getting done.	Define a smaller, easier goal. Identify fears.
The client cannot see progress.	Praise the areas where the client is benefiting from progress.
The client is stopping for fast food.	Encourage the client to build up calming cues in their car.
The client cannot resist stopping for fast food.	Encourage the client to find a different route from work to home.
The client cannot visualize a solution.	Describe options and give the client lots of time to think about them.
The client is afraid of failure.	Empower clients to set their own pace. Make changes only when they're ready. Give clients control.
Neither the client nor the practitioner can see a solution.	Through patience and praise, the practitioner creates confidence within the client to surface solutions that fit the time and place.
PFA recovery takes place in a complex culture.	The practitioner teaches clients about addictive marketing practices and assures clients that lapses are not their fault.

25.2 ATTENTION TO LEARNING STYLES

Recent research has opened the way to new understanding about the behaviors of PFA clients. It is now easier to solve the puzzle of why clients cannot organize meals. In addition to emotional or childhood issues, blocks to starting may stem from brain fog [30], learning disabilities [31], or loss of working memory [32]. Now practitioners can find ways to compensate for these deficits by using short repetitive messages where necessary.

As described in Chapter 24, "Premises of Recovery for Adults," use of online education and mobile devices could make the practitioner more successful in a number of ways. Keep a group of clients in an email loop, a Facebook group, or a texting group—keep a channel of information and encouragement open around the clock. Group members can help one another under the supervision of the practitioner. Clients seem to be open to receiving support in this way. In a survey of patients intending to lose weight, almost 90% indicated that they would be receptive to support delivered by telephone [33].

When using electronic approaches, practitioners need to work with their organizations, their licensing boards, or professional organizations to ensure that they protect the confidentiality of their clients.

A survey of patients of general practitioners indicated that "over 80% perceived advice on healthy eating and physical activity to be useful or very useful, and were likely to follow weight-loss recommendations; 78% were in favor of regular review. Patients indicated they would be less likely to see a dietitian or to attend information sessions, and unlikely to take weight-loss medication" [34]. Quality of practitioner/patient communication was found to have a positive impact on fruit and vegetable consumption [35]. This evidence seems to indicate that clients are open to advice on food.

Challenge	Solution
Attention deficit	Deliver short repetitive messages.
Learning disability	Meal pictures.
Cravings	Divert the mind at the moment of a cravings flare-up.
Decision-making	Being with the group via a handheld device in complex situations can help the client with decision-making. Platforms such as text, email, or online groups provide connection virtually 24 hours per day.
Memory loss	Having information on a handheld device can compensate for memory loss.
Low self-esteem	Using electronic information in addition to in-person sessions means that the practitioner can do more to support recovery.

There are a number of ways to reach the PFA client in both real and virtual environments. The website www.foodaddictionresources.com was created to augment this textbook. It contains educational handouts and links to resources such as online groups, practitioners who work by phone, and residential treatment centers. The handouts are designed to be parsed out in small doses. Some handouts such as "Food Addiction Cost/Benefit Checklist" might be reviewed periodically as the client is likely to see new and different progress each time. Repetition is valuable for several reasons. The client's cognitive abilities might have improved, making it possible to absorb a greater portion of the material. The client might have had experiences with lapses or with successes that could make the material more interesting and relevant. Clients benefit from insights and comments on handouts as recovery progresses.

Practitioners may find that they are helping clients through painful realizations about compromised cognitive abilities. The client might have been labeled learning disabled or "slow" and might have missed educational or career opportunities as a result [36–38]. They may have endured ridicule from peers and frustration from parents at their inability to make academic progress. As they emerge from brain fog and work at cognitive restoration activities, they might find that they're quite bright or at least have solid normal intelligence. The practitioner can offer specific support in this circumstance. Reassurance that teachers, parents, caregivers, and other adults did not know that processed foods could create learning disabilities will help the client forgive those who misunderstood. Gently encouraging the client to look for training and educational opportunities could also be helpful.

Short handouts give practitioners the opportunity to orient clients with a combined auditory and visual approach. The handouts can be broken down into slides for presentations. Carrying printed handouts or personal devices with downloaded handouts helps compensate for impaired memory.

Accommodating the level of cognitive function through pacing, small messages, repetition, and handouts from www.foodaddictionresources.com will give the practitioner the satisfaction of watching clients make progress as well as the pleasure of praising their accomplishments.

25.3 WEIGHT LOSS IS NOT THE PRIMARY TARGET

The PFA model offers a fresh opportunity for healing for clients. Many PFA clients are overweight, and they may have low self-esteem from being unable to meet and maintain weight-loss goals in programs that were not designed for recovery from PFA [17]. Explaining why addiction recovery may be a more effective approach can help clients overcome the shame of failed weight-loss attempts. This new information could give the client a boost of self-confidence that could turn into the foundation for recovery.

Even though fat loss is normally a delightful consequence of recovery from PFA, there are quite a few reasons to avoid dwelling on weight loss for the PFA client. The first is that clients are likely to be sensitive to weight issues [10]. Also, talking about weight may encourage clients to think that they are in a weight-loss program. This could set them up for believing that when they attain a certain weight, they can go back to consuming addictive foods. Being able to resume use of addictive substances is a common misconception among some PFA clients. The perception that there is a level of safe use of PF can lead to full relapses for PFA clients. This may be a risk for PFA clients because recovery separates them from social rituals in Westernized cultures. Clients may also interpret discussion of weight as judgment, which can reduce trust in the practitioner [2].

Framing recovery as a function of brain health avoids cuing clients into a weight-loss–associated fear of failure. Framing recovery as a way of being and way to discover personal resilience helps them find meaning and purpose in life.

As a corollary, focusing on weight may result in clients missing or at least downplaying the value of important recovery benefits from:

- Control of eating behavior
- Emotional stability
- Mood improvement
- Improvement in cognitive function
- Better energy
- Mental clarity
- Release from cravings
- Reduced inflammation
- Resolution of infections
- Joint pain
- Improvements in the metabolic syndrome, including diabetes, blood pressure, cholesterol, etc. [39–41]

These results are not typically promoted with weight-loss programs so it is important to reframe the effort as primarily recovery of neurofunction and general health so clients ascribe full value to their recovery. Emphasizing recovery of mental, physical, emotional, and behavioral health helps to distinguish the lifelong nature of recovery from PFA from the short-term goal of weight loss. Here are some approaches to this issue:

- Memories of weight-loss programs may trigger an urge to restrict, which is a setup for relapse in a PFA model through the mechanism of increased cravings [42,43].
- Dwelling on weight loss could encourage clients to frame exercise as a weight-loss measure rather than for improved sleep [44] and cognitive function [45].
- Research shows that framing exercise as "fat burning" increases postexercise food consumption [46]. This is as opposed to framing exercise as a craving reducer or mood enhancer.
- Focusing on brain stabilization can motivate clients to resist calorie restriction and instead stick to complete, fully portioned meals.
- Learning how the food plan supports mental health and control over eating behavior is key [40].

Focusing on weight loss also keeps clients tied to harmful cultural and media marketing representations of disordered body images. It encourages comparison with impossible ideals, which in turn can lead to low self-esteem [47]. Although encouraging clients to get rid of their scales and reduce television time can be a slow process, these are valuable steps in leaving debilitating weight and body obsession behind.

Maintaining a virtual environment that is free from reference to weight loss is a valuable resource for recovery. By using the Internet and mobile devices to deliver education, the practitioner can overcome the barrier of body shame, which might prevent the client from accessing in-person treatment. The shame and trauma of being overweight in a culture that idealizes the thin, even underweight figure is significant [17]. Services accessed from mobile devices allow the client to heal from the trauma of obesity more easily than if the client were facing people in-person in an overweight body. Clients can more easily establish strong self-esteem independently of considerations about the shape of their body [10]. When they reenter the physical world from their online world, it is with conditioning as a confident person without a weight problem.

25.4 EXPLORING THE WORLD OF PFA

Health practitioners have not been immune to the obesity epidemic. The pervasiveness of processed foods and fattening foods in the public food supply has reached about two thirds of Americans. Losing weight is now seen to be very difficult. It is possible that people have normal control over their eating and are still overweight. Practitioners who are in this position can treat PFA with confidence. Treatment attributes call for compassion and skill that are independent of weight status. Overweight/obese practitioners may benefit from extra effort to gain the client's trust, as research shows that obese practitioners are less trusted by PFA clients [11,12]. This is similar to smoking cessation counselors who still smoke. PFA clients are challenged to trust in people in general [17]. Practitioners have also been found to feel more competent in the treatment of obesity if they themselves are of a normal weight or have successfully lost weight [48]. Practitioners can put aside any awkwardness they may feel and assure clients that treatment can be effective.

1. Regardless of personal history with food, practitioners may want to explore the process of organizing abstinent meals for themselves. A primary reason is that it is educational. The experience may help the practitioner persuade clients that they can have a pleasurable life even though they eat differently from their culture. Practitioners will enjoy having a repertoire of tips and inspirational stories to guide PFA clients through difficult situations. Practitioners also need to overcome the history of weight-loss failures that might have led the PFA client to distrust professionals in general. These goals could be made easier if the practitioner has personal experience in organizing abstinent meals.
2. Practitioners may also explore the world of PFA by attending meetings of Overeaters Anonymous, Food Addicts Anonymous, and Food Addicts in Recovery Anonymous.
3. Some personal experience with mindfulness and mindful eating would also be valuable to share with clients.

Identification with the behavior of the practitioner can promote a positive attitude toward the practitioner [49]. The pressure to conform to the obesogenic culture means that the client is searching diligently for a reason to fit in with old friends, family, and business colleagues [50]. A counselor who sets the example of occasional use might be effective if the goal is reduced harm [13].

Comparing PFA to other drug usage situations helps illuminate this argument. Alcohol and tobacco are two drugs that are approached differently in terms of both public perception and treatment approaches. A recovery practitioner might conceivably drink socially and still be an effective alcohol counselor unless they are alcoholic. There does not appear to be a safe level for tobacco consumption, and most smoking cessation programs discourage any tobacco product use or at minimum the appearance of being a smoker (smells, visible products that might be a trigger and reduce confidence of the client). The important thing is the compassion and skill of the practitioner.

The practitioner who undertakes an abstinent food plan may be rewarded in unexpected ways. Nonaddicted practitioners can be suffering from subconscious impairments stemming from even infrequent and minimal use. Going through withdrawal and attaining sobriety from processed foods could be a rewarding effort for the practitioner. Being able to share personal stories of benefits may encourage confidence in the practitioner/client relationship and motivate the client to work to attain the benefits of recovery.

25.4.1 Enjoy Unexpected Opportunities

Treating PFA offers the opportunity to create valuable, unexpected results with clients. Lifetime abstinence or reduced use of processed foods is a new approach. As such, it creates the potential for surprising benefits for the PFA client and for the people around the client. This is a pleasant aspect of PFA recovery for practitioners. The challenge comes in helping clients balance the pleasure of health that comes from abstaining from processed foods against the inconvenience of eating differently from mainstream culture.

In addition to the client, there are four populations that present opportunities for practitioners to realize unexpected and delightful results: (1) clients' household members; (2) preaddicted clients; (3) other eating disorders; and (4) normally weighted clients.

A source of unexpected benefits may be the client's household members. One way to think about the household of a PFA client is that it has had processed foods in it, which the children have likely accessed. So, removing processed foods from their diet may yield delightful results such as improved mood, academics, sleep, and behavior. Valuable results can come from educating about processed diet–related diseases regardless of whether household members meet the DSM 5 SUD criteria for addiction or are overweight [51].

Addressing the whole household serves the client in several ways [52]. An educated household creates a better sense of "normal" for the client, which is calming and reassuring, given that the client is exposed to destabilizing sights, sounds, and smells of processed food consumption outside the home. It also reduces stress for the PFA client. Processed foods are associated with physical illness, as well as mood swings, including irritability regardless of the presence of addiction [40,53]. These illnesses and disordered moods are stressful for the client to manage in close relationships within the household. This is especially true for children and interpersonal adult relationships [54]. The website www.foodaddictionresources.com gives the practitioner a number of handouts for the client to share with household members. Treating the whole household could yield many benefits.

A client who might experience unexpected results is the situation where preaddiction is found but the client is normally weighted. This is a situation in which the client may only meet one or two of the DSM 5 SUD criteria. In light of the intense exposure to processed food cues in obesogenic cultures, it could be rewarding to educate these clients about the harmful properties of processed foods and set them on a course of avoidance of processed foods and cues. This is justified not only on the grounds of arresting the progression of the addiction but also because processed foods have generally harmful properties aside from addictive properties [32,55]. Practitioners may be able to persuade a preaddicted client to try out an abstinent food plan on a trial basis. Even the preaddicted client may feel better in terms of more energy, better mood, less bloating, etc., on an unprocessed food plan. If the client is not ready, planting the seed may nonetheless yield rewards in the future.

It is also valuable to avoid missing the seriousness of PFA in normally weighted clients. It is tempting to say that a person has their food under control if they're not overweight. Cravings, obsession, compromised cognitive function, and disordered moods can be present regardless of weight status. These syndromes may be distressing enough to drive sufferers to seek help. The practitioner can have confidence by using the assessment criteria developed in Part II of the textbook when evaluating a new client, regardless of weight.

Practitioners may also look for opportunities to apply principles of PFA recovery in eating disorders such as anorexia, bulimia, and binge eating disorder (BED). Depression and anxiety can be present in these cases, and depression and anxiety are linked to processed foods. Encouraging the elimination of processed foods for other disorders could improve outcomes. Practitioners can also work to avoid missing PFA in other eating disorders such as anorexia, bulimia, and BED. Like food addiction, these are also neurodisorders that could benefit from the stabilizing properties of an unprocessed nonaddictive food plan [56,57]. Considering the evidence for addictive properties for a range of processed foods, it would seem beneficial for the disordered eating client to avoid them. The mistake would be to attempt to establish positive attitudes toward food and normal eating behavior without eliminating mood-altering processed foods.

25.5 OPTIMIZING ABSTINENCE

Regardless of which population is being helped by abstinence/reduced use, there is constant cultural pressure to consume processed foods. The culture exerts pressure to allow exceptions to the food plan at business, social, and family events. This pressure presents a challenge for practitioners. A bite here and there may present a low risk for mild cases. In more severe cases, where more than six of the DSM 5 SUD criteria are present, clients may be unable to judge consequences. At the same time, they may be more cue reactive and thereby at increased risk of relapse. With experience, practitioners will develop approaches to advising clients about the risk of taking a bite.

The disease may require the client to step away from mainstream obesogenic practices including the sharing of processed food at business, social, and family gatherings [58]. Given low self-esteem, the client may find it very difficult to be so different from their social, family, and work circles [59]. Under these kinds of pressures, the practitioner may be tempted to "allow" the client risky exposure to processed foods and cues. Occasional use in a "reduced harm" model may be appropriate in mild cases. However, in cases of severe addiction as determined by the number of DSM 5 SUD criteria met and as assessed by the severity rating in the Addiction Severity Index, the practitioner faces a greater challenge. Although the best solution may be to be unwavering regarding the maintenance of abstinence and cue avoidance, the reality is that lapses are likely. Reassuring the client and gently illuminating consequences may work better in a sustainable and comfortable level of abstinence.

The practitioner may feel pressured to "allow" use on special occasions such as the splurge allowed by Weight Watchers [60]. It might feel acceptable to "allow" an unstable client to do their own grocery shopping or attend a highly triggering social event under the rationale that these activities are so normal and common in our obesogenic culture. It's difficult to reconcile the need to reduce risk with the need to be social [10,13,61]. Borrowing from the drug addiction paradigms, clients can be taught to judge whether they're safe to attend events depending on whether they're hungry, angry, lonely, or tired (HALT); strength of recovery; number of years; and enhanced self-awareness. Maintaining the goals of consistent manageable abstinence from processed foods, addictive food additives, and food cues will contribute to success.

As practitioners gain experience with the range of severity of PFA, it may become apparent that long-term treatment is justified. Especially in the case of clients who developed food addiction in childhood, crucial periods of emotional and behavioral development may have been missed. Many months may be needed to address issues such as reestablishing sensation in the physical body, healthy relationship management, and the ability to experience pleasure. As with alcohol and drug addiction, lifetime support can be warranted. As discussed in Chapter 24, "Premises of Recovery for Adults," it is important not to cut treatment short. It may take months for a client with limited cognitive functioning to develop protective routines for the complex tasks of making abstinent meals and avoiding triggering cues and situations. In a short program, such a client might emerge a failure. However, with enough time, encouragement, and simple examples, food-addicted clients could build a strong recovery for the long term.

25.6 WEAVING EDUCATION ABOUT PFA INTO EXISTING PRACTICES

In many practices, brief educational interventions with patients will be sufficient to start the process of eliminating processed foods from their diets. Patients/clients who seem unable to implement an unprocessed food plan may benefit from more in-depth support. They can be referred or can be supported in-house with counseling.

For non–diet-related practitioners, sharing educational handouts with patients is a good place to start. Such handouts may be found at http://www.foodaddictionresources.com/handouts.html. Handouts on food plans are under Section 3. In practices that are not equipped to support lifestyle changes, referrals may be made to the practitioners listed at http://www.foodaddictionresources.com/resources.html.

In diet-related practices addressing obesity, diabetes, cardiovascular disease, and Alzheimer's, existing staff may already be supporting clients in long-term lifestyle changes. In this case, clients who seem unable to adhere meaningfully to diet recommendations may benefit from information about PFA. Abstinence and cue avoidance may be the keys to quelling cravings, developing impulse control, and successfully resisting temptation in clients who have a history of noncompliance to diet recommendations. Because PFA is a complex disease that responds to specialized approaches, persistently noncompliant patients may need to be referred for treatment.

For some eating disorder (ED) practices, suggestions such as abstinence may be somewhat novel. ED approaches such as intuitive eating and mindfulness are sometimes used to help clients eat processed foods in moderation. Intuitive eating and mindfulness could be helpful to food-addicted clients, so these treatment modalities transfer well into PFA. It is easy to adjust the purpose of intuitive eating and mindfulness to helping clients counteract cues to crave with a goal of achieving a degree of abstinence. ED practitioners are likely to be delighted that application of abstinence guidelines brings serenity to struggling clients. Only slight adjustments to existing ED practices can adapt practices to the treatment of PFA.

In practices serving the mentally ill, it is probable that long-term counseling and group support are already in place. In these situations, practitioners can gradually introduce the information found at www.foodaddictionresources.com.

Drug addiction professionals might be surprised at the number of treatment elements that are common to both PFA and drug addiction. Abstinence/reduced use, cue avoidance, relapse prevention, support for building healthy behaviors, recovery of careers, and relationship repair are familiar territory to drug addiction practitioners. Learning about PFA may help SUD counselors prevent drug addiction from shifting to PFA in the course of recovery.

All practices can teach patients and clients about PFA. Clients will be grateful to have a new perspective on their struggles with food.

25.7 CONCLUSION

This chapter, "Avenues to Success for the Practitioner," has touched on several opportunities to improve outcomes. Adopting a deeply compassionate and encouraging attitude will create a safe environment. Pacing the rate of learning to accommodate compromised cognitive function will yield steady progress at skill acquisition and self-confidence. Avoiding a focus on weight loss will help clients focus on a broad range of valuable results. Becoming a good model by personally working a nonaddictive, unprocessed food plan is also helpful to establish trust, confidence, and expertise. Looking for opportunities to treat aggressively and avoid undertreating will be appreciated. PFA is a broad-reaching disease, but with the right approaches it can be put into remission.

REFERENCES

1. Jarcho, J.M., et al., Neural activation during anticipated peer evaluation and laboratory meal intake in overweight girls with and without loss of control eating. *NeuroImage*, 2015; **108**: 343–53.
2. Gudzune, K.A., et al., Patients who feel judged about their weight have lower trust in their primary care providers. *Patient Educ Couns*, 2014; **97**(1): 128–31.
3. Voon, V., Cognitive biases in binge eating disorder: The hijacking of decision making. *CNS Spectr*, 2015; **20**(6): 566–73.
4. Wang, J., et al., Childhood/adolescent obesity and long term cognitive consequences during aging. *J Comp Neurol*, 2015; **523**(10): 1587.

5. Yau, P.L., et al., Preliminary evidence of cognitive and brain abnormalities in uncomplicated adolescent obesity. *Obesity (Silver Spring)*, 2014; **22**(8): 1865–71.
6. Zhu, N., et al., Cognitive function in a middle aged cohort is related to higher quality dietary pattern 5 and 25 years earlier: The CARDIA study. *J Nutr Health Aging*, 2015; **19**(1): 33–8.
7. Turk, M.W., et al., Randomized clinical trials of weight loss maintenance: A review. *J Cardiovasc Nurs*, 2009; **24**(1): 58–80.
8. Micali, N., et al., Frequency and patterns of eating disorder symptoms in early adolescence. *J Adolesc Health*, 2014; **54**(5): 574–81.
9. Pavan, C., et al., Overweight/obese patients referring to plastic surgery: Temperament and personality traits. *Obes Surg*, 2013; **23**(4): 437–45.
10. Coelho, J.S., et al., Reactivity to thought-shape fusion in adolescents: The effects of obesity status. *Pediatr Obes*, 2013; **8**(6): 439–44.
11. Puhl, R.M., et al., The effect of physicians' body weight on patient attitudes: Implications for physician selection, trust and adherence to medical advice. *Int J Obes (Lond)*, 2013; **37**(11): 1415–21.
12. Bleich, S.N., et al., Impact of non-physician health professionals' BMI on obesity care and beliefs. *Obesity (Silver Spring)*, 2014; **22**(12): 2476–80.
13. Boswell, R.G. and H. Kober, Food cue reactivity and craving predict eating and weight gain: A meta-analytic review. *Obes Rev*, 2016; **17**(2): 159–77.
14. Seacat, J.D., S.C. Dougal, and D. Roy, A daily diary assessment of female weight stigmatization. *J Health Psychol*, 2016; **21**(2): 228–40.
15. Phelan, S.M., et al., Impact of weight bias and stigma on quality of care and outcomes for patients with obesity. *Obes Rev*, 2015; **16**(4): 319–26.
16. Danese, A. and M. Tan, Childhood maltreatment and obesity: Systematic review and meta-analysis. *Mol Psychiatry*, 2014; **19**(5): 544–54.
17. Ratcliffe, D. and N. Ellison, Obesity and internalized weight stigma: A formulation model for an emerging psychological problem. *Behav Cogn Psychother*, 2015; **43**(2): 239–52.
18. Tomasi, D., et al., Overlapping patterns of brain activation to food and cocaine cues in cocaine abusers: Association to striatal D2/D3 receptors. *Hum Brain Mapp*, 2015; **36**(1): 120–36.
19. Ventura, T., et al., Neurobiologic basis of craving for carbohydrates. *Nutrition*, 2014; **30**(3): 252–6.
20. Carr, D., M.A. Friedman, and K. Jaffe, Understanding the relationship between obesity and positive and negative affect: The role of psychosocial mechanisms. *Body Image*, 2007; **4**(2): 165–77.
21. Lifshitz, F. and J.Z. Lifshitz, Globesity: The root causes of the obesity epidemic in the USA and now worldwide. *Pediatr Endocrinol Rev*, 2014; **12**(1): 17–34.
22. O'Brien, K.S., et al., The relationship between weight stigma and eating behavior is explained by weight bias internalization and psychological distress. *Appetite*, 2016; **102**: 70–6.
23. Brownell, K.D. and K.E. Warner, The perils of ignoring history: Big tobacco played dirty and millions died. How similar is big food? *Milbank Q*, 2009; **87**(1): 259–94.
24. Drewnowski, A., et al., Food environment and socioeconomic status influence obesity rates in Seattle and in Paris. *Int J Obes (Lond)*, 2014; **38**(2): 306–14.
25. Sharma, S., M.F. Fernandes, and S. Fulton, Adaptations in brain reward circuitry underlie palatable food cravings and anxiety induced by high-fat diet withdrawal. *Int J Obes (Lond)*, 2013; **37**(9): 1183–91.
26. Iemolo, A., et al., Withdrawal from chronic, intermittent access to a highly palatable food induces depressive-like behavior in compulsive eating rats. *Behav Pharmacol*, 2012; **23**(5–6): 593–602.
27. Colantuoni, C., et al., Evidence that intermittent, excessive sugar intake causes endogenous opioid dependence. *Obes Res*, 2002; **10**(6): 478–88.
28. Gearhardt, A.N., W.R. Corbin, and K.D. Brownell, Development of the Yale Food Addiction Scale Version 2.0. *Psychol Addict Behav*, 2016; **30**(1): 113–21.
29. Palmeira, L., et al., Finding the link between internalized weight-stigma and binge eating behaviors in Portuguese adult women with overweight and obesity: The mediator role of self-criticism and self-reassurance. *Eat Behav*, 2017; **26**: 50–54.
30. Theoharides, T.C., et al., Brain "fog," inflammation and obesity: Key aspects of neuropsychiatric disorders improved by luteolin. *Front Neurosci,* 2015; **9**: 225.
31. Ptacek, R., et al., Attention deficit hyperactivity disorder and eating disorders. *Prague Med Rep*, 2010; **111**(3): 175–81.
32. Noble, E.E. and S.E. Kanoski, Early life exposure to obesogenic diets and learning and memory dysfunction. *Curr Opin Behav Sci*, 2016; **9**: 7–14.
33. Yoong, S.L., et al., A cross-sectional study assessing Australian general practice patients' intention, reasons and preferences for assistance with losing weight. *BMC Fam Pract,* 2013; **14**: 187.

34. Tan, D., et al., Weight management in general practice: What do patients want? *Med J Aust*, 2006; **185**(2): 73–5.
35. Baumann, M., et al., Impact of patients' communication with the medical practitioners, on their adherence declared to preventive behaviours, five years after a coronary angiography, in Luxembourg. *PLoS One,* 2016; **11**(6): e0157321.
36. Ali, S.M. and M. Lindstrom, Socioeconomic, psychosocial, behavioural, and psychological determinants of BMI among young women: Differing patterns for underweight and overweight/obesity. *Eur J Public Health,* 2006; **16**(3): 325–31.
37. Feng, X. and A. Wilson, Getting bigger, quicker? Gendered socioeconomic trajectories in body mass index across the adult lifecourse: A longitudinal study of 21,403 Australians. *PLoS One,* 2015; **10**(10): e0141499.
38. Gonzalez-Casanova, I., et al., Individual, family, and community predictors of overweight and obesity among Colombian children and adolescents. *Prev Chronic Dis,* 2014; **11**: E134.
39. Lindeberg, S., Paleolithic diets as a model for prevention and treatment of Western disease. *Am J Hum Biol*, 2012; **24**(2): 110–15.
40. Logan, A.C. and F.N. Jacka, Nutritional psychiatry research: An emerging discipline and its intersection with global urbanization, environmental challenges and the evolutionary mismatch. *J Physiol Anthropol*, 2014; **33**: 22.
41. Guh, D.P., et al., The incidence of co-morbidities related to obesity and overweight: A systematic review and meta-analysis. *BMC Public Health,* 2009; **9**: 88.
42. Moreno-Dominguez, S., et al., Impact of fasting on food craving, mood and consumption in bulimia nervosa and healthy women participants. *Eur Eat Disord Rev*, 2012; **20**(6): 461–7.
43. Stice, E., K. Burger, and S. Yokum, Caloric deprivation increases responsivity of attention and reward brain regions to intake, anticipated intake, and images of palatable foods. *NeuroImage*, 2013; **67**: 322–30.
44. Kline, C.E., et al., Consistently high sports/exercise activity is associated with better sleep quality, continuity and depth in midlife women: The SWAN sleep study. *Sleep*, 2013; **36**(9): 1279–88.
45. Annesi, J.J. and G.A. Tennant, Mediation of social cognitive theory variables in the relationship of exercise and improved eating in sedentary adults with severe obesity. *Psychol Health Med*, 2013; **18**(6): 714–24.
46. Fenzl, N., K. Bartsch, and J. Koenigstorfer, Labeling exercise fat-burning increases post-exercise food consumption in self-imposed exercisers. *Appetite*, 2014; **81**: 1–7.
47. Culbert, K.M., S.E. Racine, and K.L. Klump, Research review: What we have learned about the causes of eating disorders – A synthesis of sociocultural, psychological, and biological research. *J Child Psychol Psychiatry*, 2015; **56**(11): 1141–64.
48. Bocquier, A., et al., Overweight and obesity: Knowledge, attitudes, and practices of general practitioners in France. *Obes Res*, 2005; **13**(4): 787–95.
49. McConnell, A.R., et al., Forming implicit and explicit attitudes toward individuals: Social group association cues. *J Pers Soc Psychol*, 2008; **94**(5): 792–807.
50. Munt, A.E., S.R. Partridge, and M. Allman-Farinelli, The barriers and enablers of healthy eating among young adults: A missing piece of the obesity puzzle: A scoping review. *Obes Rev*, 2017; **18**(1): 1–17.
51. Thuan, J.F. and A. Avignon, Obesity management: Attitudes and practices of French general practitioners in a region of France. *Int J Obes (Lond)*, 2005; **29**(9): 1100–6.
52. Mogul, A., M.B. Irby, and J.A. Skelton, A systematic review of pediatric obesity and family communication through the lens of addiction literature. *Child Obes*, 2014; **10**(3): 197–206.
53. Sarris, J., et al., Nutritional medicine as mainstream in psychiatry. *Lancet Psychiatry*, 2015; **2**(3): 271–4.
54. Salwen, J.K., et al., Childhood abuse, adult interpersonal abuse, and depression in individuals with extreme obesity. *Child Abuse Negl*, 2014; **38**(3): 425–33.
55. Myles, I.A., Fast food fever: Reviewing the impacts of the Western diet on immunity. *Nutr J*, 2014; **13**: 61.
56. Davis, C., et al., Binge eating disorder and the dopamine D2 receptor: Genotypes and sub-phenotypes. *Prog Neuropsychopharmacol Biol Psychiatry*, 2012; **38**(2): 328–35.
57. Spinella, M. and J. Lyke, Executive personality traits and eating behavior. *Int J Neurosci*, 2004; **114**(1): 83–93.
58. Powell, K., et al., The role of social networks in the development of overweight and obesity among adults: A scoping review. *BMC Public Health*, 2015; **15**: 996.
59. Westermann, S., et al., Social exclusion and shame in obesity. *Eat Behav*, 2015; **17**: 74–6.
60. Watchers, W. You can eat that! 2017 [cited 2017 June 17]; Available from: https://www.weightwatchers.com/util/art/index_art.aspx?tabnum=1&art_id=88341&sc=3025
61. Murdaugh, D.L., et al., fMRI reactivity to high-calorie food pictures predicts short- and long-term outcome in a weight-loss program. *NeuroImage*, 2012; **59**(3): 2709–21.

26 Adaptation of APA Practice Guidelines for SUD to Processed Food Addiction

Carrie L. Willey
Shades of Hope Treatment Center
Buffalo Gap, TX

Joan Ifland
Food Addiction Training, LLC
Cincinnati, OH

CONTENTS

The practice guidelines for the treatment of clients with processed food addiction (PFA) are modeled on the *Practice Guideline for the Treatment of Patients with Substance Use Disorders* published by the American Psychiatric Association (APA) [1]. The structure of topics described here for PFA practice guidelines parallels that of the APA's substance use disorder (SUD) guidelines. Modeling this Chapter on the APA practice guidelines thus follows the concept used in Part II of this textbook, where PFA manifestations are organized and described according to the APA's DSM 5 SUD diagnostic criteria.

The approach of modeling the PFA practice guidelines on the APA SUD practice guidelines was chosen for several reasons. Practitioners may become comfortable with PFA as an SUD when the close parallels between the two syndromes are shown through the PFA guidelines that follow. Practitioners are already aware of SUDs and have already incorporated treatments for SUD clients based on the primary focus of their practices. The parallel with SUD will help practitioners decide how to approach treatment of PFA within the context of their own practice structure. Some practitioners will feel comfortable providing counseling, guidance, and group support if they are already providing those services to drug-addicted clients, eating-disordered clients, or clients who are working to overcome mental, emotional, or behavioral challenges. General practitioners may be most comfortable with brief interventions and referrals. Practitioners focused on treating the metabolic syndrome may provide diet-related counseling for mild cases while referring more severely affected clients who need help with psychosocial comorbidities.

These PFA practice guidelines have been developed by two practitioners who are active in educating about and treating food addiction. In the course of education, the authors have received income related to some of the practices described in the guidelines. The development of these guidelines was not supported financially by any commercial organization.

Because PFA is a young field, much of the evidence supporting the guidelines is adapted from the fields of obesity, eating disorders, SUDs, and nutrition. Parts I and II of this textbook are annotated with this type of research. These guidelines refer back to Parts I and II for detailed evidence supporting the guidelines. Observations were gained from a residential facility, an online training, the food addiction 12-step fellowships, as well as from the popular writings of food addiction practitioners such as Tennie McCarty, Kay Sheppard, Rhona Epstein, Ann Katherine, Natalie Gold, and Joan Ifland.

It is not the intent of the guidelines to be a stand-alone document. Many of the concepts used in the guidelines have been discussed in detail in previous chapters of the textbook. Of importance, Part I of the textbook describes the evidence for abstinent food plans as well as PFA as an SUD with extensive consequences. Discussion of these concepts will not be repeated here. The guidelines thus proceed from the premise that PFA is an SUD and that abstinence from processed food is a practice guideline. Part II of this textbook describes the evidence that chronic overeaters manifest the characteristics of SUD according to the DSM 5 SUD diagnostic criteria. Part II also describes the process of assessment using the Addiction Severity Index (ASI). So these guidelines do not cover diagnosis and assessment. The guidelines proceed from the premise that the practitioner has already conducted a diagnosis and assessment. PFA treatment is aimed at recovering from the DSM 5 SUD manifestations described in Part II.

Similar to the APA's practice guidelines for SUD, these practice guidelines for the treatment of clients with PFA are not intended to serve as a standard of medical care. As the APA guidelines state, a standard of medical care is determined for individuals based on the data available for that client (p. 5) [1]. The PFA guidelines can be expected to change as research generates new findings in the field of addiction to processed foods. PFA is a complex condition, and adherence to these guideline does not ensure a successful outcome for every individual. These guidelines are not exhaustive. PFA can affect individuals broadly and specialized treatment could be needed. Practitioners' decisions about what to include in a recovery plan will depend on the information about comorbidities collected and the services available to the client [2].

26.1 HOW TO USE THE GUIDELINES

The PFA guidelines cover a wide range of material that practitioners can adapt to their own practices. Accordingly, some material will be more useful than other. As described in Part II of this textbook, PFA clients may manifest a wide range of physical, mental, emotional, and behavioral comorbidities. Practitioners will approach these comorbidities with their own range of skills and capabilities. Sources of referral will complement practitioners' own training to give PFA clients the diversity of services they need.

Section II of this Chapter follows on the general treatment principles described in the APA guidelines. It provides a general discussion of the formulation and implementation of a treatment plan as it applies to individual clients. As noted, diagnosis and assessment are not covered here, as they are the subject of Part II of this textbook. The APA's general treatment principles include:

APA SUD Subject Title (p. 8–12) [1]	PFA Adaptation
Goals	26.2.1. The "Goals" section describes abstinence and relapse prevention in PFA.
Assessment	This has been covered in Part II of this textbook.
Psychiatric Management	26.2.2. The "Recovery Management" section lays out areas of treatment such as retention and relapse prevention.
Specific Treatments	26.2.3. The "Specific Treatments" section describes a variety of recovery modalities practitioners may employ to help clients regain functioning.
Formulation and Implementation of a Treatment Plan	26.2.4. The section "Formulation of a Treatment Plan" delineates the elements of a plan to achieve abstinence, adherence, and treatment for comorbidities.
Treatment Settings	26.2.5. The "Treatment Settings" section gives practitioners options for finding help for PFA clients from hospitalization to 12-step groups.
Clinical Features Influencing Treatment	26.2.6. The section "Clinical Features Influencing Treatment" alerts practitioners to characteristics of PFA clients that could inform treatment in a specific direction. These include social, cultural, and personal factors that could be taken into consideration when choosing approaches to and settings for treatment.

Note: PFA, processed food addiction; APA, American Psychiatric Association; SUD, substance use disorder.

26.2 GENERAL TREATMENT PRINCIPLES

Diagnosis and assessment have been covered in Part II of the textbook.

26.2.1 Goals

Goals of treatment may be summarized as keeping the client in treatment long enough to impart skills needed to avoid relapsing and to regain the ability to fulfill functioning in life. These goals are adapted from the APA *Practice Guidelines for the Treatment of Patients with Substance Use Disorders* (p. 17–18) [1].

26.2.1.1 Treatment Retention and Substance Use Reduction or Abstinence

The ideal outcome for a PFA client is abstinence from a broad range of processed food products, as well as harmful use of drugs and alcohol. Processed foods include sweeteners, flour, gluten, excessive salt, dairy, processed fats, and caffeine. See Chapter 6 of this textbook for a discussion of abstinence. PFA clients may find it difficult to accept that broad abstinence is a worthwhile goal, particularly before learning about the consequences of lapsing. Even if abstinence is developed over time by eliminating processed foods sequentially rather than entirely, PFA clients can still begin to realize results from partial abstinence. As they experience results, they can gain the motivation to continue to eliminate groups of processed foods.

Practitioners work with clients to help them identify improvements in physical, mental, emotional, behavioral, relationship, and family functioning. For example, reductions in stops for fast food and substitution of unprocessed meals may be achievable even though complete abstinence is beyond the abilities of the client. The client can feel more energy through the hours following an unprocessed meal and gain motivation. Keeping the PFA client focused on the broad range of benefits while teaching skills to manage availability of unprocessed meals in Westernized environments can help clients maintain enthusiasm for continuing to build their recovery programs.

26.2.1.2 Reduction in the Frequency and Severity of Substance Use Episodes

Reduction in the frequency and volume of consumption of processed foods is a primary goal of recovery from PFA. PFA clients are educated about the risks of exposure to priming substances that can be hidden in foods prepared commercially or even by friends and family. PFA clients also learn to avoid prolonged exposure to food cues and to relationship stressors. In Westernized cultures, PFA clients may be often exposed to high-risk situations where processed foods are openly available [3]. Training in counteracting craving cues with calm therapies can be helpful.

Like drug-addicted clients, PFA clients are at a greater risk of relapse when the following are present:

- The first 4–8 days of withdrawal may exacerbate cravings.
- PFA clients may have been classically conditioned to crave from early childhood due to exposure to commercials for processed foods.
- Processed foods are easily available.
- Processed foods are associated with social, business, and family events.
- PFA clients experience negative affect.
- Emotional life events occur.
- Physical discomfort occurs as a consequence of processed food consumption.
- Due to avoidance of social events and mobility issues, PFA clients may experience unstructured time or boredom.
- PFA clients face daily challenges to adherence to abstinence due to the lack of availability of unprocessed meals in Westernized cultures.

Some PFA clients are at a high risk of relapse because of cuing, availability, relationship sensitivity, and mood disorders. Anticipating the inevitability of lapses can help reduce the stress of lapsing. Practitioners can teach acceptance that lapses are normal, while still working to develop skills to avoid lapsing. This can help practitioner and client alike avoid becoming discouraged when PFA clients who have achieved abstinence relapse under compounded, prolonged cuing. Practitioners can manage lapses by teaching skills to recover from a lapse. Being prepared for a lapse can help halt the downward spiral into despair and further lapses.

26.2.1.3 Improvement in Psychological, Social, and Adaptive Functioning

As can be seen in Part II of this textbook, chronic use of processed foods is associated with a broad range of physical, mental, emotional, and behavioral impairments. In the case of PFA, these impairments may manifest in early childhood. Regardless of age of onset, impairments can adversely impact psychological functioning, family systems, social activities, employment, education, financial security, and general health and well-being. Mobility may be limited by excess adipose tissue, joint pain, depression, and fatigue. The treatment of PFA will commonly include strategies for repairing the consequences of chronic processed food consumption. Practitioners may aid in developing effective coping skills in social situations, self-care, and employment venues. Because processed foods are so prevalent in Westernized cultures, the household members may need to be educated and motivated to support an abstinent lifestyle for the PFA client. As was detailed in Part II, often treatment will need to focus on co-occurring psychiatric or general medical conditions. General well-being is supported by resolution of chronic pain, depression, anxiety, impaired cognition, and impulse control disorders.

26.2.2 Recovery Management

PFA manifests in a broad of range of consequences that may require a variety of treatments. Treatments may vary for any one client over time and involve a variety of practitioners. Recovery management calls for selecting, monitoring, and coordinating components of recovery and making adjustments as needed over time. PFA chronic relapsing clients may need a long-term, at least a year, commitment to a supportive environment such as transitional living or a halfway house where the client is able to experience life's challenges and return to an environment and peers that are supportive of recovery from PFA.

The objectives of managing recovery include the following.

26.2.2.1 Motivating the Client to Change

The techniques used in motivating drug-addicted clients to change can also be used in food addiction. PFA clients can gain motivation by learning about the reasons for change, recognizing the benefit of resolving problems, gaining confidence about changing, and committing to change by choosing among options for first steps. Practitioners can share about the full range of problems identified through the diagnostic and assessment processes. Clients may be unaware of the mental, emotional, behavioral, and physical problems that could be resolved by undertaking recovery. Clients may not have been aware of the consequences of processed food use beyond weight loss. PFA clients may be reluctant to start because of a history of failures with weight loss. Clients may gain confidence about recovery from PFA as a new approach. Learning that meals are simple, quick, and easy to prepare can overcome barriers to start. It is helpful to use an empathetic, collaborative, and supportive approach to examining the client's ambivalence about undertaking what may appear to be another weight-loss attempt. Understanding the client's stage of readiness to change (precontemplation, contemplation, preparation, action, or maintenance stage) allows the practitioner to determine what motivational strategies are most appropriate for the client at that time.

26.2.2.2 Establishing and Maintaining a Therapeutic Alliance with the Client

As the APA practice guidelines for SUD point out, the strength of the therapeutic alliance has been found to be a significant predictor of psychotherapy outcome (p. 30) [1]. Obesity has been shown to be associated with trauma. It has been suggested that obesity is a protective solution to trauma [4]. Trauma resolution has been shown to benefit from a strong therapeutic relationship with the practitioner [5]. This is similar to recovery from drug addiction. As cited in the APA SUD practice guidelines, "being flexible, honest, respectful, confident, warm, and open all contributed to the development of a positive therapeutic alliance. The most effective strategies for developing such an alliance included exploration, reflection, highlighting past therapy successes, providing accurate interpretation, facilitating the expression of affect, and attending to the client's experience" [6].

PFA clients have often suffered ridicule and stigmatization as a result of the collection of adipose tissue on their bodies [7]. The loss of control over eating may have been internalized as lack of willpower, discipline, and moral fortitude. Adverse childhood experiences (ACE) are also associated with obesity [8]. As described in Chapter 16, "DSM 5 SUD Criterion 6: Interpersonal Problems," the obese person can suffer from relationship sensitivity and be adversely affected by criticism. The issue of managing the therapeutic alliance in a client with internalized stigmatization is discussed in more detail in Chapter 25, "Avenues to Success for the Practitioner." Practitioners will find avenues to success through patience, encouragement, education, and empathy. The therapeutic alliance could be productive particularly in terms of helping clients understand that lapsing is normal and that the development of PFA was not the client's fault. Acceptance of lapsing as normal and not a failure could be instrumental in retaining clients in treatment.

26.2.2.3 Assessing the Client's Safety and Clinical Status

Much of the work of assessing the client's safety and clinical status has been described in Part II of the textbook, which describes manifestations of PFA according to the DSM 5 SUD diagnostic criteria and the ASI. Chapter 18 uses the DSM 5 SUD Criterion 8, hazardous use, to describe how food addiction can lead to harmful circumstances. The discussion of hazardous use also informs the assessment conducted in Chapter 22, "The Addiction Severity Index in the Assessment of Processed Food Addiction." For PFA clients, safety can be impaired by accidents related to fatigue and brain fog; falls related to joint dysfunction; interpersonal violence; suicide ideation; consumption of foods that are contaminated, spoiled, too hot, or too cold; caretaker neglect of children; and harmful medical practices. In addition to developing abstinent meals, education and encouragement can focus on not driving while groggy, strengthening exercises, child care, and referrals to medical practitioners who empathize with obesity. Developing protection from abusive relationships is also an issue.

26.2.2.4 Managing the Client's Intoxication and Withdrawal States

Intoxication and withdrawal mostly resolve themselves in PFA similar to marijuana and cocaine. Intoxication may lead to slurred speech, grogginess, and shame.

"Brain fog" may be a barrier to clients obtaining unprocessed meals that support withdrawal from processed foods. Brain fog includes reduced cognition, inability to concentrate or multitask, and loss of short- and long-term memory [9]. Clients may need help with ordering groceries and with organizing a few hours of cooking food in order to have abstinent meals available during withdrawal. Practitioners may review the the List of Unprocessed Foods under Handouts at www.foodaddictionresources.com with clients to help them identify the foods that they like. To avoid exposing clients to the compounded food cuing found in grocery stores, practitioners can help by identifying local grocery shopping services and referring clients to them. Some clients may benefit from having the practitioner even call in the order or show the client how to create an account at the store's website.

Clients should be encouraged to clear their homes of processed foods in preparation for withdrawal. This minimizes the risk that the client would use a processed food to diminish the discomfort of withdrawal. Household members should be educated about what the client is going through and dissuaded from giving the client processed foods. The client's car keys may be put into a timed lock box to prevent the client from leaving the house to get processed foods.

A compassionate attitude also helps success during withdrawal after a lapse. It is compassionate to teach PFA clients to manage the discomfort of withdrawal. Clients may have the idea that increasing the suffering of withdrawal could create a deterrent to relapsing. However, suffering through withdrawal can create a barrier to going through withdrawal after a lapse. Clients could be sick with headache, cravings, fatigue, nausea, depression, grogginess, etc. [10–12]. The value of lapses is that they have built-in negative reinforcement. Practitioners can use this to the client's advantage by acknowledging the symptoms and expressing compassion and empathy. This attitude displays kindness to the client and supports improvements in self-compassion and self-esteem. By associating the distress of withdrawal to lapses, clients can develop a natural aversion to processed foods.

26.2.2.5 Developing and Facilitating the Client's Adherence to a Treatment Plan

This is perhaps the bulk of the practitioner's job. Recovery from PFA is not commonly practiced in the greater culture, which makes finding role models difficult. The practitioner is inveighing against cultural views of PFA as a "weight loss" issue. Clients may have difficulty with learning and remembering tasks stemming from limited cognitive functioning [13]. It is possible that the majority of clients' activities center around processed foods, so they may feel lost without these activities.

There are several keys to adherence. Breaking down skill acquisition into small steps increases the chances of success and gives the client a sense of accomplishment. Education about how the environment influences the brain to crave and lose cognitive functioning while activating stress pathways helps the client avoid thinking that the program is not working at times of lapses. Animal research shows that repeat exposure to processed foods sensitizes stress pathways in the brain [14]. Processed food cues can hijack decision-making and impulse-control functions in the prefrontal cortex [13,15]. Identifying and praising results across the full spectrum of physical, mental, emotional, and behavioral health is encouraging and helps the client avoid confusing recovery with a short-term weight-loss program.

26.2.2.6 Managing and Preventing the Client's Relapse

As compared to recovery from SUD, preventing relapse in PFA recovery is complicated by the proliferation of cues and availability of processed foods in Westernized cultures. More detailed discussion of this problem is found in Chapter 25, "Avenues to Success for the Practitioner." Accidental ingestion is a risk, as food processors may hide addictive ingredients in processed food products. Relationship stressors may be a factor in PFA due to sensitivities stemming from body shame and internalized stigmatization [7]. One study found an average of three stigmatizing events per day per person in an obese/overweight population [16]. The impact of stigmatization is also discussed in Chapter 25, "Avenues to Success for the Practitioner." For PFA clients, relapses can be expected to be a feature of recovery. Practitioners can use lapses to help clients increase determination to follow their abstinent food plans. PFA clients may associate lapses with a painful sense of failure learned from inability to comply with inadequate diet plans, so education about the normalcy of lapses is valuable.

Many of the recommendations described by the APA for relapse prevention in SUD are applicable to PFA. Educating about cues, stress, and processed food consumption can give clients new insight into their eating behavior and reduce the distress of self-blame. Inventorying exposure to food cues can empower clients to make plans to avoid people, places, and things that trigger relapse. A handout for inventorying exposure to triggers is found at http://www.foodaddictionresources.com/handouts.html. Planning for management of high-risk situations through training in social skills can help.

Setting up a plan for recovery from a lapse early in recovery can be helpful. This may involve putting processed foods down the disposal or spraying them with soapy water, making an abstinent meal, logging into an online support community, meditation, exercise, reading recovery literature, etc. Lapses can be used for prevention by letting the client connect particular distress to processed foods. Processed food reactions can be varied. In the event of a lapse, the practitioner can work through the consequences of the lapse based on information gathered through the ASI. In this exercise, the client can develop a natural aversion to processed foods.

26.2.2.7 Educating the Client about PFA

Education about the role of food/media industry food cuing and addictive product formation helps the client heal from self-blame and develop strategies for achieving abstinence from processed foods. Education about the nature of cue reactivity can motivate the client to avoid cues and engage in calming activities. Education about the myriad of health problems can be surprising to PFA clients, who may not have connected negative moods and behaviors to processed foods. Learning that physical distress such as skin problems, chronic infections, and inflammation can improve on an abstinent food plan can be significant motivators to achieve abstinence and avoid lapses. For the purpose of education, the practitioner can review chapters from this textbook and can slowly introduce handouts from http://www.foodaddictionresources.com/handouts.html.

26.2.2.8 Reducing the Morbidity and Sequelae of PFA

Research shows that PFA clients are likely to present with a myriad of health problems. Practitioners will have identified these in the course of diagnosis and assessment. However, PFA clients may have experienced discrimination, ridicule, even emotional abuse from some health providers [17,18]. The experience of discrimination and condescension could have created an aversion to seeking medical care in clients. PFA clients who suffer from internalized stigmatization may not have sufficient self-esteem to care for themselves. Practitioners can be helpful by identifying health providers who are prepared to treat PFA clients with dignity, respect, and sensitivity for the problems associated with obesity. When screening other health providers, practitioners can collaborate on reinforcement of abstinence, cue avoidance, and resumption of social activities. Praise for progress can be a strong motivator for clients to improve self-care.

The resumption of careers and education should be approached cautiously. The stress of assuming a job or school could be a relapse trigger.

Practitioners can track progress toward goals of the treatment plan as a means of encouraging adherence to treatment. As the APA specifies, recovery management could be combined with specific treatments carried out in a collaborative manner with professionals of various disciplines at a variety of sites, including:

- Medical practitioners for management of physical consequences such as diabetes, hypertension, and cardiovascular disease.
- Therapists and counselors for help with ACE, abusive relationships, and self-esteem.
- Residential treatment facilities for clients who are too impaired to start.
- In-person and online self-help groups to provide community and social support. More detail about the provision of support in online communities is provided in Chapter 25, "Avenues to Success for the Practitioner."

26.2.3 Specific Treatments

26.2.3.1 Pharmacological

Limited pharmaceutical therapies are available for PFA itself. Pharmaceutical applications for binge eating have been found to be ineffective [19]. Various side effects such as depression, heart disease, memory loss, etc., are associated with pharmaceuticals to control eating. Current pharmaceutical approaches include orlistat, phentermine/topiramate, and lorcaserin [20]. Lisdexamfetamine dimesylate has been approved by the FDA specifically for moderate to severe bingeing but not for weight loss [19]. However, pharmacological approaches have not been evaluated in controlled long-term studies [21].

One issue to consider is that these drugs may have been prescribed due to the failure of weight-loss regimes or therapies to control eating without the benefit of abstinence. It is possible that control of eating could be accomplished with a PFA recovery approach of abstinence, cue avoidance, cognitive restoration, and support, thus obviating the need for pharmaceuticals.

Pharmacological treatment of psychiatric comorbidities may be warranted [22]. There may be need also for pharmaceutical treatment for physical comorbidities. Practitioners may need to help clients find service providers who are prepared to compassionately and effectively treat obese clients for the consequences of chronic overconsumption of processed foods.

26.2.3.2 Psychosocial

Along with abstinence, cue avoidance, and cognitive restoration, psychosocial interventions are the mainstay of treatment for chronic overeating of processed foods. The goals of psychosocial modules are to increase motivation, coping skills, contingency recovery, positive affect, social support, and interpersonal functioning. Processed foods commonly serve an important function in the life of a PFA client.

Shifting to a life free from processed foods gives PFA clients energy, mental clarity, and emotional stability for developing new behaviors, emotions, thoughts, and relationships.

Psychosocial treatment is at the core of recovery from PFA. PFA clients need frequent support for eating differently from mainstream culture, avoiding cues, managing relationships, and recovering from lapses against a background of internalized stigmatization. They need social skills in order to participate safely in circles where other people are eating processed foods. They need to find new and satisfying activities to fill time previously spent eating and sleeping off processed food use. PFA clients need to manage emotions without the neurological effects of processed foods. And clients need to repair personal relationships that may have suffered under mood swings, body changes, isolation, and dysfunctional eating patterns.

Because of limited applicability of pharmaceuticals to PFA, there is no discussion of the relation of psychosocial treatment to pharmacotherapy for PFA.

Types of psychosocial treatments are discussed below. Research specifically on PFA is lacking. However, there are extensive findings regarding the efficacy of a variety of treatments for weight loss and binge eating.

1. Cognitive behavioral therapies (CBTs) have been shown to be helpful in binge eating, including relapse prevention and social skills training [23]. Self-guided CBT was shown to be effective at reducing binge eating after 4 weeks, more so than interpersonal therapy (IPT) or behavioral weight loss. Improvements were sustained for the long term [24]. An 8-week CBT program was also found to decrease psychological stress in a population of post-op bariatric surgery patients. The program was less helpful with emotional overeating, relationship anxiety, and avoidance [25]. In a randomized comparison of CBT with IPT, both therapies reduced interpersonal problems [26].
2. An uncontrolled pilot study of 5 weekly group sessions and 3 weekly individual sessions showed that motivational enhancement therapy (MET) is effective in weight loss. The study suggested that evaluation of MET combined with other psychosocial treatments needs to be conducted [27].
3. A review article of controlled reduced-calorie dieting, exercise, and behavioral therapy provided in primary care found the approach to be effective at weight loss in a longer-term (12–24 months) program. However, results declined at longer follow-up. All three components of diet, exercise, and counseling were required for efficacy. More sessions correlated with greater weight loss [28]. Cue avoidance has been shown to be effective at diet adherence and improvements in cognition, more so than social pressure [29]. Community reinforcement does not seem to have been evaluated for chronic overeating. In a study of six obese African-American adolescents, contingency management was effective for weight loss when added to behavioral skills training and when caregivers were involved [30]. Mindfulness has also been shown to be effective in control of eating. See Chapter 7 of this textbook. Aversion therapy of a rubber band snapped on the wrist has also been shown to be effective at reducing consumption of junk food [31].
4. Twelve-step facilitation (TSF): Twelve-step groups are available specifically for food addiction. They include Food Addicts Anonymous and Food Addicts in Recovery Anonymous. Practitioners should supply the abstinence list to clients being referred to 12-step groups to assure adequate abstinence. Other 12-step groups such as Overeaters Anonymous, Grey Sheet, and Eating Disorders Anonymous also support recovery from progressed foods. Practitioners should ascertain that cuing of processed foods is not permitted in the meeting. Acceptance of the excluded list and the concept of abstinence from those foods is important. PFA clients may be easily swayed to eat processed foods by members of these groups who do not abstain.
5. In a randomized trial of 95 binge eaters, IPT was shown to be as effective as CBT at reducing incidents of binge eating [26]. In another study, IPT was found to be as effective

as CBT at a 2-year follow-up [32]. A review article made a similar finding [21]. However, other research has shown CBT to be more effective [24]. In light of this evidence, it seems advantageous to attempt CBT first and only use IPT if CBT fails.

6. Self-help programs include purely self-prompted help, self-administered manuals, computer-assisted therapy, professionally assisted correspondence courses, and nonprofit and commercial self-help groups. Self-help has the greatest potential use, given that so many people need treatment. However, the self-help approach has mixed results for weight loss [33] and results are unknown for PFA specifically.
7. Brief interventions are an attractive concept for PFA. Because awareness of PFA is only slowly gaining ground, it is possible that people would be able to stop cravings and regain control solely on the basis of learning about the addictive properties of processed foods. This is similar to the experience with nicotine, where the majority of smokers gradually stopped smoking in response to learning about the harmful effects of tobacco. Some people have meal management skills from having implemented a variety of weight-loss plans and would likely be able to implement a food plan that eliminates processed foods. A brief intervention could consist of sharing information about the addictive properties of processed foods and the food plan for combining unprocessed foods into meals. The handouts are in Section 3 at http://www.foodaddictionresources.com/handouts.html.
8. A review article of practices in the United Kingdom found that case management of lifestyle changes for weight loss is increasingly involving nurses in practitioner's offices. The role of the nurse in the United States is subject to agreement about responsibilities between the practitioner and the nurse. The review article reported mixed results, but the majority were positive for the role of a nurse in helping clients manage lifestyle changes [34].
9. Group therapies have been shown to be helpful in weight management [35].
10. In addition to the treatment modalities listed in the APA practice guidelines for SUD, the adapted guidelines for PFA include cognitive restoration. This is for the reason that the tasks facing PFA clients in recovery, such as meal preparation, cue avoidance, and relationship management, can be complex. Cognitive restoration is increasingly advocated for the treatment of SUD based on improvements in sustained attention and executive control [36]. Cognitive impairment is well established in binge eaters and obese populations [13,37]. Neurocognitive rehabilitation could be implemented with traditional paper and pencil testing or computer-based technology in both inpatient and outpatient settings.

26.2.4 Formulation and Implementation of a Treatment Plan

Although the long-term goals of abstinence, relapse prevention, and improved functioning do not change over time, intermediate goals can change depending on progression in skill acquisition and current demands of life. The specific therapies developed to achieve these goals may vary among clients and even for the same client at different phases of recovery. Because PFA is chronic and cuing in Westernized environments is prevalent, PFA clients may require long-term treatment and lifetime support. Clients benefit from training in identifying increases in the level of risk of relapse in order to increase access to support during those times.

Treatment plans include the following elements:

1. Recovery management as described in Part 26.2.2 of this Chapter
2. Plans for achieving abstinence or reducing the effects of processed foods
3. Strategies to adhere to the treatment program, prevent relapse, and improve functioning
4. Treatment for co-occurring mental illnesses or general medical conditions

The duration of treatment should be tailored to the individual client's needs and may vary from a few months to several years. However, due to the prevalence of cuing and availability of processed foods in Westernized cultures, it is prudent to train clients to access support for a lifetime. It is important to intensify the monitoring of use of processed foods during periods when the client is at a high risk of relapsing, including:

1. During the early stages of treatment
2. Times of transition to less intensive levels of care
3. The first year after active treatment has ceased

26.2.4.1 Managing Abstinence

Managing abstinence includes a strategy for achieving abstinence or reducing the effects or use of processed foods. Clients learn about the challenges of food prep and eating differently from mainstream culture. This topic is covered in Chapter 28, "Insights from the Field."

26.2.4.2 Enhance Adherence and Relapse Prevention

Practitioners work to enhance ongoing adherence with the treatment program, prevent relapse, and improve functioning. In working towards consistent adherence, the client faces challenges of cue avoidance and gradual development of a recovery program to include regular sleep, exercise, and cognitive restoration. More information is provided in Chapter 28, "Insights from the Field."

26.2.4.3 Treat Comorbidities

Additional treatments may be necessary for clients with a co-occurring mental illness or general medical conditions. How each practitioner approaches the treatment of comorbidities will depend on the practitioner's own competencies. The central idea is to assess comprehensively, decide what to treat in-house, and then identify compassionate, capable practitioners for referral.

26.2.5 Treatment Settings

PFA clients may receive care in a variety of settings, although options for care are still limited because PFA is an emerging condition and training for health professionals has been unavailable. For a variety of financial, mobility, body size, and health reasons, many PFA clients are unable to travel, so outpatient and online services may often be the best option.

Treatment settings vary according to the availability of resources such as medical monitoring, specialization of services and therapy, and the availability of psychiatric consultation. The primary purpose of the facility should be a match for the client's most important needs. Needs may be for medical care, education, 12-step support, peer support, or faith counseling. Because treatment best occurs in a system that encourages cessation of a range of processed foods, consideration should be given to whether the facility permits processed food cues or offers processed foods to clients. The intensity of treatment duration/participation can be determined by severity as developed in the diagnostic and assessment processes described in Part II of this textbook.

Typically, PFA clients have not been sentenced to facilities because possession and use of processed foods are not illegal.

26.2.5.1 Choosing a Treatment Setting

Determining a place for treatment can depend on many factors related to the status of the client. These include:

1. The capacity and willingness of the client to cooperate with treatment. Because of the range of processed foods and the integration of processed food use into Western cultures, PFA clients may be unwilling to cooperate in eliminating all addictive processed foods. This may preclude the value of an expensive residential program in favor of treating the client with education and motivation in an outpatient or online setting.

2. The client's ability to care for self. This is a common issue in PFA clients, as they may be caring for family members and struggle to prioritize their own needs. The difficulty arises because these same clients may be unable to take advantage of residential care because of their family commitments. Practitioners may accept that clients who are unable to care for themselves at the initiation of treatment may need a greater emphasis on recovery from codependency in early stage education.
3. The social environment of the client, which may be either supportive or high risk. Supportive home environments where household members are willing and able to avoid cuing the client are good treatment settings for PFA. Households where members are vehemently determined to use processed foods in spite of the client's needs are high risk. To reduce cuing, clients can learn to keep processed foods out of sight and avoid rooms where household members are eating processed foods. These clients need extra support in terms of daily phone calls and online communication with a support group.
4. The client's need for structure, support, and supervision to remain safe and abstinent. PFA clients may have lost the ability to structure their time because they may be watching television, sleeping, or working several low-paying jobs. This is described in Chapter 13, "DSM 5 Criterion 3: Time Spent." However, the difficulty is that clients who need the most structure may be the least able to travel due to the worsening of comorbidities such as excess adipose tissue and joint pain. In the absence of residential treatment, clients may be taught slowly to replace television with healthy activities at the same time that they are developing routines to make abstinent meals.
5. The client may need specific treatments for co-occurring general medical or psychiatric conditions. The consequences of chronic processed food use are significant. In the assessment process, practitioners determine what referrals are needed.
6. There may be a need for particular treatment that may be available only in certain settings. Some PFA clients may need dialysis or they may need protection from a violent partner. The assessment process will generate information for psychiatric and medical care. Detox can generally be accomplished at home if the client can source unprocessed groceries and combine them into abstinent meals.
7. The client may have a preference for a service. PFA clients may already be comfortable with a counselor, 12-step group, or faith partner. Practitioners can adapt these settings to treat PFA by specifying an abstinent food plan.

These factors can also be used to determine where to send a PFA client. The American Society of Addiction Medicine also publishes placement criteria at http://www.asam.org/quality-practice/guidelines-and-consensus-documents/the-asam-criteria. Practitioners can improve retention by educating clients about the broad range of benefits of recovery, by teaching the life skills needed to comfortably live in heavily cued food cultures and by situating clients in empathetic support groups.

26.2.5.2 Commonly Available Treatment Settings and Services

Settings and services used in the treatment of PFA may be considered as points along a continuum of care from most to least intensive. Practitioners should consider the possibility that cognitive impairment may be present in recently detoxified clients when determining where to refer. Consideration of cognitive limitations is important to decisions about care for PFA clients because of the complex recovery tasks of meal preparation, cue avoidance, and relationship management. The choice of a treatment setting may be influenced by availability, given that training in food addiction is spreading and more facilities may become suitable for PFA over time. Certain specialized treatment settings such as dual-diagnosis or intensive outpatient care may be adapted to PFA if the facility can offer support for an abstinent meal plan. For PFA clients, most treatment occurs in outpatient settings. This is similar to nicotine and marijuana treatment. In a treatment program, practitioners may employ counselors, therapists, support groups, and online communities.

26.2.5.2.1 *Hospitals*

Hospitalization for PFA clients is not needed for detoxification but could be needed for comorbidities. The need to treat comorbidities is determined in the assessment process described in Part II of this textbook. Partial hospitalization and intensive outpatient programs are rarely able to accommodate PFA clients. This may change with time and training in the treatment of PFA. Practitioners are more likely to employ residential, outpatient, 12-step, and online programs in the development of treatment plans for PFA clients.

26.2.5.2.2 *Residential Treatment*

Residential treatment is indicated primarily for clients whose lives and social interactions have come to focus exclusively on processed foods. These clients are too cue-reactive or lacking in substance-free environments to remain abstinent in an outpatient setting. The client must be well enough and mobile enough to travel. For these individuals, residential facilities provide a cue- and substance-free environment in which residents learn a range of food management skills for maintaining abstinence and preventing relapse. Similar to SUD programs, residential treatment programs for PFA may provide a comprehensive assessment similar to the ASI; psychoeducation; and training in self-help groups. Help with social or employment needs may be provided in-house or on referral. They typically rely on referring health professionals for aftercare. Residential treatment settings should have access to general medical and psychiatric care for individual needs.

Practitioners will need to ascertain that the facility is capable of providing a fully abstinent food plan and of protecting PFA clients from exposure to processed food cues and availability. Practitioners may ask facilities if the client can be provided meals that are abstinent from the list of excluded foods provided at www.foodaddictionresources.com. Practitioners can evaluate whether the facility is engaged in teaching clients to eat processed foods in moderation, which would disqualify it for treatment of PFA as use in moderation is contrary to the goal of abstinence from processed foods. If the facility is also treating SUDs, it is important to evaluate whether the facility is switching SUD clients to processed foods, such as substituting sugar for alcohol. This practice would also disqualify such a facility for treatment of PFA.

In the APA practice guidelines for SUD, it is specified that duration of residential treatment should be dictated by the length of time necessary for the client to meet specific criteria that suggest successful aftercare. These criteria may include:

- A demonstrated motivation to continue in outpatient treatment.
- The ability to remain abstinent even in situations where processed foods are available. Due to the proliferation of processed foods in Westernized cultures and increased likelihood of lapses, clients may need a plan to recover from a lapse.
- The availability of substance-free living, social, and workplace situations. Due to the prevalence of processed foods, this requirement may be difficult to meet. Practitioners may compromise with an increased risk of lapsing and strategies for recovering from lapses.
- Sufficient stabilization of any comorbidities so that the client can participate in counseling or group support. This may include online support, which the clients can access from a computer or mobile device.
- The availability of adequate follow-up care from therapists, counselors, and support groups, including online support.

26.2.5.2.3 *Therapeutic Communities and Community Residential Facilities*

Although therapeutic communities and halfway houses would seem to be a good fit for PFA, at this time long-term PFA recovery is limited to programs connected to residential treatment facilities. Long-term facilities are available for eating disorders and for recovery from SUD, but these facilities do not seem to be equipped to offer protection from cuing and the availability of processed foods.

They also do not have educational programs aimed at helping clients understand the nature of PFA. Abstinence from processed foods as a means of preventing overeating seems to be gaining acceptance, so the options may be expected to grow in the future.

26.2.5.2.4 Aftercare

Aftercare occurs after residential treatment and generally includes outpatient care and involvement in self-help approaches. Research on aftercare for SUD has examined different treatment models, including eclectic, medically oriented, motivational, 12-step, cognitive behavioral, group, and marital strategies. Given the chronic, relapsing nature of PFA, it is expected that aftercare will be recommended with few exceptions. In fact, as PFA is a chronic rather than an acute disease model, the different elements of care can be conceptualized as part of a continuous, long-term treatment plan.

26.2.5.2.5 Outpatient Settings

Most PFA treatment will take place in outpatient treatment settings. Outpatient treatment is appropriate in circumstances that do not require a more intensive level of care. At this time, treatment for comorbidities, but not for PFA itself, may be found in mental health clinics, integrated dual-diagnosis programs, and primary care clinics. For PFA, treatment will be limited to private practice settings where the practitioner is familiar with PFA practice guidelines. As with all referrals, practitioners should ascertain that the PFA client will receive treatment consistent with recovery from PFA, i.e., support for abstinence from processed foods and cue avoidance.

As in other treatment settings, the optimal outpatient approach is a comprehensive one that includes a variety of psychotherapeutic interventions along with behavioral monitoring. As described above in the section on specific treatments, outpatient treatments for eating disorders with strong evidence of effectiveness include CBT, MET, behavioral therapies, TSF, IPT, self-help, behavioral therapy, brief interventions, case management, and group therapy.

Many specific outpatient treatments have been designed to enhance an individual's participation in treatment and sense of self-efficacy regarding the reduction or cessation of problematic substance use. As in the case of residential and partial hospitalization programs, high rates of attrition can be problematic in outpatient settings, particularly in the early phase (i.e., the first 6 months). Because intermediate and long-term outcomes are highly correlated with retention in treatment, individuals should be strongly encouraged to remain in treatment. Practitioners should also encourage and attempt to integrate into treatment a client's participation in self-help programs where appropriate (see Section II.F.9).

26.2.5.2.6 Case Management

The goals of case management interventions are to provide advocacy and coordination of care and social services and to improve client adherence to prescribed treatment and follow-up care. Although this would be helpful for PFA clients who are homeless, live in homes with intense processed food use, or have co-occurring mental challenges that preclude the ability to prepare abstinent meals, it would be unusual to find a case worker who is trained in PFA recovery. Research shows that nurses are beginning to assume the role of case manager in developing lifestyles conducive to weight management [34].

26.2.5.2.7 Legally Mandated Treatment

Because processed foods are not illegal, legally mandated treatment for PFA is virtually nonexistent.

26.2.5.2.8 Employee Assistance Programs

Employee assistance programs (EAPs) help employees in a workplace setting. At this stage of development of PFA awareness, it is unlikely to find an EAP that provides treatment for PFA specifically. However, treatment for eating disorders may be adapted to PFA by incorporating abstinence from processed foods and cue avoidance.

26.2.6 Clinical Features Influencing Treatment

As suggested in the practice guidelines for SUDs (p. 45), practitioners should consider a number of variables with regard to PFA clients. Incorporating these variables into treatment will improve outcomes by focusing the treatment plan on key issues, which will in turn promote the well-being of the client and motivate the client to adhere to treatment.

26.2.6.1 Use of Multiple Substances

PFA is typically an addiction that incorporates a number of different processed food ingredients. These are discussed in detail in Chapter 6, "Abstinent Food Plans for Processed Food Addiction." Substances include many different sugars and sweeteners, flour, gluten, excessive salt, dairy, processed fats, caffeine, and food additives. The nature of processed food products and meals virtually ensures that multiple ingredients are ingested simultaneously. Chapter 6 provides the evidence for the addictive properties of ingredients and describes how they are combined into commercial products.

Regardless of which processed food combinations are being used, withdrawal is self-limiting and can be managed at home.

The readiness of clients to abstain from the list of addictive foods will vary considerably. Some clients who have a history of implementing weight-loss diets may be comfortable with eliminating all addictive foods and preparing unprocessed foods. Clients who are facing severe consequences may also be at an advanced stage of readiness. Some clients may be willing but lack cooking skills. Other clients may balk at the long list of foods to be eliminated and may need to work toward abstinence over time.

Practitioners can let clients start with the easiest food to eliminate and keep developing the motivation to eliminate more foods as recovery progresses. If clients are unable to give up any of the addictive foods, the practitioner can start with skill acquisition in other areas. Useful skills include preparation of unprocessed meals, cue avoidance, relationship management, mindfulness, exercise, etc. Clients who are too overwhelmed to start anywhere are candidates for residential treatment.

The ASI also surfaces information about substances that the client may be using for weight control. These may include nicotine, cocaine, amphetamines, laxatives, and diuretics. Practitioners can diagnose for the presence of SUD related to these addictive substances and treat according to the practice guidelines for SUD.

26.2.6.2 Comorbid Psychiatric and General Medical Conditions

PFA is associated with a wide range of physical, mental, emotional, and behavioral issues [38]. These are described in detail in Part II of this textbook. The descriptions of comorbidities are organized according to the DSM 5 SUD diagnostic criteria. Comorbidities are important to address, as they can impair the client's ability to prepare abstinent meals, avoid food cues, and manage relationships. As practitioners work through the DSM 5 SUD diagnostic criteria, they will discover a range of health issues. These issues help the practitioner complete the ASI, as shown in Chapter 22. The ASI can also surface helpful information about the treatment priorities of the client. Incorporating the client's preferences for the sequencing of treatment into the treatment plan can aid in motivating the client to undertake recovery.

As clients achieve abstinence, they are likely to report relief from the mood disorders discussed in this section. The practitioner can monitor improvements in mood, mental health, and behaviors. As the health problems resolve, the practitioner can use these benefits to motivate the client to adhere more closely to the treatment plan. In a synergistic pattern, the client will also be more capable of adhering to the treatment plan due to improvements in energy and cognitive functioning.

26.2.6.2.1 Psychiatric Factors

As described in Part II of this textbook, there is a high prevalence of comorbidity of PFA and other psychiatric disorders. Practitioners may not be able to distinguish the psychiatric impact of processed foods from the effects of other factors until the client has completed withdrawal and achieved comprehensive abstinence. Comprehensive abstinence is elimination of foods on the excluded list found at www.foodaddictionresources.com. The rate of resolution of PFA-related disorders has not been researched. Clinical observations suggest that the rate of improvement can vary from a few months to several years. Clients should be monitored closely for changes in medication. Specific treatment of comorbid disorders should be provided. According to the APA Practice Guidelines for SUD, in addition to pharmacotherapies specific to the client's general condition, various psychotherapies may also be indicated when a client has:

1. A co-occurring psychiatric disorder
2. Psychosocial stressors
3. Life circumstances that exacerbate PFA
4. Life circumstances that interfere with treatment

26.2.6.2.1.1 Risk of Suicide Practitioners should be aware that suicide is a risk for PFA populations. A study conducted in Germany found that 33% of obese women and 13% of obese men had engaged in suicidal behavior that did not result in a successful attempt [39]. A 10-year follow-up study of bariatric surgery clients found a substantial increase in the rate of suicide in this population [40].

26.2.6.2.1.2 Risk of Aggressive Behaviors, Including Homicide *Homicide* is not an issue in obese populations. A study of homicides found that the obese were underrepresented in that population, dying rather of natural causes. The study suggested that this might be due to the protective nature of adipose tissue and the relative isolation of obese people [41]. Exposure to violence has been found to predict BMI in the transition from adolescence to young adulthood [42]. Detailed discussions of violence may be found in Chapter 18, which describes hazardous use under DSM 5 SUD Diagnostic Criterion 8.

26.2.6.2.1.3 Sleep Disturbances Sleep problems are common in PFA clients and contribute to excessive caloric intake [43]. Clinical observations are that sleep improves on an unprocessed food plan. Possible explanations include improvements in hormones, metabolism, and inflammation [44].

26.2.6.2.1.4 Co-Occurring Psychiatric and PFA It is beyond the scope of this document to describe treatment of psychiatric disorders that co-occur with PFA. The reader can find such descriptions in the APA's practice guidelines for SUD (pp. 51–66) [1]. Schizophrenia, depressive, dipolar disorder, anxiety, attention deficit hyperactivity disorder, personality disorders, and pathological gambling can co-occur with PFA. These conditions may improve during recovery from processed food use due to recovery from the inflammatory nature of processed foods as well as improvements in nutrition.

26.2.6.2.2 Comorbid General Medical Disorders

The metabolic syndrome is associated with chronic use of processed foods. Chapter 4, "Sugar Consumption: An Important Example Whereby Recognizing Food Addiction May Prove Important in Gaining Optimal Health," describes the consequences of sugar and salt use. Practitioners can evaluate whether they can treat comorbidities or need to refer to specialists based on information discovered through the diagnostic and assessment processes.

Like drug-addicted clients, PFA clients may suffer from malnutrition [45]. A study conducted by the International Food Policy Research Institute found that obesity was related to increasing rates of malnutrition [46]. This issue will be mitigated when the client has organized meal preparation.

Adequate general medical care for PFA clients is complicated by a lack of development of procedures specific to care of the obese and by weight-based discrimination by some health-care providers.

A review article found that many health-care providers hold strong negative attitudes regarding obesity and that this can affect decision-making and care [47].

Elimination of processed food use may also be associated with changes in the metabolism of medications. Doses may need to be adjusted based on changes in weight status, blood pressure levels, blood glucose levels, etc.

26.2.6.2.3 *Pregnancy*

Poor diet and depression in obese woman has been shown to result in emotional dysregulation in their young children [48]. Rat studies have shown that offspring of junk-food–eating dams show a preference for junk food [49]. Practitioners should educate pregnant clients about the dangers of processed foods during pregnancy and lactation.

26.2.6.2.4 *Gender-Related Factors*

Women have been found to crave more than men [50]. This may be related to increased exposure to food cues. Male clients may have more challenges in sourcing unprocessed meals. They may lack meal preparation skills, and their partners may resent having to make special meals for them. Practitioners will want to carefully assess the home dynamic of food preparation regardless of gender. Education of family members about the harmful consequences of processed food use as well as methods for simple meals will help.

26.2.6.2.5 *Age*

Treatment related to food-addicted children are covered in Chapter 24, "Food-Addicted Children". This chapter is an adaptation of the APA's practice guidelines for SUD in children.

Obesity rates among the elderly are predicted to rise from 32.0% in 2000 to 37.4% in 2010 [51]. The elderly may be challenged to source unprocessed food; however, they may be motivated by education regarding the possibility that their age-related health problems could be helped by an unprocessed food plan. For example, fatigue and depression may be ascribed to aging but actually be associated with processed foods. The elderly are entitled to the same education as any client. Practitioners will need to carefully assess the capabilities of the elderly client and work with caregivers if the client is motivated to change. However, it may also be the case that the capabilities of elderly clients have diminished so significantly that processed foods may have become the most rewarding aspect of their lives [52]. Their caregivers may not be able to deny elderly clients their pleasures.

26.2.6.2.6 *Racial, Ethnic, and Cultural Factors*

Research shows that obesity is disproportionally prevalent in disadvantaged populations. Convenience, mood, family, and availability of food at home, but not nutrition, were salient factors guiding meal and snack planning in a low-income population in Pennsylvania [53]. This population may benefit from education about the low cost of healthy foods. Media campaigns claiming that it's too expensive to eat healthy may have dissuaded this population from preparing healthy foods.

26.2.6.2.7 *Gay/Lesbian/Bisexual/Transgender Issues*

A study conducted in England found that gay/lesbian/bisexual/transgender (LGBT) populations have a poorer health status in general {Elliott, 2015 #9859}. A study of data taken from the Massachusetts Youth Risk Behavior survey of adolescent sexual minorities showed more body dissatisfaction and dangerous weight control practices in that population as compared to heterosexual youth {Hadland, 2014 #9860}. It is important to assess LGBT clients carefully.

26.2.6.2.8 *Family Characteristics*

Practitioners will need to assess families for their vulnerability to processed foods {Sigman-Grant, 2015 #3922}. Neglect and abuse have been shown to correlate with the development of obesity in adults {Felitti, 1998 #9833}.

26.2.6.2.9 Social Milieu

Practitioners can ask about work, social, and entertainment settings to evaluate unavoidable exposure to cues. Online groups can provide noncuing virtual environments where clients can socialize without fear of stigmatization or cue exposure. These resources may be found at www.foodaddictionresources.com.

26.3 CONCLUSION

This chapter has given practitioners an overall view of how approaches to recovery from PFA are similar to those of other SUD such as alcoholism and drug addiction. Practitioners are aiming for similar goals of abstinence and recovery from the comorbidities of a substance-based addiction. Similar techniques and treatment structures are suggested. Practitioners will bring their own skills and experiences to the recovery process while referring clients for needs which are outside their own competencies. Above all, this chapter serves to demonstrate that PFA is a serious addiction which needs comprehensive treatment.

REFERENCES

1. American Psychiatric Association, *Practice Guidelines for the Treatment of Patients with Substance Use Disorders*. 2006, American Psychiatric Association: Washington, DC.
2. Kleber, H.D., et al., *Practice Guideline for the Treatment of Patients with Substance Use Disorders*, A.P. Association, Editor. 2006, American Psychiatric Association.
3. Lifshitz, F. and J.Z. Lifshitz, Globesity: the root causes of the obesity epidemic in the USA and now worldwide. *Pediatr Endocrinol Rev*, 2014. **12**(1): p. 17–34.
4. Felitti, V.J., et al., Obesity: problem, solution, or both? *Perm J*, 2010. **14**(1): p. 24–30.
5. Pearlman, L.A. and C.A. Courtois, Clinical applications of the attachment framework: relational treatment of complex trauma. *J Trauma Stress*, 2005. **18**(5): p. 449–59.
6. Ackerman, S.J. and M.J. Hilsenroth, A review of therapist characteristics and techniques positively impacting the therapeutic alliance. *Clin Psychol Rev*, 2003. **23**(1): p. 1–33.
7. Ratcliffe, D. and N. Ellison, Obesity and internalized weight stigma: a formulation model for an emerging psychological problem. *Behav Cogn Psychother*, 2015. **43**(2): p. 239–52.
8. Van Niel, C., et al., Adverse events in children: predictors of adult physical and mental conditions. *J Dev Behav Pediatr*, 2014. **35**(8): p. 549–51.
9. Theoharides, T.C., et al., Brain "fog," inflammation and obesity: key aspects of neuropsychiatric disorders improved by luteolin. *Front Neurosci*, 2015. **9**: p. 225.
10. Sharma, S., M.F. Fernandes, and S. Fulton, Adaptations in brain reward circuitry underlie palatable food cravings and anxiety induced by high-fat diet withdrawal. *Int J Obes (Lond)*, 2013. **37**(9): p. 1183–91.
11. Iemolo, A., et al., Withdrawal from chronic, intermittent access to a highly palatable food induces depressive-like behavior in compulsive eating rats. *Behav Pharmacol*, 2012. **23**(5–6): p. 593–602.
12. Colantuoni, C., et al., Evidence that intermittent, excessive sugar intake causes endogenous opioid dependence. *Obes Res*, 2002. **10**(6): p. 478–88.
13. Voon, V., Cognitive biases in binge eating disorder: the hijacking of decision making. *CNS Spectr*, 2015. **20**(6): p. 566–73.
14. Moore, C.F., et al., Pathological overeating: emerging evidence for a compulsivity construct. *Neuropsychopharmacology*, 2017. **42**(7): p. 1375–89.
15. Houben, K., C. Nederkoorn, and A. Jansen, Eating on impulse: the relation between overweight and food-specific inhibitory control. *Obesity (Silver Spring)*, 2014. **22**(5): p. E6–8.
16. Seacat, J.D., S.C. Dougal, and D. Roy, A daily diary assessment of female weight stigmatization. *J Health Psychol*, 2016. **21**(2): p. 228–40.
17. Matharu, K., et al., Reducing obesity prejudice in medical education. *Educ Health (Abingdon)*, 2014. **27**(3): p. 231–7.
18. deShazo, R.D., J.E. Hall, and L.B. Skipworth, Obesity bias, medical technology, and the hormonal hypothesis: should we stop demonizing fat people? *Am J Med*, 2015. **128**(5): p. 456–60.
19. Reas, D.L. and C.M. Grilo, Pharmacological treatment of binge eating disorder: update review and synthesis. *Expert Opin Pharmacother*, 2015. **16**(10): p. 1463–78.

20. Bray, G.A., Medical treatment of obesity: the past, the present and the future. *Best Pract Res Clin Gastroenterol*, 2014. **28**(4): p. 665–84.
21. Wilson, G.T., Treatment of binge eating disorder. *Psychiatr Clin North Am*, 2011. **34**(4): p. 773–83.
22. Merlo, L.J., K. Wandler, and M.S. Gold, Co-occurring addiction and eating disorders, in *The ASAM Principles of Addiction Medicine*, R.M. Ries, M.C. Shannon, D. Fiellin, R. Saitz, Editors. 2014, pp. 529–534. American Society of Addiction Medicine: Washington, DC.
23. Agras, W.S., et al., One-year follow-up of cognitive-behavioral therapy for obese individuals with binge eating disorder. *J Consult Clin Psychol*, 1997. **65**(2): p. 343–7.
24. Hilbert, A., et al., Rapid response in psychological treatments for binge eating disorder. *J Consult Clin Psychol*, 2015. **83**(3): p. 649–54.
25. Beaulac, J. and D. Sandre, Impact of a CBT psychotherapy group on post-operative bariatric patients. *Springerplus*, 2015. **4**: p. 764.
26. Tasca, G.A., et al., Outcomes of specific interpersonal problems for binge eating disorder: comparing group psychodynamic interpersonal psychotherapy and group cognitive behavioral therapy. *Int J Group Psychother*, 2012. **62**(2): p. 197–218.
27. Fioravanti, G., et al., Motivational enhancement therapy in obese patients: a promising application. *Obes Res Clin Pract*, 2015. **9**(5): p. 536–8.
28. Wadden, T.A., et al., Behavioral treatment of obesity in patients encountered in primary care settings: a systematic review. *JAMA*, 2014. **312**(17): p. 1779–91.
29. Bennett, G.A., Cognitive rehearsal in the treatment of obesity: a comparison against cue avoidance and social pressure. *Addict Behav*, 1986. **11**(3): p. 225–37.
30. Hartlieb, K.B., et al., Contingency management adapted for African-American adolescents with obesity enhances youth weight loss with caregiver participation: a multiple baseline pilot study. *Int J Adolesc Med Health*, 2015. **29**(3): p. 7.
31. Abramson, E.E. and D. Jones, Reducing junk food palatability and consumption by aversive conditioning. *Addict Behav*, 1981. **6**(2): p. 145–8.
32. Wilson, G.T., et al., Psychological treatments of binge eating disorder. *Arch Gen Psychiatry*, 2010. **67**(1): p. 94–101.
33. Latner, J.D., Self-help in the long-term treatment of obesity. *Obes Rev*, 2001. **2**(2): p. 87–97.
34. van Dillen, S.M. and G.J. Hiddink, To what extent do primary care practice nurses act as case managers lifestyle counselling regarding weight management? A systematic review. *BMC Fam Pract*, 2014. **15**: p. 197.
35. Schwartz, D.C., et al., A substance called food: long-term psychodynamic group treatment for compulsive overeating. *Int J Group Psychother*, 2015. **65**(3): p. 386–409.
36. Rezapour, T., et al., Perspectives on neurocognitive rehabilitation as an adjunct treatment for addictive disorders: from cognitive improvement to relapse prevention. *Prog Brain Res*, 2016. **224**: p. 345–69.
37. Yau, P.L., et al., Preliminary evidence of cognitive and brain abnormalities in uncomplicated adolescent obesity. *Obesity (Silver Spring)*, 2014. **22**(8): p. 1865–71.
38. Guh, D.P., et al., The incidence of co-morbidities related to obesity and overweight: a systematic review and meta-analysis. *BMC Public Health*, 2009. **9**: p. 88.
39. Wagner, B., et al., Extreme obesity is associated with suicidal behavior and suicide attempts in adults: results of a population-based representative sample. *Depress Anxiety*, 2013. **30**(10): p. 975–81.
40. Tindle, H.A., et al., Risk of suicide after long-term follow-up from bariatric surgery. *Am J Med*, 2010. **123**(11): p. 1036–42.
41. Omond, K.J., N.E. Langlois, and R.W. Byard, Obesity, body mass index, and homicide. *J Forensic Sci*, 2016. **62**(4): p. 930–33.
42. Clark, C.J., et al., Dating violence, childhood maltreatment, and BMI from adolescence to young adulthood. *Pediatrics*, 2014. **134**(4): p. 678–85.
43. Galli, G., et al., Inverse relationship of food and alcohol intake to sleep measures in obesity. *Nutr Diabetes*, 2013. **3**: p. e58.
44. Panossian, L.A. and S.C. Veasey, Daytime sleepiness in obesity: mechanisms beyond obstructive sleep apnea—a review. *Sleep*, 2012. **35**(5): p. 605–15.
45. Wells, J.C., Obesity as malnutrition: the dimensions beyond energy balance. *Eur J Clin Nutr*, 2013. **67**(5): p. 507–12.
46. Gulland, A., Malnutrition and obesity coexist in many countries, report finds. *BMJ*, 2016. **353**: p. i3351.
47. Phelan, S.M., et al., Impact of weight bias and stigma on quality of care and outcomes for patients with obesity. *Obes Rev*, 2015. **16**(4): p. 319–26.

48. Pina-Camacho, L., et al., Maternal depression symptoms, unhealthy diet and child emotional-behavioural dysregulation. *Psychol Med*, 2015. **45**(9): p. 1851–60.
49. Gugusheff, J.R., Z.Y. Ong, and B.S. Muhlhausler, The early origins of food preferences: targeting the critical windows of development. *FASEB J*, 2015. **29**(2): p. 365–73.
50. Hallam, J., et al., Gender-related differences in food craving and obesity. *Yale J Biol Med*, 2016. **89**(2): p. 161–73.
51. Arterburn, D.E., P.K. Crane, and S.D. Sullivan, The coming epidemic of obesity in elderly Americans. *J Am Geriatr Soc*, 2004. **52**(11): p. 1907–12.
52. Murray, S., C. Kroll, and N.M. Avena, Food and addiction among the ageing population. *Ageing Res Rev*, 2014. **10**(9): p. 540–52.
53. Stotts Krall, J. and B. Lohse, Interviews with low-income Pennsylvanians verify a need to enhance eating competence. *J Am Diet Assoc*, 2009. **109**(3): p. 468–73.

27 Preparing Adults for Recovery

Joan Ifland
Food Addiction Training, LLC
Cincinnati, OH

Robin Piper
Turning Point of Tampa
Tampa, FL

CONTENTS

This chapter describes a process for preparing adults to undertake recovery from processed food addiction (PFA). In prior chapters, readers learned about the model describing PFA as a substance use disorder (SUD), how to approach PFA with compassion, and what skills PFA clients need to build their recovery. With this background, readers now have the foundation to start helping PFA clients organize for recovery.

Preparing PFA clients for recovery is described in two phases.

1. Motivation
2. Organizing the client to receive support online via the Internet and over mobile devices

As is the case with any addiction, food-addicted clients can benefit from a process of motivational interviewing before starting treatment. As discussed in prior chapters, PFA clients may be taught that they can access treatment via websites and social media, over their computers, or from their mobile devices. These topics are covered in this section.

27.1 PHASE I: MOTIVATING ADULTS

Like addicts in general, food addicted clients need to be encouraged and educated before they may be ready to undertake change. This section reviews the process of motivation. Practitioners can help clients develop motivation by explaining that recovery from PFA is a new approach based on new research showing addictive adaptations in the brain related to processed foods. Regardless of how many times the PFA client has failed using a "weight loss" approach, developing a PFA recovery program can succeed.

Motivation is organized into:

- Learning about reasons for change
- Recognizing problems and benefits of resolving problems
- Gaining optimism and confidence about changing
- Committing to change through development of options (Donovan, 2013)

Often, the first barriers a PFA client faces is shame about past failure to lose weight. It may help the PFA client to explain how PFA is provoked by the food industry and why the problem is not the fault of the client. In the process of diagnosing and assessing as described in Part II of the textbook, practitioners have collected information about how PFA has manifested in the client's life. With this information, clients learn how to define the problem of PFA in their own lives by identifying behaviors described in the DSM 5 SUD diagnostic criteria. Identifying a broad range of benefits can be an effective motivator. The practitioner can also reduce barriers by going over any concerns that the client has about their ability to make changes. Talking about solutions can give clients the confidence that they will be successful and allow them to move forward. Giving clients options while explaining the value of each option will help clients make the commitment to try at least one activity. By dwelling on education and encouragement, the practitioner can increase the likelihood that clients will stay the course and recover.

Clients will present with a set of problems that have brought them into treatment. They will have an idea of why they want to change. By building a base of knowledge about PFA, clients can develop a broad base of understanding of the value of a program of recovery, perhaps beyond their initial goals. In this way, they can broaden their definition of the problem. By sharing examples of how clients have managed to change their food and avoid cues, the practitioner can help instill confidence in the client. By breaking down the process into options for small steps to begin, the practitioner can bring the client to the point of committing to take action. Of course, in all instances, the practitioner is using a collaborative tone to avoid directing or pushing the client.

27.1.1 Learning about Reasons to Move Forward and Change

Although clients may benefit broadly from physical, mental, emotional, and behavioral improvements, food-addicted clients are likely to come into treatment with a goal of weight loss or cessation of distressing eating patterns. Their framework for change may be one primarily of finding the right diet to achieve weight loss or stop bingeing. The practitioner may probe to find out how committed the client is to this view to gauge how much education might be needed to shift the client to framing the problem as one of PFA rather than just excess adipose tissue. This will guide the practitioner in educating the client about the nature of PFA as a behavioral health care challenge with extensive consequences.

Practitioners may find it helpful to introduce the client to three handouts that can help shift the client to a broader perspective:

- "Weight-Loss Schemes Can Make PFA Worse"—This handout helps clients understand what has happened such that their loss of control may have worsened.
- "How Long Will It Take to Recover?"—This handout helps clients visualize the long-term benefits of recovery as opposed to a short-term weight-loss approach.
- "Why PFA Is Hard to Recover From"—This handout helps clients understand that past failures at weight loss were possibly the result of a mismatch between problem and program rather than a personal failing.

These handouts are available from www.foodaddictionresources.com. As the client begins to reframe the problem from weight loss to recovery from PFA, the client will be able to also redefine the solution from a "diet" to a need to eliminate addictive foods and avoid triggers while working to restore cognitive function. This is a significant shift away from a goal of weight loss that could bring relief and hope to the client across a range of distressing problems.

Grounding the client in the addiction framework will also give the client reason to try again regardless of discouragement from failed attempts. The practitioner can explain that past attempts might have failed for a number of reasons:

- The food plan had addictive foods that stirred up cravings.
- Insufficient calories and hunger may have made cravings worse.
- Avoidance of food cues and stress was not sufficient to stop cravings.
- Not enough acquisition of positive recovery-focused behaviors to help stop disordered eating.

Armed with this knowledge, PFA clients may be persuaded to ascribe failure to the weight-loss framework rather than their own shortcomings. The relief from self-blame may allow the client to reduce fear of failure, move forward, and undertake a new approach.

The client may benefit from a broader perspective on the problem. Practitioners may do well to review the mental, emotional, and physical problems associated with processed food use and the risks associated with overwhelming cravings that lead to chronic overconsumption of processed foods. It may also be beneficial to educate clients about the addictive properties of sugars, gluten, excessive salt, processed fat, dairy, and caffeine. Practitioners can use the handout "Excluded Foods" from www.foodaddictionresources.com to teach clients about the types of addictive foods.

Practitioners can particularly emphasize the connection between addictive foods and the painful obsession that food-addicted clients endure. This can encourage the client to hope for relief from the obsession through abstinence, cue avoidance, and cognitive restoration. The hope for relief from mental obsession can be a surprisingly effective motivator.

Normalizing clients' experiences can be helpful. It helpful to let clients know they are not alone, they are not weird, and obsession is a normal part of addiction for any addicted person. Clients are likely to respond favorably to reinforcement that there is nothing inherently wrong with them and that they are suffering from an addiction.

Clients may not realize that it's even possible to stop cravings and obsession. They may think that they have to live with cravings and this belief may drive the fear of giving up processed foods.

It could also be helpful to review information about the impact of commercial practices as they provoke cravings. This information may be effective at helping to persuade the client that chronic overeating is not their fault. Rather, the neuroscientists employed by the food industry have trained brains to react to food and stress cues with intense cravings. These are the cravings that lead to loss of control. Cues to crave include:

- Provocative food advertising
- Product formulation to circumvent satiation
- Unrealistic body ideals that invite negative self-comparison
- Harmful diet advice that can intensify cravings through hunger
- Deceptive labeling to claim healthy benefits
- Food industry influence in government (Avena, Potenza, & Gold, 2015; Lindberg, Dementieva, & Cavender, 2011; McLaren et al., 2014; Morris, Beilharz, Maniam, Reichelt, & Westbrook, 2014)

Without understanding causality, the PFA client may remain stuck in fear of failing at another weight-loss attempt. By realizing potential causes of overeating and loss of control, clients may see a reason to change their frame of reference from simple weight loss to comprehensive addiction recovery. This helps create motivation by reducing fear of failure. Letting clients know they are not alone can be an effective approach to getting motivated for change and engagement in recovery.

27.1.2 Problem Recognition

The practitioner works with the client to focus on the aspects of the problem that are most relevant to the client. In this phase, the practitioner can review the results of any diagnostics and assessments such as conformance to the DSM 5 SUD diagnostic criteria and the Addiction Severity Index. For this purpose, the handout "DSM Diagnostic Criteria" will be helpful. The practitioner can present a comprehensive picture of the physical, mental, emotional, and behavioral characteristics of the disease and consequences as they are manifesting in the client. Clients may be aware of these problems and feel helpless to resolve them. Finding out that a range of problems could be addressed in a recovery program could bring meaningful relief to a PFA client. Knowing that most of the issues they are facing could be addressed in a comprehensive program could be very motivating.

As the practitioner pulls together a comprehensive picture of the problem, it is important that clients be consistently assured that they did not cause the problems. This reassurance is to prevent guilt, shame, and self-stigmatization (Palmeira, Pinto-Gouveia, Cunha, & Carvalho, 2017) from creating a barrier to recovery. The practitioner can reemphasize the role of commercial and emotional triggers in creating PFA and assure the client that overeating and consequences are not their fault (Cohen & Farley, 2008).

In defining the problem, the practitioner can focus on the problem of triggers that lead to cravings for processed foods and loss of cognitive abilities for the individual client. This can include the primary role of addictive foods but can also cover anxiety and stress, particularly as it comes from relationships, extreme emotions, and fatigue. The practitioner can offer training in ways to neutralize triggers so they don't progress to overeating. The client can get a picture of the scope of the triggers as a cause of overeating from the handout "Trigger Avoidance Checklist" at http://www.foodaddictionresources.com/handouts.html.

Many food-addicted clients do not associate their food use with financial issues. So the practitioner can review not just the problem of spending on volumes of processed foods but also losses associated with abandoned education, missed opportunities to be promoted, accepting low-paying jobs, and even the possibility of job loss due to processed food use.

The practitioner may also want to include the impact of a parent's PFA on children in the household. If weight problems as well as mood, behavioral, learning, or physical problems have manifested in children, the parents may be motivated to make changes to help their children.

Defining the problem as an addiction with consequences serves to explain past struggles, encourage the client to undertake a new approach, and give the client new hope for a rewarding life. It also provides clients with the opportunity to get in touch with the emotional consequences of their addiction in themselves and those they love. This takes the focus off losing weight and perceiving PFA as purely a physical problem. Framing the condition as an addiction puts recovery in the emotional and spiritual realms.

27.1.3 Optimism and Confidence about Change

In this phase of motivation, the practitioner is working to surface and address the client's fears about eliminating processed foods from their diets. To allay fears of failure, the practitioner can assure clients that the program is easy when broken down into small steps. Practitioners can teach clients that food preparation can be as simple as filling a Crock Pot, or frying ingredients, or assembling a baking tray for the oven. Often food-addicted clients have cooking skills from years of food obsession, so the practitioner can emphasize the transferability of these skills. Clients who work full-time can be assured that they can prepare their food for the week in a few hours on the weekend. A video available at Amazon.com for the United States can help show clients how to do this (https://www.amazon.com/Victory-Over-Food-Addiction-Meals/dp/B00HKVA55M/ref=sr_1_1?s=instant-video&ie=UTF8&qid=1475105480&sr=1-1&keywords=food+addiction).

Because the client is likely to have limited financial means, practitioners can review pricing of such food items as rice and beans as compared to fast food meals. The practitioner can offer fees on a sliding scale that could be adjusted when expenditures on processed foods have lessened or the client becomes well enough to work. This addresses another common fear—affordability of recovery.

Another concern may be about eating differently from household members or having to cook different meals for them. The practitioner can assure that client that changes can be brought about peacefully by slowly educating household members about the consequences of processed foods at the same time as providing unprocessed foods that they already like. Baked chicken, steak, shrimp, pork chops, rice, and beans are foods that many people like regardless of their fondness for processed foods. At http://www.foodaddictionresources.com/handouts.html, practitioners will find the handout "Unprocessed Foods." Clients can be encouraged to see how many of those foods their household might enjoy.

Clients may also be worried about enduring withdrawal. Withdrawal management can be accomplished by whatever topical methods are most comfortable. Fortunately, the acute phase of headache, fatigue, and cravings seems to be fairly short at 4–8 days. Hot and cold compresses, lots of rest, water, meditation, and movement are all helpful in managing the symptoms of withdrawal. Group support can also be helpful in successfully completing withdrawal. The practitioner can give clients the handout "Managing Withdrawal," found at http://www.foodaddictionresources.com/handouts.html. Caffeine withdrawal can be postponed for several months. The rationale for this is that caffeine withdrawal can last 2–3 weeks and involve protracted headaches and fatigue. This may be overwhelming to a newly recovering food addict. The symptoms of caffeine withdrawal may also mask the relief of finishing withdrawal from processed foods.

By talking through common concerns about starting a recovery program, the practitioner can move the client through barriers to change. Fear of failure, time and energy commitment, household reactions, and withdrawal can all be overcome through reassurance and the development of specific strategies.

27.1.4 Commitment to Change

In this phase, the practitioner can remind the client of the complex personal, family, and social forces that work to create overeating. The client can consider how difficult, if not impossible, it would be to successfully address chronic overeating without ongoing education, strategy development, and a sympathetic support group. Clients seem to respond favorably to the idea that they can carry out the process very slowly. They can take their time in thinking about what steps they're ready to take. Practitioners can assure clients that they can start the treatment program by achieving abstinence from processed foods gradually. The idea that the program is structured in small steps can enhance motivation. The practitioner can describe smaller or alternative first steps that could help improve brain function and make managing food more possible. Lapses are understood to be normal and are not considered to be a failure. If food preparation seems overwhelming, the practitioner can offer exercise, meditation, prayer, crafts, and music to reduce stress, improve mood, and increase energy in preparation for tackling food preparation.

Practitioners may consider requiring clients to contact prescribing health professionals to find out how to adjust medications in the event that underlying diet-related conditions improve.

Giving the client options to gradually undertake the easiest, most natural aspects of building a program of recovery makes a pathway for the client to proceed.

27.2 PHASE II: PRACTITIONER PREPARATION FOR OFFERING SERVICES ONLINE OR BY MOBILE DEVICE

This section is for practitioners who want to add an outreach component to their practice. It is also useful for practitioners who plan to conduct their practice over Internet, phone, text, and email functions. Practitioners start by identifying the Internet platform they wish to use. Facebook is an easy platform to use and many food-addicted clients are already familiar with how to access it. After creating a secret group e.g., the practitioner can add clients to it. If the practitioner chooses Facebook, the secret group format is recommended for reasons of confidentiality.

- For practitioners who are using Facebook, it is important to upload files as part of setting up the secret group. These include food lists and a food plan as well as lists of triggers, recovery activities, and a recovery cost–benefit check list. Or practitioners can use the handouts at www.foodaddictionresources.com.
- If using the Facebook platform, practitioners may also want to create small chat groups on focused topics such as budget, plant-based, faith, sleep, volunteering, and family/children.
- Practitioners can recommend books that can be found at www.foodaddictionbooks.com.
- Practitioners may find it easiest to set up a recurring, sliding payment function at PayPal. (www.paypal.com).
- Given the severity of PFA, practitioners may want to consider a daily conference call with clients. Clients may encounter difficulties with different types of triggers from home, work, and public environments. Being able to review stressors and release them on a daily basis can improve outcomes. Conference call facilities provide for recording calls, which makes replays available any time. A sample of a conference call company is found at www.instantteleseminar.com.
- Alternatively, practitioners can check in with clients using a periodic email blast. Daily would be optimal. Practitioners choose the most appropriate email provider and develop a client email database.

27.3 PHASE III: CLIENT PREPARATION FOR ACCESSING SERVICES ONLINE OR VIA MOBILE DEVICE

It is fairly easy to guide clients through the process of accessing services online or by mobile device.

- Help the client establish an account at whichever Internet platform or email service that the practitioner has selected. This could include Facebook, Gmail, or a texting function.
- Establish affordable, comfortable recurring payments through PayPal or defer payments until the client can undertake a job again.
- Train clients in taking pictures of their meals to upload to the Internet or attach to emails.
- Load conference call dial-in number and access code into phones.
- Establish accounts at a brain-training site such as Lumosity or Elevate.

27.4 CONCLUSION

This section has described the processes of motivating and preparing clients for recovery from PFA. The process of motivation includes defining the problem as one of addiction and shifting away from weight loss to reduce fear of failure. It also involves describing a range of physical, emotional, mental, and behavior benefits from recovery. Resolving clients' concerns about barriers to starting helps the client move forward.

Identifying services to be delivered online and by mobile device is another step in preparing to provide PFA recovery services. The practitioner can use Internet sites, telephone conference calls, text, or email. Once the practitioner has decided on which outreach platforms to use, the client can be guided through the process of accessing those platforms.

REFERENCES

Avena, N. M., Potenza, M. N., & Gold, M. S. (2015). Why are we consuming so much sugar despite knowing too much can harm us? *JAMA Intern Med, 175*(1), 145–146. doi:10.1001/jamainternmed.2014.6968.

Cohen, D., & Farley, T. A. (2008). Eating as an automatic behavior. *Prev Chronic Dis, 5*(1), A23.

Donovan, D. M. (2013). Evidence-based assessment: Strategies and measures in addictive behaviors. In B. S. McCrady & E. E. Epstein (Eds.), *Addictions: A Comprehensive Guidebook*, pp. 311–351, Oxford: Oxford University Press.

Lindberg, M. A., Dementieva, Y., & Cavender, J. (2011). Why has the BMI gone up so drastically in the last 35 years? *J Addict Med, 5*(4), 272–278. doi:10.1097/ADM.0b013e3182118d41.

McLaren, I. P., Dunn, B. D., Lawrence, N. S., Milton, F. N., Verbruggen, F., Stevens, T., … Leknes, S. (2014). Why decision making may not require awareness. *Behav Brain Sci, 37*(1), 35–36. doi:10.1017/S0140525X13000794.

Morris, M. J., Beilharz, J., Maniam, J., Reichelt, A., & Westbrook, R. F. (2014). Why is obesity such a problem in the 21st century? The intersection of palatable food, cues and reward pathways, stress, and cognition. *J Neurosci, 58*, 36–45.

Palmeira, L., Pinto-Gouveia, J., Cunha, M., & Carvalho, S. (2017). Finding the link between internalized weight-stigma and binge eating behaviors in Portuguese adult women with overweight and obesity: The mediator role of self-criticism and self-reassurance. *Eat Behav, 26*, 50–54. doi:10.1016/j.eatbeh.2017.01.006.

28 Insights from the Field

Joan Ifland
Food Addiction Training, LLC
Cincinnati, OH

H. Theresa Wright
Renaissance Nutrition
East Norriton, PA

CONTENTS

When considering the wealth of materials that would be appropriate for informational and support programs, it is useful to bring to mind the multiple goals of recovery from processed food addiction (PFA). From a neurological standpoint the goals are to reduce cue reactivity and restore cognitive functions. From a lifestyle standpoint, the goals are to establish an orderly pattern of eating while slowly reintegrating the client into healthy relationships, both with food and people. In terms of general well-being, the goal is to heal physical, mental, emotional, and behavioral disorders. Given the broad devastation of PFA, programs can be rich in a variety of educational topics.

Because PFA is a relatively young concept, no research has been conducted in the efficacies of treatment. However, practitioners in the fields of dietetics, counseling, and therapy, as well as 12-step groups, have been practicing recovery from PFA since the 1980s, using the tools of abstinence from processed foods and healing of emotional distress [1–4]. In this chapter, two practitioners with a combined 50 years of experience share their insights into how to help PFA clients.

The material can be divided into two categories:

1. Orientation to basic knowledge and skills
2. Building a healthy lifestyle

The orientation covers five basic skills. These include:

1. Basic knowledge of the symptoms of PFA as well as the broad consequences of the disease.
2. Food management abilities such as shopping, cooking, storing, and meal assembly.
3. In Westernized cue-dense cultures, the ability to avoid triggering is crucial to success.
4. For some PFA clients, cognitive restoration is important.
5. Clients should know how to identify children who might have PFA.

Because the orientation covers extensive information, clients whether new or established can benefit from repeated exposure to this basic knowledge.

Many topics are appropriate for the section on building a healthy lifestyle. Clients may be dealing with novelties on many fronts. These may be cause for celebration but also require new skills and reassurance. Clients may not have ever experienced physical health. They may be adjusting to the realization that their problems are not only genetic but also environmental. If they have been overweight for their whole lives, the transition to a normal weight can bring on memories of childhood trauma and lifelong weight-loss struggles. Even release from long-term medications for diabetes, high blood pressure, or heart disease can benefit from discussion in support groups. The professional who teaches emotional stability can bring new awareness of how to enjoy a daily routine where chaos has been the norm. Newfound behavioral control may bring the client to a desire to interact positively with their children and partners. There are many skills to be learned around the issue of protecting a recovery program against insistent or ignorant people in the client's life. Clients need ideas for how to spend the time formerly given up to television and fatigue. Artistic talents may be resurrected. Even abandoned careers and educations may be dusted off and renewed. The list goes on and on.

Whatever method practitioners choose to be in touch with their clients, whether by in-person sessions, an electronic device, text, email, or daily call, there is no end to the recovery material that clients will enjoy and benefit from.

28.1 ORIENTATION MATERIALS FOR ADULTS

Skills can be acquired through webinars, posts in an online group, emails, conference calls, texts, and in-person meetings.

The list of skills has been developed from listening to food addicts talk about the challenges to building recovery and the nature of relapse. Needed skills have also been identified from research about cognitive impairment associated with chronic processed food use [5,6]. These skills are designed to help food addicts thrive by understanding PFA, securing reliable unprocessed meals, avoiding exposure to food cues and stress associated with relapse, and actively restoring brain function. If children are in the household, there are also skills associated with teaching caregivers how to protect them from PFA. This topic is covered in Chapters 29 and 30.

28.1.1 Recognizing PFA

By understanding the symptomology, clients may also come to a deeper level of acceptance about the nature of the disease and the unlikelihood that their overeating has some other cause. Thereby, clients may develop a deeper commitment to completing the program.

In this section, clients learn to recognize the symptoms described in the DSM 5 addiction diagnostic criteria. This can help clients discern when symptoms might be returning. The client can also derive motivation and satisfaction from watching the symptoms disappear. The 11 DSM criteria can be incorporated into a daily program over 11 consecutive days, or perhaps 1 day per week for an 11-week program. By the end of the segment, clients should know how many criteria they met while active in the disease, how many criteria have faded, and how many criteria clients may still be meeting as they progress through the program. To facilitate this process, practitioners may use the handout "DSM Diagnostic Criteria" from www.foodaddictionresources.com.

Clients also learn to recognize the connection between processed foods and a wide range of diseases. Absorbing this material helps the client in several ways. It helps the client defend against minimization of the consequences of use. It also helps the client value the program. And it helps motivate clients as they manifest benefits of the program. If clients don't know that various illnesses are associated with processed foods, they lose the opportunity to develop a deeper commitment to the process.

By the end of this section, clients should know that PFA results from specific brain dysfunction, particularly cued-craving reactivity and loss of cognitive function. Based on this understanding, clients can become comfortable with the purpose of recovery as stabilizing the brain and reducing cue reactivity, while restoring cognitive functions. This is great progress away from thinking that the primary goal of the program is weight loss.

Practitioners may want to access the handout at www.foodaddictionresources.com titled "Diet-Related Diseases" to find those associated with processed foods.

The material in this section can be complex and overwhelming to clients. Repeatedly reviewing the nature of the brain dysfunction and the array of diseases associated with processed foods allows the client to gradually absorb the material. Then clients can use the information to reinforce their determination to stick with recovery as they associate painful conditions with lapses. This is especially important in obesogenic environments, where it is not generally recognized that even small quantities of processed foods can result in a variety of illnesses.

28.1.2 Conquering Basic Food Shopping and Preparation

In this section, clients learn how to secure a steady supply of unprocessed meals and snacks without overexposure to relapse cues. The scientific foundations of the food plan are discussed in Chapter 6, "Abstinent Food Plans for Processed Food Addiction," and may need adjusting for clients' medical conditions. Of great value to the process will be the ability of the practitioner and fellow group members to share pictures of the meals that clients are making. The practitioner can ask clients to bring digital pictures of their meals to in-person sessions. Pictures may be attached to emails and texts, or they may be uploaded to a platform such as Facebook. Pictures make learning much easier for clients who may be suffering from cognitive impairment. Cognitive impairment may make learning from a printed page challenging, while a picture can bring the desired meal to mind easily.

Regardless of how pictures are delivered, the practitioner is looking to see if meals meet three criteria within the limitations of each client:

1. The four basic elements of the meal are present, i.e., protein, starch, fruit/vegetable, and fat.
2. The meal excludes addictive processed foods while including the unprocessed foods. The handouts for the lists of unprocessed and excluded foods, as well as "Brief Food Plan," "Breakfast Variations," and "The Difference between Food and Drugs," can all be downloaded and copied from www.foodaddictionresources.com. Periodic review of the lists will help clients expand the variety of foods enjoyed and avoid allowing addictive foods to creep into food plans.

3. The correct portion sizes.
   a. For breakfast, 6 ounces of protein (or 3 eggs, 6 ounces of starch, 6 ounces of fruit/vegetable, and 2 teaspoons of cold-pressed oil or fat).
   b. For lunch and dinner each, 4 ounces of protein, 7 ounces of vegetable, 6 ounces of starch, and 2 teaspoons of cold-pressed oil or fat.
   c. For snack, it's 2 ounces of protein and 6 ounces of fruit/vegetable.
   d. Men need 2 ounces of extra protein at each meal and snack.

Clients who are grazers and clients who have had weight-loss surgery may need to divide meals in two and eat each meal in two sittings. Practitioners will find that clients are able to achieve these meals slowly, over time. It may take months for a client to achieve consistent portions. Practitioners can work with clients on the other five key skills, with the expectation that restoring cognitive function will eventually enable the food addict to undertake meal preparation. Some clients may not be able or willing to measure foods because measuring is a trigger to restrict calories or could trigger fear of not enough food. For these clients, the pictures will be especially helpful.

The final skill sought in meal preparation is scheduling. Clients may go through stages of struggling to pull meals together on a daily basis. After some period of time, they may gradually realize that they need to spend a few concentrated hours on free days cooking proteins and starches and assembling ingredients into meal containers. Pictures of such efforts can help individuals by creating a sense of normalcy and routine around the weekly task.

So the client develops skills in assembling meals, which includes learning the difference between addictive and nonaddictive foods, portion sizes, and the elements of a meal. The client learns to avoid highly stimulating commercial food environments. And finally, clients learn how to carve out a few hours in their week in which to prepare ingredients for the week. The use of digital pictures of meals facilitates the process significantly.

Periodically, practitioners can review the food plan with clients to bring details to memory.

1. The food plan
   a. What is a starch?
   b. What is a protein?
   c. What are low-sugar fruits?
   d. What are fats?
   e. What are vegetables?
2. Shopping routines
3. Cooking and storage routines
4. Barriers to eating on time
5. Time management
6. The importance of eliminating availability of addictive foods in the home, workplace, car, driving routes, etc.
7. Safety of children

28.1.3 Gaining Protection from Relapse Triggers

As in all addictions, relapse is a constant risk. In PFA, the risk may be elevated due to unavoidable exposure to food cues. Another factor that may affect food addicts disproportionately is the risk of stress of interpersonal interactions. Relationship sensitivity has been shown to be high in food addicts due to unfair criticism of weight issues. At the same time, the PFA client needs to negotiate with household members around the issue of processed food cues and availability in the house. Relapse is a very normal occurrence in early stage recovery because it's unrealistic for clients to obtain skills fast enough to prevent exposure to overwhelming triggers.

This section covers four basic categories of skills needed to minimize the risk of relapse. They include:

1. Relationship management
2. Avoidance of environmental triggers
3. Management of triggers in the home
4. Counteracting unavoidable exposure to cues

Five handouts on these topics can be found at www.foodaddictionresources.com; they include "Trigger Avoidance Checklist," "Availability is a Problem," "Counteracting Craving Cues," "Food Cue Management for Households," and "Recover from a Cravings Flare-up."

As can be seen, the skills needed to successfully manage relapse triggers is extensive for food addicts. At the same time, cognitive ability may be compromised. Emotional management skills may also have been diminished by the addiction. Practitioners can encourage clients to accept the nature of the disease. It is important to frame lapses as normal to avoid having clients frame lapses as failure with concomitant stress.

28.1.3.1 Managing Relationships

Practitioners will certainly have tools to offer clients in this area. For food addicts, a few handouts found at www.foodaddictionresources.com could help. The handout "How to Live with Imperfect People" describes skills that clients can use to avoid upsets from relationships. Unlike therapy groups, it can be argued that in early stage recovery, clients should be protected from confrontations with fellow addicts in group settings. Food addicts may be too sensitive to recover from perceived slights, criticisms, or just comments about them. At the same time, addicts in the early months of recovery may have mood swings that make them prone to outbursts. For these reasons, practitioners may want to adapt the guidelines found in the handout "Rules of the Road," which prohibit criticisms of fellow group members. Practitioners will certainly have their own methods for helping clients move through upsets. One suggestion is the handout "Eight Healing Questions," but there are many such tools. Clients will also appreciate the handout "What to Say to Food Pushers."

28.1.3.2 Avoiding Environmental Cues

In Westernized environments, learning to avoid processed food cues is a huge job. Because cues are so prevalent, clients will need to develop their trigger avoidance program over time. A handout that offers a roadmap for this journey is "Trigger Avoidance Checklist." When clients have inventoried the sizeable number of cues to which they're exposed, they may begin to understand why it's been so difficult to maintain a recovery program. The handout may be downloaded and copied from www.foodaddictioneducation.com.

The "Trigger Avoidance Checklist" handout is also useful to help clients determine why they have lapsed and to give them the motivation to develop routines that shield them from triggers. Tying triggers to lapses will help reduce confusion about where relapse originates. This is useful in helping clients to reduce self-blame for lapses.

A challenging task is to persuade the client to avoid grocery stores and restaurants in the pursuit of food. These environments are intensely cueing even for short periods of time. It's possible that cues in grocery stores are a cause of relapse in food addicts. In early stage recovery, clients can be encouraged to find shopping services, order and pick up from the parking lot, or ask others to do the shopping. Taking a list at a time when the store is not busy are two helpful suggestions. They can also look for smaller local grocery stores that might be less stimulating and easier to manage in a shorter time.

Food cues in the home may be the most difficult to reduce and yet at the same time may be the most provocative. Clients can use the following tasks to reduce food cuing in the home. All handouts are available to download and copy from www.foodaddictionresources.com.

1. Clients can educate household members with the handout "Diet-Related Diseases."
2. Clients can ask household members to circle the unprocessed foods they like from the handout "Unprocessed Foods." Clients can help to keep processed foods out of the house by supplying unprocessed foods that family members like.
3. Clients can also educate household members with two handouts, "Availability Is a Problem" and "Food Cue Management for Households."

28.1.3.3 Counteracting Food Cues with Cues to Calm

Because of the inevitability of encountering food cues, it is useful for clients to go through a process of associating cues, particularly nonfood smells, with calming activities. With the availability of a smell cue associated with calming activities, the client stands a good chance of being able to counteract exposure to prolonged, compounded cueing for processed foods in commercial, entertainment, family, social, and business environments.

For instructions on how to develop a cue to calm, practitioners may download and copy the handout "Counteracting Craving Cues" from www.foodaddictionresources.com. The handout walks clients through the process of associating a craft, music, meditation, prayer, or reading with a nonfood smell and a calm place. The place serves the purpose of retreat, which has been cued for calm in the event of a cravings flare-up. Clients are also shown how to use a calming routine to neutralize stress in advance of a high-risk event.

28.1.3.4 Other Trigger Management Topics

Practitioners can draw on their own backgrounds in therapy and counseling to help clients develop these capabilities.

1. Planning for social events, finding fun things to do
2. Risk management plans including meditation
3. Establishment of routines to avoid triggers
4. Brain-stabilizing activities such as exercise, meditation, crafts, etc.
5. Increasing vigilance during holidays

28.1.4 Cognitive Restoration

In this section, clients are given suggestions to help restore learning, decision-making, memory, and restraint. The handouts available at www.foodaddictionresources.com include "Three One-Minute Meditations," "Why Exercise?," "Brain Training," and "Affirmations."

Four methods of cognitive restoration are suggested. With the handouts, clients can learn the evidence behind exercise, sleep, mediation, and brain training in the role of cognitive restoration. Clients seem to be motivated by the goal of cognitive restoration. Reviewing the evidence for the role of exercise, sleep, meditation, and brain training with clients helps to reinforce the belief that these activities will yield valuable capabilities. Clients may want to go back to school, try for promotions, or resume careers, all of which are obviously facilitated by a functional brain. Client concerns about avoiding the development of dementia and Alzheimer's can serve as effective motivators.

In encouraging exercise, practitioners can also use pictures to help clients normalize a routine. Clients can be encouraged to take pictures of their exercise venues. If they exercise outside, they can take pictures of interesting sights along the way. Food addicts are challenged to sleep through the night. So practitioners may offer strategies for managing wakefulness during the night. These may include avoiding turning on screens, avoiding getting out of bed, and queueing recorded meditations before sleep to be played in the event of waking up. Cues to go to bed may be provided by text, automated calls, or emails. Clients can be educated about the restorative function of meditation to discourage giving up on sleep and getting up at night during a bout of restlessness.

Food addicts may suffer from attention deficit disorder, which can make meditation difficult. Practitioners may want to limit meditations to 1 minute. Practitioners can teach clients to ground themselves by using their senses to identify five things they can see, hear, smell, then touch in the room. Then, what are five things that they feel. They can observe an object, a room, or their own breath for 1 minute. This can be done periodically throughout the day.

Clients seem to readily accept and enjoy brain training, which is designed to improve cognitive functions such as learning, decision-making, memory, and restraint. There is evidence for the restorative abilities of www.Lumosity.com [7,8].

28.1.5 Awareness of PFA in Children

It may seem odd to include information about protecting children in basic skill acquisition for food addicts. Indeed, for the food addict with limited capabilities, this material should perhaps wait until clients are firmly established in their own recovery. However, the problem of children who are overly exposed to processed foods [9] can be viewed as a responsibility of the entire society and not just the parents of the child. It may be argued that in the extenuating circumstances of an epidemic of childhood obesity [10], cognitive impairment [11], and the metabolic syndrome in increasingly younger children [12], it is responsible to give clients at least a passing knowledge of the conditions of children as they relate to processed foods.

A thorough exploration of addicted children follows in Chapter 30. That material will help practitioners guide people who have presented with addicted children. In the current section on basic skills and education, the practitioner can limit comments to these brief points.

1. Children might put themselves in danger to obtain processed foods. These might include crossing a busy street to reach a store. A child might use a hot stove dangerously. Children may also be tempted to climb up to high cabinets to reach processed foods.
2. With patience, even picky eaters can be transitioned to unprocessed foods. This may involve waiting a few weeks after introducing unprocessed foods for the sense of taste to be restored after exposure to concentrated sweet tastes. This may also involve making new foods an adventure or a game for children.
3. Research shows cognitive impairment in obese children. Parents can work with children to restore cognitive function.
4. Children can be taught to say, "No, thank you," to adults who offer them processed foods.
5. Children may be exposed to prolonged, compounded, harmful cues for processed foods in school and caregiving environments.
6. People who provide child care can be trained in how to protect children in their charge from processed foods and cues for processed foods.
7. Other topics include
   a. Strategies for transitioning children to clean food.
   b. School-friendly lunches and snacks
   c. Educating children's caregivers and teachers
   d. Boundaries with relatives such as grandparents

The orientation materials are extensive. Because of compromised capabilities, food addicts need a lot of time, encouragement, and repetition to master the six basic skills for recovery from PFA. Food addicts will come to treatment with a range of preexisting skills, knowledge, understanding of disease consequences, cooking, trigger avoidance, cognitive abilities, and awareness of PFA in children. Practitioners can build programs to match their clients' abilities.

28.2 BUILDING A HEALTHY LIFESTYLE

Even while clients are being introduced to orientation material, they can begin to be exposed to more general topics related to a healthy lifestyle. Given the vast array of dysfunction associated with chronic overeating of processed foods, practitioners can draw helpful material from a variety of recovery backgrounds. To track progress, clients can review the handout "Food Addiction Cost/Benefit Checklist" found at www.foodaddictionresources.com. The topics listed below can be used in any order. Practitioners can schedule materials based on their perception of client needs in general or for specific guidance.

28.2.1 Daily Routines

Many food addicts need time and patience to develop daily routines. This is a worthwhile effort as routines can boost adherence to healthy recovery activities. The practitioner can prompt clients through standing channels of communication that clients can access throughout the day. To prompt and reinforce daily routines, automated texting, emailing, conference calls, or posts on the Internet can be used. Where comfortable, practitioners can set the example by communicating about their own meals, exercise, sleep, meditation, etc.

Meals Meals can be scheduled 4–5 hours apart. The snack can be scheduled into any stretch between meals. Barriers to eating meals on time may include not enough time, poor planning, poor prioritizing, work conflicts, lack of preparation, or the demands of family care. Clients may need to be taught to plan their day with enough time to prepare meals, eat, and clean up. Clients can be encouraged to make meals the night before. Clients may be so busy with children or jobs that they eat late. If late evening or nighttime eating is still occurring, clients may not have an appetite for breakfast. Chronic undereaters may struggle with wanting to eat at all. One approach is to encourage client to prepare all of their meals and snacks the night before. Clients can be trained to prepare the bulk of their week's food in a few hours over the weekend. See https://www.amazon.com/Victory-Over-Food-Addiction-Meals/dp/B00HKVA55M/ref=sr_1_1?s=instant-video&ie=UTF8&qid=1473634312&sr=1-1&keywords=food+addiction for an Amazon video that guides food addicts through meal preparation over the weekend.

Exercise Practitioners can offer clients options for exercise that will meet their lifestyles and physical capabilities. Clients may present with joint problems, which would be accommodated by seated exercises. Seated exercise videos can be found at www.youtube.com. Food addicts who have been ridiculed or accosted on the street may be reluctant to walk outdoors. Walking videos for indoors can also be found at www.youtube.com. For example, Leslie Sansone produces free walking videos at www.youtube.com with trainers who are appropriately dressed. Walking has been shown to stop cravings more than other forms of exercise. Yoga is another good form of exercise, especially stretches that are done on the floor. Water aerobics may also appeal to some clients. Clients should be encouraged to find activities that they enjoy. It is recommended that clients avoid gyms, which can trigger unfavorable body comparison as well as harmful faddish weight-loss advice from trainers.

Sleep Food addicts may struggle with establishing healthy sleep routines. They may be accustomed to staying up late to eat. They may wake up due to low blood glucose. They may have difficulty falling asleep as the result of caffeine use or elevated adrenaline levels. They may also be dehydrated. Clients need to drink enough fluids early enough in the day that they are neither dehydrated nor getting up during the night to urinate.

Healthy sleep is essential to brain health, so the practitioner may want to provide support for three activities in particular: (1) bedtime routine of snack, soothing reading or writing; (2) a healthy time to go to bed; and (3) use of recorded meditation, soothing audio material, or bedside writing materials that will help the client stay in bed for 7–8 hours even if they wake up.

The bedtime prompt may come by an email or text. It could be posted on the Internet on Facebook, or even a preprogrammed telephone call could be helpful. This is another area where the practitioner can take the lead. In the morning, clients can report how many hours they were able to rest and whether they used a recording to stay in bed. A group of helpful sleep-inducing recordings have been made by the Honest Guys at www.youtube.com. Clients should be discouraged from opening phone, computer, or television screens if they wake up during the night. Light from screens may prompt the brain to believe that it's daytime and encourage wakefulness as a result.

Prayer and Meditation Another restorative daily routine is at least a few minutes of prayer or meditation, possibly with a prayer partner by phone in the morning. One-minute meditations can be surprisingly calming to a food addict. Books about mindfulness and meditation may be found at www.foodaddictionbooks.com. The handout "Three One-Minute Meditations" can be downloaded and copied from www.foodaddictionresources.com.

Resolution of Emotional Triggers It is important to include a method to resolve strong emotions on a daily basis. This is due to findings that emotions are a leading cause of relapse and food addicts are sensitive to relationship issues [13,14]. Practitioners can encourage clients to report daily on any emotional upsets through one of the communication channels described above. Clients should choose a method to work through strong emotions. Although some practices advocate letting the client sit with emotions (rather than eat over the emotion), this would seem to be counter-indicated, given that stress been shown to be a leading cause of overeating [15]. Processing and resolving issues from the past may decrease the triggers to overeat [16,17].

Stress Management It is possible that PFA has progressed in the food addict in response to unmanaged stress [18]. Reviewing stress levels periodically, if not daily, will help clients reduce this source of relapse. Techniques to reduce stress through more generous scheduling, deletion of excessive activities, the addition of more helpers, or boundary setting with people can all help.

Service A routine of service can be very helpful to recovery. Clients can be encouraged to use standing channels of communication to support other members of the practice.

Conference Calls As part of the outreach component of a practice, health professionals may want to set up a conference call facility through a website such as www.instantteleseminar.com. The calls can be arranged independently of the practitioner's participation by scheduling clients to lead the call. The following agenda is suggested:

a. A friendly greeting from the practitioner or leader to each client. It's possible that no one has asked these clients about their day. So a simple inquiry can bear good results in terms of letting the client know that someone is interested in their well-being. They also may be able to refrain from acting out during the day if they know they can talk about a problem during their check-in.
b. A short meditative reading.
c. The leader may pick a topical reading. Readings may follow any of the themes described in this section. Or clients may pick readings that address concerns of the moment.
d. The leaders discusses the reading.
e. Open the call for discussion. Because of the telephone format, the leader may want to keep the meeting orderly by calling on participants to share. The leader can go down the list of callers in the order that they joined the meeting, making clear that anyone can pass.
f. Close the meeting with closing statements or a one-word check-out by each participant.
g. No cross talk except by the leader. Criticisms are not allowed to avoid triggering relationship sensitivities.
h. Confidentiality is protected.

28.2.2 Assessment of Progress

Food addicts can find reassurance and motivation from periodic assessments of their progress. Practitioners can use the DSM 5 diagnostic criteria to track the remission of addictive behaviors and consequences. The Addiction Severity Index may also be used for this purpose to track improvements in physical, emotional, mental, and behavioral well-being. An inventory of recovery from diet-related diseases can also be a powerful motivator. Handouts for tracking can be found at www.foodaddictionresources.com.

28.2.3 The Difference between Recovery from PFA and Weight Loss

Food addicts may come into recovery with a long history of futile attempt to lose weight. The glamor industry, which idealizes media figures who could be considered to be at an unhealthy low weight, also promotes negative self-comparison in food-addicted populations. Health professionals and family members may have judged the food addict harshly for their failure to control their weight. As the result of these numerous factors, addicts may have developed crippling self-loathing. Addressing the origins and fallacies of weight-loss failure can bring healing to food addicts as they understand that failing to lose weight was not their fault.

It is valuable to dwell repeatedly on the reasons why weight-loss schemes cannot work as a primary goal of treatment. In a PFA model, brain function takes priority. The cessation of cravings and the restoration of cognitive functions are the gateway to weight loss. Practitioners can cover the six following topics in the effort to shift clients from a weight-loss model to an addiction recovery model.

Self-Forgiveness Food addicts can be taught about the role of intense cueing for food cravings practiced by the food industry through advertising, cheap prices, availability, and focus on a very young market. They can understand that their weight-loss "failures" were not their fault, but rather the fault of misguided programs. Food addicts can restore self-esteem through education about the influence of an obesogenic environment.

Avoiding the Scale Food addicts can be triggered into intense emotions that could lead to relapse from stepping on the scale. The scale is associated with the negative feelings associated with weight gain and failure of weight loss. Thus the scale can be deeply ingrained as a symbol of self-loathing. In recovery from PFA, the scale can continue to be a source of pain. Food addicts may be coming into recovery with depleted bone and muscle mass. They may have dehydration issues. In recovery, especially with the addition of exercise, clients may add significant weight from bone density, muscle development, hydration, and even the growth of organs from adequate nourishment.

So it's possible that the scale will not move, which could actually cause a client to quit the recovery program. Nonetheless, fat loss can be a source of encouragement and motivation. One method for managing this conundrum is to encourage the client to just squeeze a skin fold. Using this method, the client can feel the fat disappearing from the skin fold and at the same time feel muscle building and firming beneath the skin.

Dangers of Weight-Loss Schemes Throughout recovery, clients will be bombarded with enticements to return to the diet/weight-loss markets. It is helpful to teach food addicts about the dangers of the weight-loss market in terms of making PFA worse. Cravings can intensify under programs that encourage people to eat addictive foods, undereat, become malnourished, undergo inappropriate surgery, and/or take medications with harmful side effects. A handout, "'Weight-Loss' Schemes can Make Food Addiction Worse," describes the effects of weight-loss schemes on food addicts. The handout can be downloaded from www.foodaddictionresources.com.

Cultural and Media Body Distortions Food addicts may suffer from comparing themselves unfavorably to the distorted body images found in media. Severely underweight media figures such as actors and models may be engaging in disordered eating in order to achieve the underweight ideal. It is helpful to food addicts to understand the nature of the distorted body images so they can release themselves from the "failure" of attaining those silhouettes.

Disengagement from Weight-Loss Mentality In order for food addicts to move on in their lives without the depression associated with disordered eating, it is helpful for them to disengage from the urge to look for the next weight-loss scheme. Avoiding media outlets such as television, glamor, men's, and women's magazines will help with this effort.

Repair of Body Image This can be a deliberate effort on the part of the practitioner. Positive affirmations such as, "I have a great body right now," or, "I am super comfortable in my body," can help. References to images of women through art history can help clients see that modern media has severely distorted the ideal, possibly to support the diet industry.

28.2.4 Relationship Normalization

Relationship normalization is surprisingly crucial for long-term recovery from PFA. As seen in the description of Criterion 6 of the DSM 5 SUD diagnostic criteria in Part II, stress emanating from interpersonal relationships can a leading cause of relapse. Fortunately, food addicts gain emotional control, confidence, optimism, and a positive outlook in recovery from the example of the practitioner as well as the kindness of group members. This is one of the many reasons that practitioners may want to keep a positive, complimentary, generous tone to their programs. As clients internalize this positivity, they can employ it in rebuilding relationships. A review of DSM 5 Criterion 6 will familiarize the practitioner with the many relationship issues faced by addicts.

1. *Interpersonal Relationships as Relapse Triggers* Clients can benefit from early realization that relationships are a relapse trigger. Practitioners can equip clients with means of releasing strong emotions originating in relationships. Describing the incident in a post or email can help. Including a set of questions that help clients resolve an upset can also help.
2. *Codependency* The codependency literature can yield guidelines for PFA in their quest to disengage in harmful behaviors of people around themselves. The website www.foodaddictionbooks.com offers several of Melody Beattie's works.
3. *Healthy Reconnection* It is possible that the entire family of the PFA client has suffered from the ill effects of processed foods on mood and behavior. Low self-esteem expressed as criticism may have damaged relationships. As clients absorb the positive attitude of the practitioner and fellow clients, they will be able to extend more positive attitudes toward people in their lives.
4. *Sexual Relations* For a range of issues, clients may have avoided sex. As they become more comfortable with themselves and their bodies, they may want to engage in sex again. Practitioners can help them reengage slowly and respectfully with their partners. Practitioners should also watch that as weight falls away, clients may feel vulnerable to sexual abuse. Clients may also have the urge to act out in their new slender bodies. Practitioners should be aware that food addicts could transfer to sex addiction.
5. *Boundaries* Practitioners will want to set boundaries with clients in a group around criticism of fellow members. In light of relationship sensitivity and painful reactions to criticism, this is a healthy boundary for groups. Clients may also carry this boundary into their relationships outside the group as a means for getting some "breathing room" from upset while in early stage recovery. Clients may benefit from being empowered to set boundaries around teasing or complaining about issues such as keeping processed foods out of the house.
6. *Working with Health Professionals* As PFA recovery is a relatively new concept, clients are likely to run into inappropriate advice from their health professionals. Practitioners can encourage clients to carry copies of key handouts from www.foodaddictionresources.com

such as the list of excluded foods and the rationale for excluding them. "The Evidence for Food Addiction: A Handout for Health Professionals" may help other health practitioners see that the client has a rationale for excluding processed foods and is not behaving pathologically.

28.2.5 Healing Physically, Mentally, Emotionally, Behaviorally, and Spiritually

Physical recovery from processed foods is certainly a positive. Practitioners can review progress in recovery from abnormal blood glucose, cholesterol, and blood pressure. Clients may also experience improved digestion, circulation, muscle strength, and mobility. Practitioners may acknowledge weight loss, but be careful to discourage approaching the program as a short-term weight-loss effort.

Clients can be helped to reacquire mental capabilities. Through abstinent balanced food, cue avoidance, exercise, meditation, and healthy sleep, clients can reduce cravings and restore learning, decision-making, memory, restraint, and satiation. Practitioners can celebrate moments when clients were able to make good decisions about food and exercise restraint. Clients can learn to disassociate themselves from unhealthy thoughts.

Clients may come into the program with a history of depression, irritability, anxiety, and shame, which are based on the biochemical imbalances associated with processed foods. They may have a history of being around family members with similar emotional profiles. Thus their internal negative affect may have been reinforced by external feedback from family members. Further, they may be facing stressful medical, financial, employment, and family situations in their current life. Practitioners will want to work exercises with clients to promote forgiveness of family members, examine and release negative feelings, and evaluate self-beliefs. They will also want to teach clients to draw and enforce boundaries with family members, coworkers, and others. Monitoring for anger, anxiety, and stress will be helpful. Practitioners can devise programs for clients to be of service that can promote healing of emotional issues.

Clients can come into recovery with a range of comfort levels with spirituality. Some will be able to use spirituality comfortably to help stabilize brain function and find a purpose in life. At the other end of the spectrum, some clients will be very uncomfortable with spiritual concepts. Practitioners can use spiritual concepts without broaching religious issues. Clients may benefit from learning about their own inner wisdom and their own spiritual practices, without choosing a religion. By dwelling on the "miracles" often experienced in recovery, practitioners can help clients adhere willingly to a lifestyle that is quite different from mainstream culture.

Practitioners may be able to restore spiritual strengths in clients who had lost hope. Clients who had prayed for relief from the myriad of ailments associated with processed food use can now be helped to see the miracle of recovery. They can be encouraged to rekindle faith and dwell in gratitude. Concepts of a higher power may be adapted from 12-step fellowships. Promoting healing thoughts, gratitude, and acceptance as spiritual qualities can be helpful.

28.2.6 Recovery of Education, Careers, and Finances

As seen in the DSM 5 SUD criteria, food addicts have suffered the loss of educational and employment opportunities. Clients may present on disability due to depression and immobility. Recovery from financial difficulties may come somewhat naturally as spending on processed foods diminishes. Spending in other areas may also be reduced as the restraint center in the brain starts to function. Clients may have debts to pay off but they can derive relief from knowing that they're making progress in this area. Competent financial assistance may be essential for some clients.

For clients on disability, the ability to earn income may be limited because it puts their disability benefits at risk. Nonetheless, clients can be gently encouraged to begin exercising simple skills such as writing. They may be able to regain reading comprehension skills. Practitioners may have small volunteer jobs for clients such as welcoming new group members, encouraging group members, answering questions, etc. Gradually clients may branch out into a volunteer job for a few hours per week. As mobility returns, they may be able to babysit or care for a pet in their homes.

For clients who are holding down a job, they may improve performance and gain the confidence to apply for advancement. As their weight, fatigue, brain fog, and decision-making normalize, they may feel ready for more challenging responsibilities. The practitioner should watch for improvements and affirm them in clients. A bit of encouragement and enthusiasm can work wonders for recovering food addicts.

In terms of returning to an interrupted education, clients can start back slowly by taking an online class. Some universities are offering free courses. This might be a good place to start. Clients should be encouraged to take any decision very slowly so they don't create stress nor set themselves up for failure.

28.2.7 Evaluating other Sources of Support

PFA recovery is a complex disease and it is also a new field. Recovery benefits from expertise in the biochemistry of the disease, its interaction with the obesogenic culture, and the specifics of neurorestoration. Clients may want to augment the practitioner's service with other means of support. It is wise to help clients evaluate these means. A few guidelines are offered here.

1. Check for triggers such as displays of addictive food/drinks in recovery rooms.
2. Look for facilitators who can support abstinence from the full range of addictive food/drinks. Avoid people who advocate learning how to eat addictive foods in moderation or require the use of addictive foods.
3. Check for stress-inducing practices such as phone calls that disrupt sleep, as well as forced agendas and requirements.
4. Avoid out-of-balance foods plans, including inadequate portions/calories and support for timing of meals.
5. Look for focus on restoration of neurofunction, emotions, and behaviors as opposed to weight loss.

28.3 FUTURE RESEARCH AND CONCLUSION

As set forth in the beginning of this chapter, these suggestions are based on the observations of two practitioners. From working with PFA clients, there are virtually endless issues that arise in the course of establishing a secure lifestyle free from processed foods. Research is needed that would evaluate the many elements of recovery with the goal of guiding practitioners in setting priorities, shifting goals in response to progress, and monitoring for increases in risk of relapse.

The program materials for recovery from PFA are both rich and extensive. Food addicts not only have skills to acquire, but they also have traumas to heal from living in a judgmental culture. Practitioners will reap many rewards from patiently teaching program materials to clients who are replacing suffering with security and joy.

REFERENCES

1. Food Addicts in Recovery Anonymous. 2013. *Food Addicts in Recovery Anonymous.* Woburn, MA: Food Addicts in Recoverys Anonymous.
2. Food Addicts Anonymous. 2010. *Food Addicts Anonymous.* Port St. Lucie, FL: Food Addicts Anonymous, Inc. p. 299.
3. Carrie, W. 2005. *Beyond Our Wildest Dreams.* Rio Rancho, NM: Overeaters Anonymous.
4. Sheppard, K. 1993. *Food Addiction: The Body Knows.* Deerfield Beach, FL: Health Communications.
5. Yau, P.L., et al. Preliminary evidence of cognitive and brain abnormalities in uncomplicated adolescent obesity. *Obesity (Silver Spring)*, 2014; **22**(8): 1865–71.

6. Zhu, N., et al. Cognitive function in a middle aged cohort is related to higher quality dietary pattern 5 and 25 years earlier: the CARDIA study. *J Nutr Health Aging*, 2015; **19**(1): 33–8.
7. Ballesteros, S., et al. A randomized controlled trial of brain training with non-action video games in older adults: results of the 3-month follow-up. *Front Aging Neurosci*, 2015; **7**: 45.
8. Hardy, J.L., et al. Enhancing cognitive abilities with comprehensive training: a large, online, randomized, active-controlled trial. *PLoS One*, 2015; **10**(9): e0134467.
9. van Meer, F., et al. What you see is what you eat: an ALE meta-analysis of the neural correlates of food viewing in children and adolescents. *NeuroImage*, 2015; **104**: 35–43.
10. Ogden, C.L., et al. Trends in obesity prevalence among children and adolescents in the United States, 1988–1994 through 2013–2014. *JAMA*, 2016; **315**(21): 2292–9.
11. Bauer, C.C., et al. Child overweight and obesity are associated with reduced executive cognitive performance and brain alterations: a magnetic resonance imaging study in Mexican children. *Pediatr Obes*, 2015; **10**(3): 196–204.
12. Shashaj, B., et al. Origin of cardiovascular risk in overweight preschool children: a cohort study of cardiometabolic risk factors at the onset of obesity. *JAMA Pediatr*, 2014; **168**(10): 917–24.
13. Verdejo-Garcia, A., et al. Dysfunctional involvement of emotion and reward brain regions on social decision making in excess weight adolescents. *Hum Brain Mapp*, 2015; **36**(1): 226–37.
14. Rutters, F., et al. Acute stress-related changes in eating in the absence of hunger. *Obesity (Silver Spring)*, 2009; **17**(1): 72–7.
15. Wagner, D.D., et al. Inducing negative affect increases the reward value of appetizing foods in dieters. *J Cogn Neurosci*, 2012; **24**(7): 1625–33.
16. Petroni, M.L., et al. Psychological distress in morbid obesity in relation to weight history. *Obes Surg*, 2007; **17**(3): 391–9.
17. Felitti, V.J. Origins of addictive behavior: evidence from a study of stressful chilhood experiences. *Prax Kinderpsychol Kinderpsychiatr*, 2003; **52**(8): 547–59.
18. Yau, Y.H., and M.N. Potenza, Stress and eating behaviors. *Minerva Endocrinol*, 2013; **38**(3): 255–67.

29 Adaptation of SUD and ED Practice Parameters to Adolescents and Children with PFA

Joan Ifland
Food Addiction Training, LLC
Cincinnati, OH

CONTENTS

Obesity and eating disorders are prevalent in children in Westernized countries (Ng et al., 2014). Studies of processed food addiction (PFA) in children are emerging (Burrows et al., 2017; Gearhardt, Roberto, Seamans, Corbin, & Brownell, 2013). Intervening in families with children who are exhibiting characteristics of PFA is valuable insofar as early intervention can prevent a lifetime of struggle with weight, mood, and the metabolic syndrome. Children differ from adults in the key aspect that they live in households where adults control food cues and availability of food. Thus, family involvement is key to helping children overcome PFA.

This chapter follows the topic headings shown in two documents issued by the American Academy of Child and Adolescent Psychiatry concerning treatment of eating disorders (ED) (Lock & La Via, 2015) and substance use disorders (SUD) (Bukstein et al., 2005): *Practice Parameter for the Assessment and Treatment of Children and Adolescents with Eating Disorders* and *Practice Parameter for the Assessment and Treatment of Children and Adolescents with Substance Use Disorders*. The adapted subject headings are shown below. Practice guidelines for pediatric obesity and its consequences are also adapted from the Children's Hospital Association (Estrada et al., 2014), the Endocrine Society (August et al., 2008), and an expert committee of pediatric obesity centers (Barlow, 2007).

AACAP Subject Headings for Treatment of Pediatric SUD and ED	Adapted for PFA
Background	
Presentation	PFA in children manifests according to the DSM 5 SUD diagnostic criteria.
Epidemiology	Manifestations of PFA are growing among children. These include obesity, metabolic, mood, mental, and behavioral syndromes.
Etiology and Risk Factors	Risk factors for PFA are similar to those for SUD and obesity. They include adverse childhood experiences (ACE) such as trauma, loss of a parent, neglect, and weight teasing. Obese parents and poverty are also risk factors.
Comorbidity	Comorbidities in PFA can include depression, anxiety, PTSD, poor impulse control, and behavioral disorders, as well as the metabolic syndrome.
Prevention (SUD)	Consistently providing unprocessed, nonaddictive foods, emotionally supportive attention, and exercise as an alternative to screen time could prevent development of PFA. Limiting exposure to cuing is also important.
Recommendations	
Confidentiality (SUD)	This is less of an issue in PFA because processed food substances are not illegal.
Screen all children (ED) Screen all older children (SUD)	Brief screening can use DSM 5 SUD criteria failed attempts to cut back, unintended use, failure to fulfill roles at school or home, use in spite of knowledge of consequences.
Follow a positive screen with a comprehensive evaluation (ED). Adolescents with SUDs should receive thorough evaluation for comorbid psychiatric disorders (SUD).	A comprehensive evaluation can generally follow the topics of the Addiction Severity Index (ASI) as described in Chapter 22.
Severe acute physical signs and medical complications need to be treated (ED). Comorbid conditions should be appropriately treated (SUD).	The ASI surfaces immediate needs for medications, therapy, managed withdrawal, and training of parents in methods to provide unprocessed, nonaddictive foods. Treatment depends on availability of services and the motivation of caregivers.
Psychiatric hospitalization, day program, partial hospitalization programs, and residential programs for eating disorders in children should be considered only when outpatient interventions have been unsuccessful or are unavailable (ED). Adolescents with SUDs should be treated in the least restrictive setting that is safe and effective. Programs and interventions should provide or arrange for posttreatment aftercare (SUD).	It is likely that most PFA will be resolved at home with education and support from individual and family counselors, online support groups, and in-person groups. Hospitalization for caregivers with PFA can follow the guidelines in Chapter 26, "Adaptation of APA Practice Guidelines for SUD to Processed Food Addiction."
Treatment of eating disorders in youth usually involves a multidisciplinary team that is developmentally aware, sensitive, and skilled in the care of children and adolescents with eating disorders (ED). Family therapy or significant family/parental involvement in treatment should be a component of treatment of SUDs. Programs/interventions should attempt to provide comprehensive services in other domains (e.g., vocational, recreational, medical, family, and legal) (SUD).	The broad range of skills for treatment of children with SUD as well as BED are similar to those required for children with PFA. Children may need help with schoolwork, cognitive restoration, exercise routines, medical problems, and family relationships. Legal problems are not likely. Professionals who provide long-distance services by telephone are available at http://www.foodaddictionresources.com/resources.html.

(Continued)

AACAP Subject Headings for Treatment of Pediatric SUD and ED	Adapted for PFA
Outpatient psychosocial interventions are the initial treatment of choice for children and adolescents with eating disorders (ED).	Psychosocial interventions are also indicated for PFA clients. There is evidence for mood disorders, trauma, and neglect in children with chronic addictive overeating.
The use of medications, including complementary and alternative medications, should be reserved for comorbid conditions and refractory cases (ED). Medication may be used for craving and withdrawal (SUD).	Medication for comorbidities is also indicated for children with PFA. Medications should be monitored closely as health conditions may resolve on an unprocessed food plan. Caregivers should be trained in how to monitor and consult with the prescribing professional. Treatment for withdrawal from processed foods is generally for headache and fatigue.
Treatment programs and interventions should develop procedures to minimize treatment dropout and to maximize motivation, compliance, and treatment completion (SUD).	Compliance with treatment has been shown to be effective for resolution of BED.
Treatment should encourage development of peer support regarding the nonuse of substances (SUD).	Peer usage is a factor in overeating.
Twelve-step approaches may be used as a basis for treatment (SUD).	Monitoring for reinforcement of dysfunctional eating is important in support groups for addictive eating.

Note: AACAP, American Academic of Child and Adolescent Psychiatry; SUD, substance use disorder; ED, eating disorder; PFA, processed food addiction; DSM 5, *Diagnostic and Statistical Manual of Mental Disorders, 5th edition*; BED, binge eating disorder.

As can be seen from the above table, practice parameters for children with ED or SUD are quite similar. Both parameters provide for a process of screening, evaluation, comprehensive treatment plans, treatment of comorbidities, support, and family therapy. PFA can be considered as having elements of both SUD and ED, which facilitates adaptation of the practice guidelines. Practitioners who are already providing comprehensive treatment for obesity, ED, or SUD can screen for PFA and educate parents about addictive foods and cues accordingly.

29.1 METHOD

The approaches described here are gathered from research related to obesity, SUD, and ED in children and adolescents. This research was collected from PubMed using the search terms *children*, *adolescents*, *obesity*, *binge-eating*, *prevalence*, and *treatment*. The research is applied to PFA based on clinical observations as well as recollections of childhood behaviors obtained from adults who self-identify as PFA clients. Very little research has been conducted on PFA in adolescents and children. However, the need for new approaches to childhood obesity; the existence of treatment parameters for obesity, SUD, and ED in children and adolescents; as well as the strength of the research describing PFA in this textbook point to the value of describing treatment approaches to PFA in children and adolescents.

29.2 CLINICAL PRESENTATION

Children experience PFA in ways that are sometimes similar to those of adults insofar as children's behaviors can be organized along the diagnostic criteria for SUD described in the DSM 5. Although the circumstances differ appreciably, children still suffer loss of control and dysfunctions in managing their lives just as adults with PFA might. Manifestations of the DSM 5 SUD diagnostic criteria in children are described below.

29.2.1 The DSM 5 SUD Diagnostic Criteria in Children as Recalled by Adult PFA Clients

Adult PFA clients are able to describe experiences as children that conform to the DSM 5 SUD diagnostic criteria. This information was observed in educational setting with self-identified PFA clients.

29.2.1.1 Criterion 1: Foods Were Eaten in Larger Amounts or for a Longer Period of Time than Intended

This may manifest in children who have been subjected to weight loss regimes by their parents. Children may have been scolded for violating rules set down for their consumption of processed foods, which could be interpreted as consuming more than intended. Children may or may not be aware of the sensation of loss of control. However, if they've been unable to meet a parent's intentions for them, this may be considered as an indication of loss of control.

29.2.1.2 Criterion 2: There Is a Persistent Desire or Unsuccessful Efforts to Cut Down or Control Food Use

Because of the weight issue, children may have gone through failed attempts to cut down in order to lose weight. The practitioner will be able to ask parents for this history.

29.2.1.3 Criterion 3: A Great Deal of Time Is Spent in Activities Necessary to Obtain Processed Foods, Eat Processed Foods, and Recover from Their Effect

PFA clients report having spent time as children looking for hidden food. They report spending time thinking about how to get food. Children may spend time walking to a store or to other homes for processed foods. They might also spend time hiding in order to eat the food. They report losing educational time and opportunities as they experience the brain fog created by consumption of processed foods.

29.2.1.4 Criterion 4: Cravings, or a Strong Desire or Urge to Eat Processed Foods

PFA clients do report being obsessed with processed foods as children. Parents may notice that children talk about processed foods frequently and express yearning for them.

29.2.1.5 Criterion 5: Recurrent Food Consumption Resulting in a Failure to Fulfill Major Role Obligations at School or Home

PFA clients recall that they failed to fulfill the role of normally weighted children. They report that their parents were ashamed of them and frustrated with them. They also report being so obsessed with processed foods that they were unable to focus on their schoolwork. Practitioners can ask parents about the presence of "learning disabilities" or failure to work up to potential that may reflect disordered thinking related to cravings.

29.2.1.6 Criterion 6: Continued Processed Food Consumption Despite Having Persistent or Recurrent Social or Interpersonal Problems Caused or Exacerbated by the Effects of Processed Food Consumption

PFA clients recount being bullied, teased, and physically abused by neighborhood children, fellow students, and family members because of their weight.

29.2.1.7 Criterion 7: Important Social or Recreational Activities are Given Up or Reduced because of Processed Food Consumption

PFA clients remember wishing that their parent's house guests would go home so that the child could eat the leftovers. They were ashamed to go to social events because of their weight. They didn't want to go places that didn't have food.

29.2.1.8 Criterion 8: Recurrent Processed Food Use in which It Is Physically Hazardous

PFA clients remember being injured by climbing up to cabinets in search of processed foods. They may have cooked sugary treats when parents were not at home. They may have consumed an entire bottle of candy-flavored medication. They recall crossing a forbidden busy street to go to the candy store.

29.2.1.9 Criterion 9: Processed Food Use Is Continued Despite Having Knowledge of a Persistent or Recurrent Physical or Psychological Problem That Is Likely to Have Been Caused or Exacerbated by Processed Food Consumption

PFA clients recollect that they knew that they were in trouble because of their weight. They're generally unaware of other physical, mental, emotional, or behavioral consequences of their consumption of processed foods.

29.2.1.10 Criterion 10: Tolerance as Defined by Either (a) a Need for Markedly Increased Amounts of Processed Foods to Achieve the Desired Effect or (b) a Markedly Diminished Effect with Continued Use of the Same Amount of Processed Foods

Adult PFA clients report increasing drive to obtain processed foods by spending time looking for hidden foods at home and walking to stores to obtain foods.

29.2.1.11 Criterion 11: Withdrawal, as Manifested by Either of the Following: (a) The Characteristic Withdrawal Syndrome for Processed Foods or (b) Processed Foods Are Consumed to Relieve or Avoid Withdrawal Symptoms

Children may become lethargic, disinterested in food, and angry during withdrawal. Headaches and stomachaches may also occur.

The DSM 5 diagnosis requires clinically significant impairment or distress and conformance to at least two of the criteria. Practitioners can use their judgment about how many of the criteria have been met and advise parents/caregivers about the severity of PFA in their child.

29.3 EPIDEMIOLOGY

Children in Westernized cultures are experiencing epidemics of diet-related diseases. Among US children and adolescents aged 2–19 years, the prevalence of obesity in 2011–2014 was 17.0% and extreme obesity was 5.8% (Ogden et al., 2016). In Kuwait, the prevalence of overweight and obesity was 50.5% in boys and 46.5% in girls (Al-Haifi et al., 2013). On a global basis, 23.8% of boys and 22.6% of girls were overweight or obese in 2013. Obesity increased in developing countries from 8.1% to 12.9% for boys and from 8.4% to 13.4% for girls between 1980 and 2013 (Ng et al., 2014). Mendez noted a decline in energy intake in children in 2003–2004 that corresponded to a plateau in increases in obesity. However, this trend was reversed in 2009–2010 (Mendez, Sotres-Alvarez, Miles, Slining, & Popkin, 2014). Rankin et al. noted that there are 42 million children under 5 years of age who are estimated to be overweight or obese. If current trends continue, an estimated 70 million children will be overweight or obese by 2025 (Rankin et al., 2016).

Comorbidities of PFA are also prevalent. In a population of US obese children aged 8–17, 34% were found to have depression (Morrison, Shin, Tarnopolsky, & Taylor, 2015). In the United States, approximately 4.4 million children aged 4–17 years were reported to have a history of ADHD diagnosis. Of these, 2.5 million (56%) were reported to be taking medication for the disorder (Center for Disease Control, 2005). Prescription medications for mood and behavior are being given to children but without extensive testing (Carlezon & Konradi, 2004). Obese children have trouble decoding emotions, which can impact social functioning (Koch & Pollatos, 2015). Micali et al. found that 11% of 13-year-olds experience extreme levels of fear of weight gain (Micali, Ploubidis, De Stavola, Simonoff, & Treasure, 2014).

29.4 ETIOLOGY AND RISK FACTORS

Children may develop PFA as a result of repeat exposure to ingestion and cuing for addictive foods in Westernized cultures (Berthoud, Zheng, & Shin, 2012; Burger & Stice, 2012; Sinha & Jastreboff, 2013). Research shows that risk factors may also include adverse childhood experiences (ACE) such as trauma, abuse, and neglect (Felitti, 1993). The child may turn to processed foods to numb feelings or to gain weight as protection against sexual abuse (Felitti, Jakstis, Pepper, & Ray, 2010). Behaviors and family characteristics can also predict chronic overeating (Evans, Fuller-Rowell, & Doan, 2012) even in newborn suckling patterns (Stice, Agras, & Hammer, 1999).

29.4.1 Repeat Ingestion and Cue Exposure

Processed foods are heavily marketed to children through intense television advertising and associative cues such as toys, clothing, and fast food outlets (Kraak & Story, 2015; Powell, Harris, & Fox, 2013; Zimmerman & Shimoga, 2014). Caregivers generally give processed foods to children, and children watch other people eat these foods. In this way, processed foods and cues surround children in Westernized cultures. Not surprisingly, evidence is emerging that shows the presence of addictive brain functioning in children as young as 3 years old (Bauer et al., 2014; Rollins, Loken, Savage, & Birch, 2014), including loss of cognitive abilities in response to food cues (van Meer, van der Laan, Adan, Viergever, & Smeets, 2015).

Children may even have cravings that are stronger than the cravings experienced by adults (Silvers et al., 2014). Shashaj et al. found that 39.3% of newly overweight children between the age of 2 and 5.8 had at least one symptom of the metabolic syndrome (Shashaj et al., 2014). Bauer et al. found reduced brain mass in obese children aged 6–8 (Bauer et al., 2014). Stice et al. found that newborn babies who suckled longer predicted obesity by age 2 (Stice et al., 1999). There is evidence that may develop in very young children, even babies.

As seen in Part I, "Fundamentals," processed foods have addictive qualities. Toddlers can be easily imprinted with product preferences (Halford, Boyland, Hughes, Oliveira, & Dovey, 2007), while the food industry may show over 500 processed food commercials in a single Saturday morning (Nestle, 1996). As processed food cravings develop in young children, irrational, harmful food choices can manifest just as they do in adults. Cravings and loss of decision-making can affect loss of control over eating in children (Verbeken, Braet, Bosmans, & Goossens, 2014). Uneducated parents and caregivers can unwittingly worsen the addiction by accommodating the child's pleading for processed foods to avoid denying the child (Baker & Altman, 2015).

29.4.2 Adverse Childhood Experiences

ACE have been found to correlate with the development of obesity as well as ED. Evans et al. found that children's BMI increased in adolescence according to their exposure to cumulative risks such as poverty, physical stressors, and family turmoil (Evans et al., 2012). Helton and Liechty found that youth investigated for maltreatment are more likely to have obesity (Helton & Liechty, 2014). Shin and Miller found that children who experienced neglect experienced higher BMI growth, and further co-occurring neglect and physical abuse were related to increased BMI at baseline in the study (Shin & Miller, 2012). King et al. found that almost half of adolescents who experienced weight-based violence engaged in unhealthy eating behaviors. With implications for treatment, the study found that unhealthy eating behaviors corresponded to less desire for a supportive intervention. The interpretation of the finding is that unhealthy eating behaviors may compensate for healthy coping strategies (King, Puhl, Luedicke, & Peterson, 2013). There is evidence that ACE increase the risk of addictive overeating.

29.4.3 Behavioral and Psychosocial Factors

Providers may be able to prevent the development of consequences of PFA by identifying behaviors that have been found to correlate with or predict chronic overconsumption of processed foods. For example, Duckworth et al. found that self-controlled fifth graders had lower BMI by eighth grade. This finding held even when controlled for gender, age, socioeconomic status, ethnicity, IQ, and happiness (Duckworth, Tsukayama, & Geier, 2010). Evans et al. made a similar finding showing that gains in BMI between the age of 9 and 13 are largely accounted for by deterioration in self-regulatory abilities in children who have experienced more cumulative risks as compared to children who did not experience gains in BMI (Evans et al., 2012). Goldschmidt et al. found that loss of control tends to remit as adolescents grow into adulthood. However, adolescents with psychosocial problems are more like to go on to develop binge eating disorder (BED) in adulthood (Goldschmidt et al., 2014). Loss of control is shown to be a factor in the development of chronic overeating.

Body dissatisfaction is a significant issue in PFA. Iannaccone et al. found that body shame was associated with vulnerability to eating problems. Body shame was the mediator between low self-esteem and disordered eating (Iannaccone, D'Olimpio, Cella, & Cotrufo, 2016). Presnell et al. found that the risk factors for body dissatisfaction were elevations in body mass, negative affect, and perceived pressure to be thin from peers (Presnell, Bearman, & Stice, 2004). Stice et al. found two distinct pathways to body dissatisfaction. The first was pressure to be thin and the second was increased adiposity (Stice, Presnell, & Spangler, 2002). For BED, Stice et al. found that dieting, pressure to be thin, modeling of eating disturbances, appearance overvaluation, body dissatisfaction, depressive symptoms, emotional eating, body mass, low self-esteem, and low social support predicted BED onset with 92% accuracy (Stice et al., 2002). In obesity, Stice et al. found that self-reported dietary restraint, radical weight-control behaviors, depressive symptoms, and perceived parental obesity predicted the onset of obesity (Stice, Presnell, Shaw, & Rohde, 2005). In a longitudinal study of depression, Stice et al. found that body image and eating disturbances predicted onset of depression in female adolescents (Stice et al., 2000). Body dissatisfaction is seen to be an important factor in the development of chronic overeating.

Risk factors can appear at birth. Stice et al. found that body weight and time spent suckling at birth predicted disordered eating in childhood. The risk of disordered eating increased during the first 5 years of life and correlated with maternal body dissatisfaction, internalization of the thin ideal, dieting, bulimic symptoms, and maternal and paternal body mass (Stice et al., 1999). Practitioners may find that viewing early childhood obesity as an addiction to processed foods yields improvements in outcomes.

29.4.4 Family Characteristics

Epstein et al. found that food reinforcement and parental obesity independently predict obesity among adolescents (Epstein, Yokum, Feda, & Stice, 2014). In a review article, Heerwagon found that fetal exposure to excess blood lipids, particularly saturated fatty acids, could affect a number of gene pathways of metabolic importance, including those for energy storage, oxidation, growth, death, differentiation, and inflammation (Heerwagen, Miller, Barbour, & Friedman, 2010). Shin and Miller et al. found an association of obesity with parental obesity and education, and family income (Shin & Miller, 2012).

29.4.5 Sexual Minorities

Hadland et al. found that a third of sexual minority youth engage in hazardous weight control behaviors (Hadland, Austin, Goodenow, & Calzo, 2014).

29.4.6 Ethnicity

Huh et al. found that European-American girls were not at risk for developing obesity through adolescence but that African-American and Latino girls were more likely to transition from overweight to obese (Huh, Stice, Shaw, & Boutelle, 2012).

29.5 COMORBIDITY

Extensive comorbidities are found in children who are repeatedly exposed to ingestion of processed foods and cues for processed foods in the development of PFA. There is evidence for mood disorders, cognitive impairment, and behavioral problems in children, as well as the metabolic syndrome. The evidence is described below.

29.5.1 Mood

Mood disorders are associated with drug addiction in general and with chronic use of processed foods resulting in obesity. Marmorstein et al. found that correlations between obesity and depression were more likely early in adolescence than later. Depression in early adolescence predicted obesity in late adolescence. Obesity in late adolescence predicted depression in early adulthood in girls (Marmorstein, Iacono, & Legrand, 2014). Presnell et al. found that depression predicted bulimia, which in turn predicted depression. This is interpreted as evidence that bulimia and depression can be mutually reinforcing (Presnell, Stice, Seidel, & Madeley, 2009).

In a study of 23,020 mothers and children, Jacka et al. (2013) found that children with poor diet had higher levels of internalized and externalized problems (Jacka et al., 2013). Byrne et al. found that inflammation and obesity follow depression rather than cause it. The study also found that multiple health problems can worsen depression (Byrne, O'Brien-Simpson, Mitchell, & Allen, 2015). In a study of 496 US female adolescent girls, Rohde et al. found that approximately 1 of 6 girls experienced a major episode of depression with a mean duration of 5.3 months. The incidents peaked at age 16. White racial status and young age were associated with greater feelings of worthlessness and suicidality (Rohde, Beevers, Stice, & O'Neil, 2009). Seely et al. found that the most potent predictors of depression included poor school and family function, low parental support, bulimia, and delinquency (Seeley, Stice, & Rohde, 2009). Beevers et al. found reduced cognitive control correlated with depression (Beevers, Clasen, Stice, & Schnyer, 2010). Sjoberg et al. found that obesity was significantly associated with depression and shame among 15- and 17-year-olds. Shaming experiences, parental employment, and parental separation explained the relationship (Sjoberg, Nilsson, & Leppert, 2005). Boutelle et al. found that obese status was associated with future depressive symptoms but not major depression. Overweight was not associated with depression (Boutelle, Hannan, Fulkerson, Crow, & Stice, 2010). Burton et al. found that deficits in peer support predicted increases in depressive symptoms, as did negative life events (Burton, Stice, & Seeley, 2004). In a study of South Korean children, Do et al. found that lack of sleep, excessive Internet usage, and negative life events predicted depression, suicide ideation, and obesity (Do, Shin, Bautista, & Foo, 2013). The evidence weaves processed foods, health problems, depression, bulimia, poor family function, reduced cognitive control, shame, obesity, negative life events, lack of sleep, and Internet usage into a syndrome of mood disorders associated with chronic overeating.

Body dissatisfaction has been found to be a significant factor in mood disorders. Stice et al. found that negative affect moderates the relationship between dieting and binge eating (Stice, Akutagawa, Gaggar, & Agras, 2000). In a study of Palestinian adolescents, Al Sabbah, Vereecken, Abdeen, Coats, and Maes (2009) found that although 16% of adolescents were overweight, twice that number were dissatisfied with their bodies (Al Sabbah et al., 2009). Bearman et al. found that body dissatisfaction increases the risk for depression and eating disorders (Bearman, Martinez, Stice, & Presnell, 2006). In a study of 428 US adolescent boys and girls, Bearman and Stice found that body dissatisfaction predicts depression for girls but not for boys (Bearman & Stice, 2008). Markey argued that body image plays a central role in development and should be the subject of future research (Markey, 2010). Roberts and Duong found that controlling for body image eliminated the association between depression and obesity (Roberts & Duong, 2015). Addressing body dissatisfaction can help relieve the distress of disordered eating.

29.5.2 Cognitive Impairment

Cognitive impairment in children who are faced with recovery from PFA can be a barrier to learning the skills needed to avoid processed foods and cues. In toddlers at 48 months, lower impulse control corresponded with higher BMI and increased carb consumption at snack (Levitan et al., 2014). Loss of impulse control may predispose children to excessive weight gain through early adolescence (Francis & Susman, 2009). Children who are malnourished suffer delayed development through neurological system dysfunction but also because they are found to receive less care (Engle & Fernandez, 2010). There is evidence that eating disorders predict thought-shape fusion such that children fear weight gain, body dissatisfaction, and moral wrongdoing after only thinking about eating high-calorie foods (Coelho, Siggen, Dietre, & Bouvard, 2013). Michaelides found that obese adolescents have the same cognitive impairment as obese adults (Michaelides, Thanos, Volkow, & Wang, 2012). These findings are important as adolescence should be the time when self-regulatory processes are formed. Biederman et al. found that ADHD significantly increases the risk of ED and that ED plus ADHD increased the risk of addiction morbidity and dysfunction such as depression, anxiety disorders, and disruptive behavior disorder (Biederman et al., 2007). Burger and Stice found that increased caloric intake corresponds with hyperresponsivity to processed food cues in attentional regions of the brain (Burger & Stice, 2013). Cognitive impairment can be seen to be an important issue for children who overeat chronically.

29.5.3 Behavioral

There are four areas of behavioral dysfunction that are found in chronic overeaters. These are sleep disruption, screen time, carb consumption, dieting, and social behaviors. Behavioral anomalies can start early. Mackenbach et al. found that BMI correlates with fussiness and emotional undereating in preschoolers (Mackenbach et al., 2012).

Chahal et al. found that 64% of parents reported that their child had access to one or more electronic devices in their bedroom, which is associated with shortened sleep (Chahal, Fung, Kuhle, & Veugelers, 2013). Landis found that a greater craving was associated with more daytime sleep in an adolescent population (Landis, Parker, & Dunbar, 2009).

A relationship between screen time and intake of carbohydrate intake has been found. In a cross-sectional study of 283 postpubertal adolescents, Cameron et al. found that higher carbohydrate intake mediated the relationship between TV, video gaming, and BMI (Cameron et al., 2016). Nguyen found a similar association in an adolescent population in Vietnam (Nguyen, Hong, Nguyen, & Robert, 2016).

Restricted calorie dieting is a behavior that can impact chronic overeating in adolescents. In a review article, Burger and Stice found that dieting correlated with hyperresponsivity in reward-related brain regions, which could increase cue reactivity and risk for overeating and binge eating (Burger & Stice, 2011).

Social behaviors are also a behavior in eating patterns in adolescents. Bruening et al. found that high schoolers were more likely to visit fast food outlets if their friends did (Bruening et al., 2014).

29.5.4 Physical

Physical comorbidities in obese children are rising. Children's Hospital Association found a number of comorbidities for children with obesity including hypertension, dyslipidemia, fatty liver disease, diabetes, and polycystic ovary syndrome (PCOS) (Estrada et al., 2014). In a review of studies of Australian children 0–18 years old, obesity was found to correlate with more cardiometabolic and nonalcoholic fatty liver disease risk factors (Sanders, Han, Baker, & Cobley, 2015). Comorbidities in obese children are so extensive that the Children's Hospital Association recommends training primary care providers to treat the conditions rather than refer due to limited availability of specialists (Estrada et al., 2014).

29.6 PREVENTION

Studies of obesity prevention are inconclusive (Parkin et al., 2015); however, recommendations for obesity prevention are consistent around the world. Recommendations developed in the United Kingdom include:

- Education regarding diet
- Increased physical activity
- Limits on stimulation of the consumption of processed foods
- Monitoring weight gain in infancy
- Evaluation of genetic factors (Hoey, 2014)

In Japan, recommendations were for:

- Six months of breast-feeding
- Sixty minutes per day of exercise
- Behavioral therapy
- Reduction in sedentary behavior
- Dietary and exercise education

A study based on this approach resulted in decreased adiposity (Togashi, Iguchi, & Masuda, 2013). The Endocrine Society in the US recommends intensive lifestyle modification including:

- Dietary
- Physical activity
- Behavioral approaches

In a seemingly inconsistent position, the society recommends surgery for families where lifestyle interventions have failed but only for families that are able to adhere to lifestyle modifications. Similar to the Japanese study, the society recommends breastfeeding for at least 6 months, 60 minutes of vigorous exercise daily, and early education about healthy dietary and activity habits. The society also recommends:

- Restricting the availability of unhealthy food choices in schools
- Policies to ban advertising unhealthy foods to children
- Community redesign to maximize opportunities for safe walking and bike riding to school, athletic activities, and neighborhood shopping (August et al., 2008)

These school/community initiatives might take a long time to implement. Families can be educated about how to adapt these goals at home by eliminating processed foods and television from the home while increasing family activities involving exercise and cognitive function (puzzles, reading aloud, games, etc.).

29.7 RECOMMENDATIONS

Recommendations for adapting practice parameters to PFA are bridged from evidence for the treatment of obesity and eating disorders in children. Clinical observations are derived from working with parents of pediatric PFA clients and from recollections of adult PFA clients. In addition to recommendations for treating obesity and ED, key parameters from the treatment SUD are included. These include abstinence from processed foods, avoidance of cues for processed foods, and cognitive restoration. The following discusses each recommendation as it applies to PFA.

29.7.1 CONFIDENTIALITY

Confidentiality is an issue in the treatment of adolescents who are using illegal drugs. Confidentiality is recommended to foster trust between client and practitioner. Processed foods are not illegal; however, it is often the case in households that parents have established limits and rules about the consumption of processed foods by the child with PFA. The child may be breaking these rules. The practitioner may wish to withhold this information from caregivers until it is established that the child will not be punished or chastised for seeking addictive processed foods. Motivating the adults in the household to remove processed foods from the home may be based on education about the cuing effects of availability. A handout on this topic may be found at www.foodaddictionresources.com.

29.7.2 SCREENING

The American Academy of Pediatrics is recommending that all children be screened for obesity.

These recommendations support a shift from simple identification of obesity, which often occurs when the condition is obvious and intractable, to universal assessment, universal preventive health messages, and early intervention. If primary care providers are to have an impact on the childhood obesity epidemic, then their best approach is assessment of obesity risk for all patients, with anticipatory guidance on healthy behaviors to minimize that risk (Barlow, 2007).

Given the prevalence of obesity and eating disorders among children in Westernized cultures, this recommendation is adapted to provide that all children be screened for PFA. A quick screening tool is derived from four common DSM 5 SUD criteria.

- Does the child eat even when it's against the rules and could result in punishment? (Use in hazardous conditions.)
- Does the child eat in spite of knowing that it might cause weight gain or another consequence? (Use in spite of knowledge of consequences.)
- Does anyone tease the child about weight? (Use in spite of interpersonal problems.)
- Is the child struggling in school or engaging in disruptive behavior at home? (Failure to fulfill roles.)

The DSM provides that a positive for two of these screening questions would warrant more comprehensive diagnostics according to the 11 DSM 5 PFA diagnostic criteria described above under "Clinical Presentation."

Practitioners should also screen children who exhibit the risk factors discussed above including:

- Repeat exposure to processed foods and cues
- ACE
- Mood disorders
- Eating disorders
- Cognitive impairment

- Behavior problems
- Parental obesity
- Poverty
- Comorbidities such as obesity, cardiovascular disease, diabetes, and fatty liver

29.7.3 Evaluation

If there is a positive diagnosis, the practitioner can create a treatment plan according to the Addiction Severity Index (ASI) described in Chapter 22 of this textbook. The ASI will surface the severity of physical, mental, emotional, and behavioral conditions that support recommendations for treatment. In the case of PFA, the practitioner will also be planning for the:

- Provision of nonaddictive unprocessed foods for the child
- Reduction or elimination of food cues
- Minimization of screen time
- Cognitive restoration
- Opportunities for physical activity
- Counseling in the event of need for trauma resolution

29.7.4 Treatment

The Children's Hospital Association encourages primary care provider to treat rather than refer obesity comorbidities such as diabetes, hypertension, abnormal lipids, abnormal liver enzymes, and hypertension:

However, because primary care pediatric providers often are underequipped to deal with these comorbidities, they frequently refer these patients to subspecialists. However, as a result of the US pediatric subspecialist shortage and considering that 12.5 million children are obese, access to care by subspecialists is limited (Estrada et al., 2014).

The Children's Hospital Association has developed guidelines for health providers. The full article may be found here: http://online.liebertpub.com/doi/pdf/10.1089/chi.2013.0120

The guidelines suggest screening obese children for three primary purposes:

1. To evaluate possible underlying diagnoses that may have contributed to the development of obesity
2. To identify physiological sequelae of obesity
3. To provide data for monitoring progress and response to treatment (Estrada et al., 2014)

The tests described in the guidelines are:

- Fasting lipid profile
- Fasting glucose
- Aspartate aminotransferase (AST), Alanine aminotransferase (ALT)
- Fasting insulin
- Sleep
- Blood pressure
- PCOS
- Hemoglobin A1c
- Vitamin D
- Body composition
- Glucose tolerance

Treatment practices, primarily weight management, are described for:

- Abnormal lipids
- Abnormal liver enzymes
- Hypertension
- PCOS

In the case of PFA, practitioners who are already supporting lifestyle changes can add abstinence and food cue avoidance to their existing programs. Practitioners who refer for support for lifestyle changes can specify abstinence and cue avoidance with the referral. The handouts "Excluded Foods," "Unprocessed Foods," and "Trigger Avoidance Checklist" can be found at http://www.foodaddictionresources.com/handouts.html.

29.7.5 Treatment Setting

PFA in children will most likely be resolved in a home setting. The American Psychiatric Association recommends that children be treated for ED and SUD in the least restrictive setting. In some cases, educating and supporting parents to provide unprocessed, nonaddictive foods in combination with eliminating cues will be enough to resolve harmful eating. In cases where parents are not successful at providing unprocessed meals and physical activity while reducing cues and screen time, counseling may be helpful. Where local resources are unavailable, long-distance telephone counselors are available as are online support groups. These resources may be found at http://www.foodaddictionresources.com/resources.html. These resources are for caregivers and parents and for older adolescents.

29.7.6 Interdisciplinary Teams

Based on the evaluation, practitioners may need to refer to dieticians, providers of physical activity, counselors, physical therapists, psychologists, or psychiatrists. Specialists in the field who treat through long-distance phone calls can be found at http://www.foodaddictionresources.com/resources.html. If the practitioner wishes to help develop local resources, sharing the handouts with service providers can start the process. The leader of the team educates health professionals about guidelines for abstaining from processed foods and avoiding food cues.

Any caregivers who are in a position to control cuing and availability should be included on the team. These include parents, older siblings, teachers, babysitters, extended family, caregivers in faith settings, etc. Practitioners may want to develop a list of the people who have access to the child and share educational handouts regarding the importance of not giving the child processed foods. Helpful handouts may be found at http://www.foodaddictionresources.com/handouts.html. These include:

- *Diet-Related Diseases* Caregivers may not know that a range of diseases are related to processed foods (https://drive.google.com/file/d/0B4iSL6lRp80QanRrR3VtUHBYUUk/view).
- *Excluded Foods* Caregivers benefit from knowing what foods to avoiding giving the PFA child (https://drive.google.com/file/d/0B4iSL6lRp80QM2w3eFhtY1FWVjg/view).
- *Unprocessed Foods* This handout explains what foods are safe for the child (https://drive.google.com/file/d/0B4iSL6lRp80QbmhuMzhMZm1oRHc/view).
- *Availability Is a Problem.* This handout explains how availability of processed foods can trigger cravings (https://drive.google.com/file/d/0B4iSL6lRp80QdmROZFU2Y2ZXS1U/view).
- *Trigger Avoidance Checklist* This handout helps caregivers identify where cues may be found (https://drive.google.com/file/d/0B4iSL6lRp80QZU1ldEUxY3VqVHM/view).

29.7.7 Outpatient Services

As described by the Endocrine Society, there are an estimated 12.5 million obese children in the US. Resources to treat them are limited. Primary care physicians can be trained to treat processed-food addicted children. An expert committee of pediatric professionals recommend a four-step process, which Minnesota physicians have summarized in the Minnesota Medicine Newsletter (Kuzel & Larson, 2014). It is adapted for PFA below.

1. Educate caregivers using the handout listed above under "Interdisciplinary Teams." Ask the caregiver to distribute handouts to people who have access to the child. The primary care physician may evaluate the caregiver for PFA. If the caregiver is found to have PFA, it may be beneficial to treat the caregiver first.
2. If no improvements are seen at the first follow-up visit, refer the primary caregiver to a dietician for help with shopping, meal planning, and strategies for quick meal preparation. Consult with the dietician to ensure that the handouts "Excluded Foods" and "Unprocessed Foods" are reflected in meal planning. If some improvement is seen, encourage the caregiver to continue more comprehensive abstinence, cue avoidance, and physical activity.
3. If by the third follow-up visit, there is still no improvement, include a mental health professional and a provider of physical activities on the team. It is possible that the caregiver may have cognitive impairment, trauma, or other disabilities that interfere with the caregivers' ability to organize unprocessed meals and healthy activities.
4. This stage recommends surgery and medications, which are not appropriate for food-addicted children. This is due to the risk of developing alcoholism or continuing to over-consume foods that can pass through restricted stomachs, such as ice cream and sugary drinks. A better strategy is to continue to meet with the caregiver and encourage smaller steps such as moving all of the processed foods into one cabinet to reduce cuing or replacing 20 minutes of television with a dance, stretching, or exercise video done with the child. Practitioners may find that the caregiver is also recovering from PFA and thus may become more capable with time and encouragement.

Where local expertise is not available, practitioners may refer to the resources listed at http://www.foodaddictionresources.com/resources.html.

29.7.8 Medication

Data about medication requirements is captured in the course of completing the ASI. Medications are most likely to be for comorbidities. Physical diet-related comorbidities may resolve on an unprocessed food plans so the need for mediation for comorbidities should be carefully monitored to avoid overmedicating. Caregivers of pediatric PFA clients should know how to monitor medications for elements of the metabolic syndrome. Glucose testing for diabetes and blood pressure readings for hypertension are essential. Caregivers should be trained in how to adjust medications or call the practitioner for instructions in how to adjust medications. Failing to adjust medications could result in blood glucose, or blood pressure levels that are too low.

Medications for mood and behavior also should be monitored carefully. The underlying neuro-conditions may resolve. Metabolism of medications may change. And, as weight status changes, levels of medications may need to be adjusted.

29.7.9 Adherence

Practitioners can encourage families to adhere to an unprocessed food plan and cue avoidance through identification of results and through praise for progress. Finding a support group for caregivers either online or in person is also helpful to promoting adherence to recovery from PFA. Resources may be found at http://www.foodaddictionresources.com/resources.html.

Practitioners may recall from Chapter 25, "Avenues to Success for the Practitioner," that patience and an understanding of PFA as a lapsing disease are key to helping clients over the long term. Because of the prevalence of processed foods and cues, treatment of PFA may be more likely to result in reduced harm than consistent abstinence.

29.7.10 Twelve-Step Support

Support should be recommended for the caregivers but not for children. It is the caregivers' responsibility to maintain a supply of healthy food for children in an environment that is free from cuing. Healthy activities that involve movement and intellectual stimulation can be organized by caregivers. Caregivers can supply education and encouragement for their children. Twelve-step resources for caregivers can be found at http://www.foodaddictionresources.com/resources.html.

29.8 DISCUSSION

The treatment guidelines for adolescent SUD and ED are readily bridged to treatment for PFA. The need for screening, evaluation, treatment planning, and monitoring are similar. Diet advice, exercise, reduced screen time, improved sleep, and counseling are also similarly employed.

The major difference between ED/SUD treatment and PFA is the need for abstinence from processed foods, the need to avoid cuing, and a greater need for relationship management to help children resist offers of processed foods from adults and other children.

The challenges for a parent or primary caregiver in terms of provision of foods is not much different than the case of a child who is allergic to a range of foods. Some caregivers may be more adept at keeping processed foods out of the house. These parents may also be more reliable in terms of supplying children with unprocessed foods when they're away from home. Other caregivers will be more challenged to shop for unprocessed foods and assemble them into meals. These parents will need more support, praise, and encouragement.

Similarly, some caregivers will welcome guidance to turn off the television and Internet. They will enjoy playing with their children and engaging in fun exercise such as playing, walking, swimming, sports, or dancing. Other caregivers may be limited by fatigue or extensive commitments to work. In these cases, practitioners can help parents find after school activities for the children that involve movement.

The burden of avoiding cues in Westernized cultures may seem overwhelming at first glance. Parents and caregivers can start slowly by noticing cues for processed foods at home, then gradually becoming more aware on the road. Suggested strategies are provided in Chapter 30, "Strategies for Helping Food-Addicted Children."

Practitioners are likely to find that the success of the child depends on the capabilities of their primary caregivers. In fact, it could be argued that the youngest children are dependent on the ability of their caregivers to provide unprocessed foods, a cue-free environment, and physical activity. Suggestions for educating children are provided in Chapter 30, but it is unrealistic for children to overcome PFA unless the family is creating an environment that is conducive to recovery.

Practitioners can look forward to more successful outcomes by applying classic addictive recovery approaches to children who are manifesting addictive behaviors in their consumption of processed foods.

29.9 CONCLUSION

Addiction to processed foods in children is a difficult disease to treat due to availability and cues for processed foods. However, like drug addiction, PFA responds to education, support, taking action, and cognitive restoration. Practitioners who are already engaged in treating obesity, eating disorders, and substance use disorders will find that they can adapt their approaches to PFA. The keys are to screen for loss of control over consumption and consequences, to educate about abstinent versus addictive foods, to support caregivers in reducing screen and cues in the home, and to give children more physical activities.

REFERENCES

Al-Haifi, A. R., Al-Fayez, M. A., Al-Athari, B. I., Al-Ajmi, F. A., Allafi, A. R., Al-Hazzaa, H. M., & Musaiger, A. O. (2013). Relative contribution of physical activity, sedentary behaviors, and dietary habits to the prevalence of obesity among Kuwaiti adolescents. *Food Nutr Bull, 34*(1), 6–13.

Al Sabbah, H., Vereecken, C., Abdeen, Z., Coats, E., & Maes, L. (2009). Associations of overweight and of weight dissatisfaction among Palestinian adolescents: findings from the national study of Palestinian schoolchildren (HBSC-WBG2004). *J Hum Nutr Diet, 22*(1), 40–49. doi: 10.1111/j.1365-277X.2008.00901.x.

August, G. P., Caprio, S., Fennoy, I., Freemark, M., Kaufman, F. R., Lustig, R. H., ... Montori, V. M. (2008). Prevention and treatment of pediatric obesity: an endocrine society clinical practice guideline based on expert opinion. *J Clin Endocrinol Metab, 93*(12), 4576–4599. doi: 10.1210/jc.2007-2458.

Baker, E. H., & Altman, C. E. (2015). Maternal ratings of child health and child obesity, variations by mother's race/ethnicity and nativity. *Matern Child Health J, 19*(5), 1000–1009. doi: 10.1007/s10995-014-1597-6.

Barlow, S. E. (2007). Expert committee recommendations regarding the prevention, assessment, and treatment of child and adolescent overweight and obesity: summary report. *Pediatrics, 120* (Suppl 4), S164–S192. doi: 10.1542/peds.2007-2329C.

Bauer, C. C., Moreno, B., Gonzalez-Santos, L., Concha, L., Barquera, S., & Barrios, F. A. (2014). Child overweight and obesity are associated with reduced executive cognitive performance and brain alterations: a magnetic resonance imaging study in Mexican children. *Pediatr Obes, 10*(3), 196–204. doi: 10.1111/ijpo.241.

Bearman, S. K., Martinez, E., Stice, E., & Presnell, K. (2006). The skinny on body dissatisfaction: a longitudinal study of adolescent girls and boys. *J Youth Adolesc, 35*(2), 217–229. doi: 10.1007/s10964-005-9010-9.

Bearman, S. K., & Stice, E. (2008). Testing a gender additive model: the role of body image in adolescent depression. *J Abnorm Child Psychol, 36*(8), 1251–1263. doi: 10.1007/s10802-008-9248-2.

Beevers, C. G., Clasen, P., Stice, E., & Schnyer, D. (2010). Depression symptoms and cognitive control of emotion cues: a functional magnetic resonance imaging study. *Neuroscience, 167*(1), 97–103. doi: 10.1016/j.neuroscience.2010.01.047.

Berthoud, H. R., Zheng, H., & Shin, A. C. (2012). Food reward in the obese and after weight loss induced by calorie restriction and bariatric surgery. *Ann N Y Acad Sci, 1264*, 36–48. doi: 10.1111/j.1749-6632.2012.06573.x.

Biederman, J., Ball, S. W., Monuteaux, M. C., Surman, C. B., Johnson, J. L., & Zeitlin, S. (2007). Are girls with ADHD at risk for eating disorders? Results from a controlled, five-year prospective study. *J Dev Behav Pediatr, 28*(4), 302–307. doi: 10.1097/DBP.0b013e3180327917.

Boutelle, K. N., Hannan, P., Fulkerson, J. A., Crow, S. J., & Stice, E. (2010). Obesity as a prospective predictor of depression in adolescent females. *Health Psychol, 29*(3), 293–298. doi: 10.1037/a0018645.

Bruening, M., MacLehose, R., Eisenberg, M. E., Nanney, M. S., Story, M., & Neumark-Sztainer, D. (2014). Associations between sugar-sweetened beverage consumption and fast-food restaurant frequency among adolescents and their friends. *J Nutr Educ Behav, 46*(4), 277–285. doi: 10.1016/j.jneb.2014.02.009.

Bukstein, O. G., Bernet, W., Arnold, V., Beitchman, J., Shaw, J., Benson, R. S., ... Ptakowski, K. K. (2005). Practice parameter for the assessment and treatment of children and adolescents with substance use disorders. *J Am Acad Child Adolesc Psychiatry, 44*(6), 609–621.

Burger, K. S., & Stice, E. (2011). Variability in reward responsivity and obesity: evidence from brain imaging studies. *Curr Drug Abuse Rev, 4*(3), 182–189.

Burger, K. S., & Stice, E. (2012). Frequent ice cream consumption is associated with reduced striatal response to receipt of an ice cream-based milkshake. *Am J Clin Nutr, 95*(4), 810–817. doi: 10.3945/ajcn.111.027003.

Burger, K. S., & Stice, E. (2013). Elevated energy intake is correlated with hyperresponsivity in attentional, gustatory, and reward brain regions while anticipating palatable food receipt. *Am J Clin Nutr, 97*(6), 1188–1194. doi: 10.3945/ajcn.112.055285.

Burrows, T., Skinner, J., Joyner, M. A., Palmieri, J., Vaughan, K., & Gearhardt, A. N. (2017). Food addiction in children: associations with obesity, parental food addiction and feeding practices. *Eat Behav, 26*, 114–120. doi: 10.1016/j.eatbeh.2017.02.004.

Burton, E., Stice, E., & Seeley, J. R. (2004). A prospective test of the stress-buffering model of depression in adolescent girls: no support once again. *J Consult Clin Psychol, 72*(4), 689–697. doi: 10.1037/0022-006X.72.4.689.

Byrne, M. L., O'Brien-Simpson, N. M., Mitchell, S. A., & Allen, N. B. (2015). Adolescent-onset depression: are obesity and inflammation developmental mechanisms or outcomes? *Child Psychiatry Hum Dev, 46*(6), 839–850. doi: 10.1007/s10578-014-0524-9.

Cameron, J. D., Maras, D., Sigal, R. J., Kenny, G. P., Borghese, M. M., Chaput, J. P., … Goldfield, G. S. (2016). The mediating role of energy intake on the relationship between screen time behaviour and body mass index in adolescents with obesity: the HEARTY study. *Appetite, 107*, 437–444. doi: 10.1016/j.appet.2016.08.101.

Carlezon, W. A., Jr., & Konradi, C. (2004). Understanding the neurobiological consequences of early exposure to psychotropic drugs: linking behavior with molecules. *Neuropharmacology, 47* (Suppl 1), 47–60. doi: 10.1016/j.neuropharm.2004.06.021.

Center for Disease Control. (2005). Mental health in the United States. Prevalence of diagnosis and medication treatment for attention-deficit/hyperactivity disorder—United States, 2003. *MMWR Morb Mortal Wkly Rep, 54*(34), 842–847.

Chahal, H., Fung, C., Kuhle, S., & Veugelers, P. J. (2013). Availability and night-time use of electronic entertainment and communication devices are associated with short sleep duration and obesity among Canadian children. *Pediatr Obes, 8*(1), 42–51. doi: 10.1111/j.2047-6310.2012.00085.x.

Coelho, J. S., Siggen, M. J., Dietre, P., & Bouvard, M. (2013). Reactivity to thought-shape fusion in adolescents: the effects of obesity status. *Pediatr Obes, 8*(6), 439–444. doi: 10.1111/j.2047-6310.2012.00121.x.

Do, Y. K., Shin, E., Bautista, M. A., & Foo, K. (2013). The associations between self-reported sleep duration and adolescent health outcomes: what is the role of time spent on Internet use? *Sleep Med, 14*(2), 195–200. doi: 10.1016/j.sleep.2012.09.004.

Duckworth, A. L., Tsukayama, E., & Geier, A. B. (2010). Self-controlled children stay leaner in the transition to adolescence. *Appetite, 54*(2), 304–308. doi: 10.1016/j.appet.2009.11.016.

Engle, P. L., & Fernandez, P. D. (2010). INCAP studies of malnutrition and cognitive behavior. *Food Nutr Bull, 31*(1), 83–94.

Epstein, L. H., Yokum, S., Feda, D. M., & Stice, E. (2014). Food reinforcement and parental obesity predict future weight gain in non-obese adolescents. *Appetite, 82*, 138–142. doi: 10.1016/j.appet.2014.07.018.

Estrada, E., Eneli, I., Hampl, S., Mietus-Snyder, M., Mirza, N., Rhodes, E., … Pont, S. J. (2014). Children's Hospital Association consensus statements for comorbidities of childhood obesity. *Child Obes, 10*(4), 304–317. doi: 10.1089/chi.2013.0120.

Evans, G. W., Fuller-Rowell, T. E., & Doan, S. N. (2012). Childhood cumulative risk and obesity: the mediating role of self-regulatory ability. *Pediatrics, 129*(1), e68–e73. doi: 10.1542/peds.2010-3647.

Felitti, V. J. (1993). Childhood sexual abuse, depression, and family dysfunction in adult obese patients: a case control study. *South Med J, 86*(7), 732–736.

Felitti, V. J., Jakstis, K., Pepper, V., & Ray, A. (2010). Obesity: problem, solution, or both? *Perm J, 14*(1), 24–30.

Francis, L. A., & Susman, E. J. (2009). Self-regulation and rapid weight gain in children from age 3 to 12 years. *Arch Pediatr Adolesc Med, 163*(4), 297–302. doi: 10.1001/archpediatrics.2008.579.

Gearhardt, A. N., Roberto, C. A., Seamans, M. J., Corbin, W. R., & Brownell, K. D. (2013). Preliminary validation of the Yale Food Addiction Scale for children. *Eat Behav, 14*(4), 508–512. doi: 10.1016/j.eatbeh.2013.07.002.

Goldschmidt, A. B., Wall, M. M., Choo, T. H., Bruening, M., Eisenberg, M. E., & Neumark-Sztainer, D. (2014). Examining associations between adolescent binge eating and binge eating in parents and friends. *Int J Eat Disord, 47*(3), 325–328. doi: 10.1002/eat.22192.

Hadland, S. E., Austin, S. B., Goodenow, C. S., & Calzo, J. P. (2014). Weight misperception and unhealthy weight control behaviors among sexual minorities in the general adolescent population. *J Adolesc Health, 54*(3), 296–303. doi: 10.1016/j.jadohealth.2013.08.021.

Halford, J. C., Boyland, E. J., Hughes, G., Oliveira, L. P., & Dovey, T. M. (2007). Beyond-brand effect of television (TV) food advertisements/commercials on caloric intake and food choice of 5–7-year-old children. *Appetite, 49*(1), 263–267.

Heerwagen, M. J., Miller, M. R., Barbour, L. A., & Friedman, J. E. (2010). Maternal obesity and fetal metabolic programming: a fertile epigenetic soil. *Am J Physiol Regul Integr Comp Physiol, 299*(3), R711–R722. doi: 10.1152/ajpregu.00310.2010.

Helton, J. J., & Liechty, J. M. (2014). Obesity prevalence among youth investigated for maltreatment in the United States. *Child Abuse Negl, 38*(4), 768–775. doi: 10.1016/j.chiabu.2013.08.011.

Hoey, H. (2014). Management of obesity in children differs from that of adults. *Proc Nutr Soc, 73*(4), 519–525. doi: 10.1017/s0029665114000652.

Huh, D., Stice, E., Shaw, H., & Boutelle, K. (2012). Female overweight and obesity in adolescence: developmental trends and ethnic differences in prevalence, incidence, and remission. *J Youth Adolesc, 41*(1), 76–85. doi: 10.1007/s10964-011-9664-4.

Iannaccone, M., D'Olimpio, F., Cella, S., & Cotrufo, P. (2016). Self-esteem, body shame and eating disorder risk in obese and normal weight adolescents: a mediation model. *Eat Behav, 21*, 80–83. doi: 10.1016/j.eatbeh.2015.12.010.

Jacka, F. N., Ystrom, E., Brantsaeter, A. L., Karevold, E., Roth, C., Haugen, M., … Berk, M. (2013). Maternal and early postnatal nutrition and mental health of offspring by age 5 years: a prospective cohort study. *J Am Acad Child Adolesc Psychiatry, 52*(10), 1038–1047. doi: 10.1016/j.jaac.2013.07.002.

King, K. M., Puhl, R. M., Luedicke, J., & Peterson, J. L. (2013). Eating behaviors, victimization, and desire for supportive intervention among adolescents in weight-loss camps. *Eat Behav, 14*(4), 484–487. doi: 10.1016/j.eatbeh.2013.08.004.

Koch, A., & Pollatos, O. (2015). Reduced facial emotion recognition in overweight and obese children. *J Psychosom Res, 79*(6), 635–639. doi: 10.1016/j.jpsychores.2015.06.005.

Kraak, V. I., & Story, M. (2015). Influence of food companies' brand mascots and entertainment companies' cartoon media characters on children's diet and health: a systematic review and research needs. *Obes Rev, 16*(2), 107–126. doi: 10.1111/obr.12237.

Kuzel, R., & Larson, J. (2014). Treating childhood obesity. *Minn Med, 97*(1), 48–50.

Landis, A. M., Parker, K. P., & Dunbar, S. B. (2009). Sleep, hunger, satiety, food cravings, and caloric intake in adolescents. *J Nurs Scholarsh, 41*(2), 115–123. doi: 10.1111/j.1547-5069.2009.01262.x.

Levitan, R. D., Rivera, J., Silveira, P. P., Steiner, M., Gaudreau, H., Hamilton, J., … Meaney, M. J. (2014). Gender differences in the association between stop-signal reaction times, body mass indices and/or spontaneous food intake in pre-school children: An early model of compromised inhibitory control and obesity. *Int J Obes (Lond), 39*(4), 614–619. doi: 10.1038/ijo.2014.207.

Lock, J., & La Via, M. C. (2015). Practice parameter for the assessment and treatment of children and adolescents with eating disorders. *J Am Acad Child Adolesc Psychiatry, 54*(5), 412–425. doi: 10.1016/j.jaac.2015.01.018.

Mackenbach, J. D., Tiemeier, H., Ende, J., Nijs, I. M., Jaddoe, V. W., Hofman, A., … Jansen, P. W. (2012). Relation of emotional and behavioral problems with body mass index in preschool children: the Generation R study. *J Dev Behav Pediatr, 33*(8), 641–648. doi: 10.1097/DBP.0b013e31826419b8.

Markey, C. N. (2010). Invited commentary: why body image is important to adolescent development. *J Youth Adolesc, 39*(12), 1387–1391. doi: 10.1007/s10964-010-9510-0.

Marmorstein, N. R., Iacono, W. G., & Legrand, L. (2014). Obesity and depression in adolescence and beyond: reciprocal risks. *Int J Obes (Lond), 38*(7), 906–911. doi: 10.1038/ijo.2014.19.

Mendez, M. A., Sotres-Alvarez, D., Miles, D. R., Slining, M. M., & Popkin, B. M. (2014). Shifts in the recent distribution of energy intake among U.S. children aged 2–18 years reflect potential abatement of earlier declining trends. *J Nutr, 144*(8), 1291–1297. doi: 10.3945/jn.114.190447.

Micali, N., Ploubidis, G., De Stavola, B., Simonoff, E., & Treasure, J. (2014). Frequency and patterns of eating disorder symptoms in early adolescence. *J Adolesc Health, 54*(5), 574–581. doi: 10.1016/j.jadohealth.2013.10.200.

Michaelides, M., Thanos, P. K., Volkow, N. D., & Wang, G. J. (2012). Translational neuroimaging in drug addiction and obesity. *Ilar J, 53*(1), 59–68.

Morrison, K. M., Shin, S., Tarnopolsky, M., & Taylor, V. H. (2015). Association of depression & health related quality of life with body composition in children and youth with obesity. *J Affect Disord, 172*, 18–23. doi: 10.1016/j.jad.2014.09.014.

Nestle, M. (1996). *Food Politics*. New York: Random House.

Ng, M., Fleming, T., Robinson, M., Thomson, B., Graetz, N., Margono, C., … Gakidou, E. (2014). Global, regional, and national prevalence of overweight and obesity in children and adults during 1980–2013: a systematic analysis for the Global Burden of Disease Study 2013. *Lancet, 384*(9945), 766–781. doi: 10.1016/s0140-6736(14)60460-8.

Nguyen, P. V., Hong, T. K., Nguyen, D. T., & Robert, A. R. (2016). Excessive screen viewing time by adolescents and body fatness in a developing country: Vietnam. *Asia Pac J Clin Nutr, 25*(1), 174–183. doi: 10.6133/apjcn.2016.25.1.21.

Ogden, C. L., Carroll, M. D., Lawman, H. G., Fryar, C. D., Kruszon-Moran, D., Kit, B. K., & Flegal, K. M. (2016). Trends in obesity prevalence among children and adolescents in the United States, 1988–1994 through 2013–2014. *JAMA, 315*(21), 2292–2299. doi: 10.1001/jama.2016.6361.

Parkin, P., Connor Gorber, S., Shaw, E., Bell, N., Jaramillo, A., Tonelli, M., & Brauer, P. (2015). Recommendations for growth monitoring, and prevention and management of overweight and obesity in children and youth in primary care. *CMAJ, 187*(6), 411–421. doi: 10.1503/cmaj.141285.

Powell, L. M., Harris, J. L., & Fox, T. (2013). Food marketing expenditures aimed at youth: putting the numbers in context. *Am J Prev Med, 45*(4), 453–461. doi: 10.1016/j.amepre.2013.06.003.

Presnell, K., Bearman, S. K., & Stice, E. (2004). Risk factors for body dissatisfaction in adolescent boys and girls: a prospective study. *Int J Eat Disord, 36*(4), 389–401. doi: 10.1002/eat.20045.

Presnell, K., Stice, E., Seidel, A., & Madeley, M. C. (2009). Depression and eating pathology: prospective reciprocal relations in adolescents. *Clin Psychol Psychother, 16*(4), 357–365. doi: 10.1002/cpp.630.

Rankin, J., Matthews, L., Cobley, S., Han, A., Sanders, R., Wiltshire, H. D., & Baker, J. S. (2016). Psychological consequences of childhood obesity: psychiatric comorbidity and prevention. *Adolesc Health Med Ther, 7*, 125–146. doi: 10.2147/ahmt.s101631.

Roberts, R. E., & Duong, H. T. (2015). Does major depression affect risk for adolescent obesity? *J Affect Disord, 186*, 162–167. doi: 10.1016/j.jad.2015.06.030.

Rohde, P., Beevers, C. G., Stice, E., & O'Neil, K. (2009). Major and minor depression in female adolescents: onset, course, symptom presentation, and demographic associations. *J Clin Psychol, 65*(12), 1339–1349. doi: 10.1002/jclp.20629.

Rollins, B. Y., Loken, E., Savage, J. S., & Birch, L. L. (2014). Measurement of food reinforcement in preschool children. Associations with food intake, BMI, and reward sensitivity. *Appetite, 72*, 21–27. doi: 10.1016/j.appet.2013.09.018.

Sanders, R. H., Han, A., Baker, J. S., & Cobley, S. (2015). Childhood obesity and its physical and psychological co-morbidities: a systematic review of Australian children and adolescents. *Eur J Pediatr, 174*(6), 715–746. doi: 10.1007/s00431-015-2551-3.

Seeley, J. R., Stice, E., & Rohde, P. (2009). Screening for depression prevention: identifying adolescent girls at high risk for future depression. *J Abnorm Psychol, 118*(1), 161–170. doi: 10.1037/a0014741.

Shashaj, B., Bedogni, G., Graziani, M. P., Tozzi, A. E., DiCorpo, M. L., Morano, D., … Manco, M. (2014). Origin of cardiovascular risk in overweight preschool children: a cohort study of cardiometabolic risk factors at the onset of obesity. *JAMA Pediatr, 168*(10), 917–924. doi: 10.1001/jamapediatrics.2014.900.

Shin, S. H., & Miller, D. P. (2012). A longitudinal examination of childhood maltreatment and adolescent obesity: results from the National Longitudinal Study of Adolescent Health (AddHealth) Study. *Child Abuse Negl, 36*(2), 84–94. doi: 10.1016/j.chiabu.2011.08.007.

Silvers, J. A., Insel, C., Powers, A., Franz, P., Weber, J., Mischel, W., … Ochsner, K. N. (2014). Curbing craving: behavioral and brain evidence that children regulate craving when instructed to do so but have higher baseline craving than adults. *Psychol Sci, 25*(10), 1932–1942. doi: 10.1177/0956797614546001.

Sinha, R., & Jastreboff, A. M. (2013). Stress as a common risk factor for obesity and addiction. *Biol Psychiatry, 73*(9), 827–835. doi: 10.1016/j.biopsych.2013.01.032.

Sjoberg, R. L., Nilsson, K. W., & Leppert, J. (2005). Obesity, shame, and depression in school-aged children: a population-based study. *Pediatrics, 116*(3), e389–e392. doi: 10.1542/peds.2005-0170.

Stice, E., Agras, W. S., & Hammer, L. D. (1999). Risk factors for the emergence of childhood eating disturbances: a five-year prospective study. *Int J Eat Disord, 25*(4), 375–387. doi: 10.1002/(SICI)1098-108X(199905)25:4<375::AID-EAT2>3.0.CO;2-K.

Stice, E., Akutagawa, D., Gaggar, A., & Agras, W. S. (2000). Negative affect moderates the relation between dieting and binge eating. *Int J Eat Disord, 27*(2), 218–229. doi: 10.1002/(SICI)1098-108X(200003)27:2<218::AID-EAT10>3.0.CO;2-1.

Stice, E., Presnell, K., Shaw, H., & Rohde, P. (2005). Psychological and behavioral risk factors for obesity onset in adolescent girls: a prospective study. *J Consult Clin Psychol, 73*(2), 195–202. doi: 10.1037/0022-006x.73.2.195.

Stice, E., Presnell, K., & Spangler, D. (2002). Risk factors for binge eating onset in adolescent girls: a 2-year prospective investigation. *Health Psychol, 21*(2), 131–138.

Togashi, K., Iguchi, K., & Masuda, H. (2013). Prevention and treatment of obesity in children. *Nihon Rinsho, 71*(2), 310–314.

van Meer, F., van der Laan, L. N., Adan, R. A., Viergever, M. A., & Smeets, P. A. (2015). What you see is what you eat: an ALE meta-analysis of the neural correlates of food viewing in children and adolescents. *NeuroImage, 104*, 35–43. doi: 10.1016/j.neuroimage.2014.09.069.

Verbeken, S., Braet, C., Bosmans, G., & Goossens, L. (2014). Comparing decision making in average and overweight children and adolescents. *Int J Obes (Lond), 38*(4), 547–551. doi: 10.1038/ijo.2013.235.

Zimmerman, F. J., & Shimoga, S. V. (2014). The effects of food advertising and cognitive load on food choices. *BMC Public Health, 14*, 342. doi: 10.1186/1471-2458-14-342.

30 Strategies for Helping Food-Addicted Children

Joan Ifland
Food Addiction Training, LLC
Cincinnati, OH

CONTENTS

30.1 INTRODUCTION

The specter of children addicted to processed foods is disturbing, but a variety of research points to its possibility. Fortunately, the research also suggests avenues for recovery.

Caregivers may be unaware of what they might be doing to contribute to their children's problems. Many adults would be very willing to protect their children if they only knew what to do. To this end, it is worthwhile to educate adults about the link between common pediatric health problems and the addictive use of processed foods by their children. There is evidence that when processed foods are removed from children's diets, behavioral and physical health problems may fade (Khan et al., 2015). Bright, agreeable, healthy children may emerge from under the distressing effects of processed foods.

Caregivers' confusion and distress may be compounded by a weight gain in the child (Ogden, Carroll, Kit, & Flegal, 2012). Attempts to control the child can result in the development of eating disorders in the child if caregivers employ authoritarian approaches such as punishing and criticizing (Kakinami, Barnett, Seguin, & Paradis, 2015). Added to these factors are the challenges that the addicted child meets in food- and cue-dense environments such as school and other homes (Terry-McElrath, Turner, Sandoval, Johnston, & Chaloupka, 2014). Helping children gain control of eating is not easy because the processed food industry targets the youngest markets (Nestle, 2013; Scully et al., 2015). This chapter suggests issues related to the need for protocols to teach caregivers help addicted children. The suggestions and issues described in this chapter are bridged from evidence to observations of the difficulties that parents face when working to help their children recover from processed food addiction (PFA). There is no research directly evaluating methods for helping children recover from PFA. This chapter relies on evidence from approaches to treating eating disorders (ED) and substance use disorders (SUD) in adolescents. It targets areas of concern such as neglect and trauma, based on evidence that these experiences predict obesity, eating disorders, and SUD as well as common comorbidities such as depression and body dissatisfaction (Dube, Anda, Felitti, Edwards, & Croft, 2002; Dube et al., 2003; Felitti et al., 1998). This chapter builds on Chapter 29, which describes practice parameters for PFA in children. Whereas Chapter 29 suggests approaches for practitioners, this chapter is focused on helping primary caregivers.

30.1.1 Models for Food Intolerances

Models exist for dealing with food intolerances in children. These come from a number of sources such as food allergies. They also come from the development of special gluten-free diets for celiac disease (Ciacci et al., 2005) and from research showing a role for food additives in ADHD (Boris & Mandel, 1994). Households may adopt special diets for religious reasons. A household might adhere to a vegan diet for moral reasons. So fortunately, there is precedent for managing food addiction in children with a special nonaddictive diet.

The striking difference between the special-diet child and the food-addicted child is the very presence of the addiction, as discussed in the "Evidence" section below, especially the evidence for cue-reactive cravings (Stice, Yokum, Burger, Epstein, & Small, 2011) and the prevalence of food cues in Westernized cultures (Lifshitz & Lifshitz, 2014). Addictions in adults are a mental illness of cue-reactive cravings with loss of cognitive function and increased stress (Volkow, Koob, & McLellan, 2016). This is as opposed to a physical illness such as celiac disease. In the case of food allergies or other special diets, the child retains reasoning and learning capabilities. These children can be expected to effectively learn the dangers of particular foods and have the clarity to decline the offer of allergic foods outside of the home. Food-addicted children may have lost these capabilities, as chronic overconsumption of processed foods has been associated with loss of cognitive abilities (Miller, Lee, & Lumeng, 2014).

30.1.2 Characteristics of Externally Cued Cravings

As will be described in the review of evidence, in the case of food addiction, the child suffers from processed food cravings (Silvers et al., 2014), food cue reactivity (Burger & Stice, 2014a), and loss of cognitive abilities (Miller et al., 2014). These are significant barriers to teaching addicted children to avoid addictive foods and to successfully maintain abstinence in Western cultures where processed food cues and availability can activate the loss of control (Morris, Beilharz, Maniam, Reichelt, & Westbrook, 2015). The challenge of keeping an addicted child free from cravings is daunting but manageable. The key is to provide the child's caregivers with relevant education, support, and skills. The basic approach is the same for children as it is for adults. Avoid addictive foods, avoid heavily cued environments, and engage in brain stabilizing activities.

Several concepts can be helpful when considering how best to approach the addicted child. The first is that exposure to cueing drives the intensity of the craving. The greater the exposure, the greater the craving (Powell, Harris, & Fox, 2013). The second is that cravings can be counteracted. With training, a craving can be quelled without giving into the impulse to act on it and losing control (Boutelle & Bouton, 2015). So, like adults, the path to helping children is to minimize exposure to processed foods and cues and maximize recovery activities.

Difficulties arise when children need to be in environments without their caregivers. Child care arrangements, school, playdates, parties, family events, and faith organizations are examples where cues for processed foods have been found to be rife and the value of a reinforcing context such as a home or setting is lost (Trask, Schepers, & Bouton, 2015). School environments have been found to be associated with food cues (Grenard et al., 2013). Teachers may use sweets and coupons for fast food to reward students (Terry-McElrath et al., 2014). Vending machines and sweets in classmates' packed lunches may also provoke overwhelming cravings (Drewnowski & Rehm, 2014). These are obstacles to resolving cravings in a child.

30.1.3 Importance of Food-Addicted Children

Children exhibit many of the consequences of chronic processed food use. Symptomology is appearing at younger and younger ages including heart disease, fatty liver, depression, overweight, learning disabilities, and mood disorders (Armstrong et al., 2016). The epidemic of overweight children is no longer just a US problem (Ogden et al., 2016) but is spreading around the world (Ng et al., 2014). At the same time, effective solutions are elusive. It is possible that past attempts to help children "lose weight" have failed because the presence of food addiction has been missed, and therefore the core problem of cravings and loss of decision-making capabilities in the child's brain were not addressed.

The goal is to avoid controlling the child and focus instead on processed food availability and cues in the home environment (Neumark-Sztainer, 2005). An additional risk of failure and damage to personality development may derive from thinking that only one child in a family system needs help because that one child has a "weight" problem (Wansink & van Kleef, 2014). Making processed foods available to normally weighted children while forcing the overweight child to abstain is a recipe for failure, as cue reactivity in the addicted child can be activated by the sight of consumption by siblings (Werthmann et al., 2011).

30.1.4 Strengths of "Strategies for Helping Food-Addicted Children"

"Strategies for Helping Food-Addicted Children" stands on research developed in earlier chapters. This chapter's strengths are also in evidence showing that addictions are "caught" from environments (Lioutas & Tzimitra-Kalogianni, 2015; Lobstein et al., 2015). Stanton Peele recounts the story of the Roman general who received a letter from one of his soliders asking which town he should move to. The general suggested that moving to the wine-drinking town would result in a wasted life (Peele, 1992). This chapter focuses on processed food availability and cues in environments.

30.1.5 Limitations of Food-Addicted Children

The practices described herein have not been subjected to rigorous scientific evaluation; rather, they are bridged from evidence for practices in ED, SUD, and obesity in adolescents and adults.

There are a number of topics that are not covered in this chapter because they have already been discussed in detail earlier in the textbook. This includes evidence for the relationship between processed foods and physical, emotional, and behavioral problems. This chapter also does not include the most basic information about the food plan, as this has been covered in Chapter 6, "Abstinent Food Plans for Processed Food Addiction." The practitioner will have covered this with adults in the treatment section for adults. In fact, this chapter on children assumes that the adults have acquired food management skills and are practicing an unprocessed food plan for themselves, as described earlier in Part III of the textbook.

30.2 EVIDENCE

As seen in Chapter 29, there is evidence for an epidemic of PFA in children with comorbidities of obesity, endocrine issues, mood disorders, and adverse childhood experiences (August et al., 2008; Barlow, 2007; Ng et al., 2014). The epidemic has continued for several decades without an apparent solution. Primary care physicians have been found to avoid diagnosing obesity and are being urged to routinely screen for it (O'Brien, Holubkov, & Reis, 2004). Guidelines for treatment have been developed regarding exercise, diet, reduced screen time, and resolution of comorbidities (August et al., 2008; Barlow, 2007; Kuzel & Larson, 2014).

There is significant evidence for PFA in children. The evidence comes primarily from research showing obsessional behaviors and neuroanomalies in reaction to processed foods in children

(Rollins, Loken, Savage, & Birch, 2014; van Meer, van der Laan, Adan, Viergever, & Smeets, 2015). Chronic exposure of children to advertising and availability is evidence for the etiology of food addiction in children (Gebauer & Laska, 2011; Scully et al., 2012; Temple, 2016). This section bridges what is known about treating obesity, SUD, and ED to suggest how research findings might be applied to helping children with PFA.

This chapter builds on the foundation of evidence presented in earlier chapters of this textbook. The research on food addiction is extensive as it is derived from research into obesity, SUD, and ED. These three topics have engaged researchers globally for decades, thus generating a significant body of research. Evidence from the textbook that underpins this chapter is summarized below.

Evidence Presented by Chapter	Significance for Food-Addicted Children
4. "Sugar Consumption: An Important Example Whereby Recognizing Food Addiction May Prove Important in Gaining Optimal Health"	Describes evidence for the role of sugar and salt in comorbidities found in obese children.
5. "Sugar and Fat Addiction"	Describes evidence for the ways in which the brain adapts to processed foods including evidence from studies conducted with adolescent girls.
6. "Abstinent Food Plans for Processed Food Addiction"	Describes evidence for the foods involved in the development of food addiction and recovery from food addiction for children.
7. "Mindfulness Therapies for Food Addiction"	Supports the value of bridging cognitive restoration techniques from adults to children.
14. "DSM 5 SUD Criterion 4: Cravings"	Describes the role of cues in triggering cravings and loss of control.
24. "Premises of Recovery for Adults"	Describes the evidence for abstinence, cue-avoidance, and cognitive restoration in recovery from food addiction.
25. "Avenues to Success for the Practitioner"	Supports approaches of collaboration, patience, and compassion.
26. "Adaptation of APA Practice Guidelines for SUD to Processed Food Addiction"	Describes evidence for methods to treat adults.
27. "Preparing Adults for Recovery"	Primary caregivers may need to be treated before food-addicted children.
28. "Insights from the Field"	Education has a role in helping food-addicted children, as well.
29. Adaptation of SUD and ED Practice Parameters to Adolescents and Children with PFA	Describes • Epidemiological evidence for PFA in children • Evidence for pediatric risk factors including neglect, poverty, and trauma • Methods for assessment, evaluation, and treatment planning for pediatric PFA • Evidence for physical, mood, behavioral, and cognitive comorbidities in obese children as well as adolescents with eating disorders • Organization of health services using abstinence from processed foods and cue avoidance.

Note: SUD, substance use disorder; APA, American Psychiatric Association; ED, eating disorder; PFA, processed food addiction.

Thus, this section of evidence will not cover, e.g., the evidence for the effectiveness of abstinence from processed foods (Chapter 6) and avoidance of cues in recovery from PFA (Chapter 14). Of particular importance, this section does not present the evidence for cognitive impairment in obese children, as this has been covered in Chapter 29. However, this chapter does present the evidence for cue reactivity in children, as the evidence for cue reactivity informs recommendations for cue avoidance in recovery from food addiction in children.

This "Evidence" section for helping children recover from PFA is organized into the following categories.

Topic	Evidence
Obesogenic Environment, Cuing, and Addictive Neuroanomalies	Exposure of children to cuing and availability is a factor in the etiology of PFA. Cue avoidance is an element in recovery.
Influence of Family on Development of PFA	Caregivers' dieting behavior and attention to children are factors. Normalization of children's weight is a motivator in parents.
Family Recovery	Involvement of primary caregivers is important to helping children recover.
Approaches to Recovery	Abstinence, cue avoidance, and therapy, especially CBT. Therapy, exercise, cue control, reduced screens are shown to be helpful.

Note: CBT, cognitive behavioral therapy.

30.2.1 Obesogenic Environment, Cuing, and Addictive Neuroanomalies

Much of the evidence for food addiction in children comes from brain-imaging research showing a relationship between addictive neuroanomalies in children's brain and cues for processed foods. Berthoud describes it as follows:

> The power of food cues targeting susceptible emotions and cognitive brain functions, particularly of children and adolescents, is increasingly exploited by modern neuromarketing tools. Increased intake of energy-dense foods high in fat and sugar is not only adding more energy, but may also corrupt neural functions of brain systems involved in nutrient sensing as well as in hedonic, motivational and cognitive processing. (Berthoud, 2012)

30.2.1.1 Cue Reactivity

Bruce et al. found that obese children were hyperresponsive to food stimuli as compared to healthy-weight children. Of importance to the pediatric PFA model, unlike healthy-weight children, brain activations in response to food stimuli in obese children failed to diminish significantly after eating (Bruce et al., 2010). Burger and Stice made a similar finding that excess energy intake correlates positively with increased activity in attentional, gustatory, and reward regions of the brain when anticipating palatable food. They note that while hyperresponsivity of these regions may increase risk of overeating, it is unclear whether the hyperresponsivity is an initial vulnerability factor or a result of previous overeating (Burger & Stice, 2013). In a follow-up study, they found that habitual soft drink intake promotes hyperresponsivity of regions encoding salience/attention toward brand specific cues and hyporesponsivity of inhibitory regions while anticipating intake (Burger & Stice, 2014b).

Even before the development of signs of obesity, youth at risk for obesity show elevated reward circuitry responsivity in general, coupled with elevated somatosensory region responsivity to food. This may lead to overeating that produces blunted dopamine signaling and elevated responsivity to food cues (Stice, Yokum, Burger, et al., 2011). Genetics can pay a role both in cases of hyporeactivity of dopamine pathways to cues and in the case of hyperreactivity (Stice, Burger, & Yokum, 2015; Stice & Dagher, 2010). These two conditions can be seen as two distinct routes to addictive overeating, i.e., either because of overstimulation or because of a drive to stimulate underactive dopamine production.

In another approach with similar results, Hofmann et al. studied event-related potentials in obese versus lean juveniles in response to appetizing food images. The results showed impulsivity as a general risk factor by increasing food-cue salience in response to cues. Dietary restraint showed paradoxical effects in patients, making them more vulnerable to visual food-cues (Hofmann, Ardelt-Gattinger,

Paulmichl, Weghuber, & Blechert, 2015). Batterink et al. found similar results in an functional MRI (fMRI) study of obese versus lean adolescents showing increased sensitivity of reward pathways and hypoactivity in impulse control in obese adolescents (Batterink, Yokum, & Stice, 2010). Increased stress, salience, and reduced inhibition are characteristics of SUD in adults (Volkow et al., 2016).

30.2.1.2 Food Cues in Environments

Food cue reactivity can be seen as a stimulation for addictive overeating. Grenard et al. studied what kinds of cues are associated with processed food and drink use in adolescents. Cues include:

- Being at school
- Being with friends
- Feeling lonely or bored
- Craving a drink or snack
- Being exposed to food cues
- Exercising with sweet drink consumption
- TV with sweet snacks but not with salty snacks or sweet drinks (Grenard et al., 2013)

Scully et al. found a prevalence of advertising for processed food and drink on Irish television in spite of new rules to restrict such advertising (Scully et al., 2015).

In a study using momentary associations, Borgogna et al. looked at whether specific electronic mechanisms mediated the relationship between media exposure and cravings for processed foods. Their research found that non-Hispanic adolescents showed stronger associations between television exposure and cravings for sweet snacks, salty snacks, and sweetened drinks. In Hispanic adolescents, there was an association between phone messaging and cravings for sweet snacks, salty snacks, and sweetened drinks. Males showed stronger associations between video game use and cravings for salty snack cravings (Borgogna et al., 2014).

In a study of 50 adolescents seeking hospital-based weight-loss treatment, those with food addiction, as assessed by the Yale Food Addiction Scale, reported more binge days, more frequent food cravings, higher eating, weight and shape concerns, more symptoms of depression, and higher attentional and motor impulsivity (Meule, Hermann, & Kubler, 2015).

30.2.1.3 Poverty/Discrimination as an Environmental Factor

Fuller-Rowell et al. found more evidence for factors in the environment that can influence the development of chronic overeating. In an analysis of mediating factors, it was found that 13% of the effect of poverty on poor health is explained by perceived discrimination. The findings suggest that social-class discrimination is one important mechanism behind the influence of poverty on physical health (Fuller-Rowell, Evans, & Ong, 2012).

30.2.1.4 Availability in Obesogenic Environments

A factor that hinders recovery from food addiction is availability of processed foods. The American Psychiatric Association, in their practice guidelines for the treatment of SUD, recommend curtailing exposure to availability until addicted clients are less cue-reactive and able to exercise restraint (American Psychiatric Association, 2006). In a study of availability of processed foods to adolescents in convenience stores near high schools, Gebauer and Laska found that all stores had less healthful impulse purchase items available (e.g., candy), while only 46% carried healthier impulse items (e.g., fruit). Most stores (97%) had food/beverage advertising (Gebauer & Laska, 2011).

In data drawn from the National Health and Nutrition Examination Survey (NHANES), Drewnowski and Rehm found that children and adults source sugar primarily from stores (65%–75%) and through drinks (42.4%) (Drewnowski & Rehm, 2014).

30.2.1.5 Dieting

There is evidence that restricting calories can exacerbate the addictive neuroanomalies associated with chronic overeating. Fasting and calorie restriction have been shown to predict binge eating and bulimia over 1- to 5-year follow-up (Stice, Davis, Miller, & Marti, 2008).

Duration of acute caloric deprivation correlates positively with activation in brain regions implicated in attention, reward, and motivation in response to images, anticipated receipt, and receipt of palatable food (e.g., anterior cingulate cortex, orbitofrontal cortex, putamen, and precentral gyrus, respectively). Youth in a longer-term negative energy balance likewise show greater activation in attention (anterior cingulate cortex, ventral medial prefrontal cortex), visual processing (superior visual cortex), reward (caudate), and memory (hippocampus) regions in response to receipt and anticipated receipt of palatable food relative to those in neutral or positive energy balance (Stice et al., 2013).

However, weight loss can be protective of developing eating disorders. Stice et al. found that if dieting is successful, the incidence of bulimia is reduced (Stice, Martinez, Presnell, & Groesz, 2006).

30.2.1.6 Food

Food choices among children are important to examine. Extensive evidence for addictive properties in processed foods is described in Chapter 6, "Abstinent Food Plans for Processed Food Addiction." Additional research pertains specifically to adolescents. Feldstein et al. found that overweight adolescents' brains responded addictively to sweetened beverages but not low-calorie beverages. The response correlated with insulin resistance (Feldstein Ewing et al., 2016). In a treatment-seeking population of bulimic adolescents, Fitzsimmons-Craft et al. found that loss of control was the source of distress, rather than amount of food consumed (Fitzsimmons-Craft et al., 2014). Loss of control is a central characteristic of addiction, as described in the first three of the DSM 5 SUD diagnostic criteria (American Psychiatric Association, 2013).

In a study of 906 Kuwaiti youths, Al-Haifi et al. found that consumption of breakfast, vegetables, fast food, potatoes, cakes, doughnuts, and sweets was associated with overweight and obesity (Al-Haifi et al., 2013). In an analysis of the US Department of Agriculture's 1989–1991 Continuing Survey of Food Intakes, Munoz et al. found that 30% of youth met recommendations for fruit, grain, meat, and dairy, while 36% met recommendations for vegetables. Only 1% of youth met all US dietary recommendations and 16% did not meet any of the recommendations (Munoz, Krebs-Smith, Ballard-Barbash, & Cleveland, 1997).

In a randomized cross-over study of late-adolescent girls, Hoertel et al. found that breakfast reduced cravings and increased dopamine production, especially breakfasts with higher levels of protein (Hoertel, Will, & Leidy, 2014). In an fMRI/questionnaire study of adolescent girls, Leidy et al. made a similar finding with regard to reductions in appetite and increases in satiety after a high-protein breakfast (Leidy, Lepping, Savage, & Harris, 2011). In a questionnaire study of fifteen 14-year-olds, a breakfast of solids versus a liquid breakfast was found to be more satisfying and lead to less consumption at a lunch buffet (Leidy, Bales-Voelker, & Harris, 2011).

30.2.2 Influence of Family on Development of PFA

There is evidence that caregivers, especially parents, influence the development of obesity and ED in their children. Preferences for processed foods are learned by familiarization, associative conditioning, and by observing the eating behavior of others. Parents' feeding strategies are used to influence what and how much children eat (Anzman, Rollins, & Birch, 2010).

Research demonstrates that tendencies to gain weight can start in infancy. In a 1-year study of 110 breastfeeding mother–infant dyads, Anzman-Frasca et al. found that greater observed negative reactivity in infants predicted more child weight gain when mothers had lower parenting self-efficacy. Lower mother-reported self-regulation also predicted weight gain in children (Anzman-Frasca,

Stifter, Paul, & Birch, 2013). Anzman et al. found that healthy versus unhealthy food preferences can be learned during the suckling period through flavor transmission (Anzman et al., 2010).

In a longitudinal study of 197 white, non-Hispanic girls and their parents, Anzman et al. assessed inhibitory control and parent's restrictive feeding practices every 2 years from age 5 to 15. Findings were that lower inhibitory control predicted higher weight status and that this was exacerbated by parent's restrictive feeding practices (Anzman & Birch, 2009).

In older children, Linville et al. found that maternal thin ideal internalization significantly predicted future increases in adolescent bulimic symptoms (Linville, Stice, Gau, & O'Neil, 2011).

Males have also been found to influence eating patterns. Goldschmidt et al. found that girls' binge eating was associated with their male friends' and fathers' binge eating but not with their female friends' or mothers' binge eating (Goldschmidt et al., 2014).

Outside of the family, peer support is associated with depression. Depression has been shown to be a factor in disordered eating (Presnell, Stice, Seidel, & Madeley, 2009). Deficits in parental support but not peer support predicted future increases in depressive symptoms and onset of major depression. In contrast, initial depressive symptoms and major depression predicted future decreases in peer support but not parental support (Stice, Burton, & Shaw, 2004).

30.2.3 Family Influence on Recovery

Research consistently finds a role for families, and especially primary caregivers, in recovery from addictive eating in children. In a review article, Birch and Anzman-Frasca et al. found that familiarization and associative learning are influential in teaching children to choose healthy foods over obesogenic foods (Birch & Anzman-Frasca, 2011). In a data-collection study of 321 low-income mothers and their preschool children, Speirs et al. found that families with a strong family sense of coherence that view challenges as predictable, understandable, worthy of engaging, and surmountable were practicing healthy child behaviors (Speirs, Hayes, Musaad, VanBrackle, & Sigman-Grant, 2016).

Research has demonstrated that parents are concerned about food environments for their children. In a telephone interview study of Australian parents, Kelly et al. found that 83% of parent's highest level of concern was for the positioning of food at supermarket checkouts. Parents did not trust the industry to protect children from food marketing at a rate of 91%. Parental awareness of nonbroadcast media food marketing such as print, radio, and premium offers to children was low. Nonetheless 81% of parents believed that the government should restrict the use of nonbroadcast media marketing of unhealthy food to children. The study found that children have significant interest in advertised food products. Among parents of younger children, 65% reported that their child asked for advertised food products, as compared with 48% of parents of adolescents (Kelly, Chapman, Hardy, King, & Farrell, 2009).

Parents are also concerned about weight-based victimization that their children may experience (Puhl, Luedicke, & Depierre, 2013).

Weight issues may be the primary reason that families seek treatment. Dhingra et al. studied parents' motivation for initiating weight-loss treatment for their children. The most common motivations found were:

- Parent-reported adolescent physical health problem
- Parent perception of adolescent weight category
- Parent priority of adolescent weight loss
- Parent perception of discrepancy between adolescent current and ideal weight (Dhingra, Brennan, & Walkley, 2011)

From the child's perspective, skin problems may also be a motivator to remove processed foods from the diet (Cordain et al., 2002).

Researchers are consistent in findings that families need comprehensive support to help their children overcome addictive eating that manifests as obesity and other disordered eating. In a review article, Altman and Wilfley found support for the use of multicomponent lifestyle interventions, with family-based behavioral therapy and parent-only behavioral treatment being the most widely supported treatment types. The authors note that additional research is needed to test a stepped care model for treatment and to establish the ideal number and length of sessions, duration, and intensity of treatments for long-term sustainability of healthy weight management (Altman & Wilfley, 2015).

In another review article, Neumark-Sztainer identified four roles for parents in the effort to teach children to eat healthy foods:

- Role-model healthful behaviors
- Provide an environment that makes it easy for children to make healthful choices
- Focus less on weight and more on behaviors and overall health
- Provide a supportive environment for children to enhance communication

The author goes on to point out that families need to be proactive in obesogenic environments, which work against healthy weight and positive body images in children and adolescents. However, families cannot do it on their own and need support (Neumark-Sztainer, 2005).

In a study of contingency management in a population of African-American adolescents, success was achieved with caregiver participation but not without the participation (Hartlieb et al., 2015).

30.2.4 Approaches to Recovery

As the above research shows, families are the focus of recovery for children. And a range of interventions are indicated. Researchers argue that efforts at prevention and treatment must address the multifactorial causes and consequences of pediatric obesity (Merlo & Yardley, 2011). And an 8-year longitudinal study of adolescents indicates that nonobese children can be reactive to food cues and therefore should be included in treatment. The study found that subthreshold eating disorders are more prevalent than threshold eating disorders and are associated with marked impairment (Stice, Marti, Shaw, & Jaconis, 2009).

A Cochrane Review of 37 obesity studies of 27,946 children 6–12 years old found that very different programs seemed to be equally effective in reducing obesity. Here are the program elements that were found to be effective.

- School curriculum that includes healthy eating, physical activity, and body image
- Increased sessions for physical activity and the development of fundamental movement skills throughout the school week
- Improvements in nutritional quality of the food supply in schools
- Environments and cultural practices that support children eating healthier foods and being active throughout each day
- Support for teachers and other staff to implement health promotion strategies and activities (e.g., professional development, capacity building activities)
- Parent support and home activities that encourage children to be more active, eat more nutritious foods and spend less time in screen-based activities (Waters et al., 2011)

Specific techniques have been evaluated for effectiveness.

30.2.4.1 Education

Research shows that education of mothers is effective. In a 1-year study of 160 breastfeeding mother–newborn dyads, Anzman et al. found that mothers who were given a multicomponent educational intervention had babies who gained less weight than mothers who were given less education. The intervention was two nurse home visits to educate about how to soothe a nonhungry baby without using food and how to read hunger and satiety cues when introducing solids (Paul et al., 2011). Observational studies support the hypothesis that these early periods of rapid transition and development show promise as targets for childhood obesity prevention research (Anzman et al., 2010).

30.2.4.2 Source and Type of Support

Puhl et al. evaluated obese adolescents' preferences for sources of support with weight-based victimization. Participants indicated their preferences for specific strategies including:

- Inclusion in peer activities
- Confronting the bully
- Telling an adult
- Improving antibullying policies

Overweight children show preferences for who they would like to help them with weight-based victimization.

- Friends (66%)
- Peers (58%)
- Teachers (55%)
- Physical education teachers/coaches (44%)
- Parents (43%) (Puhl, Peterson, & Luedicke, 2013a)

This study has potential implications for who should be included on the team helping the child.

Rankin et al. point out the need to address significant psychiatric disorders and psychological problems. Their study points out that it remains unclear as to whether psychiatric disorders and psychological problems are a cause or a consequence of childhood obesity, or whether common factors promote both obesity and psychiatric disturbances in susceptible children and adolescents. A cohesive and strategic approach to tackle the obesity epidemic is necessary to combat this increasing trend, which is compromising the health and well-being of the young generation and seriously impinging on resources and economic costs (Rankin et al., 2016).

30.2.4.3 Needed Research

Shrewsbury et al. point to the need to focus on the transition from adolescent obesity to adult obesity. The researchers point out an absence of published intervention programs/policies, clinical guidance, and expert opinion this topic (Shrewsbury, Baur, Nguyen, & Steinbeck, 2014).

30.2.4.4 Cognitive Behavioral Therapy

Cognitive behavioral therapy (CBT) has been shown to be effective in treating addictions through decreased activity in reward pathways and increased activity in impulse control (Zilverstand, Parvaz, Moeller, & Goldstein, 2016). The obesogenic environment may engender distorted thinking that could be helped by CBT. For example, in a study of obese versus lean adolescents, eating pathology, but not obesity status or gender, predicted trait thought shape fusion (TSF). TSF is a phenomenon associated with perceptions of weight gain, body dissatisfaction, and moral wrongdoing after merely thinking about consumption of high-caloric foods (Coelho, Siggen, Dietre, & Bouvard, 2013).

An MRI study showed the efficacy of attempts to control cravings through cognitive control. In responses to images of processed foods, Silvers et al. found that children and young adults (age 6–23) can control cravings when instructed to visualize images of processed foods as moving farther away. Older participants showed fewer cravings suggesting that children may outgrow strong cravings. With effort, all participants reported less craving. Greater body mass predicted less regulation-related prefrontal activity, particularly among children (Silvers et al., 2014).

In a meta-analytic review of the efficacy of programs to reduce disordered eating in adolescents, Stice et al. found larger effects in programs that were:

- Selected versus universal
- Interactive versus didactic
- Multisession versus single session
- Solely offered to females versus both sexes
- Offered to participants over 15 years of age versus younger ones
- Delivered by professional interventionists versus endogenous providers

Programs with body acceptance and dissonance-induction content and without psychoeducational content and programs evaluated in trials using validated measures and a shorter follow-up period also produced larger effects (Stice & Shaw, 2004). Rodriguez found that a cognitive dissonance-based eating disorder prevention program was equally effective for Asian, Hispanic, and white participants (Rodriguez, Marchand, Ng, & Stice, 2008).

In a similar review of programs addressing obesity, Stice et al. found greater efficacy in:

- Children and adolescents (vs. preadolescents)
- Females
- Programs that were relatively brief
- Programs that solely targeted weight control versus other health behaviors (e.g., smoking)
- Programs evaluated in pilot trials
- Programs wherein participants were required to self-select into the intervention (Stice, Shaw, & Marti, 2006)

Stice et al. also conducted a meta-analytic review of programs addressing depression in adolescents. Larger effects emerged for:

- Programs targeting high-risk individuals
- Samples with more females
- Samples with older adolescents
- Programs with a shorter duration
- Programs with homework assignments
- Programs delivered by professional interventionists (Stice, Shaw, Bohon, Marti, & Rohde, 2009)

Marchand et al. found that a similar intervention for depression was effective for all ethnic groups attending including Asian, Latino, and European-Americans (Marchand, Ng, Rohde, & Stice, 2010).

In a randomized trial of 481 girls with a mean age of 17 years, Stice et al. found that body dissatisfaction education showed significantly greater reductions in eating disorder risk factors and bulimic symptoms than healthy weight, expressive writing, and assessment-only participants (Stice, Shaw, Burton, & Wade, 2006). A similar study randomized 306 girls with a mean age of 15.7 years to body dissatisfaction training by high-school staff versus a brochure. Compared to the brochure, the training decreased:

- Thin-ideal internalization
- Body dissatisfaction
- Dieting attempts
- Eating disorder symptoms (Stice, Rohde, Gau, & Shaw, 2009)

When considering approaches to PFA in children, it is useful to bear in mind the size of populations that may need help. Estimates are of 12.5 million US obese children (Ogden et al., 2016). Stice et al. found that CBT delivered by bibliotherapy (self-help books) was effective as well as the least expensive method for reducing risk of depression at 1- and 2-year follow-ups (Stice, Rohde, Gau, & Wade, 2010). Bibliotherapy with online support may be a realistic way to reach millions of addictive overeaters.

The enduring effects of programs is important. In a study of 401 girls with body dissatisfaction, Stice et al. evaluated a dissonance-based thin-ideal internalization reduction program versus a healthy weight control program. Dissonance participants showed a 60% reduction in risk for eating pathology onset, and healthy weight participants showed a 61% reduction in risk for eating pathology onset and a 55% reduction in risk for obesity onset relative to assessment-only controls through 3-year follow-up (Stice, Marti, Spoor, Presnell, & Shaw, 2008).

30.2.4.5 Sleep

In a Hispanic population, Drescher et al. found that parental reports of total sleep time (TST) were found to be the most closely associated with BMI z-score. Decreased TST and increased caffeine intake and screen time may result in higher obesity risk in the adolescent population (Drescher, Goodwin, Silva, & Quan, 2011). In a study of 5032 Chinese elementary school children, Ren et al. found that excessive time spent on academic-related activities outside school hours, inadequate sleep, physical inactivity, and higher levels of screen viewing were major contributors to obesity (Ren, Zhou, Liu, Wang, & Yin, 2017).

Jones and Fiese found that sleep was the only protective routine that correlated with normal weight in a study of 337 families of preschoolers (Jones & Fiese, 2014).

30.2.4.6 Screens

In an analysis of data from the NHANES 2009–2010, Siddarth et al. found that for children, screen-viewing (TV/computer) time was the only significant factor that correlated with obesity. For adolescents, eating habits were the only significant predictor. (Siddarth, 2013).

The finding for a role for screen in obese children has held in developing countries. Nguyen et al. found a correlation between more than 2 hours of screen time per day and obesity in Vietnam (Nguyen, Hong, Nguyen, & Robert, 2016) and Chen et al. as well as Li et al. made similar findings for Chinese students (Chen, Li, Song, Ma, & Wang, 2016; Li et al., 2015). And, Decelis et al. found the same to be the case on Malta in a study of 1126 Maltese children (Decelis, Jago, & Fox, 2014).

30.2.4.7 Exercise

Exercise has been found to be helpful in mood. In a longitudinal study of 496 adolescent girls followed over 6 years, Jerstad et al. found a bidirectional relation between exercise and depression. Physical activity significantly reduced risk for future increases in depressive symptoms and risk for onset of major–minor depression. The findings imply that interventions that increase physical activity may reduce risk for depression (Jerstad, Boutelle, Ness, & Stice, 2010). In a study of 138 8–17 year-olds, Selewski administered a self-questionnaire about health condition. In multivariate analysis, patients with BMI >/= 99th percentile had worse scores for depressive symptoms, anger, fatigue, and mobility. Conversely, parent-reported exercise was associated with better scores for depressive symptoms, anxiety, and fatigue (Selewski et al., 2013).

However, children face barriers to exercise. Edwards et al. found that physical distance, social isolation, lack of community offerings, and transportation were identified as key barriers to physical activity in a rural setting (Edwards, Theriault, Shores, & Melton, 2014). Physical pain can also be a barrier. Paulis et al. found an association between being overweight in childhood and musculoskeletal pain (Paulis, Silva, Koes, & van Middelkoop, 2014).

30.2.4.8 Trauma

In a meta-analysis of 41 studies, Danese and Tan found that childhood trauma is associated with adult obesity (Danese & Tan, 2014). Children who have developed obesity as a result of chronic overeating have been found to suffer weight-based violence. In a study of 361 overweight children aged 14–18 in a weight-loss camp using an online questionnaire, findings indicated that:

- Sixty-four percent of the children reported weight-based victimization at school.
- The risk of weight-based victimization increased with body weight.
- Most participants reported weight-based victimization enduring for 1 year (78%).
- Thirty-six percent were teased/bullied for 5 years.
- Peers (92%) and friends (70%) were the most commonly reported perpetrators.
- Adult perpetrators included physical education teachers/sport coaches (42%), parents (37%), and teachers (27%).
- Weight-based victimization was most frequently reported in the form of verbal teasing (75%–88%).
- Relational victimization (damage to social reputation) (74%–82%).
- Cyberbullying (59%–61%).
- Physical aggression (33%–61%).
- Weight-based victimization was commonly experienced in multiple locations at school (Puhl, Peterson, & Luedicke, 2013b).

Another study found similar results using a different approach. Physical educators expected inferior abilities for overweight students compared to nonoverweight students. Poorer performance expectations were limited to overweight female targets' physical activity, which has implications for students' physical health, academic achievement, and social development (Peterson, Puhl, & Luedicke, 2012).

These findings indicate a need to determine that overweight and obese children are safe during treatment.

30.2.4.9 Surgery

Bariatric surgery is not indicated for food addicts because of the risk of transferring the addiction from processed foods to drugs or alcohol (Bak, Seibold-Simpson, & Darling, 2016) and because of poorer psychosocial outcomes in food addicts (Brunault et al., 2016).

30.2.5 Conclusion

In addition to evidence described in earlier chapters of the textbook, this section discusses evidence that informs approaches to helping children recovery from addictive overeating. The findings demonstrate that children suffer from food cue reactivity, which points to a role for food cue avoidance in recovery from pediatric PFA. The findings also show that families are influential both in terms of the development of PFA in children and in their recovery. This suggests that children would benefit from the involvement of their families in recovery. And finally, in addition to education of adolescents, there are a number of ways to address recovery including CBT, increased exercise, reduced screen time, attention to weight-based victimization, and trauma resolution.

30.3 PREMISES OF TREATMENT FOR ADDICTED CHILDREN

Strategies for Helping Food-Addicted Children depends on an understanding of the orientation of the treatment model. Some of the premises of treatment for children will be familiar from the premises of treatment for adults including severity, risk of relapse, the potential for relationship sensitivity, as well as the need for relationship management skills to maintain boundaries with processed food "pushers." For food-addicted children, there is an addiction set of premises—that the child needs protection from processed foods and cues. A premise is that the disease of food addiction could be severe even in young children due to a young age of onset, the range of substances used, comorbidities, and intense exposure to processed food cues in fast food outlets, television, and school. Extensive symptomology can be similar including impairments in cognitive function, social relationships, academic pursuits, behavior, as well as diminished physical, emotional, and mental well-being. Although similar in nature to adults, symptoms manifest as appropriate for children. The practitioner may also find extensive conformance to DSM 5 SUD criteria. The criteria have been adapted to the lives of children and are provided below.

Another premise is that there is a high risk of relapse in cases of prolonged cue exposure and accidental ingestion. Even a young child may have already experienced trauma and developed relationship sensitivity from being ridiculed by peers and possibly neglected or rejected by family members. The protocols emphasize avoiding punishing, ridiculing, criticizing, or judging the child. An important premise is that the child will need to develop some relationship management skills related to declining offers of processed foods in their environments.

The premises of treatment are similar between adults and children and include a presumption of severity, a high risk of relapse, and cognitive impairment. The difference between the premises for adults versus children are that the adult assumes the role of providing nonaddictive foods to the child. And the adult maintains an environment for the child that is free from processed food cues.

30.4 APPLICATION

Even though educational interventions have been shown to be effective in recovery from obesity, depression, and eating disorders (Stice, Shaw, et al., 2009; Stice et al., 2006; Stice, Shaw, & Marti, 2007), the day-to-day management of recovery from chronic overeating falls to children's primary caregivers. Addictions are difficult to understand under the best of circumstances, but for caregivers who are breaking new ground in terms of helping children overcome PFA, it can be daunting.

The evidence for the neurological nature of addictive eating points to a need for multilevel interventions for food, cue exposure, cognitive restoration, and trauma resolution that go beyond simple behavioral approaches. Researchers call for program evaluations that examine the biochemical effects of complex interventions, especially in low- and middle-income countries (Lee & Gibbs, 2013). Given that the epidemic has spread to 12.5 million US children and solutions for children overextend health resources (August et al., 2008), recovery from PFA will most likely be implemented by literally millions of caregivers. Resources for complex interventions involving in-person treatment by trained health professionals are limited, so it would seem that the appropriate approach is to translate the evidence into simple methods that are realistic for primary caregivers to implement. Research shows that support groups and face-to-face meetings, but not counseling, are preferred settings for programs (Ling, Robbins, & Hines-Martin, 2016).

This section describes two stages for helping parents. A third stage of educating children about PFA is covered in the section "Future Research Needs."

"Stage 1: Enhancing Motivation in Caregivers" progresses through six steps (Donovan, 2013):

1. Sharing the problem
2. Making the recommendation to change
3. Finding out if it's worth it to change
4. Addressing concerns
5. Redefining roles
6. Offering options

"Stage 2: Training Caregivers in Childhood Addiction Management" covers:

1. Learning about what's happening in the child's body
2. Identifying and managing cravings

Stage 3. Teaching children about PFA is covered under "Future Research Needs."

30.4.1 Stage I: Enhancing Motivation in Caregivers

Educating about the benefits of "clean" eating can motivate caregivers to choose treatment. Caregivers may welcome the idea that when a child gets through withdrawal, cognitive functions may be improved (Marwitz, Woodie, & Blythe, 2015). Caregivers may be interested to learn that physical limitations, emotional swings, and erratic behaviors may improve along with academic and athletic abilities (Verbeken, Braet, Bosmans, & Goossens, 2014; Zamzow et al., 2014). In recovery, the child might pass from isolation, to acceptance, and even on to popularity (Martarelli, Borter, Bryjova, Mast, & Munsch, 2015).

30.4.1.1 Step 1 in Motivation: Describing the Problem

In the assessment, the practitioner wants to explore the issues identifies in Chapter 22, "The Addiction Severity Index in the Assessment of Processed Food Addiction," and Chapter 29, "Adaptation of SUD and ED Practice Parameters to Adolescents and Children with PFA." Although behavioral and brain imaging research has found evidence for food addiction in children, the science has not yet progressed to the point of developing a validated pediatric assessment tool (Verbeken, Braet, Lammertyn, Goossens, & Moens, 2012).

In the absence of any assessment tools for food addiction in children, the "state of the art" in assessing children for food addiction could be considered to be an adaptation of the DSM 5 substance use disorder criteria for alcohol (American Psychiatric Association, 2013). There are arguments to be made on both sides of such an adaptation and clearly research is needed to validate the approach. For the purposes of this textbook, practitioners can share with caregivers their findings of severity in terms of the number of DSM 5 SUD diagnostic criteria that the child has met.

30.4.1.1.1 Assessing Severity of Cognitive Impairment

For assessment of cognitive capabilities in children suspected of having food addiction, standardized assessments would be appropriate. In some cases, school-based testing, which typically involves an IQ assessment (e.g., WISC-V) and an evaluation of academic achievement (e.g., WIAT-III or Woodcock-Johnson IV), may be able to identify areas of cognitive impact. However, negative findings on these tests would not conclusively rule out the presence of cognitive impairment. If these approaches prove insufficient, a more comprehensive neuropsychological assessment may be required, which would better identify impairments in the areas of memory, attention/executive skills, and processing speed.

In the case of a finding of severity, practitioners are ready to educate caregivers about the disease of food addiction and how the child might benefit from recovery.

30.4.1.2 Step 2 in Motivation: Making the Recommendation to Change

As the practitioner prepares to make a recommendation for the caregivers to change food practices, he or she will be aware of the environment in the home, particularly regarding history of weight loss attempts in the household. The practitioner can sympathize with the frustration of trying so hard to be successful with approaches that have been shown to be unworkable (Foster, Makris, & Bailer, 2005).

Secondly, from the history, the practitioner will have an idea of the capabilities of the adults. This is an important task, as research shows that children of obese mothers show a lower quality of mother–child attachment, which raises the possibility of neglect (Keitel-Korndorfer et al., 2015). Obese caregivers were also shown to engage less in a family weight-loss program (Maximova, Ambler, Rudko, Chui, & Ball, 2015) and to quit due to stigma and denial (Kelleher et al., 2017).

Motivating Clients through the Recommendation to Change	
Health	A variety of problems may resolve.
Adaptable	Followers can adapt the foods to their own preferences, allergies, and cultures.
Variety	There is variety in the proteins, vegetables, fruits, starches, oils, and seasonings on the food list.
Easy	Shopping and preparation methods are easy.
Simple	The food plan is simple and easy to prepare.
Support	Online and 12-step support groups are available.
Affordable	Ingredients are inexpensive. Reduced spending comes from restaurants, medical, and lost time at work.
Researched	There is a significant body of literature showing an association between a range of diseases and processed foods (Kiecolt-Glaser et al., 2015; Koball et al., 2016; Levin et al., 2014; Manzel et al., 2014; Yau, Kang, Javier, & Convit, 2014).

30.4.1.3 Step 3 in Motivation: Increasing Awareness: Is the Change Worth It?

Making a worthwhile case for adopting an unprocessed food plan can be challenging for the practitioner because such food plans are not in widespread use. Thusly, caregivers may not be familiar with the potential improvements in general health. Benefits for the individual include mental clarity, relief from irritability, depression, and anxiety; emotional stability, increased energy, lowered blood pressure and cholesterol; relief from stomachaches, headaches, and joint aches; reduced allergies and infections; heart disease and diabetes, exaggerated PMS, etc. (Guh et al., 2009).

Clients may derive motivation from writing down their family history of medical problems, including emotional, behavioral, physical, and even spiritual struggles.

Awareness is growing of the connection between processed foods and a broad range of health problems. The handout "Diet-Related Diseases" is designed to help clients imagine the benefits that their household might enjoy if unprocessed foods are made available while processed foods are removed. The handout may be found at www.foodaddictionresources.com.

Increasing Awareness: Is the Change Worth It?	
Mood	Processed foods are associated with diminished pleasure pathways in the brain. This may result in disordered moods, which may be improved on an unprocessed food plan.
Learning	Research shows that processed foods are associated with impairment in learning and decision-making (Smeets, Charbonnier, van Meer, van der Laan, & Spetter, 2012).
Behavior	Children may exhibit calmer behavior (Leung et al., 2014).
Energy	Caring for children while fatigued is stressful.
Prevention	A number of lifelong disorders have been shown to begin in family systems (Krahnstoever Davison, Francis, & Birch, 2005). Eating disorders, obesity, and metabolic syndrome may be prevented.

30.4.1.4 Step 4 in Motivation: Exploring Caregivers' Concerns

Caregivers are likely to present for treatment with a variety of barriers to eliminating processed foods from the home (Brown, Dolisca, & Cheng, 2015; Grossklaus & Marvicsin, 2014; Kelleher et al., 2017; Ling et al., 2016). Reassurance and education are the keys to winning the caregiver over to a belief that the program can be implemented and that it would be valuable to do so. Identifying caregivers' fears and being empathetic are helpful approaches. Caregivers often express fear that their child's new eating habits will make them "different" from other children. They may fear that the task of preparing food is too great.

It is important that the practitioner explain strategies that avoid unrealistic control of the child. This reduces the risk of developing disordered eating in the child. The practitioner can help caregivers get over barriers related to social fears by gently pointing out that it is possible that their children are already suffering weight-based victimization (Puhl et al., 2013b). An unprocessed food plan can alleviate many of these differences and could result in children being more acceptable to peers (Chang & Halgunseth, 2015).

When the practitioner has reviewed the potential benefits of an unprocessed food plan, caregivers may realize that they would like to provide this food plan to their families, but they may also have concerns. It is important to talk through these concerns and offer reassurance that this food plan is manageable.

Answering Clients' Concerns

Time	With practice, most of the cooking for the week can be done in a few hours on the weekend. As relationships with children improve, kids can take responsibility for some of the food preparation.
Energy	Caregivers who are suffering from fatigue may not have the energy to prepare meals. They may need help initially and fatigue may improve.
Cooperation	Caregivers may be concerned about resistance from their children. Caregivers with low self-esteem who are accustomed to giving into children's demands may need support to effectively implement this position.
Partners	Adults may view the attitude of their partner as a barrier. Education can help.
Availability	Caregivers may balk because they think their children will just get processed foods elsewhere. This makes it all the more valuable if children have unprocessed foods at home.
Teasing	Caregivers may fear teasing from other adults, especially grandparents. The practitioner can rehearse boundary-setting with caregivers to help with this issue.
Restaurants	Clients may think that they can no longer go into restaurants. The practitioner can teach clients how to choose unprocessed foods from a menu.
Cost	Clients may think that "unprocessed" is an expensive way to eat. Practitioners can reassure clients that unprocessed foods are actually cheap.
Special occasions	Clients may be concerned about what foods they could have for special occasions. They can learn how to make special foods from unprocessed ingredients.
Deserving	Sometimes blocks to recovery are subtle and unspoken. Clients with low self-esteem may not believe they deserve to have successful children.

30.4.1.5 Step 5 in Motivation: Redefining Self-Concepts

In this stage of motivation, practitioners can explore how caregivers view their role in helping their children recover. Caregivers may have a range of negative feelings about their children's feeding routines and be frustrated and judgmental (Radoszewska, 2014). The practitioner has the opportunity to clarify and simplify roles: food supplier, educator, cue manager, model, and physical activity provider.

Simplifying Adult Roles

Food supplier	Adults can help their children stay abstinent by keeping unprocessed foods available (Neumark-Sztainer, 2005).
Educator	Education has been shown to be effective in helping girls adapt healthier food habits (Stice, Marti, Spoor, et al., 2008).
Cue manager	Children are more likely to be successful when exposure to food cuing is curtailed (Werthmann, Jansen, & Roefs, 2014).
Modeling	The caregiver is providing a consistent model in terms of ordered eating of balanced, on-time meals. All children in the household are being treated equally (Wansink & van Kleef, 2014).
Recovery activities	Physical activities. The caregiver can also help the child providing activities that promote cognitive restoration. Exercise, art projects, and music are all activities that can help with recovery (Aletraris, Paino, Edmond, Roman, & Bride, 2014; Oh & Taylor, 2013).

30.4.1.6 Step 6 in Motivation: Offering a Menu of Options to Caregivers

Offering the client a menu of options helps make the client feel in control and increases the likelihood that the client will take action. Here are some ways to help the client get started.

1. Learn about the difference between addictive and nonaddictive foods.
2. Talk to family members about the diseases associated with processed foods and the potential benefits of changing food to each family member.
3. Ask household members to circle the foods that they like from the nonaddictive list.
4. Make a nonaddictive foods shopping list.

5. Move the processed foods in the house to one cabinet and set a quit date for removing them from the house.
6. Make a plan for reducing food cuing in the house. Think about reducing exposure to television, magazines, diet books, cookbooks, etc.
7. Pick out physical activity videos from YouTube such as exercise, yoga, walking, or dancing.

30.4.2 Stage II: Training Caregivers in Childhood Addiction Management

Once a caregiver has become motivated to help children with food addiction, the practitioner can begin giving the caregiver insight into children's behaviors.

30.4.2.1 Step 1: Learn What's Happening in the Child's Body

With the right strategies, caregivers can enlist the child's natural body chemistry to help the child fight food addiction. A few biochemical reactions illustrate the strategy. In the first week of unprocessed foods, gut bacteria repopulate (David et al., 2014). Bacteria that break down unprocessed foods replace the dysfunctional organisms. So when the child eats processed foods after a week of withdrawal, there are no bacteria to break it down and the full negative impact will be felt.

Blood glucose can also stabilize (Frassetto, Schloetter, Mietus-Synder, Morris, & Sebastian, 2009). In a processed food diet, the pancreas and adrenal glands are producing insulin and cortisol, respectively, to keep glucose stable. This is uncomfortable and if the child is allowed to experience this a few times, the child will begin to avoid the unpleasant sensation.

Processed foods are also associated with a surge of craving neurotransmitters. This can result in a feeling of "brain fog" (Theoharides, Stewart, Hatziagelaki, & Kolaitis, 2015), which can make the child groggy and unable to focus on work. At the same time, research shows that cognitive centers in the brain cease functioning in the presence of this flood of craving chemicals so the child cannot perform at school (Miller et al., 2014). This can be disconcerting and the child will develop the motivation to avoid it. The caregiver's role is to educate the child about the connection between the processed food and the mental difficulties.

30.4.2.2 Step 2: Identifying and Managing Cravings

As caregivers themselves go through withdrawal and begin to enjoy the release from cravings (Innamorati et al., 2014), they may learn how processed foods and cues create cravings and intense urges. On their own, children cannot be expected to win against cravings. The compounded and prolonged exposure to food cues creates cravings that are too insistent and powerful for a child to resist. They need the help of a cue-free home environment and the example of their caregivers (Stice, Yokum, Burger, et al., 2011; Stice, Yokum, Zald, & Dagher, 2011).

Research on techniques to quell cravings in children is limited to a laboratory study showing that children can use visualization to reduce cravings (Silvers et al., 2014) and adolescent girls can use reappraisal techniques to reduce cravings (Giuliani & Pfeifer, 2014). For the purposes of this discussion, evidence for other techniques is bridged from research in adults in SUD and food cravings. The technique for adults and the proposed adaptation for children are shown below.

Craving Control in Adults	Craving Control in Children
Thinking of benefits of not eating the processed food (Yokum & Stice, 2013)	Write out the physical, mental, emotional, and behavioral benefits
Mindfulness (see Chapter 7)	Describe this object verbally
Mindfulness of environment (see Chapter 7)	Describe the environment verbally
Music (Mathis & Han, 2017)	Music
Crafts, coloring books, art (Aletraris et al., 2014)	Age-appropriate crafts
Exercise/walking (Oh & Taylor, 2013)	Playground/walking
Smells (Sayette & Parrott, 1999)	Associate cues with calming activities, especially with a smell

30.5 FUTURE RESEARCH NEEDS

As readers may have seen, the field of helping children recover from food addiction is not just young; it is in its infancy. This section proposes issues that would benefit from research, refinement, and evaluation, as well as educational approaches that could also be developed and studied.

30.5.1 Issues that Would Benefit from Research

30.5.1.1 Approaches to Food Cues

Can children avoid food cues and can parents teach children methods for coping with cues? Decisions about how to help the youngest food addicts may be seem complex because of the many types of addictive foods and the many opportunities for children to be exposed to cues for them. The risk of food cue reactivity in children may vary from day to day as it does with adults. On stressful busy days with distractions, on days of heavy cue exposure, or in the event of accidental ingestion, cue reactivity could be greater. One of the challenges of addiction recovery plans is to match severity with degree of treatment. In the case of food addiction in children, the consequences of failing to manage cued cravings could be significant.

30.5.1.2 Accommodating Cued Cravings

What are reasonable demands on children regarding avoidance of cues for processed foods? It's not reasonable for a child to turn down sweets after hours and hours of prolonged compounded cueing in a classroom, lunchroom, and after-school activity. Would education, training in counteracting cues, provision of clean food, and personal experiences with the consequences of processed foods give children a chance of withstanding moderate or mild food stimulation?

30.5.1.3 The Nature of Support

Would young children benefit from support groups for recovery from PFA? "Strategies for Helping Food-Addicted Children" concerns the need to educate children and their caregivers about food addiction, consequences, withdrawal, abstinence, and relapse. It is tragic that such education is necessary in young children. The closest precedent is found in drug and alcohol-addicted adolescents. The adolescent addict can be treated in support groups and special schools. These do not exist for the food-addicted child but recovery can still be effectuated in the home.

30.5.1.4 Normalizing a Nonaddictive Food Plan

It is common for homes to have adapted a particular food plan. There are kosher homes, vegan homes, vegetarian homes, as well as cultural homes such as a Chinese home that has mostly fish, rice, and vegetables, or a Muslim home that follows the traditions set out in the Koran. Is it possible to "normalize" a home that follows an unprocessed food plan?

30.5.1.5 Avoiding Eating Disorders

The topic of the food-addicted family is fraught with the ever-present danger of creating eating disorders in children through harmful attempts to control eating. While the caregiver is charged with protecting children from harm, adults tread a fine line between positive actions such as educating and setting boundaries with other caregivers versus potentially harmful actions such as making the child responsible for events that are beyond the ability of young children to control. How to prevent the development of eating disorders when teaching elimination of processed foods?

30.5.2 Educational Approaches for Evaluation: How Should Caregivers Teach Children about Food Addiction?

A child with PFA might benefit from knowing about Westernized food cultures, abstinence, withdrawal, and lapses as they pertain to recovery. How should such an educational program be structured and how could it be adapted to different ages? Here are some of the issues that would be subjected to development, research, evaluation, and refinement.

Lapses could be less distressing and unpredictable if PFA-affected children understand why they lose control when exposed to processed foods and cues. Education and cognitive reappraisal programs have been shown to help adolescents reduce body dissatisfaction (Stice, Durant, Rohde, & Shaw, 2014), bulimia (Stice, Marti, Shaw, & O'Neil, 2008), obesity (Stice, Yokum, et al., 2015), and depression (Stice, Rohde, Seeley, & Gau, 2010). However, no studies have evaluated educational programs for children with PFA.

This section describes the need for research to develop, evaluate, and refine educational programs for children with PFA.

30.5.2.1 How to Teach Children about the Brain Mechanisms of Food Addiction

With an understanding of the mechanisms of food addiction, even a young child might be able to reduce the risk of relapse. First, the child could better defend against the obesogenic culture through food and cue avoidance. Secondly, the child can understand why lapses are not the child's fault, thus avoiding the trauma and shame of failure.

30.5.2.1.1 What Should Children Learn about Cue Reactivity?

As discussed in the description of evidence for PFA in children, children demonstrate cue reactivity (Burger & Stice, 2013), which can be worsened by stress and sleep deprivation (Labree et al., 2015). In adults, CBT for SUD has been shown to decrease hyperreactivity in dopamine pathways while increasing reactivity in impulse control pathways (Zilverstand et al., 2016). Can CBT be applied to cue reactivity in children?

30.5.2.1.2 Would It Help Children to Learn that

- No one chooses to become addicted. No one consciously or deliberately becomes a food addict, especially not children.
- Control without abstinence is unrealistic. Without eliminating addictive processed foods, it is unreasonable to expect a child to control addictive neuroreactivity such as intense cravings and loss of restraint.
- Consequences are only partially genetic. The consequences of processed food abuse are not predominantly genetic. The addictive response can develop through a process of Pavlovian conditioning from natural neurotransmitter responses to cues for addictive processed foods (Suri et al., 2001; Temple, 2016).
- Lapses reignite the addiction. Cravings, loss of restraint, and consequences are reactivated if processed food use is resumed even in small amounts, or if there is prolonged, compounded exposure to cues, or if the child is stressed.

30.5.2.2 Would Learning about Consequences Motivate Children to Abstain?

Children may be suffering from a range of consequences. What should they know about consequences and at what age?

- Excess fat tissue
- Diabetes
- Cognitive function
- Irritable bowel syndrome
- Immune system
- Allergies
- Heart disease
- Skin

Would children become attached to abstinence if they connect meaningful results with avoidance of processed foods, or would they still be vulnerable to cue reactivity?

30.5.2.3 Can Children Learn about Similarities between Drugs and Addictive Foods?

Children are being taught in school about drugs. Could comparing the drug-like properties of processed foods to addictive substances help children understand why processed foods should be avoided?

The function of food is to...	Do processed foods generally perform this function?
Nourish	No
Provide amino acids, essential fats, or fiber	No
Provide vitamins or minerals	No
Sustain growth	No

The actions of recreational drugs	Do processed foods do this?
Provide a high	Yes
Provide a crash	Yes
Addict through cravings	Yes
Create a withdrawal syndrome	Yes
Require abstinence as an effective treatment	Yes
Have 12-step societies for lifetime recovery	Yes
Promote compulsive use to the detriment of the user	Yes
Require progressively greater quantities to get "high"	Possibly
Are mood altering	Yes

30.5.2.4 What Should Children Know about the Food Culture?

Caregivers can teach their children about the similarities between the processed food industry and the tobacco industry in terms of availability, advertising, cheap prices, and targeting the youngest possible consumer (Brandt, 2007; Nestle, 2013). Would this help children understand why processed foods are available in the culture even though they are harmful, or would it be stressful?

30.5.2.5 How Can Children Be Motivated to Abstain?

Abstinence may seem like punishment to a child. Could this be shifted by teaching children about the benefits of abstinence? Could abstinence effectively be associated with better energy, grades at school, perhaps improved athletic performance, weight loss, reduced cravings, etc.? The child might also save money and time, as well as avoid dangerous attempts to obtain processed foods. Would this reduce the risk of relapse? Would these benefits be meaningful to a child, and at what age? Is it possible that if handled with care and patience, children could appreciate abstinence?

30.5.2.6 What Should Children Know about Withdrawal?

Withdrawal symptomology in children is not well known. It is not known whether children experience headaches, intensified cravings, fatigue, lethargy, or stomachaches as has been observed in adults (p. 785) (Gold & Shriner, 2013). See Chapter 21 of this textbook under DSM 5 Criterion 11 for more information about withdrawal symptoms in adults. The acute phase of withdrawal is believed to be 3–8 days.

It would seem helpful for adults in the household to complete withdrawal before the children. Gentleness is a key element in managing a child's withdrawal. The caregiver who has just gone through withdrawal may be better able to empathize with the physical and emotional symptoms of withdrawal. Children may experience strong negative emotions in the course of withdrawal. Children may refuse to eat at all during withdrawal.

30.5.2.7 What Can Children Be Taught about Withdrawal?

Both caregiver and child can learn from the withdrawal experience. Watching for symptoms and educating the child arc ways to benefit from the withdrawal experience. Research may be able to answer questions such as, can the distress of withdrawal be a deterrent to consuming processed foods, or does fear of withdrawal act to compel consumption? What kind of support do caregivers need if the child refuses to eat during withdrawal or displays strong emotions?

30.5.2.8 What Can Children Be Taught about Lapses?

A lapse occurs after a person has completed withdrawal and then reintroduces an addictive food. What kinds of strategies would reduce the risk of lapsing? What is reasonable in terms of keeping processed foods and cues out of the home? What approaches might work to reduce cue exposure at school? Do caregivers need to avoid social events such as special events and parties and for how long? Can children be taught that lapsing is normal, while encouraging them to resist lapsing but also avoid perfectionism? Is it reasonable to expect that children can learn to refuse offers of processed foods from adults? What could be the role of consequences in teaching children not to consume processed foods? How can adults reduce stress triggers in children? Do children need help with adjusting to smaller bodies and losing the sense of protection that excess adipose tissue might bring?

30.5.2.9 What Is Reasonable in Relapse Prevention?

It could be unrealistic to expect that caregivers can completely protect a child against cues. Processed foods proliferate in Westernized cultures (Lifshitz & Lifshitz, 2014). Adults such as grandparents are sometimes determined for a variety of reasons to persuade grandchildren to eat processed foods. What would be effective in such an environment? The following approaches might be helpful but they need to be evaluated.

30.5.2.9.1 Educate about Rationalizing Thoughts

If the child can recognize that a rationalization is occurring, the child might be able to resist the temptation.

30.5.2.9.2 Educate about What Processed Foods Are

There are many kinds of processed foods (Moss, 2013).

30.5.2.9.3 Identify Vulnerable Points

Children may need extra support during vulnerable times such as exams, a fight with a friend, criticism from a teacher, or not making a team. How can caregivers help?

30.5.2.9.4 Rehearse the Child

Would it be effective to engage in role-playing to teach children how to ask for what they need?

30.5.2.9.5 Coach Children about Adult Motivations

Can children understand that adults may have their own reasons for encouraging children to eat processed foods?

30.5.2.9.6 Research Menus

Would it help to discuss what children will be able to eat at restaurants and events and what they need to take from home?

30.5.2.9.7 Feed Children before They Go Out

Would children be more likely to resist if they're not hungry?

30.5.2.10 Recovering from a Lapse

Given the prevalence of food cues (Lifshitz & Lifshitz, 2014) and the presence of cue reactivity in children (Stice, Yokum, Burger, et al., 2011), it seems probable that children will come home sick from having eaten processed foods. How can caregivers help children recover from a lapse? Would it help to review factors such as cues, stress, and availability leading up to the lapse? Or are these concepts too difficult and confusing for children? Can caregivers turn a lapse into a positive experience by attaching consequences to the lapse? Should caregivers let the consequence be the child's teacher? Or should parents maintain efforts to reduce cuing and triggers in the child's life? Would it help to encourage children to see themselves as independent from the actions of their peers (Story, Neumark-Sztainer, & French, 2002)? How important is it for children to learn to say no to adults? How should caregivers follow up with adults who are offering processed foods to PFA-affected children?

30.6 CONCLUSION

It is possible to gain the benefits of recovery from food addiction for children. Children can gain tremendous strengths from the lessons of withdrawal, abstinence, and lapses. The key for caregivers is to stay steadfast in the roles of supplier and educator while avoiding the roles of controller or punisher. Clients can reread their handouts periodically to remind themselves of why they buy clean foods. Clients can protect themselves against drifting by becoming active in the volunteer activities that the practitioner can provide. Considering the agony of leaving food-addicted children untreated; it is well worth the effort to guide caregivers through the process of helping their children put the disease into remission.

REFERENCES

Aletraris, L., Paino, M., Edmond, M. B., Roman, P. M., & Bride, B. E. (2014). The use of art and music therapy in substance abuse treatment programs. *J Addict Nurs, 25*(4), 190–196. doi:10.1097/jan.0000000000000048.

Al-Haifi, A. R., Al-Fayez, M. A., Al-Athari, B. I., Al-Ajmi, F. A., Allafi, A. R., Al-Hazzaa, H. M., & Musaiger, A. O. (2013). Relative contribution of physical activity, sedentary behaviors, and dietary habits to the prevalence of obesity among Kuwaiti adolescents. *Food Nutr Bull, 34*(1), 6–13.

Altman, M., & Wilfley, D. E. (2015). Evidence update on the treatment of overweight and obesity in children and adolescents. *J Clin Child Adolesc Psychol, 44*(4), 521–537. doi:10.1080/15374416.2014.963854.

American Psychiatric Association. (2006). *Practice Guidelines for the Treatment of Patients with Substance Use Disorders*. Washington, DC: American Psychiatric Association.

American Psychiatric Association. (2013). *The Diagnostic and Statistical Manual of Mental Disorders, Fifth Edition* (Vol. 5). Washington, DC: American Psychiatric Association.

Anzman-Frasca, S., Stifter, C. A., Paul, I. M., & Birch, L. L. (2013). Infant temperament and maternal parenting self-efficacy predict child weight outcomes. *Infant Behav Dev, 36*(4), 494–497. doi:10.1016/j.infbeh.2013.04.006.

Anzman, S. L., & Birch, L. L. (2009). Low inhibitory control and restrictive feeding practices predict weight outcomes. *J Pediatr, 155*(5), 651–656. doi:10.1016/j.jpeds.2009.04.052.

Anzman, S. L., Rollins, B. Y., & Birch, L. L. (2010). Parental influence on children's early eating environments and obesity risk: Implications for prevention. *Int J Obes (Lond), 34*(7), 1116–1124. doi:10.1038/ijo.2010.43.

Armstrong, S., Lazorick, S., Hampl, S., Skelton, J. A., Wood, C., Collier, D., & Perrin, E. M. (2016). Physical examination findings among children and adolescents with obesity: An evidence-based review. *Pediatrics, 137*(2), e20151766. doi:10.1542/peds.2015–1766.

August, G. P., Caprio, S., Fennoy, I., Freemark, M., Kaufman, F. R., Lustig, R. H., … Montori, V. M. (2008). Prevention and treatment of pediatric obesity: An endocrine society clinical practice guideline based on expert opinion. *J Clin Endocrinol Metab, 93*(12), 4576–4599. doi:10.1210/jc.2007-2458.

Bak, M., Seibold-Simpson, S. M., & Darling, R. (2016). The potential for cross-addiction in post-bariatric surgery patients: Considerations for primary care nurse practitioners. *J Am Assoc Nurse Pract, 28*(12), 675–682. doi:10.1002/2327-6924.12390.

Barlow, S. E. (2007). Expert committee recommendations regarding the prevention, assessment, and treatment of child and adolescent overweight and obesity: Summary report. *Pediatrics, 120*(Suppl. 4), S164–S192. doi:10.1542/peds.2007-2329C.

Batterink, L., Yokum, S., & Stice, E. (2010). Body mass correlates inversely with inhibitory control in response to food among adolescent girls: An fMRI study. *NeuroImage, 52*(4), 1696–1703. doi:10.1016/j.neuroimage.2010.05.059.

Berthoud, H. R. (2012). The neurobiology of food intake in an obesogenic environment. *Proc Nutr Soc, 71*(4), 478–487. doi:10.1017/s0029665112000602.

Birch, L. L., & Anzman-Frasca, S. (2011). Learning to prefer the familiar in obesogenic environments. *Nestle Nutr Workshop Ser Pediatr Program, 68*, 187–196; discussion 196–189. doi:10.1159/000325856.

Borgogna, N., Lockhart, G., Grenard, J. L., Barrett, T., Shiffman, S., & Reynolds, K. D. (2014). Ecological momentary assessment of urban adolescents' technology use and cravings for unhealthy snacks and drinks: Differences by ethnicity and sex. *J Acad Nutr Diet, 115*(5), 759–766. doi:10.1016/j.jand.2014.10.015.

Boris, M., & Mandel, F. S. (1994). Foods and additives are common causes of the attention deficit hyperactive disorder in children. *Ann Allergy, 72*(5), 462–468.

Boutelle, K. N., & Bouton, M. E. (2015). Implications of learning theory for developing programs to decrease overeating. *Appetite, 93*, 62–74. doi:10.1016/j.appet.2015.05.013.

Brandt, A. (2007). *The Cigarette Century: The Rise, Fall, and Deadly Persistence for the Product that Defined America*. New York, NY: Basic Books.

Brown, L., Dolisca, S. B., & Cheng, J. K. (2015). Barriers and facilitators of pediatric weight management among diverse families. *Clin Pediatr (Phila), 54*(7), 643–651. doi:10.1177/0009922814555977.

Bruce, A. S., Holsen, L. M., Chambers, R. J., Martin, L. E., Brooks, W. M., Zarcone, J. R., … Savage, C. R. (2010). Obese children show hyperactivation to food pictures in brain networks linked to motivation, reward and cognitive control. *Int J Obes (Lond), 34*(10), 1494–1500. doi:10.1038/ijo.2010.84.

Brunault, P., Ducluzeau, P. H., Bourbao-Tournois, C., Delbachian, I., Couet, C., Reveillere, C., & Ballon, N. (2016). Food addiction in bariatric surgery candidates: Prevalence and risk factors. *Obes Surg, 26*(7), 1650–1653. doi:10.1007/s11695-016-2189-x.

Burger, K. S., & Stice, E. (2013). Elevated energy intake is correlated with hyperresponsivity in attentional, gustatory, and reward brain regions while anticipating palatable food receipt. *Am J Clin Nutr, 97*(6), 1188–1194. doi:10.3945/ajcn.112.055285.

Burger, K. S., & Stice, E. (2014a). Greater striatopallidal adaptive coding during cue-reward learning and food reward habituation predict future weight gain. *NeuroImage, 99*, 122–128. doi:10.1016/j.neuroimage.2014.05.066.

Burger, K. S., & Stice, E. (2014b). Neural responsivity during soft drink intake, anticipation, and advertisement exposure in habitually consuming youth. *Obesity (Silver Spring), 22*(2), 441–450. doi:10.1002/oby.20563.

Chang, Y., & Halgunseth, L. C. (2015). Early adolescents' psychosocial adjustment and weight status change: The moderating roles of gender, ethnicity, and acculturation. *J Youth Adolesc, 44*(4), 870–886. doi:10.1007/s10964-014-0162-3.

Chen, L., Li, Q., Song, Y., Ma, J., & Wang, H. J. (2016). Association of physical activities, sedentary behaviors with overweight/obesity in 9–11 year-old Chinese primary school students. *Beijing Da Xue Xue Bao, 48*(3), 436–441.

Ciacci, C., Iovino, P., Amoruso, D., Siniscalchi, M., Tortora, R., Di Gilio, A., … Mazzacca, G. (2005). Grown-up coeliac children: The effects of only a few years on a gluten-free diet in childhood. *Aliment Pharmacol Ther, 21*(4), 421–429. doi:10.1111/j.1365-2036.2005.02345.x.

Coelho, J. S., Siggen, M. J., Dietre, P., & Bouvard, M. (2013). Reactivity to thought-shape fusion in adolescents: The effects of obesity status. *Pediatr Obes, 8*(6), 439–444. doi:10.1111/j.2047-6310.2012.00121.x.

Cordain, L., Lindeberg, S., Hurtado, M., Hill, K., Eaton, S. B., & Brand-Miller, J. (2002). Acne vulgaris: A disease of Western civilization. *Arch Dermatol, 138*(12), 1584–1590.

Danese, A., & Tan, M. (2014). Childhood maltreatment and obesity: Systematic review and meta-analysis. *Mol Psychiatry, 19*(5), 544–554. doi:10.1038/mp.2013.54.

David, L. A., Maurice, C. F., Carmody, R. N., Gootenberg, D. B., Button, J. E., Wolfe, B. E., … Turnbaugh, P. J. (2014). Diet rapidly and reproducibly alters the human gut microbiome. *Nature, 505*(7484), 559–563. doi:10.1038/nature12820.

Decelis, A., Jago, R., & Fox, K. R. (2014). Physical activity, screen time and obesity status in a nationally representative sample of Maltese youth with international comparisons. *BMC Public Health, 14*, 664. doi:10.1186/1471-2458-14-664.

Dhingra, A., Brennan, L., & Walkley, J. (2011). Predicting treatment initiation in a family-based adolescent overweight and obesity intervention. *Obesity (Silver Spring), 19*(6), 1307–1310. doi:10.1038/oby.2010.289.

Donovan, D. M. (2013). Evidence-based assessment: Strategies and measures in addictive behaviors. In B. S. McCrady & E. E. Epstein (Eds.), *Addictions: A comprehensive guidebook*, pp. 311–351. Oxford: Oxford University Press.

Drescher, A. A., Goodwin, J. L., Silva, G. E., & Quan, S. F. (2011). Caffeine and screen time in adolescence: Associations with short sleep and obesity. *J Clin Sleep Med, 7*(4), 337–342. doi:10.5664/jcsm.1182.

Drewnowski, A., & Rehm, C. D. (2014). Consumption of added sugars among US children and adults by food purchase location and food source. *Am J Clin Nutr, 100*(3), 901–907. doi:10.3945/ajcn.114.089458.

Dube, S. R., Anda, R. F., Felitti, V. J., Edwards, V. J., & Croft, J. B. (2002). Adverse childhood experiences and personal alcohol abuse as an adult. *Addict Behav, 27*(5), 713–725.

Dube, S. R., Felitti, V. J., Dong, M., Chapman, D. P., Giles, W. H., & Anda, R. F. (2003). Childhood abuse, neglect, and household dysfunction and the risk of illicit drug use: The adverse childhood experiences study. *Pediatrics, 111*(3), 564–572.

Edwards, M. B., Theriault, D. S., Shores, K. A., & Melton, K. M. (2014). Promoting youth physical activity in rural southern communities: Practitioner perceptions of environmental opportunities and barriers. *J Rural Health, 30*(4), 379–387. doi:10.1111/jrh.12072.

Feldstein Ewing, S. W., Claus, E. D., Hudson, K. A., Filbey, F. M., Yakes Jimenez, E., Lisdahl, K. M., & Kong, A. S. (2016). Overweight adolescents' brain response to sweetened beverages mirrors addiction pathways. *Brain Imaging Behav, 11*(4), 925–935. doi:10.1007/s11682-016-9564-z.

Felitti, V. J., Anda, R. F., Nordenberg, D., Williamson, D. F., Spitz, A. M., Edwards, V., … Marks, J. S. (1998). Relationship of childhood abuse and household dysfunction to many of the leading causes of death in adults. The Adverse Childhood Experiences (ACE) Study. *Am J Prev Med, 14*(4), 245–258.

Fitzsimmons-Craft, E. E., Ciao, A. C., Accurso, E. C., Pisetsky, E. M., Peterson, C. B., Byrne, C. E., & Le Grange, D. (2014). Subjective and objective binge eating in relation to eating disorder symptomatology, depressive symptoms, and self-esteem among treatment-seeking adolescents with bulimia nervosa. *Eur Eat Disord Rev, 22*(4), 230–236. doi:10.1002/erv.2297.

Foster, G. D., Makris, A. P., & Bailer, B. A. (2005). Behavioral treatment of obesity. *Am J Clin Nutr, 82*(1 Suppl), 230s–235s.

Frassetto, L. A., Schloetter, M., Mietus-Synder, M., Morris, R. C., Jr., & Sebastian, A. (2009). Metabolic and physiologic improvements from consuming a paleolithic, hunter-gatherer type diet. *Eur J Clin Nutr, 63*(8), 947–955. doi:10.1038/ejcn.2009.4.

Fuller-Rowell, T. E., Evans, G. W., & Ong, A. D. (2012). Poverty and health: The mediating role of perceived discrimination. *Psychol Sci, 23*(7), 734–739. doi:10.1177/0956797612439720.

Gebauer, H., & Laska, M. N. (2011). Convenience stores surrounding urban schools: An assessment of healthy food availability, advertising, and product placement. *J Urban Health, 88*(4), 616–622. doi:10.1007/s11524-011-9576-3.

Giuliani, N. R., & Pfeifer, J. H. (2014). Age-related changes in reappraisal of appetitive cravings during adolescence. *NeuroImage, 108*, 173–181. doi:10.1016/j.neuroimage.2014.12.037.

Gold, M. S., & Shriner, R. L. (2013). Food addictions. In P. M. Miller (Ed.), *Principles of Addiction: Comprehensive Addictive Behaviors and Disorders* (Vol. 1). Waltham, MA: Elsevier.

Goldschmidt, A. B., Wall, M. M., Choo, T. H., Bruening, M., Eisenberg, M. E., & Neumark-Sztainer, D. (2014). Examining associations between adolescent binge eating and binge eating in parents and friends. *Int J Eat Disord, 47*(3), 325–328. doi:10.1002/eat.22192.

Grenard, J. L., Stacy, A. W., Shiffman, S., Baraldi, A. N., MacKinnon, D. P., Lockhart, G., … Reynolds, K. D. (2013). Sweetened drink and snacking cues in adolescents: A study using ecological momentary assessment. *Appetite, 67*, 61–73. doi:10.1016/j.appet.2013.03.016.

Grossklaus, H., & Marvicsin, D. (2014). Parenting efficacy and its relationship to the prevention of childhood obesity. *Pediatr Nurs, 40*(2), 69–86.

Guh, D. P., Zhang, W., Bansback, N., Amarsi, Z., Birmingham, C. L., & Anis, A. H. (2009). The incidence of co-morbidities related to obesity and overweight: A systematic review and meta-analysis. *BMC Public Health, 9*, 88. doi:10.1186/1471-2458-9-88.

Hartlieb, K. B., Naar, S., Ledgerwood, D. M., Templin, T. N., Ellis, D. A., Donohue, B., & Cunningham, P. B. (2015). Contingency management adapted for African-American adolescents with obesity enhances youth weight loss with caregiver participation: A multiple baseline pilot study. *Int J Adolesc Med Health, 29*(3). doi:10.1515/ijamh-2015-0091.

Hoertel, H. A., Will, M. J., & Leidy, H. J. (2014). A randomized crossover, pilot study examining the effects of a normal protein vs. high protein breakfast on food cravings and reward signals in overweight/obese "breakfast skipping," late-adolescent girls. *Nutr J, 13*, 80. doi:10.1186/1475-2891-13-80.

Hofmann, J., Ardelt-Gattinger, E., Paulmichl, K., Weghuber, D., & Blechert, J. (2015). Dietary restraint and impulsivity modulate neural responses to food in adolescents with obesity and healthy adolescents. *Obesity (Silver Spring), 23*(11), 2183–2189. doi:10.1002/oby.21254.

Innamorati, M., Imperatori, C., Balsamo, M., Tamburello, S., Belvederi Murri, M., Contardi, A., … Fabbricatore, M. (2014). Food Cravings Questionnaire-Trait (FCQ-T) discriminates between obese and overweight patients with and without binge eating tendencies: The Italian version of the FCQ-T. *J Pers Assess, 96*(6), 632–639. doi:10.1080/00223891.2014.909449.

Jerstad, S. J., Boutelle, K. N., Ness, K. K., & Stice, E. (2010). Prospective reciprocal relations between physical activity and depression in female adolescents. *J Consult Clin Psychol, 78*(2), 268–272. doi:10.1037/a0018793.

Jones, B. L., & Fiese, B. H. (2014). Parent routines, child routines, and family demographics associated with obesity in parents and preschool-aged children. *Front Psychol, 5*, 374. doi:10.3389/fpsyg.2014.00374.

Kakinami, L., Barnett, T. A., Seguin, L., & Paradis, G. (2015). Parenting style and obesity risk in children. *Prev Med, 75*, 18–22. doi:10.1016/j.ypmed.2015.03.005.

Keitel-Korndorfer, A., Sierau, S., Klein, A. M., Bergmann, S., Grube, M., & von Klitzing, K. (2015). Insatiable insecurity: Maternal obesity as a risk factor for mother-child attachment and child weight. *Attach Hum Dev, 17*(4), 399–413. doi:10.1080/14616734.2015.1067823.

Kelleher, E., Davoren, M. P., Harrington, J. M., Shiely, F., Perry, I. J., & McHugh, S. M. (2017). Barriers and facilitators to initial and continued attendance at community-based lifestyle programmes among families of overweight and obese children: A systematic review. *Obes Rev, 18*(2), 183–194. doi:10.1111/obr.12478.

Kelly, B., Chapman, K., Hardy, L. L., King, L., & Farrell, L. (2009). Parental awareness and attitudes of food marketing to children: A community attitudes survey of parents in New South Wales, Australia. *J Paediatr Child Health, 45*(9), 493–497. doi:10.1111/j.1440-1754.2009.01548.x.

Khan, N. A., Raine, L. B., Drollette, E. S., Scudder, M. R., Kramer, A. F., & Hillman, C. H. (2015). Dietary fiber is positively associated with cognitive control among prepubertal children. *J Nutr, 145*(1), 143–149. doi:10.3945/jn.114.198457.

Kiecolt-Glaser, J. K., Jaremka, L., Andridge, R., Peng, J., Habash, D., Fagundes, C. P., … Belury, M. A. (2015). Marital discord, past depression, and metabolic responses to high-fat meals: Interpersonal pathways to obesity. *Psychoneuroendocrinology, 52*, 239–250. doi:10.1016/j.psyneuen.2014.11.018.

Koball, A. M., Clark, M. M., Collazo-Clavell, M., Kellogg, T., Ames, G., Ebbert, J., & Grothe, K. B. (2016). The relationship among food addiction, negative mood, and eating-disordered behaviors in patients seeking to have bariatric surgery. *Surg Obes Relat Dis, 12*(1), 165–170. doi:10.1016/j.soard.2015.04.009.

Krahnstoever Davison, K., Francis, L. A., & Birch, L. L. (2005). Reexamining obesigenic families: Parents' obesity-related behaviors predict girls' change in BMI. *Obes Res, 13*(11), 1980–1990. doi:10.1038/oby.2005.243.

Kuzel, R., & Larson, J. (2014). Treating childhood obesity. *Minn Med, 97*(1), 48–50.

Labree, W., van de Mheen, D., Rutten, F., Rodenburg, G., Koopmans, G., & Foets, M. (2015). Differences in overweight and obesity among children from migrant and native origin: The role of physical activity, dietary intake, and sleep duration. *PLoS One, 10*(6), e0123672. doi:10.1371/journal.pone.0123672.

Lee, A., & Gibbs, S. E. (2013). Neurobiology of food addiction and adolescent obesity prevention in low- and middle-income countries. *J Adolesc Health, 52*(2 Suppl 2), S39–S42. doi:10.1016/j.jadohealth.2012.06.008

Leidy, H. J., Bales-Voelker, L. I., & Harris, C. T. (2011). A protein-rich beverage consumed as a breakfast meal leads to weaker appetitive and dietary responses v. a protein-rich solid breakfast meal in adolescents. *Br J Nutr, 106*(1), 37–41. doi:10.1017/s0007114511000122.

Leidy, H. J., Lepping, R. J., Savage, C. R., & Harris, C. T. (2011). Neural responses to visual food stimuli after a normal vs. higher protein breakfast in breakfast-skipping teens: A pilot fMRI study. *Obesity (Silver Spring), 19*(10), 2019–2025. doi:10.1038/oby.2011.108.

Leung, C. Y., Lumeng, J. C., Kaciroti, N. A., Chen, Y. P., Rosenblum, K., & Miller, A. L. (2014). Surgency and negative affectivity, but not effortful control, are uniquely associated with obesogenic eating behaviors among low-income preschoolers. *Appetite, 78*, 139–146. doi:10.1016/j.appet.2014.03.025.

Levin, B. E., Llabre, M. M., Dong, C., Elkind, M. S., Stern, Y., Rundek, T., … Wright, C. B. (2014). Modeling metabolic syndrome and its association with cognition: The northern Manhattan study. *J Int Neuropsychol Soc, 20*(10), 951–960. doi:10.1017/s1355617714000861.

Li, L., Shen, T., Wen, L. M., Wu, M., He, P., Wang, Y., … He, G. (2015). Lifestyle factors associated with childhood obesity: A cross-sectional study in Shanghai, China. *BMC Res Notes, 8*, 6. doi:10.1186/s13104-014-0958-y.

Lifshitz, F., & Lifshitz, J. Z. (2014). Globesity: The root causes of the obesity epidemic in the USA and now worldwide. *Pediatr Endocrinol Rev, 12*(1), 17–34.

Ling, J., Robbins B.L., & Hines-Martin, V. (2016). Perceived parental barriers to and strategies for supporting physical activity and healthy eating among head start children. *J Community Health, 41*(3), 593–602. doi:10.1007/s10900-015-0134-x.

Linville, D., Stice, E., Gau, J., & O'Neil, M. (2011). Predictive effects of mother and peer influences on increases in adolescent eating disorder risk factors and symptoms: A 3-year longitudinal study. *Int J Eat Disord, 44*(8), 745–751. doi:10.1002/eat.20907.

Lioutas, E. D., & Tzimitra-Kalogianni, I. (2015). 'I saw Santa drinking soda!' Advertising and children's food preferences. *Child Care Health Dev, 41*(3), 424–433. doi:10.1111/cch.12189.

Lobstein, T., Jackson-Leach, R., Moodie, M. L., Hall, K. D., Gortmaker, S. L., Swinburn, B. A., … McPherson, K. (2015). Child and adolescent obesity: Part of a bigger picture. *Lancet, 385*(9986), 2510–2520. doi:10.1016/s0140-6736(14)61746-3.

Manzel, A., Muller, D. N., Hafler, D. A., Erdman, S. E., Linker, R. A., & Kleinewietfeld, M. (2014). Role of "Western diet" in inflammatory autoimmune diseases. *Curr Allergy Asthma Rep, 14*(1), 404. doi:10.1007/s11882-013-0404-6.

Marchand, E., Ng, J., Rohde, P., & Stice, E. (2010). Effects of an indicated cognitive-behavioral depression prevention program are similar for Asian American, Latino, and European American adolescents. *Behav Res Ther, 48*(8), 821–825. doi:10.1016/j.brat.2010.05.005.

Martarelli, C. S., Borter, N., Bryjova, J., Mast, F. W., & Munsch, S. (2015). The influence of parent's body mass index on peer selection: An experimental approach using virtual reality. *Psychiatry Res, 230*(1), 5–12. doi:10.1016/j.psychres.2015.05.075.

Marwitz, S. E., Woodie, L. N., & Blythe, S. N. (2015). Western-style diet induces insulin insensitivity and hyperactivity in adolescent male rats. *Physiol Behav, 151*, 147–154. doi:10.1016/j.physbeh.2015.07.023.

Mathis, W. S., & Han, X. (2017). The acute effect of pleasurable music on craving for alcohol: A pilot crossover study. *J Psychiatr Res, 90*, 143–147. doi:10.1016/j.jpsychires.2017.04.008.

Maximova, K., Ambler, K. A., Rudko, J. N., Chui, N., & Ball, G. D. (2015). Ready, set, go! Motivation and lifestyle habits in parents of children referred for obesity management. *Pediatr Obes, 10*(5), 353–360. doi:10.1111/ijpo.272.

Merlo, L. J., & Yardley, H. L. (2011). Pediatric obesity epidemic: Problem and solutions. *Curr Pharm Des, 17*(12), 1145–1148.

Meule, A., Hermann, T., & Kubler, A. (2015). Food addiction in overweight and obese adolescents seeking weight-loss treatment. *Eur Eat Disord Rev, 23*(3), 193–198. doi:10.1002/erv.2355.

Miller, A. L., Lee, H. J., & Lumeng, J. C. (2014). Obesity-associated biomarkers and executive function in children. *Pediatr Res, 77*(1–2), 143–147. doi:10.1038/pr.2014.158.

Morris, M. J., Beilharz, J., Maniam, J., Reichelt, A., & Westbrook, R. F. (2015). Why is obesity such a problem in the 21st century? The intersection of palatable food, cues and reward pathways, stress, and cognition. *J Neurosci*, 58, 36–45. doi:10.1016/j.neubiorev.2014.12.002.

Moss, M. (2013). *Salt, sugar, fat: How the food giants hooked us,* Random House, New York.

Munoz, K. A., Krebs-Smith, S. M., Ballard-Barbash, R., & Cleveland, L. E. (1997). Food intakes of US children and adolescents compared with recommendations. *Pediatrics*, *100*(3 Pt 1), 323–329.

Nestle, M. (2013). *Food Politics.* Berkeley, CA: University of California Press.

Neumark-Sztainer, D. (2005). Preventing the broad spectrum of weight-related problems: Working with parents to help teens achieve a healthy weight and a positive body image. *J Nutr Educ Behav, 37*(Suppl 2), S133–S140.

Ng, M., Fleming, T., Robinson, M., Thomson, B., Graetz, N., Margono, C., … Gakidou, E. (2014). Global, regional, and national prevalence of overweight and obesity in children and adults during 1980–2013: A systematic analysis for the Global Burden of Disease Study 2013. *Lancet*, *384*(9945), 766–781. doi:10.1016/s0140-6736(14)60460-8.

Nguyen, P. V., Hong, T. K., Nguyen, D. T., & Robert, A. R. (2016). Excessive screen viewing time by adolescents and body fatness in a developing country: Vietnam. *Asia Pac J Clin Nutr, 25*(1), 174–183. doi:10.6133/apjcn.2016.25.1.21.

O'Brien, S. H., Holubkov, R., & Reis, E. C. (2004). Identification, evaluation, and management of obesity in an academic primary care center. *Pediatrics, 114*(2), e154–e159.

Ogden, C. L., Carroll, M. D., Kit, B. K., & Flegal, K. M. (2012). Prevalence of obesity and trends in body mass index among US children and adolescents, 1999–2010. *JAMA*, *307*(5), 483–490. doi:10.1001/jama.2012.40.

Ogden, C. L., Carroll, M. D., Lawman, H. G., Fryar, C. D., Kruszon-Moran, D., Kit, B. K., & Flegal, K. M. (2016). Trends in obesity prevalence among children and adolescents in the United States, 1988–1994 through 2013–2014. *JAMA*, *315*(21), 2292–2299. doi:10.1001/jama.2016.6361.

Oh, H., & Taylor, A. H. (2013). A brisk walk, compared with being sedentary, reduces attentional bias and chocolate cravings among regular chocolate eaters with different body mass. *Appetite*, *71*, 144–149. doi:10.1016/j.appet.2013.07.015.

Paul, I. M., Savage, J. S., Anzman, S. L., Beiler, J. S., Marini, M. E., Stokes, J. L., & Birch, L. L. (2011). Preventing obesity during infancy: A pilot study. *Obesity (Silver Spring)*, *19*(2), 353–361. doi:10.1038/oby.2010.182.

Paulis, W. D., Silva, S., Koes, B. W., & van Middelkoop, M. (2014). Overweight and obesity are associated with musculoskeletal complaints as early as childhood: A systematic review. *Obes Rev*, *15*(1), 52–67. doi:10.1111/obr.12067.

Peele, S. (1992). *The Truth about Addiction and Recovery*. New York, NY: Fireside.

Peterson, J. L., Puhl, R. M., & Luedicke, J. (2012). An experimental assessment of physical educators' expectations and attitudes: The importance of student weight and gender. *J Sch Health*, *82*(9), 432–440. doi:10.1111/j.1746-1561.2012.00719.x.

Powell, L. M., Harris, J. L., & Fox, T. (2013). Food marketing expenditures aimed at youth: Putting the numbers in context. *Am J Prev Med*, *45*(4), 453–461. doi:10.1016/j.amepre.2013.06.003.

Presnell, K., Stice, E., Seidel, A., & Madeley, M. C. (2009). Depression and eating pathology: Prospective reciprocal relations in adolescents. *Clin Psychol Psychother*, *16*(4), 357–365. doi:10.1002/cpp.630.

Puhl, R. M., Luedicke, J., & Depierre, J. A. (2013). Parental concerns about weight-based victimization in youth. *Child Obes*, *9*(6), 540–548. doi:10.1089/chi.2013.0064.

Puhl, R. M., Peterson, J. L., & Luedicke, J. (2013a). Strategies to address weight-based victimization: Youths' preferred support interventions from classmates, teachers, and parents. *J Youth Adolesc*, *42*(3), 315–327. doi:10.1007/s10964-012-9849-5.

Puhl, R. M., Peterson, J. L., & Luedicke, J. (2013b). Weight-based victimization: Bullying experiences of weight loss treatment-seeking youth. *Pediatrics*, *131*(1), e1–e9. doi:10.1542/peds.2012-1106.

Radoszewska, J. (2014). Perception of the child's obesity in parents of girls and boys treated for obesity (preliminary study). *Dev Period Med*, *18*(2), 148–154.

Rankin, J., Matthews, L., Cobley, S., Han, A., Sanders, R., Wiltshire, H. D., & Baker, J. S. (2016). Psychological consequences of childhood obesity: Psychiatric comorbidity and prevention. *Adolesc Health Med Ther*, *7*, 125–146. doi:10.2147/ahmt.s101631.

Ren, H., Zhou, Z., Liu, W. K., Wang, X., & Yin, Z. (2017). Excessive homework, inadequate sleep, physical inactivity and screen viewing time are major contributors to high paediatric obesity. *Acta Paediatr*, *106*(1), 120–127. doi:10.1111/apa.13640.

Rodriguez, R., Marchand, E., Ng, J., & Stice, E. (2008). Effects of a cognitive dissonance-based eating disorder prevention program are similar for Asian American, Hispanic, and White participants. *Int J Eat Disord*, *41*(7), 618–625. doi:10.1002/eat.20532.

Rollins, B. Y., Loken, E., Savage, J. S., & Birch, L. L. (2014). Measurement of food reinforcement in preschool children. Associations with food intake, BMI, and reward sensitivity. *Appetite*, *72*, 21–27. doi:10.1016/j.appet.2013.09.018.

Sayette, M. A., & Parrott, D. J. (1999). Effects of olfactory stimuli on urge reduction in smokers. *Exp Clin Psychopharmacol*, *7*(2), 151–159.

Scully, M., Wakefield, M., Niven, P., Chapman, K., Crawford, D., Pratt, I. S., … Morley, B. (2012). Association between food marketing exposure and adolescents' food choices and eating behaviors. *Appetite*, *58*(1), 1–5. doi:10.1016/j.appet.2011.09.020.

Scully, P., Macken, A., Leddin, D., Cullen, W., Dunne, C., & Gorman, C. O. (2015). Food and beverage advertising during children's television programming. *Ir J Med Sci*, *184*(1), 207–212. doi:10.1007/s11845-014-1088-1.

Selewski, D. T., Collier, D. N., MacHardy, J., Gross, H. E., Pickens, E. M., Cooper, A. W., … Gipson, D. S. (2013). Promising insights into the health related quality of life for children with severe obesity. *Health Qual Life Outcomes*, *11*, 29. doi:10.1186/1477-7525-11-29.

Shrewsbury, V. A., Baur, L. A., Nguyen, B., & Steinbeck, K. S. (2014). Transition to adult care in adolescent obesity: A systematic review and why it is a neglected topic. *Int J Obes (Lond)*, *38*(4), 475–479. doi:10.1038/ijo.2013.215.

Siddarth, D. (2013). Risk factors for obesity in children and adults. *J Investig Med*, *61*(6), 1039–1042. doi:10.2310/JIM.0b013e31829c39d0.

Silvers, J. A., Insel, C., Powers, A., Franz, P., Weber, J., Mischel, W., … Ochsner, K. N. (2014). Curbing craving: Behavioral and brain evidence that children regulate craving when instructed to do so but have higher baseline craving than adults. *Psychol Sci*, *25*(10), 1932–1942. doi:10.1177/0956797614546001.

Smeets, P. A., Charbonnier, L., van Meer, F., van der Laan, L. N., & Spetter, M. S. (2012). Food-induced brain responses and eating behaviour. *Proc Nutr Soc*, *71*(4), 511–520. doi:10.1017/S0029665112000808.

Speirs, K. E., Hayes, J. T., Musaad, S., VanBrackle, A., & Sigman-Grant, M. (2016). Is family sense of coherence a protective factor against the obesogenic environment? *Appetite*, *99*, 268–276. doi:10.1016/j.appet.2016.01.025.

Stice, E., Burger, K., & Yokum, S. (2013). Caloric deprivation increases responsivity of attention and reward brain regions to intake, anticipated intake, and images of palatable foods. *NeuroImage*, *67*, 322–330. doi:10.1016/j.neuroimage.2012.11.028.

Stice, E., Burger, K. S., & Yokum, S. (2015). Reward region responsivity predicts future weight gain and moderating effects of the TaqIA Allele. *J Neurosci*, *35*(28), 10316–10324. doi:10.1523/jneurosci.3607-14.2015.

Stice, E., Burton, E. M., & Shaw, H. (2004). Prospective relations between bulimic pathology, depression, and substance abuse: Unpacking comorbidity in adolescent girls. *J Consult Clin Psychol*, *72*(1), 62–71. doi:10.1037/0022-006X.72.1.62.

Stice, E., & Dagher, A. (2010). Genetic variation in dopaminergic reward in humans. *Forum Nutr*, *63*, 176–185. doi:10.1159/000264405.

Stice, E., Davis, K., Miller, N. P., & Marti, C. N. (2008). Fasting increases risk for onset of binge eating and bulimic pathology: A 5-year prospective study. *J Abnorm Psychol*, *117*(4), 941–946. doi:10.1037/a0013644.

Stice, E., Durant, S., Rohde, P., & Shaw, H. (2014). Effects of a prototype internet dissonance-based eating disorder prevention program at 1- and 2-year follow-up. *Health Psychol*, *33*(12), 1558–1567. doi:10.1037/hea0000090.

Stice, E., Marti, C. N., Shaw, H., & Jaconis, M. (2009). An 8-year longitudinal study of the natural history of threshold, subthreshold, and partial eating disorders from a community sample of adolescents. *J Abnorm Psychol*, *118*(3), 587–597. doi:10.1037/a0016481.

Stice, E., Marti, N., Shaw, H., & O'Neil, K. (2008). General and program-specific moderators of two eating disorder prevention programs. *Int J Eat Disord*, *41*(7), 611–617. doi:10.1002/eat.20524.

Stice, E., Marti, C. N., Spoor, S., Presnell, K., & Shaw, H. (2008). Dissonance and healthy weight eating disorder prevention programs: Long-term effects from a randomized efficacy trial. *J Consult Clin Psychol*, *76*(2), 329–340. doi:10.1037/0022-006x.76.2.329.

Stice, E., Martinez, E. E., Presnell, K., & Groesz, L. M. (2006). Relation of successful dietary restriction to change in bulimic symptoms: A prospective study of adolescent girls. *Health Psychol*, *25*(3), 274–281. doi:10.1037/0278-6133.25.3.274.

Stice, E., Rohde, P., Gau, J., & Shaw, H. (2009). An effectiveness trial of a dissonance-based eating disorder prevention program for high-risk adolescent girls. *J Consult Clin Psychol*, *77*(5), 825–834. doi:10.1037/a0016132.

Stice, E., Rohde, P., Gau, J. M., & Wade, E. (2010). Efficacy trial of a brief cognitive-behavioral depression prevention program for high-risk adolescents: Effects at 1- and 2-year follow-up. *J Consult Clin Psychol*, *78*(6), 856–867. doi:10.1037/a0020544.

Stice, E., Rohde, P., Seeley, J. R., & Gau, J. M. (2010). Testing mediators of intervention effects in randomized controlled trials: An evaluation of three depression prevention programs. *J Consult Clin Psychol*, *78*(2), 273–280. doi:10.1037/a0018396.

Stice, E., & Shaw, H. (2004). Eating disorder prevention programs: A meta-analytic review. *Psychol Bull*, *130*(2), 206–227. doi:10.1037/0033-2909.130.2.206.

Stice, E., Shaw, H., Bohon, C., Marti, C. N., & Rohde, P. (2009). A meta-analytic review of depression prevention programs for children and adolescents: Factors that predict magnitude of intervention effects. *J Consult Clin Psychol*, *77*(3), 486–503. doi:10.1037/a0015168.

Stice, E., Shaw, H., Burton, E., & Wade, E. (2006). Dissonance and healthy weight eating disorder prevention programs: A randomized efficacy trial. *J Consult Clin Psychol*, *74*(2), 263–275. doi:10.1037/0022-006x.74.2.263.

Stice, E., Shaw, H., & Marti, C. N. (2006). A meta-analytic review of obesity prevention programs for children and adolescents: The skinny on interventions that work. *Psychol Bull*, *132*(5), 667–691. doi:10.3945/ajcn.113.069443.

Stice, E., Shaw, H., & Marti, C. N. (2007). A meta-analytic review of eating disorder prevention programs: Encouraging findings. *Annu Rev Clin Psychol*, *3*, 207–231. doi:10.1146/annurev.clinpsy.3.022806.091447.

Stice, E., Yokum, S., Burger, K., Rohde, P., Shaw, H., & Gau, J. M. (2015). A pilot randomized trial of a cognitive reappraisal obesity prevention program. *Physiol Behav*, *138*, 124–132. doi:10.1016/j.physbeh.2014.10.022.

Stice, E., Yokum, S., Burger, K. S., Epstein, L. H., & Small, D. M. (2011). Youth at risk for obesity show greater activation of striatal and somatosensory regions to food. *J Neurosci*, *31*(12), 4360–4366. doi:10.1523/jneurosci.6604-10.2011.

Stice, E., Yokum, S., Zald, D., & Dagher, A. (2011). Dopamine-based reward circuitry responsivity, genetics, and overeating. *Curr Top Behav Neurosci*, *6*, 81–93. doi:10.1007/7854_2010_89.

Story, M., Neumark-Sztainer, D., & French, S. (2002). Individual and environmental influences on adolescent eating behaviors. *J Am Diet Assoc*, *102*(3 Suppl), S40–S51.

Suri, R. E., & Schultz, W. (2001). Temporal difference model reproduces anticipatory neural activity. *Neural Comput*, *13*(4), 841–862.

Temple, J. L. (2016). Behavioral sensitization of the reinforcing value of food: What food and drugs have in common. *Prev Med*, *92*, 90–99. doi:10.1016/j.ypmed.2016.06.022.

Terry-McElrath, Y. M., Turner, L., Sandoval, A., Johnston, L. D., & Chaloupka, F. J. (2014). Commercialism in US elementary and secondary school nutrition environments: Trends from 2007 to 2012. *JAMA Pediatr*, *168*(3), 234–242. doi:10.1001/jamapediatrics.2013.4521.

Theoharides, T. C., Stewart, J. M., Hatziagelaki, E., & Kolaitis, G. (2015). Brain "fog," inflammation and obesity: Key aspects of neuropsychiatric disorders improved by luteolin. *Front Neurosci*, *9*, 225. doi:10.3389/fnins.2015.00225.

Trask, S., Schepers, S. T., & Bouton, M. E. (2015). Context change explains resurgence after the extinction of operant behavior. *Rev Mex Anal Conducta*, *41*(2), 187–210.

van Meer, F., van der Laan, L. N., Adan, R. A., Viergever, M. A., & Smeets, P. A. (2015). What you see is what you eat: An ALE meta-analysis of the neural correlates of food viewing in children and adolescents. *NeuroImage*, *104*, 35–43. doi:10.1016/j.neuroimage.2014.09.069.

Verbeken, S., Braet, C., Bosmans, G., & Goossens, L. (2014). Comparing decision making in average and overweight children and adolescents. *Int J Obes (Lond)*, *38*(4), 547–551. doi:10.1038/ijo.2013.235.

Verbeken, S., Braet, C., Lammertyn, J., Goossens, L., & Moens, E. (2012). How is reward sensitivity related to bodyweight in children? *Appetite*, *58*(2), 478–483. doi:10.1016/j.appet.2011.11.018.

Volkow, N. D., Koob, G. F., & McLellan, A. T. (2016). Neurobiologic advances from the brain disease model of addiction. *N Engl J Med*, *374*(4), 363–371. doi:10.1056/NEJMra1511480.

Wansink, B., & van Kleef, E. (2014). Dinner rituals that correlate with child and adult BMI. *Obesity (Silver Spring)*, *22*(5), E91–E95. doi:10.1002/oby.20629.

Waters, E., de Silva-Sanigorski, A., Hall, B. J., Brown, T., Campbell, K. J., Gao, Y., … Summerbell, C. D. (2011). Interventions for preventing obesity in children. *Cochrane Database Syst Rev* 12, CD001871. doi:10.1002/14651858.CD001871.pub3.

Werthmann, J., Jansen, A., & Roefs, A. (2014). Worry or craving? A selective review of evidence for food-related attention biases in obese individuals, eating-disorder patients, restrained eaters and healthy samples. *Proc Nutr Soc*, *74*(2): 99–114. doi:10.1017/s0029665114001451.

Werthmann, J., Roefs, A., Nederkoorn, C., Mogg, K., Bradley, B. P., & Jansen, A. (2011). Can(not) take my eyes off it: Attention bias for food in overweight participants. *Health Psychology*, *30*, 561–569.

Yau, P. L., Kang, E. H., Javier, D. C., & Convit, A. (2014). Preliminary evidence of cognitive and brain abnormalities in uncomplicated adolescent obesity. *Obesity (Silver Spring)*, *22*(8), 1865–1871. doi:10.1002/oby.20801.

Yokum, S., & Stice, E. (2013). Cognitive regulation of food craving: Effects of three cognitive reappraisal strategies on neural response to palatable foods. *Int J Obes (Lond)*, *37*(12), 1565–1570. doi:10.1038/ijo.2013.39.

Zamzow, J., Culnan, E., Spiers, M., Calkins, M., Satterthwaite, T., Ruparel, K., … Gur, R. (2014). B-37 The Relationship between body mass index and executive function from late childhood through adolescence. *Arch Clin Neuropsychol*, *29*(6), 550. doi:10.1093/arclin/acu038.125.

Zilverstand, A., Parvaz, M. A., Moeller, S. J., & Goldstein, R. Z. (2016). Cognitive interventions for addiction medicine: Understanding the underlying neurobiological mechanisms. *Prog Brain Res*, *224*, 285–304. doi:10.1016/bs.pbr.2015.07.019.

31 Conclusion
Nurturing the Sapling

Joan Ifland
Food Addiction Training, LLC
Cincinnati, OH

Harry G. Preuss
Georgetown University Medical Center
Washington, DC

Marianne T. Marcus
University of Texas Health Science Center School of Nursing
Houston, TX

CONTENTS

Food addiction is a young, vigorous science. It's an emerging disease concept just breaking onto the global scene of obesity and other metabolic diseases. Food addiction as a disease model is made more appealing by extensive scientific evidence that consistently lines up the manifestations of chronic overeating with the characteristics of drug addiction. From the presence of malfunctioning neurons, to multiple consequences, to the business practices of corporations that sell addictive substances, and to the epidemiological patterns of use in undereducated populations, processed food use looks like drug abuse. This textbook illuminates the similarities starting with the fundamentals of the science, through assessment using the DSM 5 substance-related addiction diagnostic criteria, and ending with recovery protocols of abstinence, cue avoidance, cognitive restoration, and long-term support.

The textbook offers an explanation for a phenomenon that would otherwise be quite puzzling. Whereas historically, a few individuals here and there may have experienced chronic overeating, the scarcity and expense of fattening food curtailed the spread of the syndrome. This is not the case today. Fattening, addictive processed foods abound thanks to "improvements" in growing methods for addictive crops such as corn and methods to refine those crops into substances such as high fructose corn syrup, which appears to provoke the neuroadaptations characteristic of drug addiction. The food addiction model explains the consequences of the shift from a relatively scarce unstable supply of unprocessed foods to a consistently abundant supply of fattening addictive foods.

31.1 CHALLENGES

As with any scientific breakthrough, the food addiction model has ardent detractors. As was the case with tobacco, the processed food industry as well as policy-makers from the states that produce crops for addictive foods, discredit the concept of food addiction. Corn, wheat, sugar, and dairy enjoy powerful political protection. Cynics could also argue that vested interests in the health care and "weight loss" industries profit from the extensive consequences of processed food abuse and so might turn a blind eye to the benefits of recovery from processed foods. Media also profits from advertising for processed foods and so has a conflict of interest in promoting information about abstinence from processed foods as a mean for normalizing eating patterns.

An example of a barrier to the acceptance of food addiction is the *Wastebook*, collected by US Senator Jeff Flake. The *Wastebook* characterizes a study of the relative addictive properties of processed foods as wasted federal spending (Flake, 2016; Schulte, Avena, & Gearhardt, 2015).

These powerful barriers raise a key question. How will the food addiction model grow in the face of vested interests in chronic overeating?

The answers are numerous but each avenue is paved with stumbling blocks. The tobacco experience serves as a useful example of how a powerful industry came under effective regulation. In the case of tobacco, a number of sources came together at various stages to increase public awareness of the dangers of smoking. Gradually, the rate of smokers dropped from 65% of adults in the mid-1900s to 25% by the end of the century (Brandt, 2007).

Compared to the task facing reduction of harmful use of processed foods, the campaign against tobacco had many advantages. Of primary importance is that tobacco has never been confused with anything essential to life. Breathing is essential but is not confused with smoking. By contrast, consumption of addictive processed foods is deeply confused with indispensable eating. It is easy to distinguish smoke from clean air, but it is not easy for most people to distinguish harmful addictive processed foods from nourishing nonaddictive unprocessed foods.

Another way in which combatting food addiction is more difficult than tobacco is the relative size of the industries. The tobacco industry was quite a bit smaller than is the processed food industry. The relative size of the processed food industry will challenge regulation.

Another significant difference between tobacco and processed foods is that the products implicated in the antitobacco campaign were clear. However, in the case of processed foods, there are a variety of crops in use including sugar cane, sugar beets, corn, wheat, gluten grains, flour, dairy, cocoa leaves, coffee beans, nuts, high-sugar fruits, and potatoes. This issue can be expected to impede meaningful regulation of processed foods.

As is the case with any addiction, education, regulation, and taxation are the keys to control. From an educated public comes the boycott of harmful products, the demand for regulation, the implementation of local controls, and the protection of children. On a positive note, the smoking experience in the US provides a roadmap for recovery on a macro basis from epidemics of addictions fostered by the tobacco industry. Tobacco regulations include banning of advertising, controlled points of sale, removal of vending machines, prohibition of sales to minors, and heavy taxation. Added to this was the successful pursuit of damages through the courts. The precedents are helpful in setting a public policy agenda for processed foods.

31.2 ADVANTAGES

Consideration of a campaign against food addiction as a disease concept does have some advantages over tobacco.

31.2.1 Educational Channels

Fortunately, channels of education about food addiction are much broader in the 2010s than was the case in the mid-1900s when tobacco use was at its highest. Social media, independent news outlets, self-publishing, and websites all provide effective means for educating about abstinence from processed foods as a means for controlling cravings, gaining normal eating patterns, and putting a range of diet-related diseases into remission. The downside to these educational outlets is that they can contain amateurish or misleading information. Social media sites may try to attract a following by minimizing the amount of foods that need to be eliminated or by focusing on short-term weight loss rather than long-term recovery of mental, emotional, behavioral, and physical health. Popular understanding is possible as people in recovery use social media to learn about abstaining from addictive foods as a way out of compulsive overeating. Research helps to make a compelling case, as do stories of recovery.

Health professionals can encourage recovering food addicts to write popular books. Based on the popularity of books such as *Sugar, Fat, Salt* by Michael Moss (2013), *Wheat Belly* by William Davis (2014), and *Grain Brain* by David Perlmutter (2014), there does seem to be a market for information about the harmful effects of processed foods. The barriers to self-publishing have been virtually eliminated by promotors of blogs and e-books such as Kindle. Thus food addicts in recovery can popularize the concept by writing their stories using accessible self-publishing avenues. As awareness spreads, social media can encourage voters to express their wishes for more regulation of promotion and availability of processed foods, especially in school environments.

31.2.2 Experience

Another possible advantage is 20+ years of experience with failed weight-loss protocols. In general, public awareness of the failure of weight-loss approaches is helping people focus on healthy eating rather than damaging weight-loss schemes. Experience with Adkins-style imbalanced food plans also seems to have created a healthy skepticism about extreme diets. The enduring popularity of diets similar to abstinent food plans such as the Paleo diet is encouraging. Another avenue of help for the field of food addiction may come from awareness that weight loss has failed. As research has been published to support this failure, eating disorder professionals have gradually shifted advice from weight loss to health eating. Speaking out against the failure, even harm of the weight loss industry could help.

31.2.3 Strength of Motivation

On the positive side, food addicts may be more willing than other addicts to undertake recovery. This is due to the benefit of losing adipose tissue and escaping from the burden of harsh judgment in media-driven Western cultures. Food addicts also may have strong skill sets for elimination diets from years of extreme weight-loss dieting such as the grapefruit and hard-boiled egg diet.

People may be motivated to try new approaches to diet-related recoveries based on limited options for recovering health in the form of pharmaceuticals and surgery. Enough time has passed that a growing segment of the public is realizing that pharmaceuticals and surgery are not real answers to some health problems. As baby-boomers age and retire, they may become more interested in methods to prolong a healthy life. They may also form a market for education about how to help their children and grandchildren avoid the consequences of processed foods.

31.2.4 Similarity to Alcoholic Anonymous

The support for change could eventually come from a grassroots movement of people who have recovered from the effects of processed foods. This would be similar to the model of Alcoholic

Anonymous, which over decades was able to effectively spread the word about abstinence as a means of recovering from alcoholism. Although alcoholism has not been eradicated, treatment is available and suffering has been reduced.

31.2.5 Sophisticated Science

Another advantage to the effort to contain the epidemic of processed food use is that science has made tremendous strides in the understanding of addictions and of chronic overeating. This is so for addictions in general, as well as the similarities between drug addiction and chronic overuse of processed foods. Findings have proliferated. Growing clarity about the roles of cuing and cognitive impairment as well as cravings are available to guide recovery programs and focus efforts on protocols that yield results. Researchers can continue to build findings and interpret findings for the public.

Another source of support for curtailing the business practices of the food industry comes from an instinctual desire to protect children. As adults undertake to stop abusing processed foods, they may become aware of the addictive properties of the food and form an awareness that the addiction, rather than a personal failing, is responsible for the failure to cut back use.

Although the sources of support for the disease concept of addiction to processed foods may grow over time, the process will be prolonged. It is not likely to be universally successful. The experience with tobacco has shown that addictions can be intractable even in the face of public health campaigns. Modern cultures seem unable to abstain from addictive harmful products. This seems to be so, regardless of the extent of harm. Alcohol and tobacco seem to have a permanent, albeit harmful, function in Westernized cultures. Cannabis is gradually claiming a similar role in the United States. Even with heavy sanctions, illegal drug use flourishes. Processed foods will likely be on this list for the long term.

Hoping for meaningful public policies to curtail processed food use seems inappropriate in the face of powerful forces promoting its use. As with all addictive substances, recovery from processed foods will likely be confined to people who find education and support at a time when they're motivated to act upon it. This points to prioritizing the creation of opportunities for people to find out about addiction to processed foods and to access recovery communities. As people achieve recovery, it is possible that popular support for curtailment of advertising and availability could follow, especially in terms of marketing to children. In the much longer term, it is possible that legal action through the courts could provide restitution for damages incurred through deceptive advertising of processed foods. Damages could also be a source of funding for research and educational programs.

31.3 FUTURE RESEARCH

Food addiction enjoys a firm foundation due in large part to the fields of obesity and addiction research. Without brain imaging, human, and animal research, the case for the existence of chronic overeating as an addiction would be much less compelling. Indeed, as researchers write about the disease, they rely on neuroimaging research as well as animal studies that demonstrate similarities to classic drug behavior including tolerance and withdrawal. Key research is needed in food addiction.

31.3.1 Withdrawal

Of perhaps the greatest urgency in research would be large-scale withdrawal studies in humans. Demonstration of prospective withdrawal, with reintroduction of specific single foods, would establish withdrawal syndromes for each of the processed foods under consideration. These would include sugar, high-fructose corn syrup, gluten, excessive salt, processed fats, and dairy. A withdrawal syndrome for caffeine has been established (American Pyschiatric Association, 2013, pp. 506–508).

Because processed foods are formulated in combinations, it would also be helpful to establish withdrawal syndromes for common combinations such as HFCS, with processed fat, gluten, and excessive salt as would be found in baked goods. The most common fast food combinations (pizza, burger and fries, tacos) would also benefit from establishing a withdrawal syndrome. This research would be useful in the effort to curtail marketing of these foods to children. The results could also help people manage withdrawal.

31.3.2 Course of Recovery

Although the 12-step societies report comprehensive recovery from processed food abuse, no research has been performed on the progress of recovery. Physical recovery from high blood pressure, diabetes, dyslipidemia, and excess adipose tissue have not been conducted. Recovery from mood, mental, and behavioral disorders also needs to be established, especially the use of cognitive restoration techniques such as mindfulness. Such research could serve to support health professionals in recommending recovery protocols. They could also be valuable in motivating food addicts to undertake recovery.

31.3.3 Neurofunction

Research in the field of addiction could translate into findings for food addiction.

> Key questions that remain are what genetic factors load these mini circuits, how the environment conveys epigenetic influences on these circuits, and how these circuits recover or do not recover with abstinence and treatment. Resolving these questions should provide biomarkers for prevention, behavioural windows of development for prevention, novel behavioural and pharmaceutical treatments, and ultimately a neurobiological understanding of recovery. (Koob & Volkow, 2016)

Understanding the progress of recovery of cognitive functions, as well as desensitization of craving pathways, could be very helpful in developing more precise guidelines for key issues in recovery from food addiction. A primary question in recovery from food addiction is how much cue avoidance is needed. In cue-dense Western cultures, cue avoidance is a burden. Yet cues have been shown to be a leading cause of relapse. Being able to thread a safe passage through the cues of Westernized life is important to recovering food addicts. Gaining insight into how food addiction is passed genetically would be very useful in terms of advising food addicts who want to conceive children. Although food addiction seems to be a disease of environment rather than genetics, understanding genetic components could encourage parents to prepare safe environments for genetically vulnerable children.

31.3.4 Process Addiction versus Substance Addiction

A burning issue that needs to be clarified is whether food addiction is a behavioral-/process- or substance-based disorder. In spite of evidence for the addictive properties of processed foods, academic articles continue to classify the addiction as behavioral. It can be discouraging when food addiction stubbornly remains classified as a behavioral disorder when it seems so clear that addictive substances are being ingested.

> The three stages of the addiction cycle are pervasive and form common domains in non-drug addictions, also known as *process addictions* (Smith DE 2012) such as pathological gambling, binge-eating disorder, compulsive buying, and internet addiction disorder (Koob GF 2013). Non-drug addictions elaborate self-regulation failures similarly to drug addictions, with transitions from impulsivity to compulsivity and a chronic relapsing trajectory. (Koob & Volkow, 2016)

Research showing withdrawal, course of recovery, neurofunction and substance use will help practitioners and policy-makers develop appropriate responses to food addiction.

31.4 CONCLUSION

Food addiction has come a long way and has a long way to go. With the availability of this textbook, it is now possible for practitioners to obtain the tools they need to take a fresh approach to chronic overeating as a substance-use disorder. With the solid empirical data and descriptions of food addictions, practitioners now have solid ground to stand on as they advocate for recognition of food addiction as a serious mental illness. They also may have the courage of their convictions to work with clients on the extensive life-alterations that recovery from food addiction entails.

Ignoring food addiction as a possibility is no longer justified. A group of food addiction researchers replied to the suggestion that the food addiction model be abandoned with these words:

> If found to be applicable to a considerable population with obesity, a food-addiction model may not only help clarify findings in obesity but, importantly, could also lead to new interventions for preventing and treating obesity, facilitated by decades of research in substance addiction. If we are to prematurely dismiss such a potentially important model on the basis of limited studies, we could miss important opportunities to improve health worldwide. (Avena, Gearhardt, Gold, Wang, & Potenza, 2012)

With the availability of this textbook, practitioners and food addicts alike have a well-supported pathway to recovery from food addiction in terms of understanding, assessing, and providing the education and support that a food addict would need to recover. As the disease is comprehensively devastating, so is the satisfaction of helping a food addict to emerge from the shadow of the disease.

As the epidemic of obesity rages on and becomes even worse at the high end of the range of severity, more practitioners are recognizing that weight loss is not an answer. Pharmaceuticals and surgery have not been consistently reliable answers. In the face of a worsening situation and the dwindling list of possible solutions, the food addiction model has gained a foothold. From a foundation of thousands of studies of obesity and addiction coupled with decades of practical experience in 12-step fellowships and pioneering food addiction practitioners, today's health professionals can proceed with confidence in the application of classic drug addiction protocols. Giving clients hope, helping them devise plans, and celebrating milestones with them can replace frustration with satisfaction for today's health professional in the battle against chronic overeating.

REFERENCES

American Pyschiatric Association. (2013). *Diagnostic and Statistical Manual V.*

Avena, N. M., Gearhardt, A. N., Gold, M. S., Wang, G. J., & Potenza, M. N. (2012). Tossing the baby out with the bathwater after a brief rinse? The potential downside of dismissing food addiction based on limited data. *Nat Rev Neurosci, 13*(7), 514; author reply 514. doi: 10.1038/nrn3212-c1.

Brandt, A. (2007). *The cigarette century: The rise, fall, and deadly persistence of the product that defined America.* New York: Basic Books.

Davis, W. (2014). *Wheat belly.* New York: Rodale.

Flake, J. (2016). *Wastebook: The farce awakens.* Retrieved from https://www.flake.senate.gov/public/_cache/files/03714fa3-e01d-46a1-9c19-299533056741/wastebook---the-farce-awakens.pdf

Koob, G. F., & Volkow, N. D. (2016). Neurobiology of addiction: A neurocircuitry analysis. *Lancet Psychiatry, 3*(8), 760–773. doi: 10.1016/s2215-0366(16)00104-8.

Moss, M. (2013). *Salt, sugar, fat: How the food giants hooked us.*

Perlmutter, J. S. (2014). *Grain brain: The surprising truth about wheat, carbs, and sugar—Your brain's silent killers.* New York: Little, Brown and Company.

Schulte, E. M., Avena, N. M., & Gearhardt, A. N. (2015). Which foods may be addictive? The roles of processing, fat content, and glycemic load. *PLoS One, 10*(2), e0117959. doi: 10.1371/journal.pone.0117959.

Index

D

E

F

G

H

I

J

L

M

R

S